Medical Terminology

Learning Through Practice

Medical Terminology
Learning Through Practice

Paula Bostwick, RN, MSN, CENP

Parkview Behavioral Health

Mc Graw Hill Education

MEDICAL TERMINOLOGY

Published by McGraw-Hill Education, 2 Penn Plaza, New York, NY 10121. Copyright ©2020 by McGraw-Hill Education. All rights reserved. Printed in the United States of America. No part of this publication may be reproduced or distributed in any form or by any means, or stored in a database or retrieval system, without the prior written consent of McGraw-Hill Education, including, but not limited to, in any network or other electronic storage or transmission, or broadcast for distance learning.

Some ancillaries, including electronic and print components, may not be available to customers outside the United States.

This book is printed on acid-free paper.

1 2 3 4 5 6 7 8 9 LWI 21 20 19

ISBN 978-1-260-54770-2
MHID 1-260-54770-1

Cover Image: ©MedicalRF.com

All credits appearing on page or at the end of the book are considered to be an extension of the copyright page.

The Internet addresses listed in the text were accurate at the time of publication. The inclusion of a website does not indicate an endorsement by the authors or McGraw-Hill Education, and McGraw-Hill Education does not guarantee the accuracy of the information presented at these sites.

mheducation.com/highered

About the Author

PAULA MANUEL BOSTWICK, RN, MSN, CENP, is an author, educator, and clinician. She is currently the Director of Inpatient and Psychiatric Emergency Services at Parkview Behavioral Health. Paula has been involved with nursing education for more than 20 years and enjoys preparing nursing students for the NCLEX. She has previously served as a nursing department chair, nurse manager, and critical care nurse. She earned her BSN from Indiana State University and MSN from Ball State University. Paula and her husband Charles have two children, CJ and Bailey Rae.

Dedication

This book is dedicated to my husband and best friend, Charles, and to our children, CJ and Bailey Rae, for their love, patience, and understanding. Thank you for all of your love and support. I love you.

—Paula Bostwick

Brief Contents

Contents

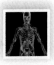

Preface

Medical Terminology: Learning Through Practice is designed to direct your study of medical terminology by guiding you through an organized approach to step-by-step learning. Author Paula Bostwick has invested her time, research, and talents to help you succeed in learning medical terminology.

The format of each chapter is designed to guide you through steps that lead to a full understanding of medical terminology. The chapters are divided into seven sections:

1. Major Structure and Function Terms
2. Word Building
3. Diagnostic, Procedural, and Laboratory Terms
4. Pathological Terms
5. Surgical Terms
6. Pharmacological Terms
7. Abbreviations

Furthermore, within each section there is a four-part exercise progression. This progression offers self-study questions that lead to an in-depth understanding of the material:

1. Pronounce and Define
2. Spell and Define
3. Understand
4. Apply

Using the Practice Sections and Exercise Progression

Each time you come to a Practice section, cover the left-hand column with a blank sheet of paper. As you proceed through the review, attempt to fill in each blank before revealing the answers. Move the paper down just far enough to see the answer. If you are correct, move on to the next blank. If you are not correct, reread the material in the copy above and make a flash card for the word you missed. Studying the flash cards at the end of each section will help you learn all the key terms in the chapter. (Later in the Preface, you can read about StudyWise, McGraw-Hill's app that will help you take your studying to another level!)

Once you have progressed through the Practice section, quiz yourself using the exercise progression. The exercise progression includes pronunciation exercises, spelling exercises, multiple choice questions, labeling exercises, matching exercises, and case studies to test your comprehension of the material.

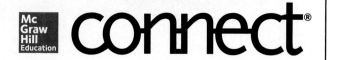

Students—study more efficiently, retain more and achieve better outcomes. Instructors—focus on what you love—teaching.

SUCCESSFUL SEMESTERS INCLUDE CONNECT

FOR INSTRUCTORS

You're in the driver's seat.

Want to build your own course? No problem. Prefer to use our turnkey, prebuilt course? Easy. Want to make changes throughout the semester? Sure. And you'll save time with Connect's auto-grading too.

65%
Less Time Grading

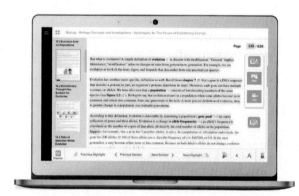

They'll thank you for it.

Adaptive study resources like SmartBook® help your students be better prepared in less time. You can transform your class time from dull definitions to dynamic debates. Hear from your peers about the benefits of Connect at **www.mheducation.com/highered/connect**

Make it simple, make it affordable.

Connect makes it easy with seamless integration using any of the major Learning Management Systems—Blackboard®, Canvas, and D2L, among others—to let you organize your course in one convenient location. Give your students access to digital materials at a discount with our inclusive access program. Ask your McGraw-Hill representative for more information.

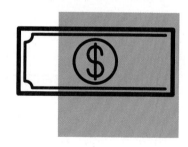

©Hill Street Studios/Tobin Rogers/Blend Images LLC

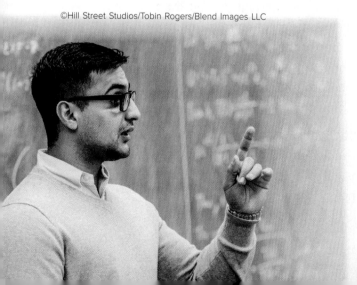

Solutions for your challenges.

A product isn't a solution. Real solutions are affordable, reliable, and come with training and ongoing support when you need it and how you want it. Our Customer Experience Group can also help you troubleshoot tech problems—although Connect's 99% uptime means you might not need to call them. See for yourself at **status.mheducation.com**

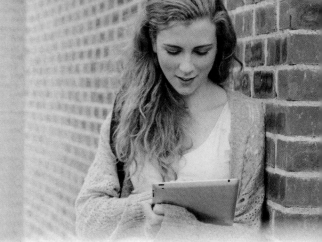

Effective, efficient studying.

Connect helps you be more productive with your study time and get better grades using tools like SmartBook, which highlights key concepts and creates a personalized study plan. Connect sets you up for success, so you walk into class with confidence and walk out with better grades.

> " I really liked this app—it made it easy to study when you don't have your text-book in front of you. "
>
> - Jordan Cunningham, Eastern Washington University

Study anytime, anywhere.

Download the free ReadAnywhere app and access your online eBook when it's convenient, even if you're offline. And since the app automatically syncs with your eBook in Connect, all of your notes are available every time you open it. Find out more at **www.mheducation.com/readanywhere**

No surprises.

The Connect Calendar and Reports tools keep you on track with the work you need to get done and your assignment scores. Life gets busy; Connect tools help you keep learning through it all.

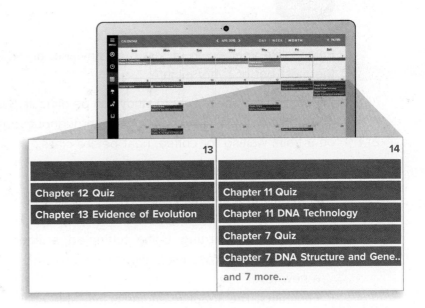

Learning for everyone.

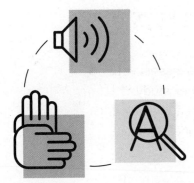

McGraw-Hill works directly with Accessibility Services Departments and faculty to meet the learning needs of all students. Please contact your Accessibility Services office and ask them to email accessibility@mheducation.com, or visit **www.mheducation.com/about/accessibility.html** for more information.

Highlights of the Book

Engaging four-color design will draw the students' attention to key concepts.

- More than 400 enhanced photos and line art images bring medical terminology to life.
- Prefixes and suffixes are each covered in their own chapters.
- Each learning outcome is correlated to a section number to direct focus on key content.
- Progressed exercises appear throughout the text, correlated to each major section, in the format of Structure and Function terms, Word Building terms, Diagnostic terms, Pathological terms, Surgical terms, Pharmacological terms, and Abbreviations. Using pronunciation, spelling, labeling, multiple choice, matching, and case study questions, these exercises enhance student learning.
- Summary table in every chapter restates the learning outcomes and provides corresponding summary points for each.
- End-of-chapter exercises are built using the exercise progression introduced throughout the text.

Student Resource

StudyWise

Personalize your exam or test prep anytime, anywhere. Life is busy. Squeeze the most out of every minute.

Scheduling a block of time to study can be difficult. StudyWise allows you to take advantage of those little opportunities throughout your day: during a work break, on a train, waiting for coffee, right before class.

With StudyWise you get:

- **A mobile-first solution.** StudyWise is available for iOS via the App Store and for Android via Google Play.
- **Personalized learning.** Using cutting-edge algorithms designed by our data scientists, StudyWise takes the former flashcard-style approach of studying to a new level.
- **Flexibility.** The adaptive engine is available offline meaning that students can use StudyWise even when their mobile devices are not connected to the Internet. Whether you are using a McGraw-Hill solution or not, StudyWise can help your students prepare for their next exam.
- **Two modes of use:**
  - Targeted. You choose the topic, StudyWise dynamically assesses your knowledge, directing you to specific content that needs further study.
  - Review. Gives you the chance to revise the content you've already studied, ensuring you have mastered it in time for the next big test, quiz, or assignment.

Instructors' Resources

You can rely on the following materials to help you and your students work with the material in the book; all are available in the Instructor's Resources under the Library tab in *Connect* (available only to instructors who are logged in to *Connect*.)

Supplement	Features
Instructor's Manual	• Lecture Outlines • Lesson Plans • Answer Keys
PowerPoint Presentations	• Key Concepts • Accessible
Electronic Testbank	• Computerized and *Connect* • Word version • Questions are tagged with Learning Objectives, level of difficulty, and level of Bloom's Taxonomy
Tools to Plan Course	• Sample Syllabi • Asset Map—recap of the key instructor resources as well as information on the content available through *Connect*

Want to learn more about this product? Attend one of our online webinars. To learn more about them, please contact your McGraw-Hill Learning Technology Representative. To find your McGraw-Hill representative, go to www.mheducation.com and click the dropdown for "Support & Contact," select "Higher Education," and then click the "GET STARTED" button under the "Find Your Sales Rep" section.

Need help? Contact the McGraw-Hill Education Customer Experience Group (CXG). Visit the CXG website at www.mhhe.com/support. Browse the FAQs (Frequently Asked Questions) and product documentation, and/or contact a CXG representative.

Acknowledgments

A special thank you to all of those on our team who participated in this book. Your creativity, insight, and patience are truly appreciated and treasured.

We would like to especially thank Thomas Timp, Managing Director; William Lawrensen, Executive Portfolio Manager; Michelle Flomenhoft, Senior Product Developer; Yvonne Lloyd, Business Product Manager; Valerie Kramer, Marketing Manager; Jessica Portz and Brent dela Cruz, Project Managers; Egzon Shaqiri, designer; and Melissa Homer, Content Licensing Specialist.

Thank you to the following reviewers for their perceptive comments and suggestions:

LaTavia Bowman, LPN, *Helms College*

Diane Bridge, EdS, MSN, RN, *Liberty University*

Sandra Brightwell, MEd, RHIA, FAHIMA, *Central Arizona College*

Kenya Brooks, EdM, CMA(AAMA), LRT, CPT(ASPT), *Delgado Community College*

Pamela Burton, *Ivy Tech Community College*

Nancy Dancs, BS, PT, MS, *Waukesha County Technical College*

Sarah Darrell, BSN, RN, CNOR, *Ivy Tech Community College*

Antoinette Deshaies, RN, BSPA, *Glendale Community College*

Andrea Doctor, RN, *University of District of Columbia*

Paul Falkenstein, MS, PA-C, *Northern Virginia Community College*

Tina Gambhir, *Northern Virginia Community College*

Traci Gentry, RN, *Southcentral Kentucky Community and Technical College*

Susan Grant, RN, MS, EdD, *Harper College*

Janis Grimland, RN, *Hill College*

Julia Halterman, *Eastern Mennonite University*

David Holt, *Long Beach City College*

Susan Horn, BS, *Central Arizona College*

Roop Jayaraman, *Central Michigan University*

Garry Johnson, RN, BSN, MSN, DHSc, CCRN, CMSRN, *Evergreen Valley College*

Colleen Lace, BLS, AA, LPN, *Moraine Park Technical College*

Amie Mayhall, MBA, *Olney Central College*

Ann Mills, MS, *Minnesota West Community and Technical College*

Donna Pritchard, RHIT, LPN, *Ozarks Technical Community College*

Amber Samaniego, CMA(AAMA), *Everett Community College*

Amber Schappaugh, MA, RMA(AMT), *Midstate College*

Mark Schubert, RT, *Tidewater Community College*

Yolanda Smith, EdD, MSN, RN, *Oakwood University*

Charlene Thiessen, CMT, AHDI-F, *GateWay Community College*

Cheryl Travelstead, BS, AS, ASS, RT(R) (BD), *Tidewater Community College*

Ji Yang, *California College San Diego*

Lisa Young, RN, BSN, MA Ed, *Southcentral Kentucky Community and Technical College*

—Paula Bostwick

Getting to Know Your Text

Learning Outcomes

Each chapter opens with learning outcomes that prepare students for the information presented.

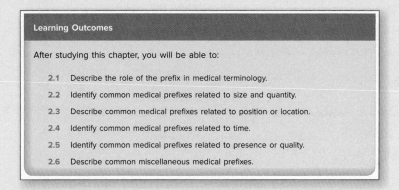

Combining Forms

The combining forms section introduces the important word parts used to build terms.

Combining Form	Meaning
aer/o	air, gas
ather/o	plaque, fatty substance (inside of a blood vessel)
blast/o	immature cells
calc/o, calci/o	calcium
chondrio, chondro	cartilage, grainy, gritty
chyl/o	chyle, a digestive juice
chym/o	chyme, semifluid production of chyme in the stomach
cyst/o, cysti	bladder, cyst, cystic duct
cyt/o	cell
ethm/o	ethmoid bone
gluc/o	glucose
glyc/o	sugars
hydr/o	hydrogen, water
ket/o, keton/o	ketone, acetone
lip/o	fat (outside of a blood vessel)
nucle/o	nucleus
plasma, plasmo	formative, plasma
salping/o	tube
sider/o	iron
somat/o	body
squam/o	scale, squamous (meaning scaly)
syring/o	tube

Practice

A section of terms is introduced in each chapter. The terms are combined with fill-in-the-blank exercises to aid in comprehension.

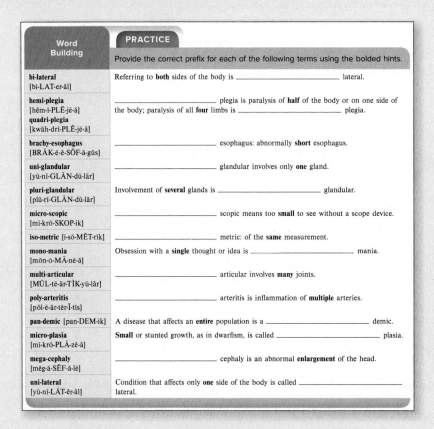

Word Building	PRACTICE
	Provide the correct prefix for each of the following terms using the bolded hints.
bi-lateral [bī-LAT-er-ăl]	Referring to **both** sides of the body is _____ lateral.
hemi-plegia [hĕm-ĭ-PLĒ-jē-ă] **quadri-plegia** [kwăh-drĭ-PLĒ-jē-ă]	_____ plegia is paralysis of **half** of the body or on one side of the body; paralysis of all **four** limbs is _____ plegia.
brachy-esophagus [BRĂK-ē-ĕ-SŎF-ă-gŭs]	_____ esophagus: abnormally **short** esophagus.
uni-glandular [yū-nĭ-GLĂN-dū-lăr]	_____ glandular involves only **one** gland.
pluri-glandular [plū-rĭ-GLĂN-dū-lăr]	Involvement of **several** glands is _____ glandular.
micro-scopic [mī-krŏ-SKOP-ik]	_____ scopic means too **small** to see without a scope device.
iso-metric [ī-sŏ-MĔT-rĭk]	_____ metric: of the **same** measurement.
mono-mania [mŏn-ō-MĀ-nē-ă]	Obsession with a **single** thought or idea is _____ mania.
multi-articular [MŬL-tē-ăr-TĬK-yū-lăr]	_____ articular involves **many** joints.
poly-arteritis [pŏl-ē-ăr-tĕr-Ī-tĭs]	_____ arteritis is inflammation of **multiple** arteries.
pan-demic [pan-DEM-ik]	A disease that affects an **entire** population is a _____ demic.
micro-plasia [mī-krŏ-PLĀ-zē-ă]	**Small** or stunted growth, as in dwarfism, is called _____ plasia.
mega-cephaly [mĕg-ă-SĔF-ă-lē]	_____ cephaly is an abnormal **enlargement** of the head.
uni-lateral [yū-nĭ-LĂT-ĕr-ăl]	Condition that affects only **one** side of the body is called _____ lateral.

Exercise Progression: Pronounce and Define

List of terms is accompanied by pronunciation guides. This exercise offers students a chance to practice pronouncing medical terms.

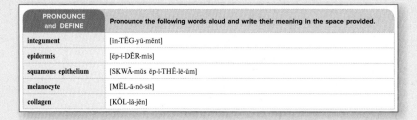

PRONOUNCE and DEFINE	Pronounce the following words aloud and write their meaning in the space provided.
integument	[ĭn-TĔG-yū-mĕnt]
epidermis	[ĕp-ĭ-DĔR-mĭs]
squamous epithelium	[SKWĀ-mŭs ĕp-ĭ-THĒ-lē-ŭm]
melanocyte	[MĔL-ă-nō-sīt]
collagen	[KŎL-lă-jĕn]

Exercise Progression: Spell and Define

Self-test exercises focus on the proper spelling of medical terms.

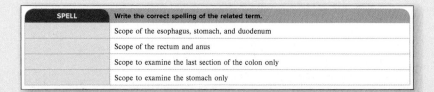

SPELL	Write the correct spelling of the related term.
	Scope of the esophagus, stomach, and duodenum
	Scope of the rectum and anus
	Scope to examine the last section of the colon only
	Scope to examine the stomach only

Exercise Progression: Understand

This feature is geared toward the ability to understand and apply medical terms.

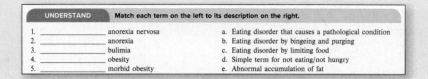

Exercise Progression: Apply

Using short case study scenarios, this feature directs students to apply knowledge learned throughout the chapter.

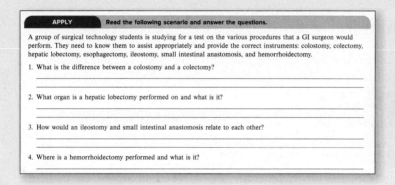

From the Perspective Of

This feature describes health care professionals who benefit from in-depth medical terminology knowledge.

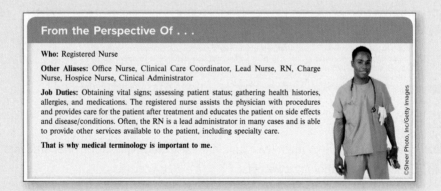

Study Tips

Tips are geared toward enhancing knowledge of medical terminology.

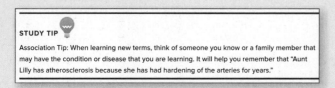

Did You Know?

This feature emphasizes interesting facts surrounding medical terminology topics.

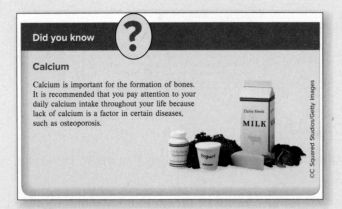

Chapter Summary

Easy-to-use tables summarize the Learning Outcomes included in each chapter.

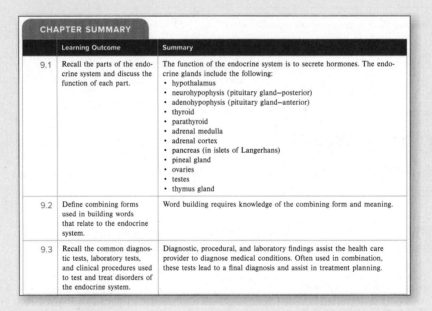

CHAPTER SUMMARY		
	Learning Outcome	Summary
9.1	Recall the parts of the endocrine system and discuss the function of each part.	The function of the endocrine system is to secrete hormones. The endocrine glands include the following: • hypothalamus • neurohypophysis (pituitary gland–posterior) • adenohypophysis (pituitary gland–anterior) • thyroid • parathyroid • adrenal medulla • adrenal cortex • pancreas (in islets of Langerhans) • pineal gland • ovaries • testes • thymus gland
9.2	Define combining forms used in building words that relate to the endocrine system.	Word building requires knowledge of the combining form and meaning.
9.3	Recall the common diagnostic tests, laboratory tests, and clinical procedures used to test and treat disorders of the endocrine system.	Diagnostic, procedural, and laboratory findings assist the health care provider to diagnose medical conditions. Often used in combination, these tests lead to a final diagnosis and assist in treatment planning.

Chapter Review

Multiple choice, matching, labeling, fill-in-the-blank, and case study questions offer students reinforcement of medical terminology concepts.

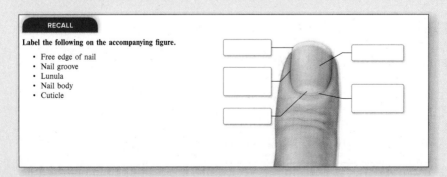

CHAPTER 1

Learning Terminology, Word Roots, and Combining Forms

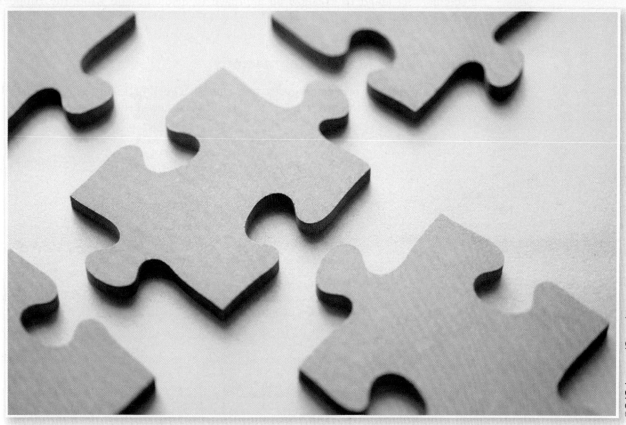

©OJO Images/Getty Images

Learning Outcomes

After studying this chapter, you will be able to:

1.1 Discuss the history of medical terminology and how terms are developed.

1.2 Describe the importance of pronunciation and spelling in medical terminology.

1.3 Illustrate the four word parts used to build medical terms.

1.4 Identify how word roots and combining forms build medical terms.

1.5 Describe the process of pluralizing terms.

1.6 Recognize and use medical terminology and its different forms.

LO 1.1 The Language of Medicine

Many everyday terms that we use to describe our health and our medical care go back to the early history of civilization. People who followed after them gave names to parts of the body, to illnesses, and to the treatments they used (Figure 1-1).

Some of these names survive in the roots and words still used today in medical terminology. For example, the ancient Greeks thought of the disease we call "cancer" as something eating at a person on the inside, and so named the condition *karkinos,* meaning both crab and cancer. Medical terminology began its standardization when Hippocrates (460–377 BC), a Greek physician sometimes referred to as "the father of medicine," set about to organize an approach to medicine and wrote the Hippocratic Oath (Figure 1-2).

Derivation of Medical Terminology

Many medical terms originate directly from ancient Greek or Latin terms. Word building became and remains the primary way to describe even new medical discoveries.

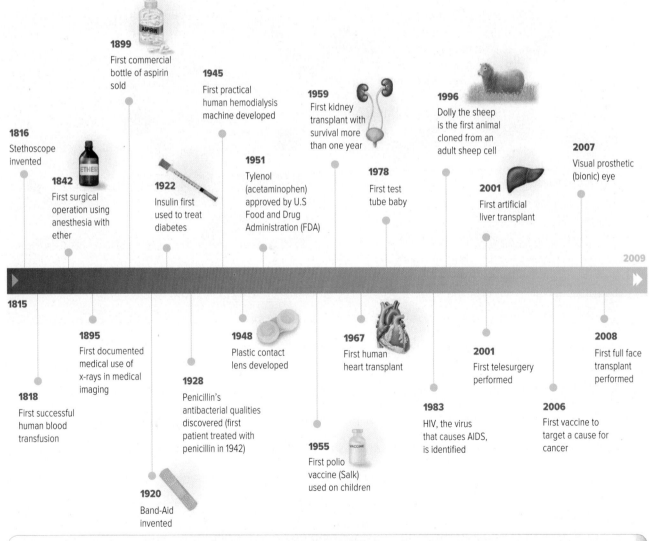

Figure 1-1 Timeline of major medical events/discoveries in medicine

So, a suffix, *-tomy,* which means "cutting," may be used in modern procedures where we do not think of "cutting"; for instance, *phlebotomy* is defined as incision into a vein, but the basic meaning is still the original one, "cutting." Throughout this text, you will learn the parts of words and the ways of combining them that will enable you to understand medical terminology.

Languages other than English form words in the same way. For example, the word *nerve* is derived from the Latin *nervus.* In Spanish, the word *nervio* also is derived from the same Latin word.

Practice

As you begin each "Practice" section in this chapter, cover the left-hand column and answer all the questions below without removing the cover. Then, uncover and check your answers. Remember to also create flash cards to practice learning the medical terms.

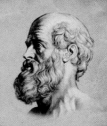

Hippocratic Oath

"I swear by Apollo, the physician, and Aesculapius, and Health, and Allheal, and all the gods and goddesses, that, according to my ability and judgment, I will keep this oath and stipulation, to reckon him who taught me this art equally dear to me as my parents, to share my substance with him and relieve his necessities if required; to regard his offspring as on the same footing with my own brothers, and to teach them this art if they should wish to learn it, without fee or stipulation, and that by precept, lecture, and every other mode of instruction, I will impart a knowledge of the art to my own sons and to those of my teachers, and to disciples bound by a stipulation and oath, according to the law of medicine, but to none other.

I will follow that method of treatment which, according to my ability and judgment, I consider for the benefit of my patients, and abstain from whatever is deleterious and mischievous. I will give no deadly medicine to anyone if asked, nor suggest any such counsel; furthermore, I will not give to a woman an instrument to produce abortion.

With purity and holiness I will pass my life and practice my art. I will not cut a person who is suffering with a stone, but will leave this to be done by practitioners of the work. Into whatever houses I enter I will go into them for the benefit of the sick and will abstain from every voluntary act of mischief and corruption; and further from the seduction of females or males, bond or free.

Whatever, in connection with my professional practice, or not in connection with it, I may see or hear in the lives of men which ought not to be spoken abroad, I will not divulge, as reckoning that all such should be kept secret.

While I continue to keep this oath unviolated, may it be granted to me to enjoy life and the practice of the art, respected by all men at all times, but should I trespass and violate this oath, may the reverse be my lot.

©Rijksmuseum, Amsterdam

Figure 1-2 The Hippocratic Oath

Word Building	PRACTICE
	Provide the correct word in the following sentences.
ligament	The modern term for the Latin *ligamentum* is _____.
kardia	The historical derivation of the modern *cardi/o* is _____.
tendo	The historical derivation of the modern tendon is _____.
gene	The modern term for the Greek *genos* is _____.
nerve	The modern term for the Latin *nervus* is _____.
arteria	The historical derivation of the modern artery is _____.
vein	The modern term for the Latin *vena* is _____.
cella	The historical derivation of the modern cell is _____.
sinus	The historical derivation of the modern sinus is _____.
hernia	The modern term for *hernia* is _____.

Modern-Day Compound Words in English

Although the basis of medical terminology comes from many Greek or Latin terms, there is also an association with modern-day concepts of compound words. Young students learn compound words in elementary school, so we are no doubt familiar with them and use them every day. The concept is simple: combining two words to create one that also combines or forms a new meaning related to the two words. For instance, the bolded words in the following sentences are compound words:

The art group gathered **downtown.**
The medical assistant escorted the patient **into** the exam room.

downtown = down + town
into   = in + to

Separately, each of the words has its own meaning, but when combined, a new meaning is created that explains two concepts with just one word, or defines a process or direction in more detail.

Medical terminology works the same way. Once the word parts themselves are learned, it becomes a process of combining them together to convey multiple concepts into one word.

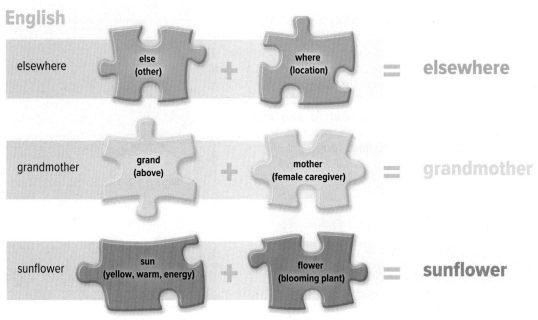

English

elsewhere — else (other) + where (location) = elsewhere

grandmother — grand (above) + mother (female caregiver) = grandmother

sunflower — sun (yellow, warm, energy) + flower (blooming plant) = sunflower

Medical Terminology

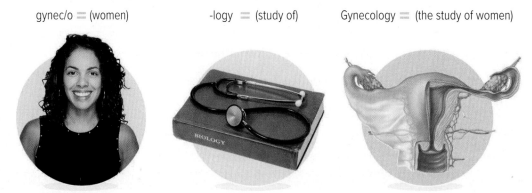

gynec/o = (women)   -logy = (study of)   Gynecology = (the study of women)

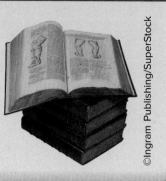
PRONOUNCE	Pronounce the following terms aloud.
gynecology	[gī-nĕ-KOL-ō-jē, ji-]
hepatitis	[hep-ă-TĪ-tis]
pulmonary	[PŬL-mō-nār-ē]
bilateral	[bī-LAT-er-ăl]

SPELL	Write the correct modern term of the historical term given.
genos	_____
kardia	_____
hernia	_____
nevus	_____
vena	_____

UNDERSTAND Match the function of the following terms.

1. _____ first languages of medicine
2. _____ compound words
3. _____ Hippocrates
4. _____ ancient word for cancer

a. *karkinos*
b. Roman and Greek
c. "the father of medicine"
d. grandfather, inside

APPLY Answer the following question.

Explain how medical terms are similar to compound words.

_____

_____

Accurate

Summary of Treatment

Date	Source	Physician	Description
			Date of injury
5/20/17	1–17	M.Howard	ER – complained of left wrist, arm pain. Fell from a ladder at work. No head injury. Severe wrist pain, probable fracture. Send for x-rays.
5/20/17	1–25	Fine	X-ray, left forearm – Colles type fracture with comminution and intraarticular extension of the distal radius. There is deformation. X-ray, left shoulder – normal.
5/23/17	1–102	J.Howard	Admission – broken left wrist, Medications Celebrex, Synthroid, Coumadin, Diazepam. Previous Surgeries: rotator cuff repair.

Inaccurate

Summary of Treatment

Date	Source	Physician	Description
			Date of injury
5/03/17	4–20	Smith	Phone- pt call for **autopsy** results. Negative for cancer per Dr. Smith.
6/31/17	4–00	Goldberg	Surgery- **open/closed** reduction of Right forearm fx. Pt states no loss of feeling in **left** fin**d**ers. Reports pain in **medial lateral** thumb.
7/01/17	3–??	Fine	ER- complained of left wrist neuralgia, describing "pins and needles" and **cephalga** with **dyskinesha**

Figure 1-3 Medical record: (A) correct documentation; (B) misspellings and incorrect grammar (terms for which corrections are needed are in red)

LO 1.2 Spelling and Pronunciation of Medical Terms

Misspellings and mispronunciations in a medical setting can result in life-threatening situations. A misspelled or a misunderstood abbreviation for a medicine dosage can have very serious consequences (Figure 1-3). Aside from the possibility of written mistakes, people in health care must check and recheck verbal instructions.

Learning how to spell and pronounce medical terms is a matter of practice. Familiarizing yourself with correct spellings of terms is a matter of seeing the terms over and over again and writing them out, over and over again. Pronouncing a word aloud each time you see the pronunciation will help you become familiar with the sound of the word. (*Note:* Not everyone agrees on every pronunciation, and there may be regional variations. If your instructor has a particular preference, follow that preference.) Also, use your own medical dictionary as a reference when you have a question. It is a good idea to know some basic terms in other languages such as Spanish when you work in an area where many people mainly speak that language.

Eponyms are terms formed from names, such as Parkinson's disease. In normal English style, such terms use an apostrophe followed by an *s*. However, some medical associations have decided to drop the apostrophe and/or leave out the *s* in eponyms so that Parkinson disease is now the preferred spelling in certain situations.

In this text, there are two ways to help you learn to pronounce words. First, we capitalize one syllable of all words with two or more syllables so you can tell where the heaviest accent falls. For example, the word *femoral* is pronounced "FEM-or-al," with the accent on the first syllable. (Sometimes when there are more than three syllables, two syllables are stressed.) Next, we add marks, called **diacritical marks.** A diacritical mark is used by placing a special mark above the vowel to indicate a special pronunciation and to guide you in pronouncing the word. Vowels are either long or short, as shown in Table 1-1.

As you work your way through the book, always practice pronouncing each term as you read it, either aloud or silently. It will help you build confidence when you actually have to pronounce the word aloud.

TABLE 1-1	Pronunciation Guide	
Vowels	**Long (¯) or Short (˘)**	**Pronunciation Examples**
a	long ā	pace, plate
a	short ă	rap, cat, bar
e	long ē	easy, beat
e	short ĕ	ever, pet
i	long ī	I, line, bite
i	short ĭ	kitten, pit
o	long ō	boat, rose, wrote
o	short ŏ	pot, hot
u	long ū	cute, cube
u	short ŭ	cut, put

Word Building

PRACTICE

Provide an example for each of the following vowel sounds.

I, line, bite	long ī _____.
pot, hot	short ŏ _____.
ever, pet	short ĕ _____.
pace, plate	long ā _____.
cut, put	short ŭ _____.
cute, cube	long ū _____.
easy, beat	long ē _____.
kitten, pit	short ĭ _____.
boat, rose, wrote	long ō _____.
rap, cat, bar	short ă _____.

PRONOUNCE

Pronounce the following terms aloud.

hyperthermia	[hī-per-THER-mē-ă]
osteoarthritis	[ŎS-tē-ō-ăr-THRĪ-tĭs]
metastasis	[mĕ-TĂS-tă-sĭs]
splenomegaly	[splēn-ō-MĔG-ă-lē]

SPELL	Write which syllable of the given word is emphasized.
femoral	_____
dermatitis	_____
osteoma	_____
anesthesia	_____
polyuria	_____

| UNDERSTAND | Match the following vowel sounds to their respective terms. |

1. _____ long ū   a. pet
2. _____ long ō   b. crime
3. _____ short ŏ   c. tot
4. _____ long ī   d. cute
5. _____ short ĕ   e. coat

| APPLY | Answer the following questions. |

1. Create four word examples that have a short ĭ. Look up your word in a dictionary and write the pronunciation for each word after.

   Example: *mortify* [MŌR-tĭ-fī]

   _____
   _____
   _____
   _____

2. Construct four word examples that have a long ō. Look up your words in a dictionary and write the pronunciation for each word.

   _____
   _____
   _____

LO 1.3 Forming Medical Terms

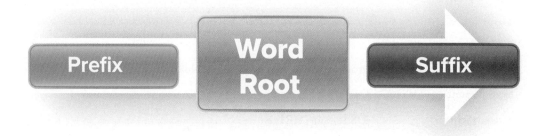

Many medical terms are formed from two or more of the following four basic word parts that are the foundation for medical terminology:

1. A **word root** is the portion of the word that contains its basic meaning. For example, the word root *cardi* means "heart." Some other examples of common medical word roots are

   dent, tooth   *laryng,* larynx
   gastr, stomach   *rhin,* nose

2. **Combining forms** are the word root and a combining vowel that connects or *links* two parts whenever two consonants come together (as in *laryngoplasty,* which is made up of the combining form *laryng-,* the combining vowel *o,* and the suffix *-plasty*). For example, the word root *cardi* and the combining vowel *o* can form words that relate to the basic meaning "heart," such as *cardiology,* the medical practice involved with studying, diagnosing, and treating disorders of the heart.

   Some other examples of words formed from combining forms are:

   laryng/o **laryngoscope**
   gastr/o **gastrology**
   rhin/o **rhinoplasty**

3. **Prefixes** are word parts attached to the *beginning* of a word or word root that modify its meaning. For example, the prefix *peri-,* meaning "around, near, surrounding," helps to form the word *pericardium,* meaning "around or surrounding the heart." (Common medical prefixes are discussed in Chapter 2 as well as in the body system chapters.)

   Some other examples of words formed from prefixes are:

   disinfection: dis-, apart + *infection,* infection = removal of infection or sterilization
   retroperitoneum: retro-, behind + *peritoneum,* peritoneum = the space behind the peritoneum

4. **Suffixes** are word parts attached to the *end* of a word or word root that modify its meaning. For example, the suffix *-oid,* meaning "like or resembling," helps to form the word *fibroid,* meaning "made of fibrous tissue."

   Some other examples of words formed from suffixes are:

   acrophobia: acro-, height, tip + *-phobia,* fear = fear of heights
   electrolysis: electro-, electricity, electric + *-lysis,* destruction of = the destruction of using electric current

STUDY TIP

Begin making flash cards of word roots, prefixes, and suffixes so that you can mix and match to learn new words as you progress through the text. Try matching different prefixes/suffixes with new word roots and then pronounce the "new term."

Word Building	PRACTICE
	Fill in the correct word elements in each of the following statements.
peri-colic [PER-i-KOL-ik]	_____ colic is around the colon. (prefix)
dent-algia [den-TAL-jē-a]	dent _____ is the term for tooth pain. (suffix)
dys-menorrhea [dĭs-mĕn-ōr-Ē-ă]	_____ menorrhea is painful menses. (prefix)
hepato-megaly [HĔP-ă-tō-MĔG-ă-lē]	hepato _____ means enlarged liver. (suffix)
hypo-tension [HĪ-pō-TĔN-shŭn]	_____ tension means abnormally low blood pressure. (prefix)
epi-gastric [ĕp-ĭ-GĂS-trĭk]	_____ gastric is the area above the stomach. (prefix)
phlebo-tomy [flĕ-BŎT-ō-mē]	phleb _____ is incision (or going into) the vein. (suffix)

Did you know

"O"

Did you know that **/o** is used 70% of the time as a combining vowel in medical terms. (When in doubt, use **o** to see if the term looks correct, then look it up to make sure!)

Laryng(o)plasty   Cardi(o)logy   Oste(o)arthritis

PRONOUNCE	Pronounce the following terms aloud.
retroperitoneum	[RE-trō-PER-ĭ-tō-nē-ŭm]
disinfection	[dis-in-FEK-shŭn]
epigastric	[ĕp-ĭ-GĂS-trĭk]
phlebotomy	[flĕ-BŎT-ō-mē]

SPELL	Write the correct spelling for each related term.
incision into the vein	_____
enlarged liver	_____
around the colon	_____
painful menses	_____

UNDERSTAND — Match the following to the appropriate definition.

1. _____ suffix
2. _____ word root
3. _____ combining vowel
4. _____ prefix

a. in front of a word root
b. used to link word parts together
c. after word root
d. main structure of term

APPLY — Answer the following questions.

1. Using the previous examples in this chapter of word roots, prefixes, and suffixes, try creating some medical terms by matching them together. List four "words."

   _____
   _____
   _____

2. Using a medical dictionary (book or online version), check to see if the words that you created are real medical terms. If so, write their definitions. If not, write a term that closely matches and its definition.

   _____
   _____
   _____
   _____

LO 1.4 Word Roots and Combining Forms

The word root is the foundation or base for each medical term. It is the basis for what a person is trying to relate in this new language. When constructing medical terms, the word root is commonly the focus and the first part of the word to begin building with. When trying to deconstruct an unfamiliar term, the suffix should be the first place to start to figure out its definition. Once the suffix has been identified, go to the beginning of the word and read from left to right to identify the meaning of the term.

All medical terms have a word root that gives the essential meaning to the word. For example, *cardi-* is a root word meaning "heart." In the word *cardiopathy,* the combining form is *cardi/o* = heart and a suffix of a condition, *-pathy.*

The **combining vowel** is a vowel that ties the word root and the associated prefix and/or suffix together. Word roots are almost always seen including (and as) a combining form, which always includes a vowel. Although there is no rule to which vowel is used, the vowel *o* is used approximately 70% of the time. Many times when the suffix begins with a vowel, the same vowel is used as the combining form.

Many prefixes and suffixes are used over and over to match different word roots to create a different meaning. The prefixes and suffixes may be used more often to mix and match medical terms. For instance, a cardiologist and a neurologist both share the same suffix, *-ist,* which means "one who studies or specializes in." However, they are two different kinds of specialists. A cardiologist is "one who studies the heart" and a neurologist is "one who studies nerves." *Cardi/o* and *neur/o* are combining forms; each will be discussed further in its associated systems chapter. The following three examples will help you begin to start working with word roots and combining forms. It is always a bonus that you start memorizing the words now; however, they will come up again in their respective systems chapters. **Focus on the construction of the term. If the suffix begins with a vowel, then adding an extra combining vowel is not needed.**

Example 1:

neuropathy: *neur* [nerve; = **word root**] + */o* [combining vowel] + *-pathy* [condition; = suffix]

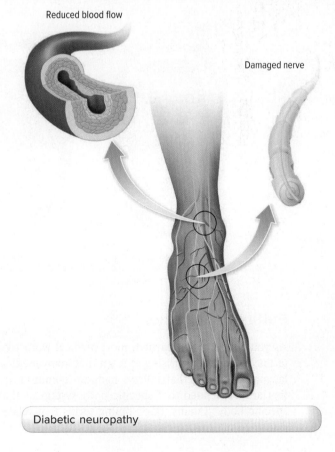

Reduced blood flow

Damaged nerve

Diabetic neuropathy

Example 2:

en**cephal**itis: *en-* [inside; = prefix] + *cephal* [head; = **word root**] + *-itis* [inflammation; = suffix]

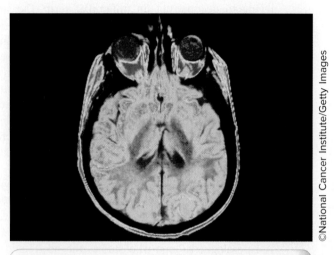

MRI and CT scan with brain inflammation (encephalitis)

©National Cancer Institute/Getty Images

Example 3:

tonsillectomy: *tonsil* [throat tissue; = **word root**] + *-ectomy* [complete removal; = suffix]. Note: If a word ends with *l*, the letter is doubled.

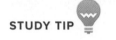

STUDY TIP

Try to use association and other learning techniques with memorization when studying the terms. It will make the process easier and help you retain the information. Create a picture in your mind of how you would "see" the term.

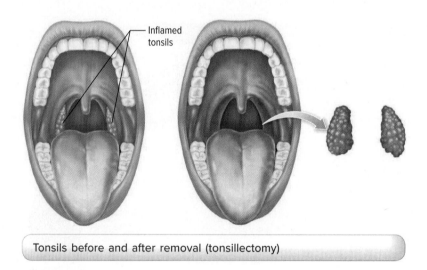

Inflamed tonsils

Tonsils before and after removal (tonsillectomy)

Putting It Together

As you have already learned, most medical word roots come directly from Greek and Latin terms. It may be surprising to learn that many medical terms are already familiar in common language. The list that follows includes common medical combining forms with meanings that are not related to a specific body system or that may apply to both general terms and specific body systems. (Combining forms that relate only to a specific body system will be discussed in later chapters.)

Some combining forms that relate to **body parts** or **elements** include:

Combining Form	Meaning
aer/o	air, gas
ather/o	plaque, fatty substance (inside of a blood vessel)
blast/o	immature cells
calc/o, calci/o	calcium
chondrio, chondro	cartilage, grainy, gritty
chyl/o	chyle, a digestive juice
chym/o	chyme, semifluid production of chyme in the stomach
cyst/o, cysti	bladder, cyst, cystic duct
cyt/o	cell
ethm/o	ethmoid bone
gluc/o	glucose
glyc/o	sugars
hydr/o	hydrogen, water
ket/o, keton/o	ketone, acetone
lip/o	fat (outside of a blood vessel)
nucle/o	nucleus
plasma, plasmo	formative, plasma
salping/o	tube
sider/o	iron
somat/o	body
squam/o	scale, squamous (meaning scaly)
syring/o	tube

STUDY TIP

When creating flash cards for study, it is important to have prefixes and suffixes separate from the word roots.

Word Building

PRACTICE

Provide the combining word element in each of the following statements.

hydro-cephaly [hī-drō-SĔF-ă-lē]	A condition characterized by excessive fluid accumulation in the brain is _____ cephaly.
chondro-cyte [KŎN-drō-sīt]	A _____ cyte is a cartilage cell.
syring-itis [sĭ-rĭn-JĪ-tĭs]	Inflammation of the eustachian tube is _____ itis.
salping-ectomy [săl-pĭn-JĚK-tō-mē]	_____ ectomy is removal of the fallopian tube.

continued on next page

Word Building	PRACTICE
	Provide the combining word element in each of the following statements.
nucleo-toxin [NŪ-klē-ō-TŎK-sĭn]	_____ toxin is a poison that acts upon a cell nucleus.
ather-oma [ăth-ĕr-Ō-mă]	_____ oma is a tumor from a fatty deposit inside a vessel.
ethmo-nasal [ĕth-mō-NĀ-săl]	Relating to the ethmoid and nasal bones is _____ nasal.
aero-gen [ĀR-ō-jĕn]	An _____ gen is a gas-producing microorganism.
somato-genic [SŌ-mă-tō-JĔN-ĭk]	Originating in the body is _____ genic.
gluco-genic [glū-kō-JĔN-ĭk]	Producing glucose is _____ genic.
glyco-penia [glī-kō-PĒ-nē-ă]	_____ penia is a sugar deficiency.
calci-penia [kăl-sĭ-PĒ-nē-ă]	_____ penia is a calcium deficiency.
lipo-blast [LĬ-pō-blăst]	An embryonic fat cell (outside a vessel) is a _____ blast.
glio-blastoma [GLĪ-ō-blăs-TŌ-mă]	A growth consisting of immature neural cells is a _____ blastoma.
plasma-pheresis [PLĂZ-mă-fĕ-RĒ-sĭs]	_____ pheresis is the separation of blood into parts.
cyto-architecture [SĪ-tō-ĂR-kĭ-tĕk-chūr]	The arrangement of cells in tissue is _____ architecture.
sidero-penia [SĬD-ĕr-ō-PĒ-nē-ă]	An abnormally low level of iron in the blood is _____ penia.
cyst-oid [SĬS-toyd]	_____ oid is bladder-shaped.
keto-genesis [kē-tō-JĔN-ĕ-sĭs]	The metabolic production of ketones is _____ genesis.
chylo-poiesis [KĪ-lō-pŏy-Ē-sĭs]	_____ poiesis is the production of chyle in the intestine.
chymo-poiesis [KĪ-mō-pŏy-Ē-sĭs]	_____ poiesis means the production of chyme.
squamo-frontal [SKWĀ-mō-FRŎN-tăl]	Relating to the squamous part of the frontal bone is _____ frontal.

PRONOUNCE	Pronounce the following terms aloud.
glioblastoma	[GLĪ-ō-blăs-TŌ-mă]
ketogenesis	[kē-tō-JĔN-ĕ-sĭs]
calcipenia	[kăl-sĭ-PĒ-nē-ă]
hydrocephaly	[hī-drō-SĔF-ă-lē]

SPELL	Write the correct spelling for each related term.
	Separation of blood into parts
	Means production of chyme
	Removal of a fallopian tube
	Inflammation of eustachian tube
	Metabolic production of ketones

UNDERSTAND	Match the following combining forms on the left to their appropriate meaning.

1. _____ lip/o
2. _____ ather/o
3. _____ cyst/o
4. _____ chondr/o
5. _____ hydr/o
6. _____ chyl/o

a. fat cell inside a vessel
b. fat cell outside a vessel
c. bladder-shaped
d. cartilage cell
e. chyle
f. fluid

APPLY	Answer the following question.

Describe in detail the difference between a word root and a combining form. Explain the basis of medical terminology.

_____
_____
_____

Sensations or Feelings

Some combining forms that relate to **sensations** *or* **feelings** include:

Combining Form	Meaning
algesi/o, algi/o, alg/o	pain
cry/o	cold
dips/o	thirst
esthesi/o	sensation, perception
kin/o, kine	movement, motion
kinesi/o, kines/o	motion
phon/o	sound, voice, speech
phot/o	light
son/o	sound
therm/o	heat

STUDY TIP

The biggest mistake that students make using combining forms is to use two vowels together in a term. Be careful that you are looking closely at the term and not using two combining form vowels.

Example:
Incorrect = cardioitis
Correct = carditis

Did you know ?

Listening to Your Insides

The first stethoscope was invented in the early 1800s, but not many physicians had them. In order to listen to the heart and lungs, they literally had to put their ear to the chest of the patient.

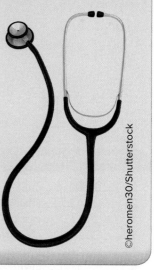

©heromen30/Shutterstock

Word Building	PRACTICE
	Provide the combining word element in each of the following statements.
cryo-cautery [KRĪ-ō-KĂW-tĕr-ē]	Destruction of tissue by freezing is _____ cautery.
photo-meter [fō-TŎM-ĕ-tĕr]	A _____ meter is an instrument for measuring light.
sono-motor [sŏn-ō-MŌ-tĕr]	_____ motor relates to movements caused by sound.
thermo-meter [thĕr-MŎM-ĕ-tĕr]	An instrument for measuring temperature is a _____ meter
algo-spasm [ĂL-gō-spăzm]	Pain caused by a spasm is an _____ spasm.
dipso-mania [dĭp-sō-MĀ-nē-ă]	_____ mania is alcoholism.
kinesio-logy [kĭ-nē-sē-ŎL-ō-jē]	The study of movement is _____ logy.
kin-esthesia [KĬN-ĕs-THĒ-zē-ă]	The perception of movement is _____ esthesia.
phono-meter [fō-NŎM-ĕ-tĕr]	A _____ meter is an instrument for measuring sound.
esthesio-metry [ĕs-thē-zē-ŎM-ĕ-trē]	Measurement of tactile sensibility is _____ metry.

PRONOUNCE	Pronounce the following terms aloud.
cryocautery	[KRĪ-ō-KĂW-tĕr-ē]
esthesiometry	[ĕs-thē-zē-ŎM-ĕ-trē]
sonomotor	[sŏn-ō-MŌ-tĕr]
kinesthesia	[KĬN-ĕs-THĒ-zē-ă]

SPELL	Write the correct spelling for each related term.
	Study of movement
	Measurement of tactile sensibility
	Destruction by freezing
	Pain caused by a spasm
	Alcoholism

UNDERSTAND

Match the following combining forms on the left to their appropriate meaning.

1. _____ cry/o
2. _____ phon/o
3. _____ phot/o
4. _____ kinesi/o
5. _____ son/o
6. _____ therm/o

a. sound, voice, speech
b. temperature
c. measuring sound
d. light
e. movement
f. freezing

APPLY

Answer the following question.

Write four words related to **sensations** or **feelings** and their definitions.

_____

_____

_____

_____

Factor or Quality

Some combining forms that relate to **factor** or **quality** include:

Combining Form	Meaning
acanth/o	spiny, thorny
andr/o	masculine
chlor/o	chlorine, green
chrom/o, chromat/o	color
crypt/o	hidden, obscure
cyan/o	blue

continued on next page

Combining Form	Meaning
eosin/o	red
erythr/o	red, redness
granul/o	granular
gyn/o, gyne, gynec/o	women
home/o, hom/o	same, constant
ichthy/o	dry, scaly, fishy
idi/o	distinct, unknown
immun/o	safe, immune
leuk/o	white
macr/o	large, long
meg/a, megal/o	large, million
melan/o	black, dark
micr/o	small, tiny
mio	smaller, less
morph/o	structure, shape
norm/o	normal
physi/o	physical, natural
pseud/o	false
scler/o	hardness, hardening
scoli/o	crooked, bent
spher/o	round, spherical
staphyl/o	grapelike clusters
sten/o	narrowness
strept/o	twisted chains, *streptococci*
terat/o	monster (as a malformed fetus)
xanth/o	yellow

Word Building	PRACTICE
	Provide the combining word element in each of the following statements.
eosino-philic [ē-ō-sĭn-ō-FĬL-ĭk]	Staining readily with certain (red) dyes is _____ philic.
micro-organism [MĪ-krō-ŌR-găn-ĭzm]	A _____ organism is a tiny organism.

xantho-derma [zăn-thō-DĔR-mă]	_____ derma is yellowish skin.
steno-cephaly [stĕn-ō-SĔF-ă-lē]	_____ cephaly is narrowness of the head.
morpho-logy [mōr-FŎL-ō-jē]	The study of the structure of animals and plants is _____ logy.
homeo-plasia [HŌ-mē-ō-PLĀ-zē-ă]	The formation of new, similar tissue is _____ plasia.
scolio-meter [skō-lē-ŎM-ĕ-tĕr]	An instrument for measuring curves is a _____ meter.
idio-pathic [ĬD-ē-ō-PĂTH-ĭk]	A disease of unknown origin is said to be _____ pathic.
pseudo-diabetes [SŪ-dō-dī-ă-BĒ-tēz]	_____ diabetes is a false test for sugar in the urine.
acanth-oid [ă-KĂN-thŏyd]	_____ oid is spine-shaped.
chromato-genous [krō-mă-TŎJ-ĕ-nŭs]	Producing color is _____ ogenous (Figure 1-4).
strepto-coccus [strĕp-tō-KŎK-ŭs]	A common organism that can cause various infections is _____ *coccus.*
leuko-blast [LŪ-kō-blăst]	A _____ blast is an immature white blood cell.
physio-therapy [FĬZ-ē-ō-THĀR-ă-pē]	Physical therapy is also called _____ therapy.
granul-oma [grăn-yū-LŌ-mă]	A small, granular lesion is a _____ oma.
erythro-clasis [ĕr-ĭ-THRŎK-lă-sĭs]	Fragmentation of red blood cells is _____ clasis.
melano-derma [MĔL-ă-nō-DĔR-mă]	Abnormal skin darkening is _____ derma.
terato-gen [TĔR-ă-tō-jĕn]	An agent that causes a malformed fetus is a _____ gen.
andro-blastoma [ĂN-drō-blăs-TŌ-mă]	_____ blastoma is a testicular tumor.
chlor-uresis [klōr-yū-RĒ-sĭs]	_____ uresis is the excretion of chloride in urine.
immuno-deficient [ĬM-yū-nō-dē-FĬSH-ĕnt]	Lacking in some essential immune function is _____ deficient.
staphylo-coccus [STĂF-ĭ-lō-KŎK-ŭs]	_____ *coccus* is a common species that is the cause of a variety of infections.

continued on next page

Word Building	PRACTICE
	Provide the combining word element in each of the following statements.
cyano-sis [sī-a-Nō-sis]	State or condition of being blue is _____ sis.
gyno-pathy [gī-NŎP-ă-thē]	_____ pathy is a disease peculiar to women.
sclero-derma [sklēr-ō-DĔR-mă]	Thickening and hardening of the skin is _____ derma.
crypto-genic [krĭp-tō-JĔN-ĭk]	_____ genic refers to obscure origin.
normo-cyte [NŌR-mō-sīt]	A normal cell is a _____ cyte.
ichthyo-toxism [ĬK-thē-ō-TŎK-sĭzm]	Poisoning by fish is _____ toxism.
sphero-cyte [SFĒR-ō-sīt]	A round red blood cell is a _____ cyte.
macro-melia [măk-rō-MĒ-lē-ă]	_____ melia is an abnormally large-sized limb.
megalo-encephaly [MĔG-ă-lō-ĕn-SĔF-ă-lē]	_____ encephaly is an abnormally large head and brain.
mio-pragia [mī-ō-PRĀ-jē-ă]	Lessened functional activity is _____ pragia.

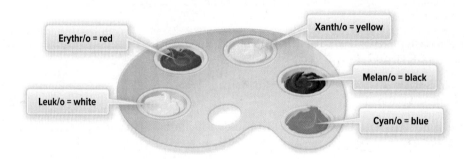

Figure 1-4 Color wheel using the combining form colors: leuk/o = white, erythr/o = red, xanth/o = yellow, melan/o = black, cyan/o = blue

PRONOUNCE	Pronounce the following terms aloud.
cryptogenic	[krĭp-tō-JĔN-ĭk]
spherocyte	[SFĒR-ō-sīt]
chloruresis	[klōr-yū-RĒ-sĭs]
eosinophilic	[ē-ō-sĭn-ō-FĬL-ĭk]

Write the correct spelling for each related term.

	Thickening of the skin
	Fragmentation of red blood
	Abnormally large head and brain
	Abnormal skin darkening
	Excretion of chloride in urine

UNDERSTAND **Match the following combining forms on the left to their appropriate meaning.**

1. _____ gyn/o   a. white
2. _____ cyan/o   b. red
3. _____ spher/o   c. large
4. _____ erythr/o   d. infectious organism
5. _____ melan/o   e. curves
6. _____ leuk/o   f. round
7. _____ scoli/o   g. black
8. _____ macr/o   h. pertaining to women
9. _____ strept/o   i. blue
10. _____ granul/o   j. granules

APPLY **Answer the following question.**

Write four words related to **factor** or **quality** and their definitions.

_____

_____

_____

_____

Condition or Condition-Related

Some combining forms that are **condition** or **condition-related** include:

Combining Form	Meaning
bacill/o	bacilli, bacteria
bacteri/o	bacteria
carcin/o	cancer
kyph/o	humpback
onch/o, onc/o	tumor
path/o	disease
pyr/o	fever, fire, heat
schist/o	split
schiz/o	split, division
spasm/o	spasm

Word Building	PRACTICE
	Provide the combining word element in each of the following statements.
patho-gen [PĂTH-ō-jĕn]	A disease-causing substance is a _____ gen.
carcino-gen [kăr-SĬN-ō-jĕn]	A _____ gen is a cancer-producing substance.
spasmo-lytic [SPĂZ-mō-LĬT-ĭk]	An agent that relieves spasms is a _____ lytic.
bacterio-genic [băk-TĔR-ē-ō-JĔN-ĭk]	_____ genic is caused by bacteria.
pyro-genic [pī-rō-JĔN-ĭk]	Causing fever is _____ genic.
kypho-scoliosis [KĪ-fō-skō-lē-Ō-sĭs]	Kyphosis combined with scoliosis is _____ scoliosis.
bacilli-form [bă-SĬL-ĭ-fōrm]	_____ form is a rod-shaped bacterium.
schizo-phrenia [skĭz-ō-FRĒ-nē-ă *or* skĭt-sō-FRĒ-nē-ă]	A spectrum of mental disorders often with a disorder in perception is _____ phrenia.
onco-lysis [ŏng-KŎL-ĭ-sĭs]	_____ lysis is destruction of a cancerous tumor.
schisto-cytosis [SHĬS-tō-sĭ-TŌ-sĭs *or* SKĬS-tō-sĭ-TŌ-sĭs]	A bladder split is a _____ cytosis.

PRONOUNCE	Pronounce the following terms aloud.
bacilliform	[bă-SĬL-ĭ-fŏrm]
schistocytosis	[SHĬS-tō-sĭ-TŌ-sĭs]
kyphoscoliosis	[KĪ-fō-skō-lē-Ō-sĭs]
pyrogenic	[pī-rō-JĔN-ĭk]

SPELL	Write the correct spelling for each related term.
	Causing fever
	Destruction of a cancerous tumor
	Relieves spasms
	Rod-shaped bacteria

1. _____ bacteri/o
2. _____ carcin/o
3. _____ pyr/o
4. _____ schist/o
5. _____ path/o
6. _____ onc/o

a. tumor
b. fever
c. bacteria
d. disease
e. cancer
f. split

APPLY | **Answer the following question.**

Write four words related to **condition** or **condition-related** and their definitions.

_____
_____
_____
_____

STUDY TIP

Association trick 1:

When thinking of the dors/o position, one trick is to think of the dorsal fin on a fish. Where is it located? On the back: *dors/o* = back/spine of the body.

Association trick 2:

What does an orthodontist do? This person straightens teeth. What would an orthopedic surgeon do? This person straightens bones. By association, what does *orth/o* mean?

Position or Location

Some combining forms that refer to **position** or **location** include:

Combining Form	Meaning
anteri/o	front
dextr/o	right, toward the right
dors/o	back
goni/o	angle
later/o	lateral, to one side
medi/o	middle, medial plane
mes/o	middle, median
orth/o	straight, normal
top/o	place, topical

Word Building

latero-duction [LĂT-ĕr-ō-DŬK-shŭn]	
dextro-cardia [DĔKS-trō-KĂR-dē-ă]	
meso-cephalic [MĔZ-ō-sĕ-FĂL-ĭk]	

PRACTICE

Provide the combining word element in each of the following statements.

Movement to one side is _____ duction.

_____ cardia is displacement of the heart to the right.

Having a medium-sized head is _____ cephalic.

continued on next page

PRACTICE

Provide the combining word element in each of the following statements.

dors-algia [dŏr-SĂL-jē-ă]	_____ algia is upper back pain.
topo-graphy [tō-PŎG-ră-fē]	_____ graphy is description of a body part in terms of a specific surface area.
gonio-meter [gō-nē-ŎM-ĕ-tĕr]	An instrument for measuring angles is a _____ meter.
ortho-dontics [ŏr-thō-DŎN-tĭks]	_____ dontics is the dental specialty concerned with straightening tooth placement (Figure 1-5).
medio-lateral [MĒ-dē-ō-LĂT-ĕr-ăl]	_____ lateral relates to the medial plane and one side of the body.

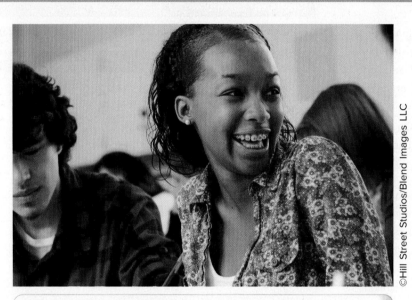

©Hill Street Studios/Blend Images LLC

Figure 1-5 Orthodontic work

PRONOUNCE

Pronounce the following terms aloud.

mediolateral	[MĒ-dē-ō-LĂT-ĕr-ăl]
goniometer	[gō-nē-ŎM-ĕ-tĕr]
dextrocardia	[DĔKS-trō-KĂR-dē-ă]

SPELL

Write the correct spelling for each related term.

	Doctor who corrects tooth placement
	Instrument that measures angles
	Body part in terms of specific area
	Upper back pain

1. _____ later/o
2. _____ dextr/o
3. _____ medi/o
4. _____ top/o
5. _____ mes/o
6. _____ orth/o

a. one side
b. surface area
c. straighten (teeth)
d. to the right
e. middle plane
f. medium-sized

APPLY | Answer the following question.

Write four words related to **position** or **location** and their definitions.

_____
_____
_____
_____

Body Processes

Some combining forms that refer to **body processes** include:

Combining Form	Meaning
crin/o	secrete
gen/o	producing, being born
hypn/o	sleep
log/o	speech, words, thought
narc/o	sleep, numbness
phag/o	eating, devouring, swallowing
somn/o, somni	sleep
spir/o	breath; breathe (Figure 1-6)

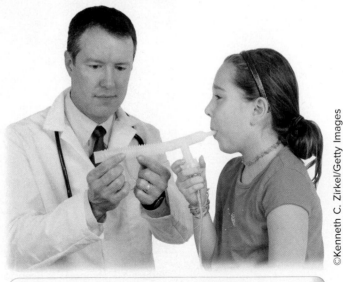

©Kenneth C. Zirkel/Getty Images

Figure 1-6 Spirometry—measuring breathing

Word Building	PRACTICE
	Provide the combining word element in each of the following statements.
hypno-genesis [hĭp-nō-JĔN-ĕ-sĭs]	Induction of sleep is _____ genesis (Figure 1-7).
somn-ambulism [sŏm-NĂM-byū-lĭzm]	_____ ambulism is sleepwalking.
crino-genic [krĭn-ō-JĔN-ĭk]	_____ genic refers to causing secretion.
phago-cyte [FĂG-ō-sīt]	A cell that ingests bacteria and other particles is a _____ cyte.
geno-blast [JĔN-ō-blăst]	_____ blast is the nucleus of a fertilized ovum.
spiro-scope [SPĪ-rō-skōp]	A _____ scope is a device for measuring lung capacity.
logo-pathy [lŏg-ŎP-ă-thē]	_____ pathy is a speech disorder.
narco-lepsy [NĂR-kō-lĕp-sē]	_____ lepsy is a sleep disorder.

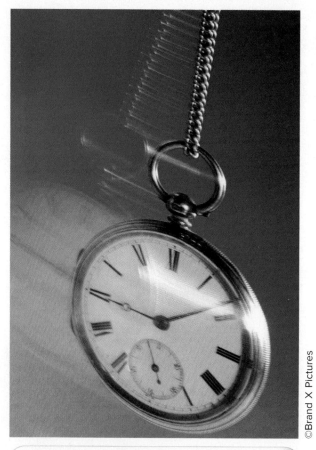

©Brand X Pictures

Figure 1-7 Hypnosis is used to control pain in addition to helping retrieve memory

PRONOUNCE	Pronounce the following terms aloud.
somnambulism	[sŏm-NĂM-byū-lĭzm]
logopathy	[lŏg-ŎP-ă-thē]
narcolepsy	[NĂR-kō-lĕp-sē]

SPELL	Write the correct spelling for each related term.
	Speech disorder
	Sleep disorder
	Inducing sleep
	Cell that ingests bacteria

UNDERSTAND

Match the following combining forms on the left to their appropriate meaning.

1. _____ crin/o   a. producing
2. _____ phag/o   b. secrete
3. _____ gen/o   c. sleep, numbness
4. _____ narc/o   d. eating
5. _____ log/o   e. sleep
6. _____ hypn/o   f. speech, words, thought

APPLY

Answer the following question.

Write four words related to **body processes** and their definitions.

_____

_____

_____

_____

STUDY TIP

When using flash cards, practice with ten cards at a time. This will help make the process less overwhelming!

Miscellaneous Combining Forms

Some **miscellaneous combining forms** include:

Combining Form	Meaning
actin/o	light
amyl/o	starch
bar/o	weight, pressure
bas/o, basi/o	base
bio	life
chem/o	chemical
chrono	time
coni/o	dust

continued on next page

Combining Form	Meaning
cycl/o	circle, cycle
dyna, dynam/o	force, energy
echo	reflected sound
electr/o	electricity
eti/o	cause
fibr/o	fiber
fluor/o	light, luminous, fluorine
fungi	fungus
galact/o	milk
ger/o, geront/o	old age
lact/o, lacti	milk
lith/o	stone
lys/o	dissolution, destruction
necr/o	death, dying
noct/i	night
nyct/o	night
pharmaco	drugs, medicine
phyt/o	plant
py/o	pus
radio	radiation, x-ray, radius
stere/o	three-dimensional
tel/o, tele/o	distant, end, complete
ton/o	tension, pressure
toxi, toxic/o, tox/o	poison, toxin
troph/o	food, nutrition

Did you know

Weighing In

The first scale dates back to 2000 BC. There are hundreds of patents for scales registered with the US Patent and Trademark Office.

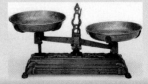

©Chepe Nicoli/ Shutterstock

etio-pathology [Ē-tē-ō-pă-THŎL-ō-jē]	The study of the cause of an abnormality or disease is _____ pathology.
litho-tomy [lĭ-THŎT-ō-mē]	_____ tomy is an operation for removal of stones.
baro-stat [BĂR-ō-stăt]	A pressure-regulating device is a _____ stat.
echo-cardiogram [ĕk-ō-KĂR-dē-ō-grăm]	An ultrasound recording of the heart is an _____ cardiogram.
tropho-cyte [TRŎF-ō-sīt]	A cell that provides nutrition is a _____ cyte.
noct-uria [nŏk-TŪ-rē-ă]	Urination at night is _____ uria.
nyctal-opia [nĭk-tă-LŌ-pē-ă]	_____ opia is reduced ability to see at night.
amylo-phagia [ĂM-ĭ-lō-FĀ-jē-ă]	_____ phagia is an abnormal craving for starch.
lacto-gen [LĂK-tō-jĕn]	An agent that stimulates milk production is _____ gen.
electro-cardiogram [ē-lĕk-trō-KĂR-dē-ō-grăm]	An _____ cardiogram is a graphic record of the heart's electrical currents.
tono-meter [tō-NŎM-ĕ-tĕr]	An instrument for measuring pressure is a _____ meter.
phyto-toxin [fī-tō-TŎK-sĭn]	_____ toxin is a substance from plants that is similar to a bacterial toxin.
cine-radiography [SĬN-ĕ-ră-dē-ŌG-ră-fē]	Imaging of an organ in motion is _____ radiography.
bi-opsy [BĪ-ŏp-sē]	_____ opsy is sampling of tissue from a living patient.
geronto-logy [jăr-ŏn-TŎL-ō-jē]	The study of the problems of aging is _____ logy.
pyo-cyst [PĪ-ō-sĭst]	A cyst filled with pus is a _____ cyst.
chemo-lysis [kĕm-ŎL-ĭ-sĭs]	_____ lysis is chemical destruction.
cycl-ectomy [sī-KLĔK-tō-mē]	Removal of a part of a ciliary body is _____ ectomy.
fungi-cide [FŬN-jĭ-sīd]	_____ cide is a substance that destroys fungi.
telo-phase [TĔL-ō-fāz]	_____ phase is a final stage of mitosis or meiosis.
necro-logy [nĕ-KRŎL-ō-jē]	Study of the cause of death is _____ logy.
actino-therapy [ĂK-tĭn-ō-THĂR-ă-pē]	_____ therapy is ultraviolet light therapy used in dermatology.

continued on next page

PRACTICE

Provide the combining word element in each of the following statements.

Word Element	Statement
dynamo-meter [dī-nă-MŎM-ĕ-tĕr]	Instrument for measuring muscular power is a _____ meter.
lys-emia [lī-SĒ-mē-ă]	_____ emia is dissolution of red blood cells.
galacto-phoritis [gă-LĂK-tō-fō-RĪ-tĭs]	Inflammation of the milk ducts is _____ phoritis.
baso-philic [BĀ-sō-FĬL-ĭk]	Having an affinity for basic dyes is _____ philic.
radio-graphy [RĀ-dē-ŎG-ră-fē]	_____ graphy is an x-ray examination.
fibro-plastic [fī-brō-PLĂS-tĭk]	_____ plastic is producing fibrous tissue.
fluoro-chrome [FLŪR-ō-krōm]	_____ chrome is fluorescent contrast medium.
chrono-metry [krō-NŎM-ĕ-trē]	Measurement of time intervals is _____ metry.
toxi-pathy [tŏk-SĬP-ă-thē]	Disease due to poisoning is _____ pathy.
pharmaco-logy [FĂR-mă-KŎL-ō-jē]	_____ logy is the science of drugs, including their sources, uses, and interactions (Figure 1-8).
stereo-logy [STĔR-ē-ŎL-ō-jē]	Study of three-dimensional aspects of a cell is _____ logy.
conio-meter [kō-nē-ŎM-ĕ-tĕr]	Device for measuring dust is a _____ meter.

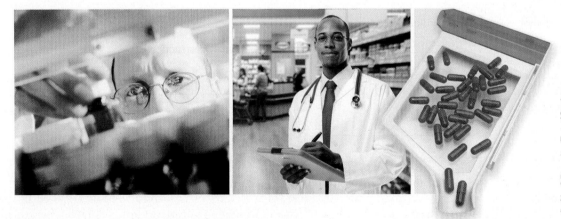

(left): ©Royalty-Free/Corbis
(middle): ©kurhan/Shutterstock
(right): ©Comstock/Alamy

Figure 1-8 Pharmacy, pharmacist, and pharmacology

PRONOUNCE	Pronounce the following reproductive terms aloud.
chemolysis	[kĕm-ŎL-ĭ-sĭs]
actinotherapy	[ĂK-tĭn-ō-THĀR-ă-pē]
etiopathology	[Ē-tē-ō-pă-THŎL-ō-jē]
basophilic	[BĀ-sō-FĬL-ĭk]

SPELL	Write the correct spelling for each related term.
	Measurement of time intervals
	Dissolution of red blood cells
	Cyst filled with pus
	Fluorescent contrast medium
	Inflammation of the milk ducts

UNDERSTAND	Match the following combining forms on the left to their appropriate meaning.

1. _____ electr/o   a. pus
2. _____ ech/o   b. drugs; medicine
3. _____ lith/o   c. light
4. _____ fluor/o   d. electricity
5. _____ py/o   e. stone
6. _____ eti/o   f. cause
7. _____ dynam/o   g. reflected sound
8. _____ troph/o   h. fiber
9. _____ pharmaco   i. food, nutrition
10. _____ fibr/o   j. force, energy

APPLY	Answer the following question.

Write four words using **miscellaneous** combining forms and their definitions.

_____

_____

_____

_____

LO 1.5 Pluralizing Terms

Most English plurals are formed by adding -s or -es to a word. This is also true of many medical terms (cancer, cancers; abscess, abscesses). However, medical terms derived from ancient Greek and Latin often use the regular plural forms from those languages (bursa, bursae; embolus, emboli). Table 1-2 shows the formation of plurals.

TABLE 1-2   Formation of Plurals

Pluralizing Rules	Singular Words	Plural Words
Add -s to words ending in any vowel or consonant except s, x, z, or y.	joint, face, angioma, cancer, muscle, paraplegic	joints, faces, angiomas, cancers, muscles, paraplegics
Add -es to words ending in s, x, or z.	abscess, reflex	abscesses, reflexes
Remove the y and add -ies to words ending in -y preceded by a consonant. When an ending y is preceded by a vowel, the usual plural suffix is -s.	vasectomy	vasectomies
Remove the x and add -ces to Latin words ending in x.	appendix, radix	appendices, radices
Add -e to Latin terms ending in a.	fossa	fossae
Remove -us and add -i to Latin words ending in us.	*Staphylococcus*	*Staphylococci*
Remove -on and add -a to Greek words ending in on; remove um and add -a to Latin words ending in um.	ganglion, datum	ganglia, data
Change -sis to -ses in Greek words ending in sis.	neurosis	neuroses

Word Building

PRACTICE

Provide the correct word in each of the following statements.

joints [jŏynts]	The plural of joint is _____.
abscess [ĂB-sĕs]	The singular form of abscesses is _____.
vasectomy [vă-SĔK-tō-mē]	The singular form of vasectomies is _____.
appendices [ă-PEN-di-sēz]	The plural of appendix is _____.
fossae [FŎS-ē]	The plural of fossa is _____.
staphylococci [STĂF-ĭ-lō-KŎK-sī]	The plural of *staphylococcus* is _____.
ganglion [GĂNG-glē-ŏn]	The singular form of ganglia is _____.
neurosis [noo-RŌ-sis]	The singular form of neuroses is _____.
angiomas *or* **angiomata** [ăn-jē-Ō-măz, ăn-jē-ō-MĂ-tă]	The plural of angioma is _____.
paraplegics [par-ă-PLĒ-jiks]	The plural of paraplegic is _____.

reflexes [RĔ-fleks-ĕz]	The plural of reflex is _____.
datum [DĀ-tŭm]	The singular form of data is _____.
cancer [KAN-ser]	The singular form of cancers is _____.
radices [RĀ-di-sēz]	The plural of radix is _____.

PRONOUNCE	Pronounce the following terms aloud.
staphylococci	[STĂF-ĭ-lō-KŎK-sī]
fossae	[FŎS-ē]
angiomas	[ăn-jē-Ō-măz]
radices	[RĀ-di-sēz]

SPELL	Write the correct plural spelling for each related term.
abscess	_____
neurosis	_____
paraplegic	_____
datum	_____
appendix	_____

UNDERSTAND	Identify which forms are singular or plural and if they are correct, and then write both forms.
Strepptococci	Incorrect spelling *Streptococci* = plural, *streptococcus* = singular
nevus	_____
cervices	_____
ganglium	_____
lobes	_____
sternums	_____

APPLY	Answer the following questions.

1. Describe which plural is used when the singular term ends in *-um*. Provide an example not listed above.
   _____
   _____
   _____

2. Describe which plural is used when the singular term ends in *-x*. Provide an example not listed above.
   _____
   _____
   _____

Using Medical Terminology and Its Different Forms

This programmed approach to learning medical terminology consists of several of the same learning components found in each of the body systems chapters.

1. Structure and function
2. Major word parts associated with the system
3. System parts in detail and word building
4. Diagnostic, procedural, and laboratory terms
5. Pathological terms
6. Surgical terms
7. Pharmacological terms

All of these components are important to the entire language of medicine. The following discussion explains how each of these components contributes so they will be familiar when you get to the systems chapters of this text.

A medical record for each patient is created with the first phone call or visit to a physician's office when information is gathered and documented (Figure 1-9). It is critical for both legal and ethical reasons that the medical record is documented any time there is communication either *with* the patient or *about* the patient with another health care provider, hospital, testing facility, and so on. Documentation is the responsibility of the health care worker involved in the communication, not just physicians. The documentation in the medical record also is used for obtaining payment for services. Although the format of the medical record and its documentation may vary, the medical terminology used is the terminology typically learned in courses such as this so that everyone accessing the medical record has the same understanding and mistakes are avoided.

Surgical, Pathological, and Pharmacological Terms

This programmed approach of medical terminology includes medical terms organized by body system, including structure and function, the main body terms, and surgical, procedural, and pharmacological terms that are associated with each body system. Many of the systems share common procedures and even medication treatments, but each functions in its own separate way.

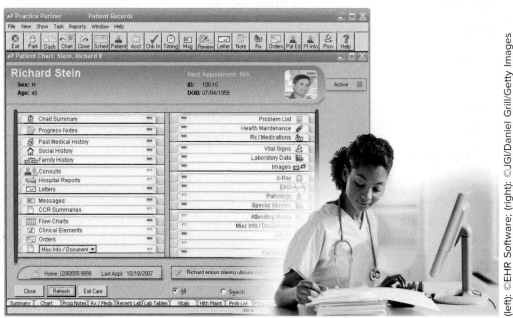

Figure 1-9 Electronic medical record

(left): ©EHR Software; (right): ©JGI/Daniel Grill/Getty Images

Abbreviations

Abbreviations are used in a variety of ways in health care. In most cases, common medical abbreviations (such as CBC for complete blood count) are so routine that the full name is almost never used. In other cases, such as in prescribing medications, the use of abbreviations has led to many medical errors. Several accrediting organizations have come out with recommendations regarding the use of certain abbreviations that have caused confusion and are no longer to be used. Following are some commonly used abbreviations. Additional abbreviations will be introduced in system chapters.

Abbreviation	Meaning
a	Before
ac	Before meals
AMI	Acute myocardial infarction
bid	Twice a day
BP	Blood pressure
c/o	Complaining of
Ca	Cancer/carcinoma
CC	Chief complaint
COPD	Chronic obstructive pulmonary disease (emphysema, chronic bronchitis)
CXR	Chest x-ray
DOB	Date of birth
Dx	Diagnosis
ECG, EKG	Electrocardiogram
Fx	Fracture
GI	Gastrointestinal
h/o	History of
HEENT	Head, ears, eyes, nose, throat
HTN	Hypertension
Hx	History
IM	Intramuscular
LAC	Laceration
LOC	Level of consciousness
mcg	Microgram
NKDA	No known drug allergies
npo	Nothing by mouth

continued on next page

Abbreviation	Meaning
po	By mouth
PRN	As needed
qid	Four times a day
SOB	Shortness of breath
tid	Three times a day
Tx	Treatment
w/o	Without
WNL	Within normal limits

With the implementation of the electronic medical record (EMR), most use of abbreviations in the patient's actual documents will cease to exist. This will alleviate confusion and help with errors. However, abbreviations are still utilized in prescription writing and shorthand notations (Figure 1-10).

SNOMED CT and ICD

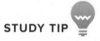

STUDY TIP

As the electronic medical record becomes more standard, abbreviations will become a thing of the past. They will be replaced with "auto-complete" sentences, voice recognition software, and other technology to make documentation easier.

SNOMED CT (Systematized Nomenclature of Medicine Clinical Terms®) is a very detailed medical terminology standard that was developed for use in electronic medical records. The purpose is to use SNOMED CT internationally for all medical coding and electronic transfer of medical data with the goal to improve patient care.

The current standard used for diagnosis coding is the *International Classification of Diseases, 11th Revision, Clinical Modification* (ICD). Eventually, when all health care records are electronic, it is expected that ICD-10-CM will be combined with SNOMED CT. The purpose, when combined, is to create the most effective foundation for future care delivery.

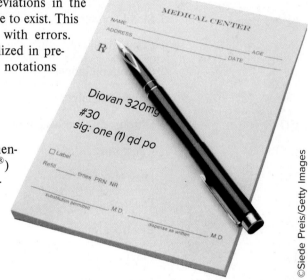

Figure 1-10 Written prescription showing abbreviations

©Siede Preis/Getty Images

Word Building	PRACTICE
	Fill in the correct words in each of the following statements.
medical record	A _____ is created with a patient's phone call or visit to a physician's office.
documented; with; about	The medical record must be _____ each time there is communication either _____ or _____ a patient.

medical record; vary; terminology; mistakes	The format of the documentation and _____ may _____. The medical _____ will typically be the same to avoid _____.
surgical; pathology	_____ procedures are treatments that require invasive cutting into the body to repair or remove a diseased part. _____ is the diagnosis of the disease or condition.
pharmacology	Dispensing of medication to treat ailments is a study called _____.
CBC	Abbreviation for complete blood count is _____.
bid; tid	_____ stands for twice per day. _____ stands for three times per day.
diagnosis	ICD-10-CM is the current standard used for _____ coding.
SNOMED CT	When all health care records are electronic, ICD-10-CM will be combined with _____.
electronic	SNOMED CT is a medical terminology standard developed for use in _____ medical records.
paper	Implementation of SNOMED CT will not take place until some time in the future because most US hospitals and physicians use _____ medical records.

SPELL — Write the correct spelling/words for each related abbreviation.

EMR	_____
ICD	_____
CBC	_____
bid	_____
tid	_____

UNDERSTAND — Match the following terms and definitions to the appropriate meaning.

1. _____ SNOMED
2. _____ ICD-10-CM
3. _____ diagnosis
4. _____ EMR

a. disease (condition) of patient
b. combined with diagnosis
c. coding for diagnosis
d. electronic format for patient medical records

APPLY — Answer the following questions.

1. What does SNOMED CT stand for?
_____
_____
_____
_____

2. Why are medical codes important and how are they used?
_____
_____
_____
_____

3. What are some possible complications or negative outcomes when using abbreviations? What are some positives?
_____
_____
_____
_____

Chapter Review

	Learning Outcome	Summary
1.1	Discuss the history of medical terminology and how terms are developed.	Medical terminology is derived from several ancient languages. It is comprised of forming words that convey a message by utilizing any of four word parts: prefix, word root, combining form, and suffix.
1.2	Describe the importance of pronunciation and spelling in medical terminology.	The nature of medicine is so important that common errors in spelling and pronunciation can cause life-threatening consequences. It is vital that the student is able to correctly pronounce and spell terms and word parts.
1.3	Illustrate the four word parts used to build medical terms.	The common word parts that are used in medical terminology are prefixes, word roots, combining forms, and suffixes. Terms can be a combination of any or all of these to form different words with different meanings.
1.4	Identify how word roots and combining forms build medical terms.	Word roots are the basic foundation of the medical term. They are often the system or body part that the term is describing. The combining form is the word root plus a combining vowel that links the word part to the suffix or prefix.
1.5	Describe the process of pluralizing terms.	Most English plurals are formed by adding -s or -es to a word. This is also true of many medical terms. However, medical terms derived from ancient Greek and Latin often use the regular plural forms from those languages.
1.6	Recognize and use medical terminology and its different forms.	This programmed approach to learning medical terminology consists of several of the same learning components found in each of the body systems chapters. 1. Structure and function 2. Major word parts associated with the system 3. System parts in detail and word building 4. Diagnostic, procedural, and laboratory terms 5. Pathological terms 6. Surgical terms 7. Pharmacological terms

RECALL

1. Relate the history of medical terminology. Explain what languages it is derived from.

_____

_____

_____

2. Illustrate how medical terms are formed.

_____

_____

_____

3. Describe in detail what word roots and combining forms are and how they are used.

_____

_____

_____

4. Relate how you would break down an unfamiliar medical term.

_____

_____

_____

UNDERSTAND

True or False: Circle the correct answer, and explain why it is true or false.

1. Medical terminology is derived from many different ancient languages.   **T**   **F**
2. There are five parts to a medical term.   **T**   **F**
3. Pronunciation is not important in medical terminology; spelling is the most important.   **T**   **F**
4. Abbreviations are always used in the medical setting and they are essential to avoid mistakes.   **T**   **F**
5. If you are an administrative worker and do not provide direct patient care, you do not have to abide by federal, state, and local legal and ethical standards.   **T**   **F**
6. Presently, SNOMED CT is used everywhere.   **T**   **F**
7. Physicians are the only health care workers responsible for medical record documentation and using correct terms/spelling.   **T**   **F**

Using the section practices, complete each term with the appropriate word part that fits the definition.

1. Cancerous tumor: _____ oma
2. Study of structure and function of immune system: _____ logy
3. White blood cell: _____ cyte
4. Condition of lateral curvature of the spine: _____ sis
5. Abnormal fear or dislike of men: _____ phobia
6. Graphic record of the electrical activity of a muscle: _____ myogram
7. Abnormally large red blood cell: _____ cyte
8. Study of the action or effects of drugs on living organisms: _____ dynamics
9. Alcoholism: _____ mania
10. The formation of cartilage: _____ genesis

Look up each term and pronounce each of the above completed terms aloud.

IMPLEMENT

Using the Dictionary: Look up each of the following words in your allied health dictionary. Pronounce each word aloud and check yourself against your dictionary's audio component. If your dictionary does not provide audio, ask your instructor to listen to your pronunciations. Then, write the plural and the definition of each word in the space provided.

1. comedo _____

_____

2. hematocrit _____

_____

3. mesothelioma _____

_____

4. laminectomy _____

_____

5. bacillus _____

_____

Using the suffix *-itis* for every term, complete the given word root/combining form. (Remember to not double vowels on combining forms. Because the suffix begins with *i*, there is usually no need to use the familiar combining form of *o*.)

Example:

cardi/o   **carditis**

1. stomat/o   a.
2. phleb/o   b.
3. cyst/o   c.
4. arthr/o   d.
5. hepat/o   e.
6. oste/o   f.

Fill in the combining form that fits the definition.

1. _____: white
2. _____: black
3. _____: red
4. _____: stones
5. _____: night
6. _____: fat (outside a vessel)
7. _____: cause (of a disease)
8. _____: sugars
9. _____: blue
10. _____: bacteria

Fill in the definition for each combining form.

1. chem/o: _____
2. erythr/o: _____
3. gero, geront/o: _____
4. lact/o: _____
5. oncho, onco: _____
6. phot/o: _____
7. scler/o: _____
8. somn/o, somni: _____
9. toxi, toxic/o, tox/o: _____
10. strept/o: _____

Using the combining form listed, create a new medical term, and then write the new term's definition.

1. lith/o _____
2. noct/o _____
3. ton/o _____
4. lys/o _____
5. bar/o _____
6. somat/o _____
7. micr/o _____

DECONSTRUCT

Break down each term into its component parts using /.

Example:

atherosclerosis	athro/scler/osis
1. pericarditis	a.
2. carcinoma	b.
3. gastroenterology	c.
4. neurofibroma	d.
5. encephalitis	e.
6. cheilosis	f.

How will you use the history of medical terminology to help you form and understand words? What ways and resources would you utilize to help break down or understand words that you don't already know?

_____

_____

Deconstruct the following words.

	Combining Form	Suffix
1. cyanosis		
2. lithogenesis		
3. fungicide		
4. electrocardiogram		
5. chondrocyte		
6. cystoid		
7. bacteriocide		
8. gynecology		

Have you trained yourself to start making flash cards? What other ways could you learn the combining forms?

_____

_____

_____

_____

CHAPTER 2

Prefixes

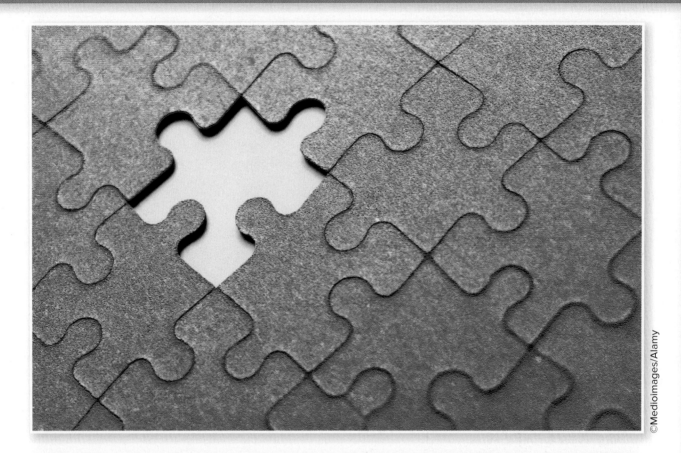

©Medioimages/Alamy

Learning Outcomes

After studying this chapter, you will be able to:

2.1   Describe the role of the prefix in medical terminology.

2.2   Identify common medical prefixes related to size and quantity.

2.3   Describe common medical prefixes related to position or location.

2.4   Identify common medical prefixes related to time.

2.5   Identify common medical prefixes related to presence or quality.

2.6   Describe common miscellaneous medical prefixes.

LO 2.1 Prefixes

As discussed in Chapter 1, medical terminology is a language of compound words matched together to define and condense phrases related to the human body, disease, and conditions. Prefixes are a common part of the English language, and therefore already familiar to use. They function much the same way in medical terminology. Word roots and/or combining forms are the base foundation for the medical term and prefixes are word parts that attach to the beginning of a combining form or word root to enhance or modify its meaning.

Prefixes tend to act like an adjective. Often, they indicate size or quantity, position, measurement, direction or location, time, or the presence or quality of a specific factor that influences the meaning of the word.

Following are some examples of how prefixes contribute to medical terminology.

Example 1:

hypertension: *hyper-* [high, excessive] + *-tension* [blood pressure] = high blood pressure

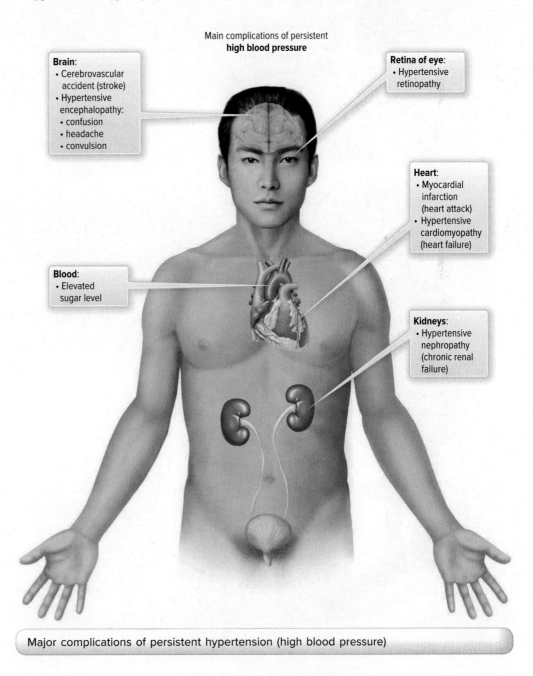

Main complications of persistent **high blood pressure**

Brain:
- Cerebrovascular accident (stroke)
- Hypertensive encephalopathy:
  - confusion
  - headache
  - convulsion

Retina of eye:
- Hypertensive retinopathy

Heart:
- Myocardial infarction (heart attack)
- Hypertensive cardiomyopathy (heart failure)

Blood:
- Elevated sugar level

Kidneys:
- Hypertensive nephropathy (chronic renal failure)

Major complications of persistent hypertension (high blood pressure)

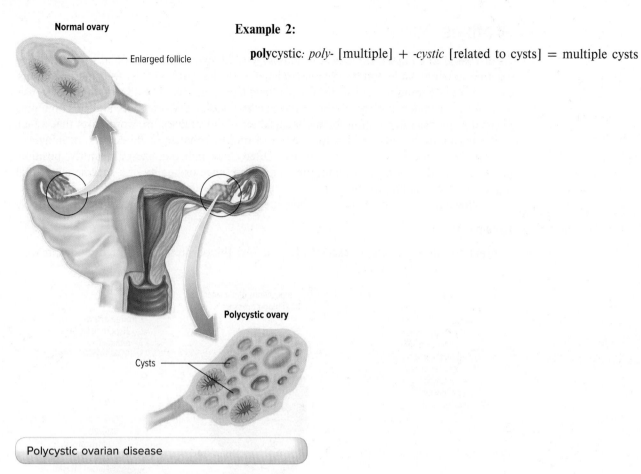

Normal ovary

Enlarged follicle

Polycystic ovary

Cysts

Polycystic ovarian disease

Example 2:

polycystic: *poly-* [multiple] + *-cystic* [related to cysts] = multiple cysts

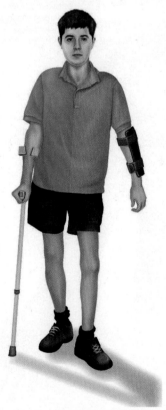

Example 3:

hemiplegic: *hemi-* [half] + *-plegia* [paralysis] = half paralysis

Hemiplegia—as noted on the green side of the body

Putting It Together

Most medical terms have a word root, which gives the essential meaning to the word. For example, *cardi-* is a root word meaning "heart." In the word *pericardia,* the prefix *peri-* is added to the word root to form the whole word meaning "surrounding (*peri-*) the heart (*cardi-*)." The word root also can appear in a combining form, which is the word root plus a combining vowel or vowels. For example, *cardiology* is formed from *cardio-* (the word root *cardi-* plus the combining vowel /*o*/) plus the suffix *-logy,* meaning "the study of the heart."

Remember!

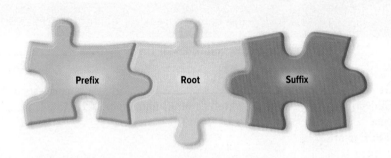

The word root is the foundation piece, and the prefix or suffix will change the meaning.

LO 2.2 Prefixes Related to Size and Quantity

Some medical prefixes that describe **size** or **quantity** include:

Prefix	Meaning
bi-, di-	twice, double
brachy-	short
hemi-	half
iso-	equal, same
mega-	large
micro-	small, microscopic
mono-	single
multi-	many
pan-, panto-	all, entire
pluri-	several, more
poly-	many
quadra-, quadri-	four
tri-	three
uni-	one, single

Practice

As you begin each practice in this chapter, cover the left-hand column and answer all the questions below without removing the cover. Then, uncover and check your answers. Remember also to create flash cards to practice learning the medical terms. At the end of each chapter, use your flash cards for study and review.

Word Building	PRACTICE
	Provide the correct prefix for each of the following terms using the bolded hints.
bi-lateral [bī-LAT-er-ăl]	Referring to **both** sides of the body is _____ lateral.
hemi-plegia [hĕm-ĭ-PLĒ-jē-ă] **quadri-plegia** [kwăh-drĭ-PLĒ-jē-ă]	_____ plegia is paralysis of **half** of the body or on one side of the body; paralysis of all **four** limbs is _____ plegia.
brachy-esophagus [BRĂK-ē-ĕ-SŎF-ă-gŭs]	_____ esophagus: abnormally **short** esophagus.
uni-glandular [yū-nĭ-GLĂN-dū-lăr]	_____ glandular involves only **one** gland.
pluri-glandular [plū-rĭ-GLĂN-dū-lăr]	Involvement of **several** glands is _____ glandular.
micro-scopic [mī-krō-SKOP-ik]	_____ scopic means too **small** to see without a scope device.
iso-metric [ī-sō-MĔT-rĭk]	_____ metric: of the **same** measurement.
mono-mania [mŏn-ō-MĀ-nē-ă]	Obsession with a **single** thought or idea is _____ mania.
multi-articular [MŬL-tē-ăr-TĬK-yū-lăr]	_____ articular involves **many** joints.
poly-arteritis [pŏl-ē-ăr-tĕr-Ī-tĭs]	_____ arteritis is inflammation of **multiple** arteries.
pan-demic [pan-DEM-ik]	A disease that affects an **entire** population is a _____ demic.
micro-plasia [mī-krō-PLĀ-zē-ă]	**Small** or stunted growth, as in dwarfism, is called _____ plasia.
mega-cephaly [mĕg-ă-SĔF-ă-lē]	_____ cephaly is an abnormal **enlargement** of the head.
uni-lateral [yū-nĭ-LĂT-ĕr-ăl]	Condition that affects only **one** side of the body is called _____ lateral.

PRONOUNCE	Pronounce the following terms aloud.
polyarteritis	[pŏl-ē-ăr-tĕr-Ī-tĭs]
isometric	[ī-sō-MĔT-rĭk]
megacephaly	[mĕg-ă-SĔF-ă-lē]
uniglandular	[yū-nĭ-GLĂN-dū-lăr]

Involves **many** joints

Abnormal **enlargement** of the head

Affects only **one** side of the body

Inflammation of **multiple** arteries

Same measurement

UNDERSTAND	Match the term on the left to its meaning on the right.

1. _____ polyarteritis
2. _____ monomania
3. _____ pandemic
4. _____ megacephaly
5. _____ bilateral
6. _____ unilateral

a. both sides (or two sides)
b. one side
c. obsession of a single thought
d. inflammation of multiple arteries
e. enlargement of the head
f. entire population

APPLY	Answer the following questions.

1. Give an example of how medical prefixes change and/or add to the entire medical term.
   _____
   _____
   _____
   _____

2. Construct four word examples with prefixes related to **size** or **quantity.**
   _____
   _____
   _____
   _____

LO 2.3 Prefixes Related to Position or Location

Some medical prefixes that describe **position** or **location** include:

STUDY TIP

Depending on your learning style, you can make different kinds of flash cards. For instance, if you are a visual learner, you may want to make one set of your flash cards with colorful pictures or diagrams on them as clues.

Prefix	Meaning
ab-, abs-	away from
ad-	toward, to
ana-	against, up, backward
apo-	derived, separated from
cata-	down
circum-	around
di-, dif-, dir-, dis-	not, separated
dia-	through

continued on next page

Prefix	Meaning
ecto-	outside or outward
endo-	within
epi-	over, above, upon
ex-	out of, away from
exo-	external, on the outside, outward
extra-	without, on the outside
infra-	positioned beneath, below, under
inter-	between
intra-	within, in
meso-	middle, median
para-	near, adjacent, beside
per-	through, intensely
peri-	around, about, near
retro-	behind, backward
sub-	less than, under, inferior, below or beneath
supra-	above, over, excessive
trans-	across, through

STUDY TIP

Everyday uses of prefixes in health care: "The patient . . .

- was admitted with left substernal chest pain."
- is having surgery due to dysfunctional uterine bleeding."
- has a history of anaphylactic shock."
- was diagnosed with bilateral breast cancer."
- is experiencing hyperglycemia."
- is here for her first prenatal visit."

Word Building

PRACTICE

Provide the correct prefix for each of the following terms using the bolded hints.

ab-duct [ăb-DŬKT]
ad-duct [ă-DŬKT]

_____ duct is to move **away** from the body;
_____ duct is to move **toward** the body.

meso-derm
[MĔZ-ō-dĕrm]

The **middle** layer of skin is the _____ derm.

sub-cutaneous
[sŭb-kyū-TĀ-nē-ŭs]

_____ cutaneous is **beneath** the skin.

supra-maxillary
[sū-pră-MĂK-sĭ-lār-ē]

_____ maxillary is **above** the maxilla.

ana-phylactic
[ĂN-ă-fĭ-LĂK-tĭk]

Exaggerated reaction to a toxin that is **against** phylaxsis is _____ phylactic.

cata-plexy
[KĂT-ă-plĕk-sē]

Sudden **extreme** muscle weakness is _____ plexy.

epi-condyle [ĕp-ĭ-KŎN-dīl]	_____ condyle: **over** or **near** the condyle.
retro-version [rĕ-trō-VĔR-zhŭn]	Turning **backward,** as of the uterus, is _____ version.
circum-oral [sĕr-kŭm-ŌR-ăl]	_____ oral means **around** the mouth.
peri-appendicitis [PĔR-ē-ă-pĕn-dĭ-SĪ-tĭs]	Inflammation of the tissue **surrounding** the appendix is _____ appendicitis.
apo-biosis [ăp-ō-bī-Ō-sĭs]	_____ biosis is the **death of a part** of a living organism.
ecto-pic [ĕk-TŎP-ĭk]	Occurring **outside** the normal place, as a pregnancy **outside** the uterus, is _____ pic.
exo-genous [ĕks-ŎJ-ĕ-nŭs]	_____ genous means produced **outside** of the organism.
extra-corporeal [ĔKS-tră-kōr-PŌR-ē-ăl]	**Outside** of the body is _____ corporeal.
dis-articulation [dĭs-ăr-tĭk-yū-LĀ-shŭn]	**Separating** a joint is _____ articulation.
endo-abdominal [ĔN-dō-ăb-DŎM-ĭ-năl]	_____ abdominal: **within** the abdomen.
endo-metrial [ĔN-dō-MĒ-trē-ăl]	_____ metrial: **within** the uterus.
intra-muscular [ĬN-tră-MŬS-kyū-lăr]	_____ muscular: **within** the substance of the muscles.
dia-placental [dī-ă-plă-SĔN-tăl]	_____ placental: passing **through** the placenta.
per-axillary [pĕr-ĂK-sĭ-lār-ē]	_____ axillary: **through** the axilla.
trans-dermal [trăns-DĔR-măl]	_____ dermal: **across/through** the skin.
ex-hale [ĕks-HĀL]; **in-hale** [ĭn-HĀL]	To breathe **out** is to _____ hale; to breathe **in** is to _____ hale.
sub-sternal [sŭb-STĔR-năl]	**Below** the sternum is _____ sternal.
intra-venous [IN-tră-VĒ-nŭs]	_____ venous refers to **into** the vein (Figure 2-1).
para-cystic [păr-ă-SĬS-tĭk]	_____ cystic refers to **near** or **next to** the bladder.

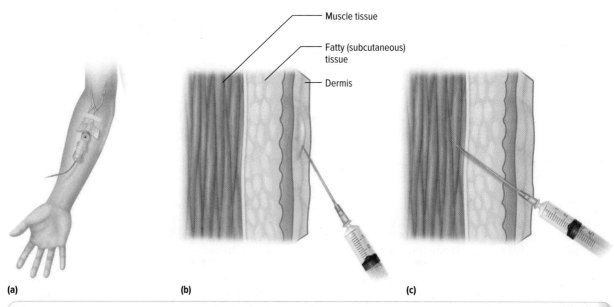

Muscle tissue

Fatty (subcutaneous) tissue

Dermis

(a)　　　　　　　　　(b)　　　　　　　　　(c)

Figure 2-1 (a) Intravenous therapy, (b) intradermal injection, and (c) intramuscular injection

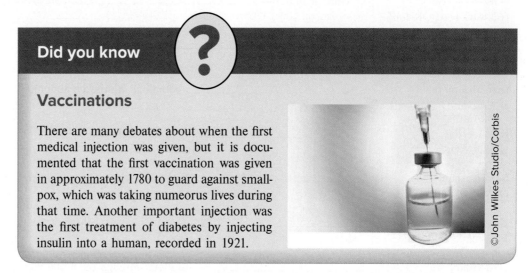

Did you know ?

Vaccinations

There are many debates about when the first medical injection was given, but it is documented that the first vaccination was given in approximately 1780 to guard against smallpox, which was taking numeorus lives during that time. Another important injection was the first treatment of diabetes by injecting insulin into a human, recorded in 1921.

©John Wilkes Studio/Corbis

PRONOUNCE	Pronounce the following terms aloud.
anaphylactic	[ĂN-ă-fĭ-LĂK-tĭk]
paracystic	[păr-ă-SĬS-tĭk]
peraxillary	[pĕr-ĂK-sĭ-lār-ē]
extracorporeal	[ĔKS-tră-kōr-PŌR-ē-ăl]

SPELL	Write the correct spelling for each related term.
	Passing **through** the placenta
	Pregnancy **outside** the uterus
	Projection **over** or **near** the condyle
	Middle layer of skin
	Refers to **near** or **next to** the bladder

Match the prefix on the left to its meaning on the right.

1. _____ ab-		a.	away from
2. _____ ad-		b.	closer to
3. _____ endo-		c.	within
4. _____ inter-		d.	between
5. _____ para-		e.	near, beside
6. _____ meso-		f.	middle, median
7. _____ epi-		g.	over, above
8. _____ ecto-		h.	outside
9. _____ sub-		i.	around
10. _____ peri-		j.	below
11. _____ ex-		k.	out of
12. _____ retro-		l.	backward

APPLY **Answer the following question.**

Construct four word examples with prefixes related to **position** or **location**.

_____

_____

_____

_____

LO 2.4 Prefixes Related to Time

Some medical prefixes that describe **time** are:

STUDY TIP

Everyday uses of prefixes in health care: "The patient . . .
- is on the postpartum unit."
- is experiencing preeclampsia."
- has a rectal prolapse."

Prefix	Meaning
ante-	before
post-	after, following
pre-	before
primi-	first
pro-	before, forward

Word Building	PRACTICE
	Provide the correct prefix for each of the following terms using the bolded hints.
ante-mortem [ĂN-tē-mŏr-tĕm]	_____ mortem: **before** death.
post-mortem [pōst-MŌR-tĕm]	_____ mortem: **after** death.

continued on next page

<table>
<tr><td colspan="2">

Word Building
</td></tr>
<tr><td colspan="2">

Provide the correct prefix for each of the following terms using the bolded hints.
</td></tr>
<tr><td>

ante-partum
[ĂN-tē-păr-tŭm]
</td><td>

_____ partum is **before** delivery or labor.
</td></tr>
<tr><td>

post-partum
[pōst-PĂR-tŭm]
</td><td>

_____ partum is **after** childbirth.
</td></tr>
<tr><td>

primi-para
[prī-MĬP-ă-ră]
</td><td>

_____ para is a woman giving birth for the **first** time.
</td></tr>
<tr><td>

pre-natal [prē-NĀ-tăl]
</td><td>

Occurring **before** a child is born (birth) is referred to as _____ natal.
</td></tr>
<tr><td>

post-natal [pōst-NĀ-tăl]
</td><td>

Occurring **after** the birth of a child is known as _____ natal.
</td></tr>
<tr><td>

pro-drome [PRŌ-drōm]
</td><td>

_____ drome: a symptom or group of symptoms that occur **before** a disease shows up.
</td></tr>
</table>

<table>
<tr><td>

PRONOUNCE
</td><td>

Pronounce the following terms aloud.
</td></tr>
<tr><td>

primipara
</td><td>

[prī-MĬP-ă-ră]
</td></tr>
<tr><td>

antepartum
</td><td>

[ĂN-tē-păr-tŭm]
</td></tr>
<tr><td>

antemortem
</td><td>

[ĂN-tē-mŏr-tĕm]
</td></tr>
</table>

<table>
<tr><td>

SPELL
</td><td>

Write the correct spelling for each related term.
</td></tr>
<tr><td></td><td>

Before delivery
</td></tr>
<tr><td></td><td>

Before death
</td></tr>
<tr><td></td><td>

Before a child is born
</td></tr>
<tr><td></td><td>

Before a disease shows up
</td></tr>
</table>

UNDERSTAND   Match the term on the left to its meaning on the right.

1. _____ antemortem   a. after death
2. _____ postmortem   b. before death
3. _____ antepartum   c. before birth
4. _____ postnatal   d. after birth
5. _____ primipara   e. before disease
6. _____ prodome   f. giving birth for first time

APPLY   Answer the following question.

Construct four word examples with prefixes related to **time**.

_____

_____

_____

_____

LO 2.5 Prefixes Related to Presence or Quality

Some medical prefixes that describe the **presence** or **quality** of a specific factor that influences the meaning of the word include:

STUDY TIP

When using flash cards, have another student read only the bolded term as a hint and see if you can remember the prefix.

STUDY TIP

Try studying medical terms in small groups of related terms either by alphabetical order, type, or similar definition. It will help you remember which prefix to use to spell each term and identify which group a term belongs to.

Prefix	Meaning
a-	without
ambi-	both, around
an-	without, no, lack
anti-	against, opposing
brady-	slow
co-, col-, com-, con-, cor-	together
contra-	against
de-	away from, cessation
dys-	abnormal, difficult, painful
eu-	well, good, normal
hyper-	above normal, overly
hypo-	below normal
mal-	bad, inadequate
re-	again, backward
semi-	half
syl-, sym-, syn-, sys-	together, union, joined
tachy-	fast
ultra-	beyond, excessive
un-	not

STUDY TIP

Everyday uses of prefixes in health care: "The patient . . .
- is euphoric."
- has a pacemaker due to persistent bradycardia."
- is experiencing tachypnea."
- was outside and experienced hypothermia."

Did you know

Modern Imaging

Newer 3D ultrasound pictures can provide detailed information. In general, ultrasound pictures are not as clear as other diagnostic imaging equipment, such as CT scan or MRI, but are used in pregnancy because they do not harm the fetus. X-rays, CT, and MRI use radiation that can injure or kill a growing baby. This is why the patient is asked before an x-ray if there is a chance she could be pregnant.

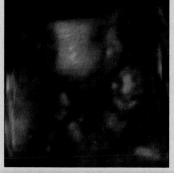

©SAG/Getty Images

Word Building	

Provide the correct prefix for each of the following terms using the bolded hints.

brady-cardia
[brăd-ē-KĂR-dē-ă]

_____ cardia is abnormally **slow** heartbeat.

tachy-cardia
[TĂK-i-KĂR-dē-ă]

_____ cardia is **rapid (fast)** heartbeat.

ambi-dextrous
[ăm-bē-DĔKS-trŭs]

Having ability on **both** the right and left sides is _____ dextrous.

hyper-active
[hī-pĕr-ĂK-tĭv]

_____ active is abnormally **high** energy.

hypo-glycemia
[HĪ-pō-glī-SĒ-mē-ă]

Low blood sugar is _____ glycemia.

re-flux [RĒ-flŭks]

_____ flux: **backward** flow.

de-myelination
[dē-MĪ-ĕ-lĭ-NĀ-shŭn]

_____ myelination: **loss** of myelin.

anti-bacterial
[ĂN-tē-băk-TĒR-ē-ăl]

Opposing the growth of bacteria is _____ bacterial.

contra-indicated
[kŏn-tră-ĬN-dĭ-kā-tĕd]

_____ indicated is **against** recommendations.

ultra-sonic
[ŭl-tră-SŎN-ĭk]

Relating to energy waves **beyond** the frequency of sound waves is _____ sonic.

co-dominant
[kō-DŎM-ĭn-ănt]

Having an **equal** degree of dominance is _____ dominant.

sym-biosis
[sĭm-bē-Ō-sĭs]

Mutual interdependence or **equally** depending on each other is _____ biosis.

eu-pepsia [yū-PĔP-sē-ă]

_____ pepsia: normal (or **good**) digestion.

dys-functional
[dĭs-FŬNGK-shŭn-ăl]

_____ functional: functioning **abnormally.**

a-sepsis [ā-SĔP-sĭs]

Without living organisms: _____ sepsis.

an-encephalic
[ăn-ĕn-sĕ-FĂL-ĭk]

_____ encephalic: **without** a brain.

mal-absorption
[măl-ăb-SŎRP-shŭn]

Inadequate absorption is _____ absorption.

semi-comatose
[sĕm-ē-KŌ-mă-tōs]

_____ comatose: **partial,** but not in a full coma.

un-conscious
[ŭn-KŎN-shŭs]

Not conscious: _____ conscious.

PRONOUNCE	Pronounce the following terms aloud.
eupepsia	[yū-PĔP-sē-ă]
anencephalic	[ăn-ĕn-sĕ-FĂL-ĭk]
symbiosis	[sĭm-bē-Ō-sĭs]
ambidextrous	[ăm-bē-DĔKS-trŭs]

SPELL	Write the correct spelling for each related term.
	Without a brain
	Loss of myelin
	Having ability on **both** the right and left sides
	Inadequate absorption
	Low blood sugar

UNDERSTAND Match the prefix on the left to its meaning on the right.

1. _____ hyper-
2. _____ hypo-
3. _____ a-
4. _____ an-
5. _____ semi-
6. _____ un-

a. below normal
b. above normal
c. without
d. lack
e. half
f. not

APPLY Answer the following question.

Construct four word examples with prefixes related to **presence** or **quality**.

_____

_____

_____

_____

LO 2.6 Additional Miscellaneous Medical Prefixes

Additional medical prefixes include:

STUDY TIP

Start good study habits early. Organizing set times in your day to study will help you feel more in control of your learning. Feeling good about what you are learning will make it more enjoyable and, more importantly, help you to retain the information.

Prefix	Meaning
auto-	self
meta-	behind, after, beyond
para-	beside, abnormal, involving two parts

PRACTICE

Provide the correct prefix for each of the following terms using the bolded hints.

auto-immune [ăw-tō-ĭ-MYŪN]	_____ immune means immunity against an individual's **own** tissue.
meta-carpals [MĔT-ă-KĂR-pălz]	The five bones **beyond** the wrist bones are the _____ carpals.
para-kinesia [păr-ă-kĭ-NĒ-zē-ă]	_____ kinesia is **partial** movement.
auto-graft [ĂW-tō-grăft]	A(n) _____ graft uses an individual's **own/self** tissue.
meta-tarsal (bones) [MĔT-ă-TĂR-săl]	_____ tarsal bones are the five bones **beyond** the ankle (in the foot).
para-cervical [păr-ă-SĔR-vĭ-kăl]	_____ cervical refers to the area **beside** the cervix or **beside** the cervical spine.

PRONOUNCE

Pronounce the following terms aloud.

parakinesia	[păr-ă-kĭ-NĒ-zē-ă]
autograft	[ĂW-tō-grăft]
paracervical	[păr-ă-SĔR-vĭ-kăl]

SPELL

Write the correct spelling for each related term.

	Beside the cervix
	Against an individual's **own/self** tissue
	Beside the cervical spine
	Partial movement

UNDERSTAND

Match the term on the left to its meaning on the right.

1. _____ autograft
2. _____ metacarpals
3. _____ metatarsals
4. _____ autoimmune
5. _____ paracervical
6. _____ parakinesia

a. bones beyond the wrist
b. bones beyond the ankle
c. partial movement
d. around/close to the cervix or cervical spine
e. one's own graft
f. immune to one's self

APPLY

Answer the following question.

Construct four word examples using **miscellaneous** prefixes.

_____
_____
_____
_____

CHAPTER SUMMARY

	Learning Outcome	Summary
2.1	Describe the role of the prefix in medical terminology.	Prefixes are descriptive word parts that appear in front of word roots. They are important to adding specifics to the foundation of the words and describe additional conditions or qualities related to word roots.
2.2	Identify common medical prefixes related to size and quantity.	Common prefixes are utilized in various systems. This is an overview of basic prefixes that add to describing size and quantity.
2.3	Describe common medical prefixes related to position or location.	It is important to condense several terms by adding a prefix that describes position and/or location.
2.4	Identify common medical prefixes related to time.	To adequately treat a patient, it is vital to use terms that can describe time. This is an overview of basic prefixes related to time.
2.5	Identify common medical prefixes related to presence or quality.	Common prefixes are utilized in various systems. This is an overview of basic prefixes that add to describing function or structure of presence or quality.
2.6	Describe common miscellaneous medical prefixes.	Some medical terminology prefixes have no other place within the structure and function of the body or its systems. This is an overview of miscellaneous medical prefixes in this category.

RECALL

1. Describe in detail how medical prefixes can change and/or add to the entire medical term.

_____

_____

_____

_____

UNDERSTAND

Utilizing chapter 2 of your textbook, fill in the blank with an appropriate prefix for each word part provided.

1. _____ lateral (both sides)
2. _____ cardia
3. _____ derm
4. _____ abdominal
5. _____ cervical
6. _____ cranial
7. _____ immune
8. _____ cyte
9. _____ version
10. _____ phylaxis
11. _____ scopic

Pronounce each of the above terms aloud.

IMPLEMENT

Complete each sentence by filling in the blank with the appropriate prefix.

1. _____ tarsals are the bones beyond the ankle.
2. _____ metrial is the lining within the uterus.
3. _____ articular means multiple joints.
4. _____ sepsis is without organisms.
5. _____ plegia is paralysis of half of the body.

Match each new term with its associating prefix definition.

1. _____ antipsychotic
2. _____ postsurgical
3. _____ unilateral
4. _____ parasympathetic
5. _____ adduction
6. _____ contralateral
7. _____ diplopia
8. _____ dysmenorrhea
9. _____ probiotic
10. _____ antibiotic

a. Against biotics (or infectious agents)
b. Move toward body
c. Against the other side
d. Beside or near the sympathetic system
e. Double vision
f. Abnormal menses
g. For biotics (infectious agents)
h. Against psychosis
i. After surgery
j. One side

For each prefix, find three words in a medical dictionary or glossary and define them.

1. mega _____ : _____
   mega _____ : _____
   mega _____ : _____
2. hyper _____ : _____
   hyper _____ : _____
   hyper _____ : _____
3. hypo _____ : _____
   hypo _____ : _____
   hypo _____ : _____
4. intra _____ : _____
   intra _____ : _____
   intra _____ : _____

DECONSTRUCT

Deconstruct each word, identifying the prefix and its meaning.

	List the prefix	Define the prefix
bipolar (example)	bi-	Both, twice, double
exocrine		
endocranium		
antidepressant		
pseudesthesia		
algesic		
litholysis		
cryolysis		

What are some tips that will help you remember the terms? How can your instructor/fellow students help you? What time of day do you like to study, and how can you develop a good study plan?

_____
_____
_____
_____

CHAPTER 3

Suffixes

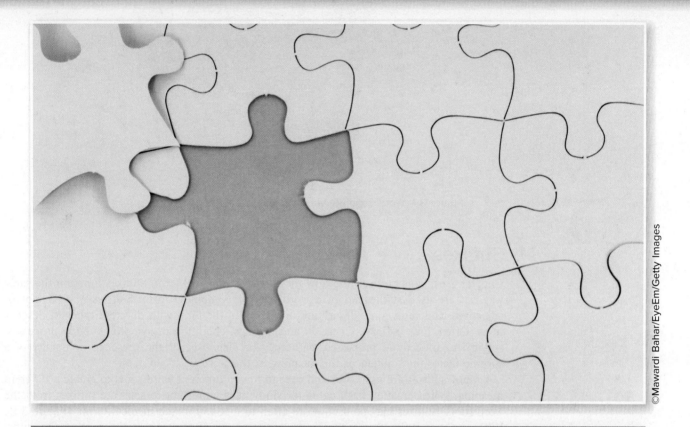

©Mawardi Bahar/EyeEm/Getty Images

Learning Outcomes

After studying this chapter, you will be able to:

3.1 Describe how suffixes are used to form medical terms.

3.2 Identify and apply common medical suffixes related to sensation and feelings.

3.3 Identify and apply common medical suffixes related to conditions or symptoms.

3.4 Identify and apply common medical suffixes related to body processes.

3.5 Identify and apply common medical suffixes related to body parts or chemical elements.

3.6 Identify and apply common medical suffixes related to surgical or procedural processes.

3.7 Identify and apply common medical suffixes related to pathology or diagnosis.

3.8 Identify and apply common miscellaneous medical suffixes.

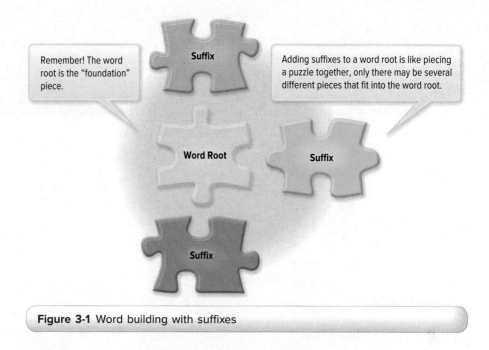

Figure 3-1 Word building with suffixes

LO 3.1 ## Suffixes

Chapter 2 explains prefixes and how they add to a medical term. Suffixes function the same way but are used at the end of a word root or combining form. Suffixes act like nouns, adjectives, and verbs, only describing or adding to the term with different types of descriptions. Often, they indicate sensation and feelings, condition or symptoms, body processes, surgical or procedural processes, pathology or diagnosis, or the presence or quality of a specific factor that influences the meaning of the word.

Many suffixes are used over and over to match different word roots to create a different meaning. When creating flash cards for study, it is important to separate suffixes from the word roots. Suffixes may be used more often to mix and match medical terms (Figure 3-1). When using a suffix, use a combing vowel such as /o to connect the root to the suffix. However, drop the combining vowel when the suffix begins with a vowel. For instance, a cardiologist and a neurologist both share the same suffix, *-logist,* which means "one who studies." However, they are two different kinds of specialists. A cardiologist is "one who studies the heart" and a neurologist is "one who studies nerves." *Cardi/o* and *neur/o* are combing forms, as discussed in Chapter 1 and will be introduced throughout the systems.

Following are some examples of how suffixes contribute to medical terminology.

Example 1:

dermat**itis**: *dermat/o-* [skin] + *-itis* [inflammation] = inflammation of the skin

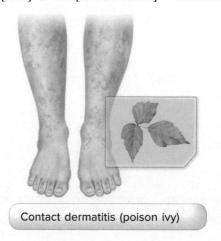

Contact dermatitis (poison ivy)

Example 2:

gastr**algia**: *gastr/o-* [stomach] + *-algia* [discomfort, pain] = stomachache/pain

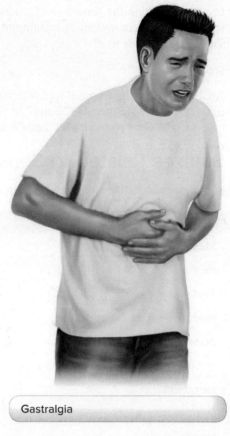

Gastralgia

Example 3:

hepato**megaly**: *hepat/o-* [liver] + *-megaly* [enlargement] = enlarged liver

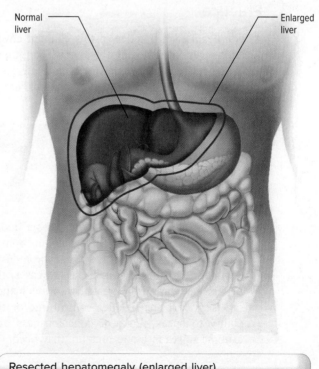

Normal
liver

Enlarged
liver

Resected hepatomegaly (enlarged liver)

Putting It Together

Using the previous examples, it should be clear to see how easy medical terminology can be. After learning the processes of prefixes, suffixes, and combining forms, the key to mastering medical terminology is learning the word roots that are associated with each system. That is all there is to it!

Review

All medical terms have a word root, which gives the essential meaning to the word. For example, *cardi-* is a root word meaning "heart." In the word *cardiopathy,* the suffix *-pathy* ("condition") is added to the word root *cardi/o* ("heart") to form the whole word, meaning "heart condition."

LO 3.2 Suffixes Related to Sensation and Feelings

Some medical suffixes that describe **sensation** or **feelings** include:

Suffix	Meaning
-algia	pain
-asthenia	weakness
-desis	binding, fusion
-dynia	pain
-esthesia	sensation
-kinesia, -kinesis	movement
-phobia	fear
-phonia	sound
-phoria	feeling, carrying

Practice

As you begin each practice in this chapter, cover the left-hand column and answer all the questions without removing the cover. Then, uncover and check your answers. For any questions you missed, review the previous material and make a flash card for each word you found difficult. At the end of each chapter, use your flash cards for study and review.

Did you know ❓

Acrophobia

Acrophobia is the most common "phobia" today and doesn't discriminate. Both men and women report a fear of heights, and it can be mild or debilitating to the person. In severe cases, the person may have to be treated with medication or else risk losing bladder control and/or the ability to speak. Loss of consciousness and extreme spikes in blood pressure may occur.

©Ingram Publishing

Provide the correct suffix for each of the following terms using the bolded hints.

brady-kinesia [brăd-ĭ-kĭn-Ē-zē-ă] **hyper-kinesis** [hī-pĕr-kĭ-NĒ-sĭs]	Decrease in **movement** is brady _____; excessive muscular movement is hyper _____.
par-esthesia [păr-ĕs-THĒ-zē-ă]	Par _____ is an abnormal **sensation,** such as tingling.
acro-phobia [ăk-rō-FŌ-bē-ă]	Acro _____: **fear** of heights.
neur-algia [nū-RĂL-jē-ă] **neuro-dynia** [nūr-ō-DĬN-ē-ă]	Nerve **pain** can be referred to as neur _____ or neuro _____.
neura-phonia [nūr-ă-FŌ-nē-ă]	Loss of **sounds** is neura _____.
neur-asthenia [nūr-ăs-THĒ-nē-ă]	Neur _____ is a condition with vague symptoms such as **weakness.**
arthro-desis [ăr-THRŎD-ĕ-sĭs *or* ăr-thrō-DĒ-sĭs]	Surgically created stiffening via **fixation** or **fusion** of a joint is arthro _____.
eu-phoria [yū-FŌR-ē-ă]	Eu _____ is a **feeling** of well-being.

Pronounce the following terms aloud.

acrophobia	[ăk-rō-FŌ-bē-ă]
neuraphonia	[nūr-ă-FŌ-nē-ă]
euphoria	[yū-FŌR-ē-ă]
arthrodesis	[ăr-THRŎD-ĕ-sĭs *or* ăr-thrō-DĒ-sĭs]

Write the correct spelling for each related term.

	Abnormal **sensation**
	Fixation or **fusion** of a joint
	Decrease in **movement**
	Loss of **sounds**

Match the correct suffix on the left to its meaning on the right.

1. _____ -asthenia   a. pain
2. _____ -esthesia   b. movement
3. _____ -phoria   c. sensation
4. _____ -kinesia   d. fear
5. _____ -algia   e. sound
6. _____ -phonia   f. feeling, carrying
7. _____ -phobia   g. weakness

1. Give an example of how medical suffixes can change and/or add to the entire medical term.

_____

_____

2. Construct four word examples with suffixes related to **sensation** and **feelings**.

_____

_____

_____

LO 3.3   Suffixes Related to Conditions or Symptoms

Some medical suffixes that describe **conditions** or **symptoms** include:

Suffix	Meaning
-cele	hernia
-cytosis	condition of cells
-ectasia, -ectasis	expansion, dilation
-edema	swelling
-ema	condition
-emesis	vomiting
-iasis	pathological condition or state, presence of
-ism	condition, disease
-itis (*pl.* -ites)	inflammation
-lepsy	seizures
-leptic	pertaining to seizures
-lithiasis	presence of stones
-mania	obsession, madness
-megaly	enlargement
-oma (*pl.* -omae)	tumor, neoplasm
-opia, -opsia	vision
-osis (*pl.* -oses)	condition, state, process
-paresis	slight paralysis, feelings of numbness and tingling
-pathy	abnormal condition, disease process
-penia	deficiency, small, fewer
-philia	attraction, affinity for
-phrenia	of the mind
-phthisis	wasting away
-physis	growing
-plegia	paralysis

Suffix	Meaning
-plegic	pertaining to paralysis
-ptosis	falling down, drooping
-rrhea	to flow or discharge
-rrhagia	excessive bleeding (amount and/or frequency)
-rrhexis	rupture
-trophic	pertaining to nutrition
-trophy	nutrition

Word Building

PRACTICE

Provide the correct suffix for each of the following terms using the bolded hints.

esophag-ectasia [ē-SŎF-ă-jĭk-TĀ-zē-ă]	**Dilation** of the passageway for food to travel to the stomach is known as an esophag _____.
dipl-opia [dĭ-PLŌ-pē-ă] **chlor-opsia** [klō-RŎP-sē-ă]	Dipl _____: double **vision;** chlor _____: condition of seeing (**vision/viewing**) objects as green.
mono-paresis [mŏn-ō-pă-RĒ-sĭs] **quadri-plegia** [kwăh-drĭ-PLĒ-jē-ă] **quadri-plegic** [kwăh-drĭ-PLĒ-jĭk]	**Paralysis** of only one extremity is mono _____; **paralysis** of all four limbs is quadri _____; a person who has **paralysis** of all four limbs is quadri _____.
epi-physis [ĕ-PĬF-ĭ-sĭs]	The **growth** plate at the ends of long bones is known as the epi _____.
erythro-cytosis [ĕ-RĬTH-rō-sī-TŌ-sĭs]	**Condition** with an abnormal number of red blood **cells** in the blood is erythro _____.
chole-lithiasis [KŌ-lē-lĭ-THĬ-ă-sĭs]	Condition of **stones** in the gallbladder is known as chole _____.
psor-iasis [sō-RĪ-ă-sĭs]	Psor _____ is a chronic skin **condition.**
dwarf-ism [DWŌRF-ĭzm]	Dwarf _____ is the **condition** including abnormally small size.
halit-osis [hăl-ĭ-TŌ-sĭs]	Halit _____ is a chronic bad breath **state.**
osteo-pathy [ŏs-tē-ŎP-ă-thē]	Osteo _____ is the term for bone **disease.**

continued on next page

Word Building	PRACTICE
	Provide the correct suffix for each of the following terms using the bolded hints.
cysto-cele [SĬS-tō-sēl]	**Hernia** of the urinary bladder is called a cysto _____.
cardio-rrhexis [kăr-dē-ō-RĔK-sĭs]	**Rupture** of the heart wall is cardio _____.
epi-leptic [ĕp-ĭ-LĔP-tĭk] epi-lepsy [ĔP-ĭ-LĔP-sē]	An epi _____ is a person with epi _____, which pertains to **seizures.**
hemat-emesis [hē-mă-TĔM-ĕ-sĭs]	Hemat _____ is the **vomiting** of blood.
megalo-mania [mĕg-ă-lō-MĀ-nē-ă] mono-mania [mŏn-ō-MĀ-nē-ă] schizo-phrenia [skĭz-ō-FRĔ-nē-ă or skĭt-sō-FRĔ-nē-ă]	Individuals with an **obsession** about themselves might be said to have megalo _____; **obsession** with one idea is mono _____; schizo _____ is a term for a common psychosis **of the mind.**
cephalo-megaly [SĔF-ă-lō-MĔG-ă-lē]	Cephalo _____ is an abnormal **enlargement** of the head.
my-oma [mī-Ō-mă] (pl.: my-omata [mī-ō-MĂ-tă])	**Tumor** of muscle tissue: my _____ (pl.: my _____).
a-trophic [ă-TRŌF-ĭk] dys-trophy [DĬS-trō-fē]	A _____: pertaining to lack of **nutrition;** dys _____: changes that result from inadequate **nutrition.**
leuko-penia [lū-kō-PĒ-nē-ă]	Condition with **fewer** or **smaller** numbers than normal of white blood cells is leuko _____.
lymph-edema [lĭmf-ĕ-DĒ-mă] nephr-itis [nĕ-FRĪ-tĭs]	Lymph _____ is **swelling** as a result of obstructed lymph glands; nephr _____ is kidney **inflammation.**
hemo-philia [hē-mō-FĬL-ē-ă]	Hemo _____ is a deficiency in the body's blood-producing mechanisms that creates a **need** or **attraction** for blood.
blepharo-ptosis [blĕf-ă-RŎP-tō-sĭs]	Blepharo _____ is a **drooping** eyelid.

PRONOUNCE	Pronounce the following terms aloud.
esophagectasia	[ē-SŎF-ă-jĭk-TĀ-zē-ă]
hemophilia	[hē-mō-FĬL-ē-ă]
myoma	[mī-Ō-mă]
cholelithiasis	[KŌ-lē-lĭ-THĪ-ă-sĭs]

	Vomiting of blood
	Drooping eyelid
	Chronic skin **condition**
	Inflammation of kidney
	Obsession with one idea

STUDY TIP

Association Tip: When learning new terms, think of someone you know or a family member that may have the condition or disease that you are learning. It will help you remember that "Aunt Lilly has atherosclerosis because she has had hardening of the arteries for years."

UNDERSTAND	Match the suffix on the left to its meaning on the right.

1. _____ -emesis   a. hemorrhage
2. _____ -mania   b. rupture
3. _____ -lithiasis   c. drooping
4. _____ -rrhagia   d. vomiting
5. _____ -rrhexis   e. disease
6. _____ -cele   f. hernia
7. _____ -pathy   g. stones
8. _____ -ptosis   h. obsession
9. _____ -phrenia   i. large/enlargement
10. _____ -philia   j. small, fewer, lack of
11. _____ -phobia   k. fear of
12. _____ -penia   l. love or attraction to
13. _____ -megaly   m. swelling
14. _____ -itis   n. inflammation
15. _____ -osis   o. condition
16. _____ -edema   p. of the mind

APPLY	Answer the following question.

Construct four word examples with suffixes related to **conditions** or **symptoms**.

_____
_____
_____
_____

LO 3.4 Suffixes Related to Body Processes

Some medical suffixes that describe **body processes** include:

Suffix	Meaning
-blast	immature, forming
-cidal, -cide	destroying, killing
-crine	secreting

continued on next page

Suffix	Meaning
-malacia	softening
-para	bearing, given birth
-parous	bearing, producing offspring
-pepsia	digestion
-phage, -phagia	eating, devouring
-phasia	speaking
-phoresis	carrying
-plasia	formation, development, growth
-plastic	forming
-pnea	breath
-poiesis	production, formation
-poietic	pertaining to production
-poietin	substance that produces
-porosis	lessening in density
-rrhage	discharging heavily
-rrhea	a flowing, a flux
-schisis	splitting
-somnia	sleep
-spasm	contraction
-stalsis	contraction
-stasis	stopping, constant, static
-stenosis	narrowing

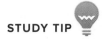

STUDY TIP

When studying, try putting your "speaking and interpreting skills" to the test. Have another person give you a term, then you create an entire sentence using that term (in context with proper pronunciations).

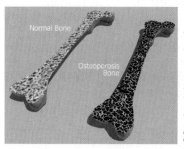

Normal Bone

Osteoporosis Bone

©Stocktrek Images, Inc./ Alamy Stock Photo

Word Building	PRACTICE
	Provide the correct suffix for each of the following terms using the bolded hints.
osteo-malacia [ŎS-tē-ō-mă-LĀ-shē-ă] **osteo-porosis** [ŎS-tē-ō-pō-RŌ-sĭs]	Osteo _____ is a gradual **softening** of bone; osteo _____ is **lessening** of bone **density** or increase of porous bone.
in-somnia [ĭn-SŎM-nē-ă]	An inability to **sleep** is called in _____.

dys-pepsia [dĭs-PĔP-sē-ă] **poly-phagia** [pŏl-ē-FĀ-jē-ă]	Dys _____ : impaired **digestion;** poly _____ : excessive **eating** or hunger.
a-phasia [ă-FĀ-zē-ă]	A loss of or reduction in **speaking** ability is called a _____ .
astro-blast [ĂS-trō-blăst]	An immature **cell** is an astro _____ .
hemo-rrhage [HĔM-ō-răj] **dysmeno-rrhea** [dĭs-měn-ōr-Ē-ă]	Hemo _____ is to **bleed** profusely; dysmeno _____ is difficult menstrual **flow.**
eu-pnea [yūp-NĒ-ă]	Easy, normal **respiration** is eu _____ .
hemo-plastic [hē-mō-PLĂS-tĭk]	Hemo _____ is forming **new** blood cells.
erythro-poiesis [ĕ-RĬTH-rō-poi-Ē-sĭs]	Erythro _____ : **formation** of red blood cells.
sui-cidal [sū-ĭ-SĪD-ăl]	Sui _____ : thoughts, plans, gestures, or attempts to **destroy oneself;** likely to kill oneself.
sui-cide [SŪ-ĭ-sīd]	Sui _____ : the act of **destroying one's own life.**
bacterio-cide [băk-TĔR-ē-ō-sīd]	Bacterio _____ : agent that **destroys** bacteria.
endo-crine [ĔN-dō-krĭn]	A gland that **secretes** hormones into the bloodstream is an endo _____ gland.
esophago-spasm [ĕ-SŎF-ă-gō-spăzm]	**Spasm** of the walls of the esophagus is esophago _____ .
peri-stalsis [pĕr-ĭ-STĂL-sĭs]	**Movement** of the intestines by contraction and relaxation of its tube to move food is peri _____ .
electro-phoresis [ē-lĕk-trō-FŌR-ē-sĭs]	Movement or **carrying** of particles in an electric field is electro _____ .
dys-plasia [dĭs-PLĀ-zē-ă]	Dys _____ : abnormal tissue **formation.**
primi-para [prī-MĬP-ăr-ă] **vivi-parous** [vī-VĬP-ă-rŭs]	Woman who has **given birth** once is a primi _____ ; **giving birth** to living young is vivi _____ .
cheilo-schisis [kī-LŎS-kĭ-sĭs]	A cleft (**split**) lip is called cheilo _____ .
homeo-stasis [HŌ-mē-ō-STĀ-sĭs]	Homeo _____ is a **state of equilibrium** in the body.
angio-stenosis [ĂN-jē-ō-stĕ-NŌ-sĭs] **esophago-stenosis** [ĕ-SŎF-ă-gō-stĕ-NŌ-sĭs]	**Narrowing** of one or more blood vessels is angio _____ ; **narrowing** of the esophagus is esophago _____ .

PRONOUNCE	Pronounce the following terms aloud.
dysplasia	[dĭs-PLĀ-zē-ă]
aphasia	[ă-FĀ-zē-ă]
osteomalacia	[ŎS-tē-ō-mă-LĀ-shē-ă]
esophagostenosis	[ĕ-SŎF-ă-gō-stĕ-NŌ-sĭs]

SPELL	Write the correct spelling for each related term.
	Gradual **softening** of bone
	Carrying of particles in an electric field
	The body's **state** of equilibrium
	Impaired **digestion**
	Agent that **destroys** bacteria

UNDERSTAND	Match the suffix on the left to its meaning on the right.

1. _____ -rrhage   a. decreased density
2. _____ -rrhea   b. speaking
3. _____ -porosis   c. destroying
4. _____ -stenosis   d. narrowing
5. _____ -cide   e. giving birth
6. _____ -para   f. eating
7. _____ -plasia   g. softening
8. _____ -malacia   h. flow
9. _____ -phagia   i. bleeding
10. _____ -phasia   j. forming

APPLY	Answer the following question.

Construct four word examples with suffixes related to **body processes**.

_____

_____

_____

_____

LO 3.5 Suffixes Related to Body Parts or Chemical Elements

Some medical suffixes that describe **body parts** or **chemical elements** include:

Suffix	Meaning
-cyte	cell
-derma	skin
-emia	blood
-emic	relating to blood
-globin, -globulin	protein
-oxia	oxygen
-plakia	plaque

Suffix	Meaning
-plasm, plasia	thing formed, growth
-uria	urine

<table>
<tr><td rowspan="2">Word Building</td><td>PRACTICE</td></tr>
<tr><td>Provide the correct suffix for each of the following terms using the bolded hints.</td></tr>
<tr><td>leuko-plakia
[lū-kō-PLĀ-kē-ă]</td><td>A white patch or plaque on the mucous membrane is a leuko _____.</td></tr>
<tr><td>sclero-derma
[sklēr-ō-DĔR-mă]</td><td>Sclero _____ is hardening of the skin.</td></tr>
<tr><td>ur-emia
[yū-RĒ-mē-ă]
ur-emic [yū-RĒ-mĭk]</td><td>Ur _____: excess urea in the blood;
ur _____: having excess urea in the blood.</td></tr>
<tr><td>thrombo-cyte
[THRŎM-bō-sīt]</td><td>A blood platelet cell is a thrombo _____.</td></tr>
<tr><td>py-uria [pī-YŪ-rē-ă]</td><td>Pus in the urine is py _____.</td></tr>
<tr><td>hemo-globin
[hē-mō-GLŌ-bĭn]
immuno-globulin
[ĬM-yū-nō-GLŎB-yū-lĭn]</td><td>Hemo _____ is protein of red blood cells;
immuno _____ is one of certain structurally related defense proteins.</td></tr>
<tr><td>an-oxia [ăn-ŎK-sē-ă]</td><td>Lack of oxygen is an _____ (Figure 3-2).</td></tr>
<tr><td>proto-plasm
[PRŌ-tō-plăzm]</td><td>A formed living thing is proto _____.</td></tr>
</table>

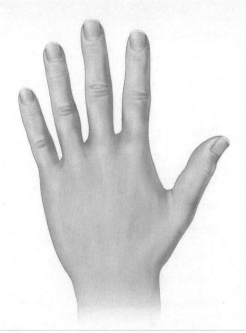

Figure 3-2 Anoxia: lack of oxygen, cyanosis: condition of being blue

PRONOUNCE	Pronounce the following words aloud and write their meaning in the space provided.
thrombocyte	[THRŎM-bō-sīt]
scleroderma	[sklēr-ō-DĔR-mă]
pyuria	[pī-YŪ-rē-ă]

SPELL	Write the correct spelling for each related term.
	Lack of **oxygen**
	Excess urea in the **blood**
	Hardening of the **skin**
	Pus in the **urine**

UNDERSTAND	Match the suffix on the left to its meaning on the right.

1. _____ -oxia   a. pertaining to urea
2. _____ -cyte   b. pertaining to skin
3. _____ -plasm   c. plaque (or patch)
4. _____ -plakia   d. living thing formation
5. _____ -uria   e. cell
6. _____ -derma   f. oxygen

APPLY	Answer the following question.

Construct four word examples with suffixes related to **body parts** or **chemical elements**.

_____

_____

_____

_____

LO 3.6 Suffixes Related to Surgical or Procedural Processes

Some medical suffixes that describe the **surgical** or **procedural processes** include:

Suffix	Meaning
-centesis	Surgical puncture to remove fluid
-ectomy	Removal of part or all of an organ or body part
-lysis	Destruction of
-lytic	Pertaining to destruction
-pexy	Fixation, usually done surgically
-plasty	Surgical repair
-rrhaphy	Surgical suturing
-static, -stasis	Maintaining a state
-stomy	Opening
-tome	Cutting instrument, segment
-tomy	Cutting operation, incision
-tripsy	Crushing

Word Building	PRACTICE
	Provide the correct suffix for each of the following terms using the bolded hints.
colo-stomy [kō-LŎS-tō-mē]	**Surgical opening** in the colon is a colo _____.
nephro-pexy [NĔF-rō-pĕk-sē]	Nephro _____ is **surgical fixation** (or pinning back in place) of a floating kidney.
rhino-plasty [RĪ-nō-plăs-tē] **hernio-rrhaphy** [HĔR-nē-ŌR-ă-fē]	Rhino _____: plastic surgery or **surgical repair** of the nose (Figure 3-3); hernio _____: **suturing** of a hernia.
hemo-static [hē-mō-STĂT-ĭk]	Hemo _____ is **stopping** blood flow within a vessel.
append-ectomy [ăp-pĕn-DĔK-tō-mē]	Append _____ is **complete removal** of the appendix (Figure 3-4).
electro-lysis [ē-lĕk-TRŎL-ĭ-sĭs]	Electro _____ is permanent **destruction** of unwanted hair.
osteo-tome [ŎS-tē-ō-tōm]	An **instrument for cutting** bone is an osteo _____.
laparo-tomy [LĂP-ă-RŎT-ō-mē]	An **incision into** the abdomen is a laparo _____.
thrombo-lytic [thrŏm-bō-LĬT-ĭk]	Thrombo _____ is **breaking down/destroying** a thrombus (blood clot).
thora-centesis [THŌR-ă-sĕn-TĒ-sĭs]	During a thora _____, **a needle is inserted** into the pleural space between the chest wall and lungs to aspirate fluid.
litho-tripsy [LĬTH-ō-trĭp-sē]	Shock wave litho _____ **breaks** kidney stones into small pieces.

STUDY TIP

These surgical suffixes will be used often and you will see them again throughout the systems because each system has some surgical interventions. Be sure to continue to make flash cards for these and keep them close so you can use them again!

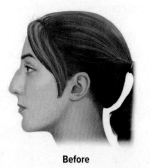 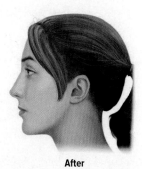

Before **After**

Figure 3-3 Rhinoplasty—notice the change in the nose

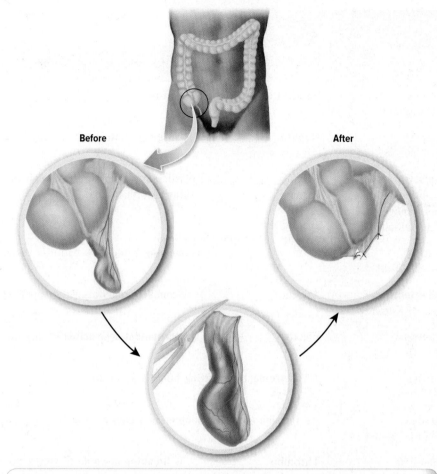

Figure 3-4 Surgical appendectomy—removal of the appendix

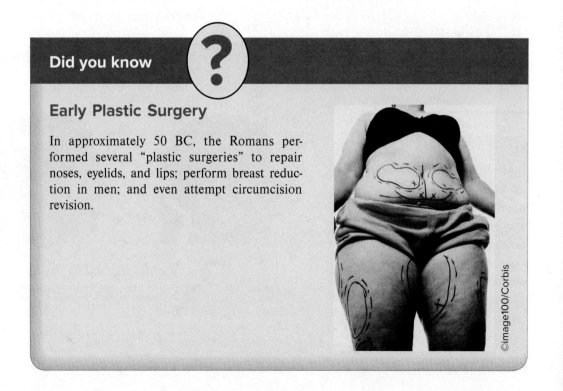

Did you know ?

Early Plastic Surgery

In approximately 50 BC, the Romans performed several "plastic surgeries" to repair noses, eyelids, and lips; perform breast reduction in men; and even attempt circumcision revision.

©image100/Corbis

PRONOUNCE	Pronounce the following terms aloud.
thrombolytic	[thrŏm-bō-LĬT-ĭk]
colostomy	[kō-LŎS-tō-mē] **(Be careful not to add an "N")**
osteotome	[ŎS-tē-ō-tōm]
herniorrhaphy	[HĔR-nē-ŌR-ă-fē]

SPELL	Write the correct spelling for each related term.
	Instrument for cutting bone
	Destroying a thrombus (blood clot)
	Surgical opening in the colon
	Suturing of a hernia
	Surgical repair of the nose

UNDERSTAND — Match the suffix on the left to its meaning on the right.

1. _____ -pexy
2. _____ -plasty
3. _____ -tomy
4. _____ -ectomy
5. _____ -rraphy
6. _____ -lysis
7. _____ -stasis

a. surgical repair
b. destruction
c. suturing
d. cutting into
e. complete removal
f. a state
g. surgical fixation

APPLY — Answer the following question.

Construct four word examples with suffixes related to **surgical** or **procedural processes**.

_____

_____

_____

_____

LO 3.7 Suffixes Related to Pathology or Diagnosis

Some medical suffixes that describe **pathology** or **diagnosis** include:

Suffix	Meaning
-crit	separate
-gen	producer
-genesis	origin
-genic	produced by
-gram	a recording
-graph	recording instrument
-graphy	process of recording (Figure 3-5)
-meter	measuring device

continued on next page

Suffix	Meaning
-metry	measurement
-opsy	view of
-pheresis	removal
-phil	attraction, affinity for
-scope	instrument for visual examination
-scopy	use of an instrument for viewing

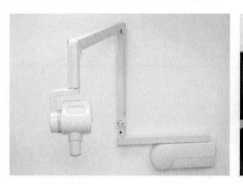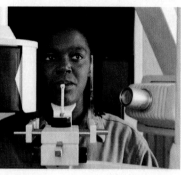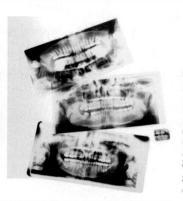

(left): ©Vitalii Berestetskyi/Shutterstock; (middle): ©Keith Brofsky/Getty Images; (right): ©Stockbyte/PunchStock

Figure 3-5 Radiogram, radiography, and radiograph

STUDY TIP

Many procedures have quick abbreviations because the medical term is very long. By remembering the abbreviations, it can help you when trying to spell the actual complete word. For instance, **EEG: E**lectro**E**ncephalo**G**ram.

Word Building	PRACTICE
	Provide the correct suffix for each of the following terms using the bolded hints.
ophthalmo-meter [ŏf-thăl-MŎM-ĕ-tĕr]	**Device for measuring** cornea curvature is an ophthalmo _____.
electroencephalo-gram [ē-LĔK-trō-ĕn-SĔF-ă-lō-grăm] **electroencephalo-graph** [ē-LĔK-trō-ĕn-SĔF-ă-lō-grăf] **echocardio-graphy** [ĔK-ō-kăr-dē-ŎG-ră-fē]	Electroencephalo _____: **record** of electrical activity in the brain (EEG); electroencephalo _____: **instrument for recording** electrical brain activity; echocardio _____: **process of recording** the size, motion, and composition of the heart.
hemato-crit [HĔM-ă-tō-krĭt] **leuko-pheresis** [lū-kō-fĕ-RĒ-sĭs]	Hemato _____ is the percentage of volume of a blood sample that is composed of cells after **separation;** the **removal** or separation of leukocytes from blood is leuko _____.

opto-metry [ŏp-TŎM-ĕ-trē]	Opto _____ is the specialty concerned with **measurement of** vision and eye function.
carcino-gen [kăr-SĬN-ō-jĕn]	A **cancer-causing** agent is a carcino _____.
patho-genesis [păth-ō-JĔN-ĕ-sĭs]	The **formation and development** of disease is patho _____.
iatro-genic [ī-ăt-rō-JĔN-ĭk]	An iatro _____ disease **develops** as a result of medical care.
bi-opsy [BĪ-ŏp-sē] **micro-scope** [MĪ-krō-skōp] **micro-scopy** [mī-KRŎS-kŏ-pē]	Bi _____: removal of living sample of tissue to **view** (Figure 3-6); micro _____: **instrument** for viewing small objects; micro _____: **use of instruments** (microscopes) for viewing small objects.
cyano-phil [SĪ-ăn-nō-fĭl]	Element that turns blue after staining is a cyano _____; literal breakdown is when exposed to blue stain, the element **reacts to** it and turns that color.

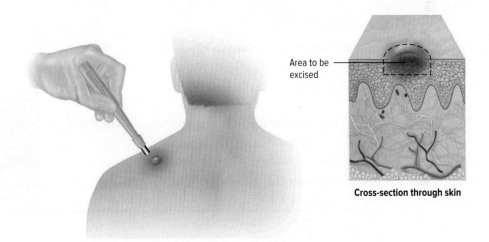

Area to be excised

Cross-section through skin

Figure 3-6 Punch biopsy instrument and procedure

PRONOUNCE	**Pronounce the following terms aloud.**
cyanophil	[SĪ-ăn-nō-fĭl]
pathogenesis	[păth-ō-JĔN-ĕ-sĭs]
hematocrit	[HĔM-ă-tō-krĭt]
leukophoresis	[lū-kō-fĕ-RĒ-sĭs]

SPELL	**Write the correct spelling for each related term.**
	Specialty concerned with **measurement of** vision and eye function
	Instrument for recording electrical brain activity
	Separation; the **removal** or separation of leukocytes
	Cells exposed to blue stain; the element **reacts to** it and turns that color
	Process of recording the size, motion, and composition of the heart by sound waves

1. _____ -meter
2. _____ -gram
3. _____ -graphy
4. _____ -graph
5. _____ -opsy
6. _____ -scope

a. process of recording something
b. the actual recording
c. the instrument used to record
d. instrument of measuring
e. view of
f. instrument to view an area

| APPLY | Answer the following question. |

Construct four word examples with suffixes related to **pathology** or **diagnosis.**

_____
_____
_____
_____

STUDY TIP

Suffixes in Health Care
Everyday uses of suffixes in health care.
"The patient . . .

- has a history of a cystocele."
- began to hemorrhage from the surgical site."
- history includes uterine dysplasia."
- had a colostomy four years ago."
- has acute appendicitis."
- is having a gastric bypass."

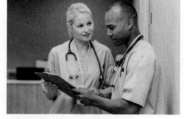

©Rido/Shutterstock

LO 3.8 Additional Miscellaneous Medical Suffixes

Some additional medical suffixes include:

Suffix	Meaning
-ad	toward
-clast, -clasis	break, fracture
-form	in the shape of
-ic	pertaining to
-ics	treatment, practice, body of knowledge
-logist	one who studies
-logy	study, practice
-oid	like, resembling
-phylaxis	protection, prevention
-plegic	pertaining to paralysis

Suffix	Meaning
-stat	agent to maintain a state of equilibrium
-tropia	turning
-tropic	turning toward
-tropy	attracted to target structures
-version	turning

Did you know

Esotropia

The brain compensates for sight disorders such as esotropia. Although it may look like the person is looking in another direction, he or she is actually able to focus and does not have double vision, like you may think. It is common today for children who are born with esotropia to have a surgical procedure that corrects the muscle weakness of the eye that controls movement for cosmetic effects.

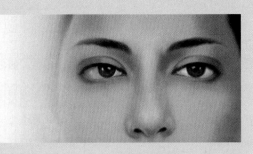

STUDY TIP

Prophylaxis is the prevention of disease. There are many ways this is done today. When thinking of the term, picture some of the preventative treatments that are used presently.

Word Building

PRACTICE

Provide the correct suffix for each of the following terms using the bolded hints.

pro-phylaxis [prō-fĭ-LĂK-sĭs]	**Prevention** of disease is pro _____ .
dermato-logy [dĕr-mă-TŎL-ō-jē] **dermato-logist** [dĕr-mă-TŎL-ō-jĭst]	Dermato _____ : **study of** skin disorders; dermato _____ : **one who studies** dermatology.
cephal-ad [SĔF-ă-lăd]	Cephal _____ means **toward** the head.
bacterio-stat [băk-TĔR-ē-ō-stăt]	Agent that **inhibits (and keeps in check)** bacterial growth is bacterio _____ .
psycho-tropic [sī-kō-TRŌP-ĭk]	Agent that treats the mind is **psycho** _____ .
neuro-tropy [nū-RŎT-rō-pē]	**Attraction to** certain contrast mediums for nervous tissue is neuro _____ .

continued on next page

Word Building

Provide the correct suffix for each of the following terms using the bolded hints.

uni-form [YŪ-nĭ-fŏrm]	Uni _____ : having the same **shape** throughout.
eso-tropia [ĕs-ō-TRŌ-pē-ă]	**Turning** inward or crossed eyes is eso _____.
osteo-clasis [ŎS-tē-ŎK-lă-sĭs]	Intentional **breaking** of a bone is osteo _____.
cardi-oid [KĂR-dē-oyd]	Cardi _____: **resembling** a heart.
gastr-ic [GĂS-trĭk]	**Relating to** the stomach is gastr _____.
orthoped-ics [ōr-thō-PĒ-dĭks]	The **study, diagnosis, and treatment** of the musculoskeletal system is orthoped _____.
retro-version [rĕ-trō-VĔR-zhŭn]	Retro _____ is a **turning backward** (said of the uterus).

PRONOUNCE	Pronounce the following terms aloud.
osteoclasis	[ŎS-tē-ŎK-lă-sĭs]
cardioid	[KĂR-dē-oyd]
cephalad	[SĔF-ă-lăd]
prophylaxis	[prō-fĭ-LĂK-sĭs]

SPELL	Write the correct spelling for each related term.
	Resembling a heart
	Turning backward (said of the uterus)
	Toward the head
	Attraction to certain contrast mediums for nervous tissue
	Intentional **breaking** of a bone

UNDERSTAND	Match the suffix on the left to its meaning on the right.

1. _____ -tropia   a. pertaining to
2. _____ -plegic   b. study of
3. _____ -ology   c. one who studies
4. _____ -ologist   d. prevention, protection
5. _____ -phylaxis   e. paralyzed
6. _____ -ic   f. turning

APPLY	Answer the following question.

Construct four word examples using **miscellaneous** medical suffixes.

_____

_____

_____

_____

CHAPTER SUMMARY

	Learning Outcome	Summary
3.1	Describe how suffixes are used to form medical terms.	Suffixes are the last of the four word parts that make up a medical term. They are used to add further clarification and/or description to the foundation body structure or function.
3.2	Identify and apply common medical suffixes related to sensation and feelings.	Word building requires knowledge of suffixes and their corresponding meanings related to sensation and feelings.
3.3	Identify and apply common medical suffixes related to conditions or symptoms.	Common word roots are associated with each body system. This is an overview of basic suffixes related to conditions or symptoms.
3.4	Identify and apply common medical suffixes related to body processes.	Function of the body includes body processes. This is an overview of suffixes for the student to start becoming familiar with basic body processes.
3.5	Identify and apply common medical suffixes related to body parts or chemical elements.	Knowledge and understanding of suffixes related to body parts or chemical elements is important to create complete medical terms that correctly describe each body part or chemical element.
3.6	Identify and apply common medical suffixes related to surgical or procedural processes.	Surgical and procedural processes are common treatment options utilized in medicine. This is an overview of the suffixes that define these components when combined with other word parts.
3.7	Identify and apply common medical suffixes related to pathology or diagnosis.	Pathology and diagnosis are two important pieces in medicine. This is an overview of basic suffixes related to describing disease processes and diagnosis of conditions.
3.8	Identify and apply common miscellaneous medical suffixes.	Some suffixes have no other place within the structure and function of the body or its systems. This is an overview of miscellaneous medical suffixes.

RECALL

1. Describe in detail how medical suffixes can change and/or add to the entire medical term.

_____
_____
_____

2. Illustrate, in your own way, how the entire medical term is created using prefixes, word roots, and suffixes.

_____
_____
_____

Utilizing chapter 3 of your textbook, fill in the blank with an appropriate suffix for each word part provided.

1. myel: _____
2. cardio: _____
3. entero: _____
4. crani: _____
5. gastr: _____

6. fibr: _____
7. brady: _____
8. blepharo: _____
9. neur: _____
10. litho: _____

Pronounce each of the above terms aloud.

Complete each sentence by filling in the blank.

1. Repair of a nose defect: rhino _____.
2. Removal of the appendix: append _____.
3. Disease of the heart: cardio _____.
4. Inflammation of the bronchi: bronch _____.
5. Bone-forming cell: osteo _____.
6. Study of the skin: dermato _____.
7. Study of tissue: histo _____.
8. Inflammation of the ovary: ovar _____.
9. Inflammation of the ear: ot _____.
10. Specialist in the treatment of nervous system disorders: neuro _____.
11. Incision into a vein: phlebo _____.
12. Study of the mind: psycho _____.
13. Removal of the kidney: nephr _____.

Match each new term with its associating suffix definition.

1. _____ acrophobia
2. _____ psychologist
3. _____ psychotropic
4. _____ tenosynovitis
5. _____ laryngoscope
6. _____ chyliform
7. _____ cardiomegaly
8. _____ diplopia
9. _____ osteoporosis
10. _____ neurasthenia

a. Resembling chyle
b. Porous bones, decreased density
c. Enlargement of the heart
d. Weakness of nerves, generalized aches and pains
e. Double vision
f. Fear of heights
g. One who studies psychology
h. Inflammation of a tendon
i. Instrument for viewing the larynx
j. Agent that treats psychosis

Break into component parts and define each part.

1. cranialgia _____

_____

2. endocranium _____

_____

3. esophagectomy _____

_____

4. pseudesthesia _____

_____

5. algesic _____

6. litholysis _____

_____

7. nephropexy _____

_____

Deconstruct the following words.

	List the Suffix	Define the Suffix
polyarteritis		
monomania		
quadriplegic		
hypodermic		
oophropexy		
rhinorrhagia		
menorrhea		
pathology		

Now that you have learned the basics of medical terminology, what will be your most difficult challenge in learning the terms and being successful in this course? How will you overcome your challenges?

_____

_____

_____

CHAPTER 4

The Human Body: An Orientation

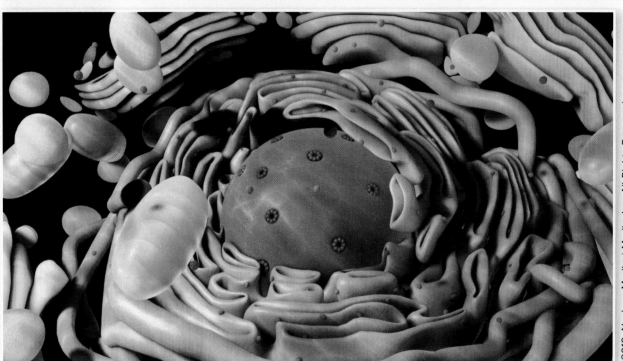

Learning Outcomes

After studying this chapter, you will be able to:

4.1 Understand the elements of human body organization and structure from the cellular to the system level.

4.2 Identify and locate the body cavities and list organs that are contained within each cavity.

4.3 Describe the directional terms, planes, regions of the body, and body positions.

4.4 Identify commonly used abbreviations related to the human body organization and regions of the body.

LO 4.1 Body Structure and Organization

The body is organized from its smallest element, the cell, to the collection of systems, with all its interrelated parts.

Cells

The entire body is made of **cells** that vary in size, shape, and function, but all cells have one thing in common: They need food, water, and oxygen to live and function. Cells (Figure 4-1) are made up of three basic parts: the *cell membrane,* which is the outer covering of the cell; the *nucleus,* which is the central portion of the cell and directs all cell activities; and the *cytoplasm,* which is the substance surrounding the nucleus that instructs cells to perform various essential tasks, such as movement and reproduction.

Cell growth can either be normal or abnormal. Later in this book you will learn how normal cell growth takes place. You will also learn about abnormal cell growth, which is a major factor in some diseases.

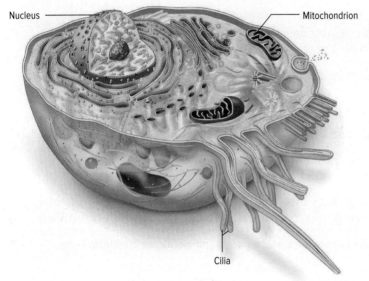

Nucleus — Mitochondrion

Cilia

Figure 4-1 Cell

Tissues

Tissues are a group of cells with specialized functions. There are four basic types of tissue within the body: connective, epithelial, muscle, and nerve. The following Practice provides a description of the types of tissues.

Organs

Groups of tissues that work together to perform a specific function are called **organs.** Examples are the kidneys, which maintain water and salt balance

Structure and Function	PRACTICE Provide the missing term(s) to complete the following sentences (may use terms more than once).
muscle [MŬS-ĕl]	_____ tissue is able to contract and expand, allowing the body to move.
connective [kŏn-NĔK-tĭv]	The fibrous substance that holds and connects body parts together is _____ tissue. Examples are bones, ligaments, and tendons.
cells [sĕlz] **tissue** [TĬSH-ū] **four**	Any group of _____ that work together to perform a single function is _____. The body has _____ types of tissue.
nerve [nĕrv]	Tissue that carries messages to and from the brain and spinal cord from all parts of the body is _____ tissue.
epithelial [ĕp-ĭ-THĒ-lē-ăl]	_____ tissue covers the internal and external body surfaces. Skin and internal organs (such as the intestines) are also _____ tissue.

in the blood, and the stomach, which breaks down food into substances that the circulatory system transports throughout the body as nourishment for its cells.

(Note: The terminology specific to each organ is provided in separate chapters on the appropriate body systems.)

Systems

When a group of organs all work together for a common purpose, a system is formed. These systems work together to support functions within the body. Figure 4-2 is an overview of the body systems.

(Note: The terminology specific to each body system is provided in separate chapters.)

Structure and Function	PRACTICE Provide the missing term(s) to complete the following sentences (may use terms more than once).
system [SĬS-tĕm]	Groups of organs that work together to perform one of the body's major functions form a _____.
integumentary [ĭn-tĕg-yū-MĔN-tă-rē]	The _____ system consists of the skin and the accessory structures derived from it (hair, nails, sweat glands, and oil glands).
musculoskeletal [MŬS-kyū-lō-SKĔL-ĕ-tăl]	The system that supports the body; protects organs; provides body movement; and includes muscles, bones, and cartilage is the _____ system.
cardiovascular [KĂR-dē-ō-VĂS-kyū-lăr]	The _____ system includes the heart and blood vessels, which pump and transport blood throughout the body, carrying nutrients to and removing waste from tissues.
respiratory [RĔS-pĭ-ră-tōr-ē *or* rĕ-SPĬR-ă-tōr-ē]	The body system that includes the lungs and airways and performs breathing is the _____ system.
nervous [NĔR-vŭs] **brain** [brān]	The _____ system regulates most body activities and sends and receives messages from the sensory organs. This system consists of the _____, spinal cord, and peripheral nerves.
urinary [YŪR-ĭ-nār-ē]	The system that includes the kidneys, ureters, bladder, and urethra is the _____ system. It eliminates metabolic waste, helps to maintain acid–base and water–salt balance, and helps regulate blood pressure.
reproductive [RĒ-prō-DŬK-tĭv]	The system that controls reproduction and heredity and is either male or female is the _____ system.
blood [blŭd]	The _____ system includes blood and all its components.
lymphatic [lĭm-FĂT-ĭk] **immune** [ĭ-MYŪN]	The _____ and _____ system includes the lymph, the glands and vessels of the _____ system, and the nonspecific and specific defense _____ system.
digestive [dī-JĔS-tĭv]	The organs that digest and excrete waste make up the _____ system.
endocrine [ĔN-dō-krĭn]	The system that includes the glands that secrete the hormones that regulate many of the body's activities is the _____ system.
sensory [SĔN-sŏ-rē]	The _____ system covers the eyes and ears and those parts of other systems that are involved in the reactions of the five senses.

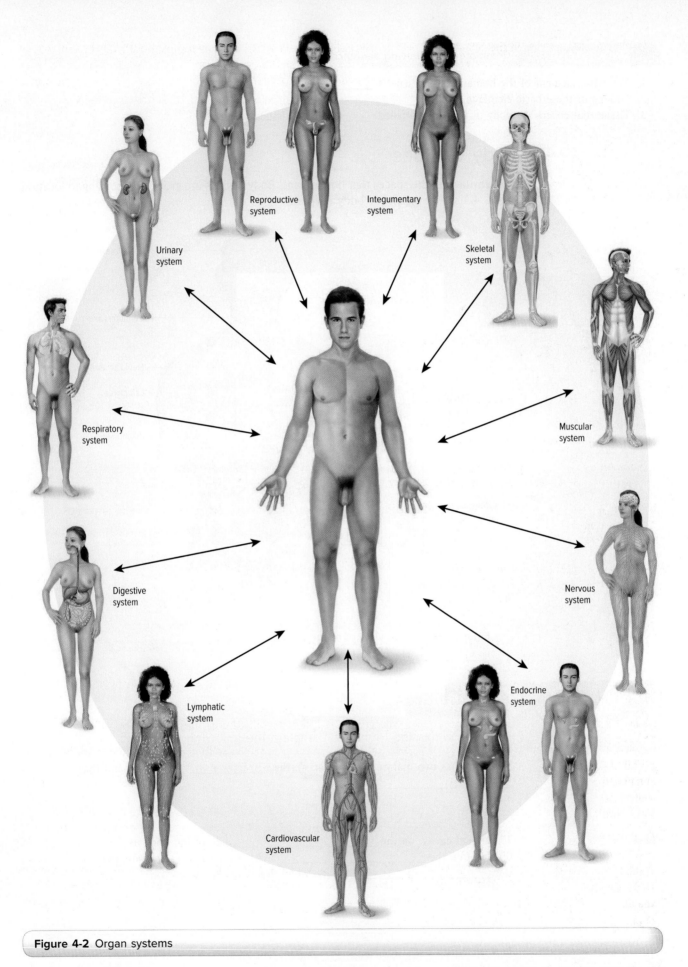

Figure 4-2 Organ systems

Reproductive system

Integumentary system

Urinary system

Skeletal system

Respiratory system

Muscular system

Digestive system

Nervous system

Lymphatic system

Endocrine system

Cardiovascular system

1. The basic element of the human body is a(n) _____.
2. Groups of these basic elements form _____.
3. Tissue that covers the body or its parts is called _____ tissue.

LO 4.2 Body Cavities

Body cavities are the spaces that hold organs. Body cavities are grouped according to location. Figure 4-3 shows the major body cavities.

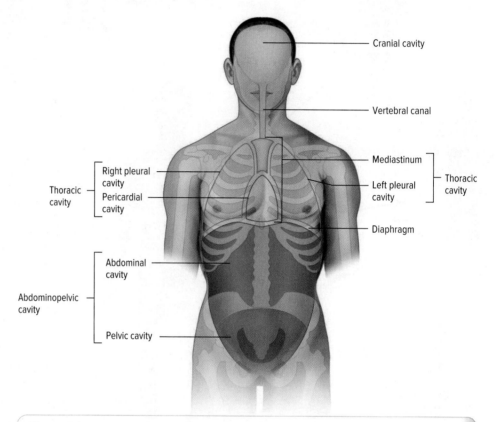

Figure 4-3 Anterior view of major body cavities

Structure and Function	**PRACTICE** Provide the missing term(s) to complete the following sentences.
dorsal [DŌR-săl] **ventral** [VĔN-trăl]	The body has two main cavities (spaces): the _____ and the _____ cavities.
back [bak] **cranial** [KRĀ-nē-ăl] **spinal** [SPĪ-năl]	The dorsal cavity, on the _____ side of the body, is divided into the _____ cavity, which holds the brain, and the _____ cavity, which holds the spinal cord.

front [frŭnt] **thoracic** [thō-RĂS-ĭk] **abdominal** [ăb-DŎM-ĭ-năl]	The ventral cavity, on the _____ side of the body, is divided into the _____ cavity, which holds the heart, lungs, and major blood vessels, and the _____ cavity, which holds the organs of the digestive and urinary systems.
diaphragm [DĪ-ă-frăm]	The _____ is the muscle that separates the thoracic and abdominal cavities.
pelvic [PĚL-vĭk]	The bottom portion of the abdominal cavity is called the _____ cavity, which contains the reproductive system.

UNDERSTAND   **Complete the following sentences.**

1. The brain is contained within the _____ cavity.
2. The muscle separating the two main parts of the ventral cavity is called the _____.
3. The spinal and cranial cavities make up the _____ cavity.
4. The space below the abdominal cavity is called the _____ cavity.
5. The system that helps eliminate fluids is the _____ system.
6. The system that breaks down food is called the _____ system.

LO 4.3   Directional Terms, Planes, and Regions

In making diagnoses or prescribing treatments, health care providers use standard terms to refer to different areas of the body. These terms describe each anatomical position as a point of reference. The anatomical position always means the body is standing erect, facing forward, with upper limbs at the sides and with the palms facing forward. The anatomical position is the position from which all other positions are derived. Figure 4-4 illustrates directional and positioning terms.

Directional Terms

Directional terms **locate** a portion of the body. Directional terms are used by health care providers to describe a position of the body. The following section provides an introduction to directional terms, planes, and regions.

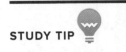

STUDY TIP

If the patient will have a procedure that requires him to be lying in the prone position, the patient is always lying on his abdomen.

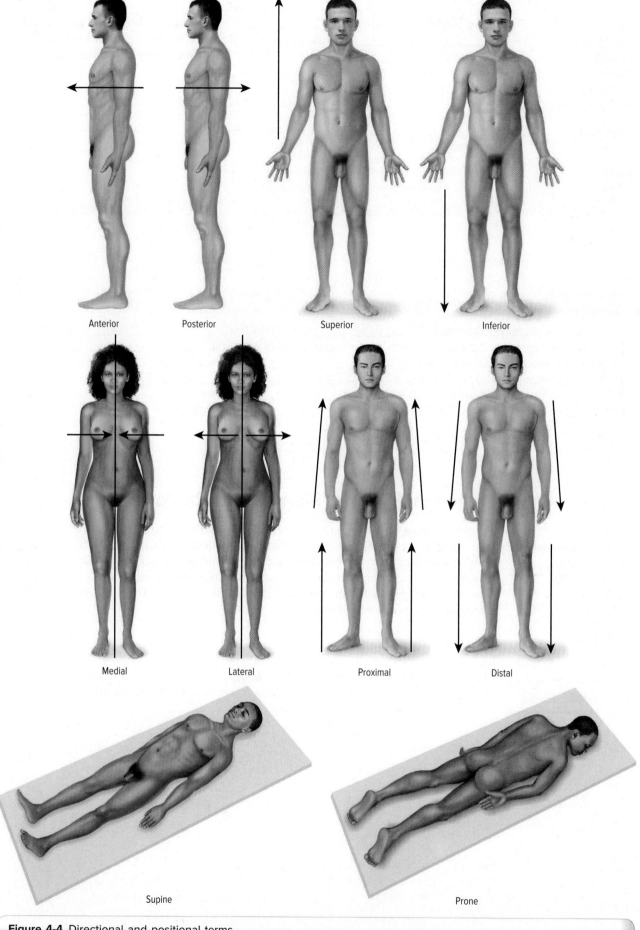

Anterior   Posterior   Superior   Inferior

Medial   Lateral   Proximal   Distal

Supine   Prone

Figure 4-4 Directional and positional terms

Combining Form	Meaning
anter/o	near or toward the front side, ventral
poster/o	near or toward the back side, behind, dorsal
ventr/o	near or toward the front side
dors/o	near or toward the back side
medi/o	middle
super/o	above
infer/o	below
proxim/o	near or at point of attachment
dist/o	far or away from point of attachment

Structure and Function	PRACTICE — Provide the missing term(s) to complete the following sentences.
anterior [ăn-TĒR-ē-ŏr] ventral [VĔN-trăl] posterior [pos-TĒR-ē-ŏr] dorsal [DŌR-săl]	The largest divisions of the body are the front side, referred to as _____ or _____, and the back side, referred to as _____ or _____.
	Some terms indicate a position relative to something else. For example:
inferior [ĭn-FĒR-ē-ŏr] superior [sū-PĒR-ē-ŏr]	_____ means below another structure, while _____ means above another structure (e.g., the stomach is superior to the large intestine).
lateral [LĂT-ĕr-ăl] medial [MĒ-dē-ăl]	_____ means to the side, as the eyes are to the nose. _____ means middle, as the nose is to the eyes.
deep [dēp] superficial [sū-pĕr-FĬSH-ăl]	Through or away from the surface is _____; at or near the surface is _____.
proximal [PRŎK-sĭ-măl]	Near the point of attachment to the trunk is _____. For example, the _____ end of the thigh bone joins the hip bone.
distal [DĬS-tăl]	Away from the point of attachment to the trunk is _____. For example, the _____ end of the thigh bone forms the knee.
supine [sū-PĪN] prone [prōn]	For examination purposes, patients are either lying on their spine facing upward (_____) or lying on their abdomen with their face down (_____).

Planes of the Body

For anatomical and diagnostic discussions, some standard terms are used for the **planes** and **positions** of the body. The planes refer to the body when it is vertical and facing front. Figures 4-5 and 4-6 illustrate the planes and positional terms of the body.

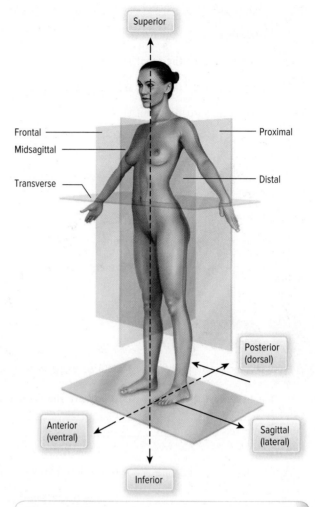

Figure 4-5 Planes of the body

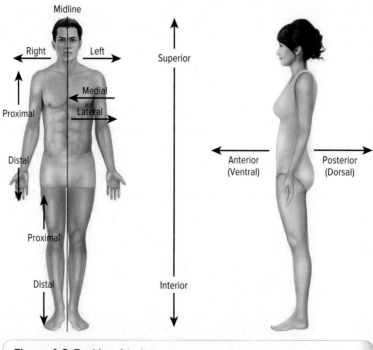

Figure 4-6 Positional terms

Structure and Function	PRACTICE
	Provide the missing term(s) to complete the following sentences.
frontal [FRŬN-tăl] **coronal** [KŌR-ŏ-năl]	The imaginary line that divides the body into anterior and posterior positions is the _____ or _____ plane.
midsagittal [mĭd-SĂJ-ĭ-tăl]	The _____ plane is the imaginary line that divides the body into equal right and left halves.
transverse [trănz-VĔRS] **(cross-sectional)**	The imaginary line that intersects the body horizontally and divides the body into upper and lower sections is the _____ plane.
sagittal [SĂJ-ĭ-tăl] **lateral** [LĂT-ĕr-ăl]	The _____ or _____ plane is parallel to the medial plane and divides the body into left and right sections.

STUDY TIP

Without adequately understanding positional terms, a health care provider may incorrectly position a patient for a procedure.

UNDERSTAND   **Circle the correct answer.**

1. The epigastric region is **above/below** the hypogastric region.
2. The heart is **above/below** the pelvic cavity.
3. The leg is **superior/inferior** to the foot.
4. The nose is **superior/inferior** to the eyes.
5. The lungs are located in the **abdominal/thoracic** cavity.
6. The **coronal/sagittal** plane divides the body horizontally.
7. The **frontal/lateral** plane is another name for the sagittal plane.
8. The wrist is **distal/proximal** to the shoulder.
9. The cranial cavity is in the **dorsal/ventral** cavity.

Regions of the Body

Health care practitioners usually refer to a specific organ, area, or bone when speaking of the upper body. In the back, the spinal column is divided into specific regions (described in a later chapter).

Doctors use two standards of terminology to describe the middle portion of the body (abdominal and pelvic cavities). Figures 4-7 and 4-8 illustrate the abdominopelvic quadrants and regions. The larger divisions, of which there are four, are called **quadrants.** The smaller divisions, of which there are nine, are called **regions.**

STUDY TIP

The hypochondriac region is the anatomic area of the upper abdomen just below (*hypo*, meaning "below") the cartilage (*chondros*, meaning "cartilage") of the ribs.

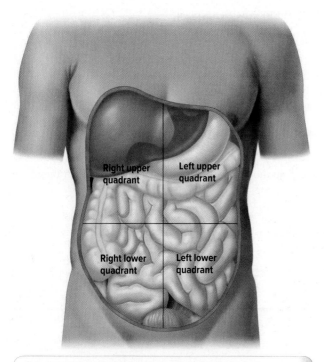

Right upper quadrant

Left upper quadrant

Right lower quadrant

Left lower quadrant

Figure 4-7 Abdominopelvic quadrants

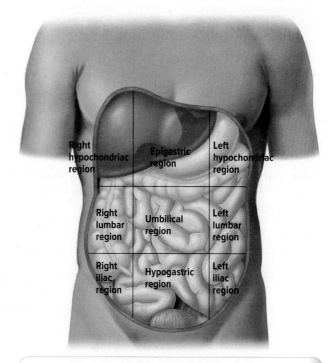

Right hypochondriac region

Epigastric region

Left hypochondriac region

Right lumbar region

Umbilical region

Left lumbar region

Right iliac region

Hypogastric region

Left iliac region

Figure 4-8 Abdominopelvic regions

Structure and Function	PRACTICE
	Fill in the missing term in each of the following sentences.
right upper quadrant (RUQ)	The area of the abdomen that contains parts of the liver, gallbladder, pancreas, and intestinal tract is the _____.
left lower quadrant (LLQ)	The _____ is the abdominal area that contains parts of the intestines and parts of reproductive organs in females.
left upper quadrant (LUQ)	The area of the abdomen that contains the stomach, spleen, and parts of the liver, pancreas, and intestines is the _____.
right lower quadrant (RLQ)	The _____ is the abdominal area that contains the appendix, parts of the intestines, and parts of the reproductive organs in females.
lumbar [LŬM-băr]	The left and right regions of the body in the back and sides between the lowest ribs and the pelvis are the _____ regions.
iliac [ĬL-ē-ăk] **inguinal [ĬN-gwĭ-năl]**	The _____ or _____ regions are the two regions near the upper portion of the hip bone.
epigastric [ĕp-ĭ-GĂS-trĭk]	The area above the stomach is the _____ region.
hypogastric [hī-pō-GĂS-trĭk]	The area just below the umbilical region is the _____ region.
umbilical [ŭm-BĬL-ĭ-kăl]	The area surrounding the navel is the _____ region.
hypochondriac [hī-pō-KŎN-drē-ăk]	The two regions just below the cartilage of the ribs, immediately over the abdomen, are the _____ regions.

1. The area above the stomach is called the _____ region.
   a. umbilical
   b. epigastric
   c. hypochondriac
   d. hypogastric

2. Another term for the area around the navel is the _____ region.
   a. epigastric
   b. iliac
   c. umbilical
   d. lumbar

3. This muscle divides the abdominal and thoracic cavities.
   a. diaphragm
   b. spinal
   c. pelvic
   d. dorsal

STUDY TIP

The client is having pain in the left lower abdominal quadrant. Where would this pain be located?

LO 4.4   Abbreviations

Common abbreviations related to the human body organization and regions of the body are given in the following table.

Abbreviation	ABBREVIATION REVIEW
	Review the definition of each abbreviation.
LLQ	left lower quadrant
LUQ	left upper quadrant
RLQ	right lower quadrant
RUQ	right upper quadrant
lat	lateral
AP	anteroposterior (from front to back)

UNDERSTAND   **Identify the meaning for each abbreviation.**

1. LLQ: _____
2. RUQ: _____
3. AP: _____
4. lat: _____

Chapter Review

CHAPTER SUMMARY

	Learning Outcome	Summary
4.1	Understand the elements of human body organization and structure from the cellular to the system level.	The body is organized from its smallest element, the cell, to the collection of systems, with all its interrelated parts. Tissues are a group of cells with specialized functions. Organs are groups of tissue that work together to perform a function.
4.2	Identify and locate the body cavities and list organs that are contained within each cavity.	Body cavities are the spaces that hold organs. Body cavities are grouped according to location.
4.3	Describe the directional terms, planes, regions of the body, and body positions.	In making diagnoses or prescribing treatments, health care providers use standard terms to refer to different areas of the body. These terms describe each anatomical position as a point of reference. The anatomical position always means the body is standing erect, facing forward, with upper limbs at the sides, and with the palms facing forward. Directional terms are used by health care providers to describe a position of the body. The planes refer to the body when it is vertical and facing front.
4.4	Identify commonly used abbreviations related to the human body organization and regions of the body.	Abbreviations are commonly used to describe the organization and regions of the body.

RECALL

1. Label the following cavities on the accompanying figure.
   - cranial
   - thoracic
   - abdominal
   - pelvic

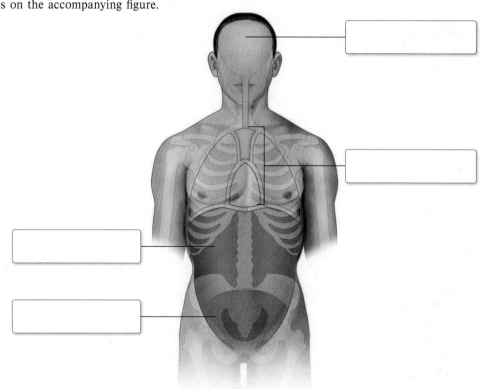

2. Label the following abdominopelvic regions on the accompanying figure.
   - hypogastric
   - left iliac
   - right iliac
   - right lumbar
   - left lumbar
   - umbilical
   - right hypochondriac
   - left hypochondriac
   - epigastric

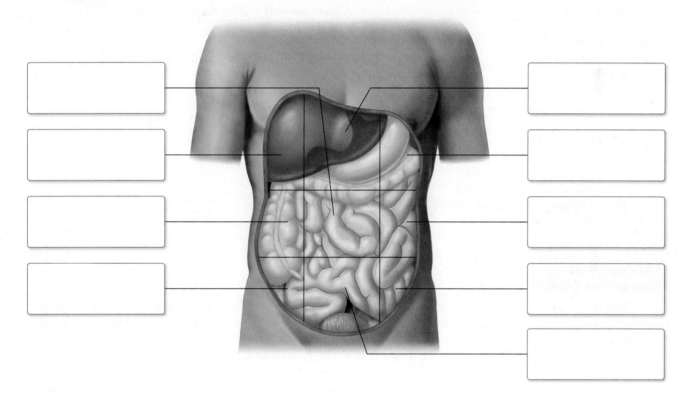

UNDERSTAND

Each of the following terms is misspelled. Write the correct spelling in the space provided and the definition for each. Say the word aloud.

1. epatelial:_____
2. limphatic:_____
3. cardeovascular: _____
4. respratory: _____
5. abdomenal:_____
6. diaphram: _____
7. thorasic: _____
8. dorsil: _____
9. soupine: _____
10. illiac:_____

Find a Match: Match the system to its function. Write the letter of the answer that best fits in the space in the left column.

1. _____
   cardiovascular system

2. _____
   digestive system

3. _____
   endocrine system

4. _____
   blood system

5. _____
   integumentary system

6. _____
   lymphatic and immune system

7. _____
   musculoskeletal system

8. _____
   nervous system

9. _____
   respiratory system

a. Performs breathing
b. Supports the body, protect organs, and provides movement
c. Sends and receives messages
d. Pumps and circulates blood to tissues
e. Consists of blood and its elements
f. Covers the body and its internal structures
g. Provides defenses for the body
h. Breaks down food
i. Regulates through production of hormones

DECONSTRUCT

Cathy Riley, a 56-year-old female, had her appendix removed. The surgeon, Dr. Tillman, explains to her family that the surgery was fairly simple. He states that Cathy was placed in the supine position and he cut through the connective tissue into the abdominopelvic cavity to remove the appendix. Dr. Tillman states that Cathy will be sore for a few days and will not be able to lay prone for about three weeks. Explain to Cathy's family what the surgeon just told them.

_____
_____
_____

Reviewing the Terms

Pronounce each of the following terms. Write the definitions on a separate sheet of paper. This review will take you through all the words you learned in this chapter. If you have difficulty with any words, make a flash card for later study. Refer to the English-Spanish and Spanish-English glossaries in the eBook.

abdominal [ăb-DŎM-ĭ-năl] **cavity**
anterior [ăn-TĒR-ē-ŏr] *or* **ventral** [VĔN-trăl]
blood [blŭd] **system**
body cavity
cardiovascular [KĂR-dē-ō-VĂS-kyū-lĕr] **system**
cell [sel]
connective [kŏn-NĔK-tĭv] **tissue**
coronal [KŌR-ŏ-năl] **plane**
cranial [KRĀ-nē-ăl] **cavity**
deep [dēp]
diaphragm [DĪ-ă-frăm]
digestive [dī-JĔS-tĭv] **system**
distal [DĬS-tăl]
dorsal [DŌR-săl] **cavity**
endocrine [ĔN-dō-krĭn] **system**
epigastric [ĕp-ĭ-GĂS-trĭk] **region**
epithelial [ĕp-ĭ-THĒ-lē-ăl] **tissue**
frontal [FRŬN-tăl] **plane**
hypochondriac [hī-pō-KŎN-drē-ăk] **regions**
hypogastric [hī-pō-GĂS-trĭk] **region**
iliac [ĬL-ē-ăk] *or* **inguinal** [ĬN-gwĭ-năl] **regions**
inferior [ĭn-FĒR-ē-ōr]
integumentary [ĭn-tĕg-yū-MĔN-tă-rē] **system**
lateral [LĂT-ĕr-ăl] **plane**
left lower quadrant [KWĂ-drănt] **(LLQ)**
left upper quadrant (LUQ)
lumbar [LŬM-băr] **regions**
lymphatic [lĭm-FĂT-ĭk] **and immune** [ĭ-MYŪN] **system**
medial [MĒ-dē-ăl]

midsagittal [mĭd-SĂJ-ĭ-tăl] **plane**
muscle [MŬS-ĕl] **tissue**
musculoskeletal [MŬS-kyū-lō-SKĔL-ĕ-tăl] **system**
nerve [NĔRV]
nervous [NĔR-vŭs] **system**
nervous [NĔR-vŭs] **tissue**
organ [ŌR-găn]
pelvic [PĔL-vĭk] **cavity**
posterior [pos-TĒR-ē-ŏr] *or* **dorsal** [DŌR-săl]
prone [prōn]
proximal [PRŎK-sĭ-măl]
reproductive [RĒ-prō-DŬK-tĭv] **system**
respiratory [RĔS-pĭ-ră-tōr-ē *or* rĕ-SPĪR-ă-tōr-ē] **system**
right lower quadrant (RLQ)
right upper quadrant (RUQ)
sagittal [SĂJ-ĭ-tăl] *or* **lateral** [LĂT-ĕr-ăl] **plane**
sensory [SĔN-sŏ-rē] **system**
spinal [SPĪ-năl] **cavity**
superficial [sū-pĕr-FĬSH-ăl]
superior [sū-PĒR-ē-ōr]
supine [sū-PĪN]
system [SĬS-tĕm]
thoracic [thō-RĂS-ĭk] **cavity**
tissue [TĬSH-ū]
transverse [trănz-VĔRS] **(cross-sectional) plane**
umbilical [ŭm-BĬL-ĭ-kăl] **region**
urinary [YŪR-ĭ-nār-ē] **system**
ventral [VĔN-trăl] **cavity**

The Integumentary System

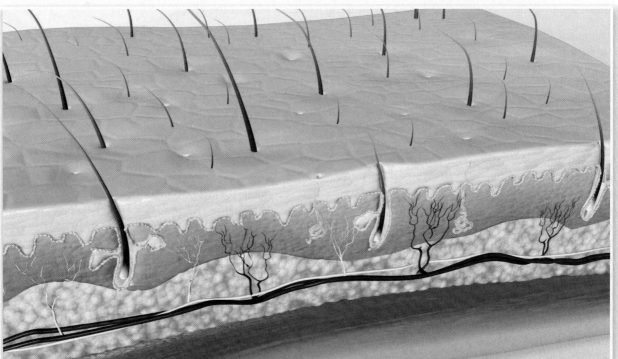

Learning Outcomes

After studying this chapter, you will be able to:

5.1 Identify parts of the skin and body membranes and discuss the function of each part.

5.2 Identify the major word parts used in building words that relate to the skin and body membranes.

5.3 Discuss common diagnostic tests, laboratory tests, and clinical procedures used in testing and treating disorders of the skin and body membranes.

5.4 Define the major pathological conditions of the skin and body membranes.

5.5 Define surgical terms related to the skin and body membranes.

5.6 Explain common pharmacological agents used in treating disorders of the skin and body membranes.

5.7 Identify common abbreviations associated with the skin and body membranes.

LO 5.1 Major Terms Describing the Structure and Function of the Skin and Body Membranes

The **integumentary system** includes the skin or **integument,** the **hair,** the **nails,** the **sweat glands** (also called the *sudoriferous glands*), and the oil-producing glands (also called the **sebaceous glands**). This system covers and protects the body, helps regulate the body's temperature, excretes some of the body's waste materials, participates in synthesis of vitamin D, and includes the body's sensors for pain and sensation.

Building Skin and Body Membranes Vocabulary

The following section provides an introduction to basic skin and body membranes' combining forms and their meanings. Review this information prior to moving to the practices.

Combining Form	Meaning
adi/o	fatty
cutan/o	skin
dermat/o, derm/o	skin
hidr/o	sweat
ichthy/o	fish, scaly
kerat/o	horny tissue
lip/o	fatty
melan/o	black, very dark
myc/o	fungus
onych/o	nail
pil/o	hair
seb/o	sebum, sebaceous glands
steat/o	fat
trich/o	hair
xanth/o	yellow
xer/o	dry

Skin

The skin is the largest organ of the body. It not only serves as an external protective covering to diseases, but it also plays a vital role in homeostasis. Figure 5-1 shows a cross section of skin with the parts of the integumentary system labeled, as well as the three layers of skin and what they contain.

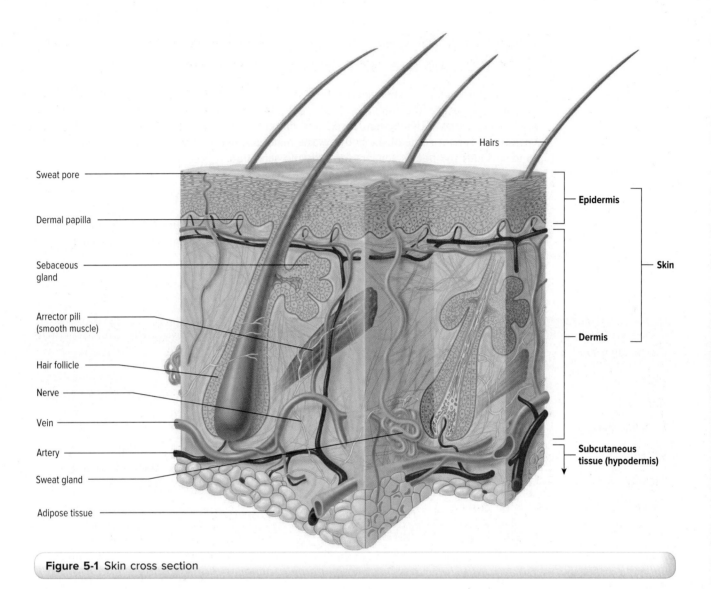

Sweat pore

Dermal papilla

Sebaceous gland

Arrector pili (smooth muscle)

Hair follicle

Nerve

Vein

Artery

Sweat gland

Adipose tissue

Hairs

Epidermis

Skin

Dermis

Subcutaneous tissue (hypodermis)

Figure 5-1 Skin cross section

Structure and Function	**PRACTICE**
	Provide the missing term(s) to complete the following sentences.
integument [ĭn-TĔG-yū-mĕnt]	The skin or _____ is the largest body organ. The average adult has about 21.5 square feet of skin. It varies in thickness depending on what part of the body it covers and what its function is in covering that part.
epidermis [ĕp-ĭ-DĔR-mĭs] **dermis** [DĔR-mĭs] **subcutaneous layer** [sŭb-kyū-TĀ-nē-ŭs] **hypodermis** [hī-pō-DĔR-mĭs]	The skin has three main parts or layers: the _____, the _____, and the _____ or _____.

outer **strata** [STRĂ-tă]	The epidermis, the _____ layer of skin, ranges from 1/200 to 1/20 of an inch thick and consists of several _____.
squamous epithelium [SKWĀ-mŭs ĕp-ĭ-THĒ-lē-ŭm] **stratified squamous** **epithelium** [STRĂT-i-fīd]	The epidermis is made up of cells called _____, a flat, scaly layer of cells. The layers that make up the squamous epithelium are called _____.
stratum corneum [KŌR-nē-ŭm]	Not all parts of the body's skin contain all the sublayers of epidermis. The top sublayer is called the _____. It consists of a flat layer of dead cells arranged in parallel rows. As new cells are produced, the dead cells are sloughed off.
keratin [KĔR-ă-tĭn]	As they die, the cells in the stratum corneum fill with _____, a water-proof barrier that keeps microorganisms out and moisture in. The keratin of the epidermis is softer than the hard keratin in nails.
	Dead skin cells on the surface fall off naturally as replacement cells rise from the base layers. Dead skin also can be removed by exfoliation or desquamation, the falling off in layers or scales. This is sometimes done for cosmetic reasons, as with exfoliation of the facial skin using an abrasive cloth or substance.
stratum germinativum [jĕr-mĭ-NĂT-ĭ-vŭm]	The bottom layer of the epidermis is called the _____. Here new cells are produced and pushed up to the stratum corneum. The epidermis itself is a *nonvascular* layer of skin, meaning that it does not contain blood vessels.
melanocytes [MĔL-ă-nō-sīts] **melanin** [MĔL-ă-nĭn]	Specialized cells called _____ produce a pigment called _____, which helps to determine skin and hair color. Melanin is essential in screening out ultraviolet rays of the sun that can harm the body's cells.
collagen [KŎL-lă-jĕn] **striae** [STRĪ-ē]	The dermis contains connective tissue that holds many capillaries, lymph cells, nerve endings, sebaceous and sweat glands, and hair follicles. These nourish the epidermis and serve as sensitive touch receptors. The connective tissue is composed primarily of _____ fibers that form a strong, elastic network. Collagen is a protein substance that is very tough, yet flexible. When the collagen fibers stretch, they form _____ or stretch marks.
adipose [ĂD-ĭ-pōs]	The subcutaneous layer is the layer between the dermis and the body's inner organs. It consists of _____ (or fatty) tissue and some layers of fibrous tissue. Within the subcutaneous layers lie blood vessels and nerves. The layer of fatty tissue serves to protect the inner organs and to maintain the body's temperature.

PRONOUNCE and DEFINE	Pronounce the following words aloud and write their meaning in the space provided.
integument	[ĭn-TĔG-yū-mĕnt]
epidermis	[ĕp-ĭ-DĔR-mĭs]
squamous epithelium	[SKWĀ-mŭs ĕp-ĭ-THĒ-lē-ŭm]
melanocyte	[MĔL-ă-nō-sīt]
collagen	[KŎL-lă-jĕn]

SPELL and DEFINE	Identify if the following terms are spelled correctly. Correct the words that are spelled incorrectly. Write the definition for each word.	
	Spelling	**Definition**
kolajen		
keratin		
melanine		
stratum jerminativum		
straie		

UNDERSTAND   Identify the term from the definition provided.

1. Outer portion of skin: _____
2. Cell in epidermis that produces melanin: _____
3. Layer below dermis: _____
4. Layer of skin containing fatty tissue: _____

APPLY   Rewrite the following information using medical terminology

The patient is experiencing stretch marks during pregnancy.

_____

_____

Hair and Nails

Hair grows out of the epidermis to cover various parts of the body. Hair serves to cushion and protect the areas it covers. The following section defines terms related to the structure and function of hair and nails. Figure 5-2 shows hair growing out of the scalp. Figures 5-3 and 5-4 illustrate the nail.

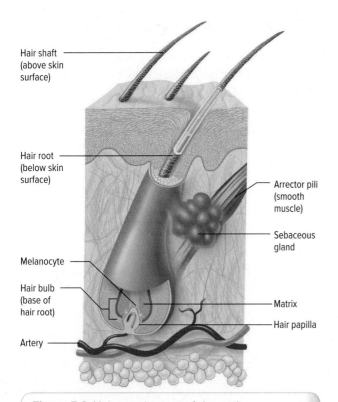

Hair shaft (above skin surface)

Hair root (below skin surface)

Melanocyte

Hair bulb (base of hair root)

Artery

Arrector pili (smooth muscle)

Sebaceous gland

Matrix

Hair papilla

Figure 5-2 Hair growing out of the scalp

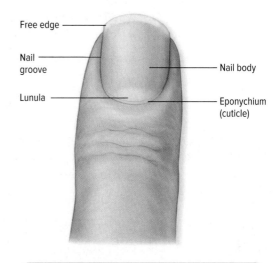

Free edge

Nail groove

Lunula

Nail body

Eponychium (cuticle)

Figure 5-3 Nail

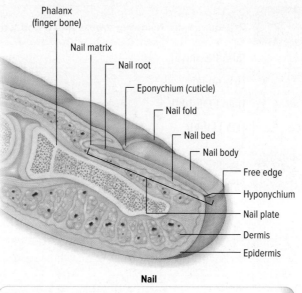

Figure 5-4 Nail cross section

Structure and Function	PRACTICE
	Provide the missing term(s) to complete the following sentences.
hair shaft **hair root**	Hair has two parts. The _____ protrudes from the skin and the _____ lies beneath the surface of the skin. The shaft is composed of outer layers of scaly cells filled with inner layers of soft and hard keratin.
hair follicle [FŎL-ĭ-kl]	Hair grows upward from the root through the _____ (tubular sacs that hold the hair fibers). The shape of the follicle determines the shape of the hair (straight, curly, wavy).
melanocyte [MĔL-ă-nō-sīt]	Hair color is determined by the presence of melanin, which is produced by the _____ in the epidermis. Gray hair occurs when melanocytes stop producing melanin.
alopecia [ăl-ō-PĒ-shē-ă]	Hair growth, thickness, and curliness are generally determined by heredity. In addition to heredity, baldness or _____ may result from disease, injury, or medical treatment (such as chemotherapy).
epilation [ep-i-lā-shŭn] **depilation** [dep-i-lā-shŭn]	A general term for removal of hair by the roots is _____ or _____. Such removal may be the result of some kind of injury or it may be done voluntarily to remove unwanted hair.
nails [nālz]	_____ are plates made of hard keratin that cover the dorsal surface of the distal bone of the fingers and toes. Nails serve as protective covering, help us grasp objects, and allow us to scratch.
lunula [LŪ-nū-lă]	Healthy nails appear pinkish because the translucent nail covers vascular tissue. At the base of most nails, a _____, or whitish half moon, is an area where keratin and other cells have mixed with air.
cuticle [KYŪ-tĭ-kl]	Nails are surrounded by a narrow band of epidermis called a _____, except at the top. The top portion grows above the level of the finger.

PRONOUNCE and DEFINE	Pronounce the following words aloud and write their meaning in the space provided.
alopecia	[ăl-ō-PĒ-shē-ă]
lunula	[LŪ-nū-lă]
hair follicle	[hār FŎL-ĭ-kl]
cuticle	[KYŪ-tĭ-kl]

SPELL and DEFINE — Identify if the following terms are spelled correctly. Correct the words that are spelled incorrectly. Write the definition for each word.

	Spelling	Definition
alopeshea		
lunula		
kyutickle		
folikle		
melanocyte		

UNDERSTAND — Identify the term from the definition provided.

1. Baldness: _____
2. Part of hair that is beneath skin: _____
3. Part of hair above skin: _____
4. Where hair shaft develops: _____
5. Half-moon-shaped area at base of nail: _____

APPLY — Read the following scenario and respond accordingly.

The medical assistant is reviewing the physician's notes with the patient. The note states that the patient is experiencing alopecia due to medication. Explain what this means to the patient.

_____

_____

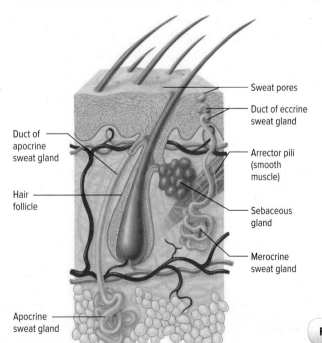

Duct of apocrine sweat gland

Hair follicle

Apocrine sweat gland

Sweat pores

Duct of eccrine sweat gland

Arrector pili (smooth muscle)

Sebaceous gland

Merocrine sweat gland

Glands

Glands are distributed throughout the body. Numerous glands are found on the hands, soles of feet, axillae, and the forehead. This section defines some of the major terms related to the structure and function of glands associated with the integumentary system. *(Note: Endocrine glands will be discussed in a separate chapter.)* Figure 5-5 shows glands found in the skin.

Figure 5-5 Glands in the skin

Structure and Function	**PRACTICE**
	Provide the missing term(s) to complete the following sentences.
	The integumentary system includes various types of glands. The following are glands in the skin:
sweat glands [swĕt glandz] **exocrine glands** [ĔK-sō-krĭn glandz] **diaphoresis** [DĪ-ă-fō-RĒ-sĭs] **pores** [pōrz]	The _____ (also called *sudoriferous glands*) are found almost everywhere on the body surface. Glands that secrete outward toward the surface of the body through ducts are called _____. The excretion of sweat is called _____. Secretions exit the body through _____, or tiny openings in the skin surface. Sweat (also called *perspiration*) is composed of water, sodium chloride, and other compounds depending on many factors, such as external temperature, fluid intake, level of activity, and hormonal levels.
eccrine glands [ĔK-rĭn glandz]	_____, or small sweat glands, are found on many places of the body. They excrete a colorless fluid that keeps the body at a constant temperature.
ceruminous glands [sĕ-RŪ-mĭn-ŭs glandz]	_____ are specialized glands in the surface of the ear that secrete *cerumen,* a waxy substance that lubricates and protects the ear.
sebaceous glands [sĕ-BĀ-shŭs glandz] **sebum** [SĒ-bŭm]	_____, located in the dermis, secrete an oily substance called _____, which is found at the base of the hair follicles. This substance serves to lubricate and protect the skin. Sebum forms a skin barrier against bacteria and fungi and also softens the surface of the skin.

PRONOUNCE and DEFINE	Pronounce the following words aloud and write their meaning in the space provided.
eccrine gland	[ĔK-rĭn gland]
sebaceous gland	[sĕ-BĀ-shŭs gland]
diaphoresis	[DĪ-ă-fō-RĒ-sĭs]
exocrine gland	[ĔK-sō-krĭn gland]
ceruminous gland	[sĕ-RŪ-mĭn-ŭs gland]

SPELL and DEFINE	Identify if the following terms are spelled correctly. Correct the words that are spelled incorrectly. Write the definition for each word.	
	Spelling	**Definition**
eksokrin		
ekrin		
seruminus		
sebaceous		
sebum		

UNDERSTAND	Identify the term from the definition provided.

1. Glands that secrete sweat: _____
2. Another term for sweating: _____
3. Glands that secrete a waxy substance in the ear: _____
4. Substance secreted into the hair follicle: _____

LO 5.2 Word Building in the Skin and Body Membranes

Word Building	PRACTICE
	Fill in the correct combining form in each of the following sentences.
adip-osis [ad-i-PŌ-sis]	Excessive accumulation of body fat is _____ osis.
dermat-itis [dĕr-mă-TĪ-tĭs]	_____ itis is inflammation of the skin.
derm-abrasion [dĕr-mă-BRĀ-zhŭn]	Surgical procedure to remove acne scars and marks using an abrasive product to remove part of the skin is _____ abrasion.
hidr-osis [hi-DRŌ-sis]	Production and excretion of sweat is _____ osis.
ichthy-osis [ik-thē-Ō-sis]	_____ osis is a congenital skin disorder characterized by dryness and peeling.
kerat-osis [kĕr-ă-TŌ-sĭs]	_____ osis is a skin lesion covered by a horny layer of tissue.
lipo-suction [LIP-ō-sŭk-shŭn]	Removal of unwanted fat by suctioning through tubes placed under the skin is _____ suction.
melan-oma [mĕl-ă-NŌ-mă]	_____ oma is a malignancy arising from cells that form melanin.
myc-osis [mī-KŌ-sis]	Any condition caused by fungus is _____ osis.
onycho-tomy [ŏn-ĭ-KŎT-ō-mē]	_____ tomy is an incision into a nail.
pilo-cystic [PĬ-lō-SĬS-tĭk]	Relating to a skin cyst with hair is _____ cystic.
sebo-rrhea [sĕb-ō-RĒ-ă]	_____ rrhea is excessive sebum caused by overactivity of the sebaceous glands.
steat-itis [stē-ă-TĪ-tis]	Inflammation of fatty tissue is _____ itis.
tricho-pathy [trĭ-KŎP-ă-thē]	_____ pathy is a disease of the hair.
xanth-oma [zan-THŌ-mă]	A yellow growth or discoloration of the skin is _____ oma.
xero-derma [ZĔR-ō-DER-mă]	Excessive dryness of the skin is _____ derma.

STUDY TIP

Melanoma is a cancer that develops in the pigment cells, called melanocytes. It can be more serious than other forms of skin cancer because it may spread to other parts of the body, causing illness and death.

PRONOUNCE and DEFINE	Pronounce the following words aloud and write their meaning in the space provided.
keratosis	[kĕr-ă-TŌ-sĭs]
mycosis	[mī-KŌ-sĭs]
trichopathy	[trĭ-KŎP-ă-thē]
steatitis	[stē-ă-TĪ-tĭs]
dermatitis	[dĕr-mă-TĪ-tĭs]

SPELL and DEFINE	Identify if the following terms are spelled correctly. Correct the words that are spelled incorrectly. Write the definition for each word.	
	Spelling	Definition
sebatorrea		
onikotome		
ickythisosis		
adiposis		
pilocsitstic		

UNDERSTAND — Identify the term from the definition provided.

1. Horny growth on the skin: _____
2. Excess pigment in the skin: _____
3. Removal of fat by suctioning: _____
4. Disease of the nail: _____
5. Condition of extreme dryness: _____

APPLY — Read the following scenario and answer the question.

You are reviewing the medical record of Lin Cave, a 38-year-old male who just left the physician's office. The physician documented the following diagnoses:

1. Hidrosis
2. Mycosis of left big toe
3. Xeroderma of right hand
4. Seborrhea
5. Trichopathy

What conditions does Mr. Cave have?

_____

_____

LO 5.3 Diagnostic, Procedural, and Laboratory Terms

Diagnostic, procedural, and laboratory findings assist the health care provider in diagnosing medical conditions. Often used in combination, these tests lead to a final diagnosis and assist in treatment planning. Figure 5-6 shows a positive Mantoux test.

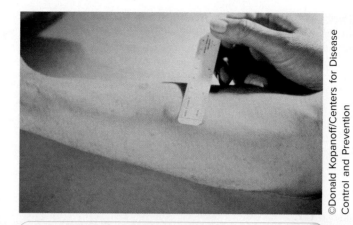

Figure 5-6 Positive Mantoux test

Diagnostic	PRACTICE
	Provide the missing term(s) to complete the following sentences.
dermatology [dĕr-mă-TŎL-ō-jē]	The field of _____ studies, diagnoses, and treats ailments of the skin. The first diagnostic test is usually visual observation of the surface of the skin.
exudate [ĔKS-yū-dāt]	Once a visual assessment has been made, the dermatologist determines which procedures and tests will help find the underlying cause of a skin problem. Samples of _____ or pus may be sent to a laboratory for examination. The laboratory can determine what types of bacteria are present. A scraping also may be taken and placed on a growth medium to be examined for the presence of fungi.
	Skin is a reliable place to test for various diseases and allergies. A suspected *allergen,* something that provokes an allergic reaction, is mixed with a substance that can be used in tests. That substance containing the allergen is called an *antigen.*
	Skin tests are typically performed in one of three ways:

patch test
 	
scratch test
 	
intradermal
[ĬN-tră-DĔR-măl]
 	
Mantoux [măn-TŪ] **test**
Purified protein derivative (PPD) test
TB tine
	1. The _____ calls for placing a suspected antigen on a piece of gauze and applying it to the skin for a designated timeframe. If a reaction results, the test is considered positive.
	2. The _____ involves scratching a suspected antigen onto the skin. Redness or swelling within ten minutes indicates a positive reaction.
	3. With an _____ test, a suspected antigen is injected between layers of skin. Infectious diseases also may be detected by this type of test. Some common intradermal tests include the following:
	  a. The _____ or _____ is used as a screening test for tuberculosis.
	  b. The _____, a screening test for tuberculosis (TB), injects the tuberculin using a tine (an instrument with a number of pointed ends).

PRONOUNCE and DEFINE	Pronounce the following words aloud and write their meaning in the space provided.
intradermal test	[ĬN-tră-DĔR-măl test]
exudate	[ĔKS-yū-dāt]
Mantoux test	[măn-TŪ test]
dermatology	[dĕr-mă-TŎL-ō-jē]

SPELL and DEFINE — Identify if the following terms are spelled correctly. Correct the words that are spelled incorrectly. Write the definition for each word.

	Spelling	Definition
eksyudat		
Mantwo		
dermatology		

UNDERSTAND — Complete the sentences by filling in the blanks.

1. Placing a suspected antigen on a piece of gauze and applying it to the skin for a designated timeframe is known as a _____.
2. Samples of _____ may be sent to a laboratory for examination.
3. Scratch tests are often used to detect _____.
4. Suspected antigens are injected between layers of skin in a(n) _____ test.

APPLY — Read the following scenario and answer the question.

You are the nurse working for Dr. Pia Turner, a dermatologist. Dr. Turner orders the following diagnostic studies for Cathy Riley, a 56-year-old female who visited the office today for multiple skin issues. Diagnostic studies ordered include:

- Culture of exudate
- Patch test
- Scratch test
- Mantoux test

Explain to Ms. Riley why the tests are ordered and how testing will occur.

_____

_____

_____

_____

LO 5.4 Pathological Terms

Pathological conditions of the skin and body membranes include lesions, diseases, and cancers. The following section presents terms associated with skin lesions. Figure 5-7 shows various types of lesions.

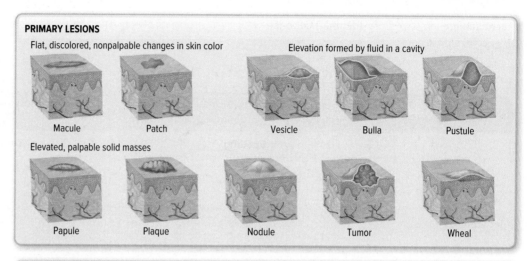

PRIMARY LESIONS

Flat, discolored, nonpalpable changes in skin color

Macule   Patch

Elevation formed by fluid in a cavity

Vesicle   Bulla   Pustule

Elevated, palpable solid masses

Papule   Plaque   Nodule   Tumor   Wheal

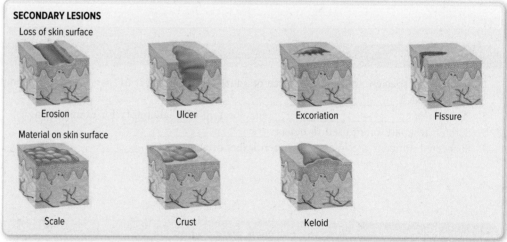

SECONDARY LESIONS

Loss of skin surface

Erosion   Ulcer   Excoriation   Fissure

Material on skin surface

Scale   Crust   Keloid

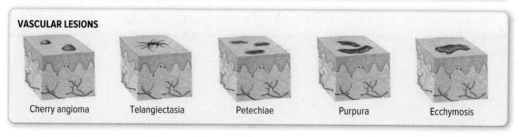

VASCULAR LESIONS

Cherry angioma   Telangiectasia   Petechiae   Purpura   Ecchymosis

Figure 5-7 Lesions

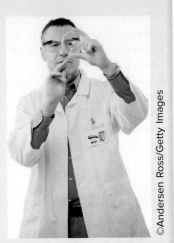
Pathological

PRACTICE

Provide the missing term(s) to complete the following sentences.

Pathological	Practice
lesions [LĒ-zhŭnz] **vascular lesions** [VĂS-kyū-lăr]	The skin is a place where abnormalities occur and where some internal diseases show dermatological symptoms. _____ are areas of tissues that are altered because of a pathological condition. *Primary lesions* appear on previously normal skin. *Secondary lesions* are abnormalities that result from changes in primary lesions. _____ are blood vessel lesions that show through the skin.
macule [MĂK-yūl] **patch** [pach] **papule** [PĂP-yūl] **nodule** [NŎD-yūl] **plaque** [plăk] **polyp** [PŎL-ĭp] **pediculated polyp** [pĕ-DĬK-yū-lā-tĕd] **sessile polyp** [SĔS-ĭl] **tumor** [TŪ-mŏr] **wheal** [hwēl]	Some common primary lesions are flat areas of discoloration, such as a _____ (freckle or flat mole) or _____. Elevated, solid masses include _____, a small elevated mass, also called a *pimple;* _____, a small patch on the skin; _____, a large pimple or a small node; _____, any mass that projects outward, either on a slender stalk (_____) or from a broad base (_____); _____, any swelling or, specifically, any abnormal tissue growth; and _____, a smooth, slightly elevated area, usually associated with allergic itching.
bulla (*pl.,* **bullae**) [BŬL-ă (BŬL-ē)] **pustule** [PŬS-tūl] **vesicle** [VĔS-ĭ-kl] **cyst** [sĭst] **pilonidal cyst** [pī-lō-NĪ-dăl] **sebaceous cyst** [sĕ-BĀ-shŭs]	A _____ is a large blister, a _____ is a small elevated mass containing pus, and a _____ is a small mass containing fluid; all are elevated skin pockets filled with fluid. A _____ may be solid or filled with fluid or gas. A _____ contains hairs and a _____ contains yellow sebum.

continued on next page

Pathological	PRACTICE
	Provide the missing term(s) to complete the following sentences.
erosion [ē-RŌ-zhŭn] **excoriation** [ĕks-KŌ-rē-Ā-shŭn] **fissure** [FĬSH-ŭr] **ulcer** [ŬL-sĕr] **decubitus** [dĕ-KYŪ-bĭ-tŭs] **pressure ulcers** **scale** [skāl]	Secondary lesions usually involve either loss of skin surface or material that forms on the skin surface. Lesions that involve loss of skin surface are an _____, a shallow area of the skin worn away by friction or pressure; an _____, a scratched area of the skin, usually covered with dried blood; a _____, a deep furrow or crack in the skin surface; and an _____, a wound with loss of tissue and often with inflammation, especially _____ or _____, which are chronic ulcers on skin over bony parts that are under constant pressure, as when someone is bed-ridden or wheelchair-bound. Pressure ulcers are staged according to depth of tissue injury.
crust **keloid** [KĒ-loyd]	Lesions that form surface material are _____, thin plates of epithelium formed on the skin's surface; _____, dried blood or pus that forms on the skin's surface; and _____, a firm, raised mass of scar tissue.

PRONOUNCE and DEFINE	Pronounce the following terms aloud and write their meaning in the space provided.
pediculated	[pĕ-DĬK-yū-lā-tĕd]
pilonidal	[pī-lō-NĪ-dăl]
wheal	[hwēl]
bulla	[BŬL-ă]
excoriation	[ĕks-KŌ-rē-Ā-shŭn]

SPELL and DEFINE	Identify if the following terms are spelled correctly. Correct the words that are spelled incorrectly. Write the definition for each word.	
	Spelling	**Definition**
dekyubitus		
keloyd		
pustule		
papyul		
makyoul		

| UNDERSTAND | Complete the sentences by filling in the blanks with the correct term. |

1. A polyp that projects upward from a slender stalk is a _____.
2. An itchy patch of raised skin is a _____.
3. A small, raised sac on the skin that contains fluid is _____.
4. The scarring that occurs after an injury or surgery is a _____.
5. Another term for a pressure sore is _____.

The physician has just examined Rose Arlia. You are reviewing the medical record information with the patient. You note that the physician has documented that Ms. Arlia has the following:

1. Vascular lesion on lower right leg
2. Macule on right hand
3. Small papule on right wrist
4. Bulla on left hand
5. Pilonidal cyst

Explain to Ms. Arlia what these conditions are.

_____

_____

_____

Did you know

Pilonidal Cyst

A pilonidal cyst was also called Jeep's syndrome due to the amount of cases found in WWII soldiers from riding in Jeeps. Cysts were formed on the tailbone due to the rough ride in Jeeps.

Symptoms, Abnormalities, and Conditions I

This section includes terms associated with skin diseases and symptoms of other diseases that appear on the skin. Figure 5-8 shows a rash caused by rubella and Figure 5-9 shows an example of petechiae.

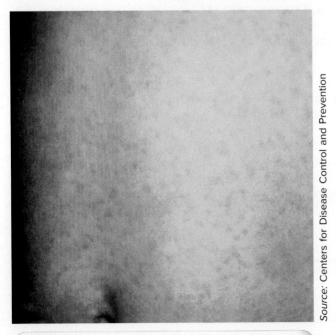

Source: Centers for Disease Control and Prevention

Figure 5-8 Rash caused by rubella—note reddened areas

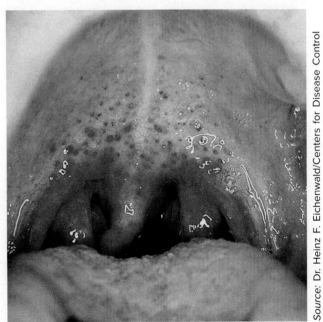

Source: Dr. Heinz F. Eichenwald/Centers for Disease Control and Prevention

Figure 5-9 Petechiae—note red blotches

Pathological	**PRACTICE I**
	Provide the missing term(s) to complete the following sentences.
rubeola [rū-BĒ-ō-lă] **rubella** [rū-BĔL-ă] **roseola** [rō-ZĒ-Ō-lă] **varicella** [văr-ĭ-SĔL-ă]	Symptoms of disease can appear on the skin. For example, common viral rashes include _____, measles with an accompanying rash; _____, disease with a rash caused by the rubella virus (also known as *German measles*); _____, disease with small, rosy patches on the skin, usually caused by a virus; and _____, disease with a rash known as chickenpox, caused by the varicella virus. Chickenpox does not usually cause harm (other than possibly scarring) in young children.
impetigo [ĭm-pĕ-TĪ-gō] **pyoderma** [pī-ō-DĔR-mă]	Infectious agents, such as staphylococci, may cause _____, which is a _____, or pus-containing, contagious skin disease. At times, staphylo-coccus infections can become deadly, as is the case with flesh-eating bacteria, a fatal type of staph infection.
tinea [TĬN-ē-ă] **ringworm** [RING-werm] **pruritus** [prū-RĪ-tŭs] **candidiasis** [kăn-dĭ-DĪ-ă-sĭs]	Fungi may cause _____ or _____, a skin condi-tion that causes intense _____, or itching. _____ is a yeast fungus that causes common rashes such as diaper rash. Other common fungi are *tinea pedis,* or athlete's foot; *tinea capitis,* scalp ringworm; and *tinea barbae,* ringworm of the beard.
dermatitis [dĕr-mă-TĪ-tĭs] **urticaria** [ŬR-tĭ-KĀR-ē-ă] **hives** [hīvz] **eczema** [ĔK-sĕ-mă, ĔG-zĕ-mă]	Skin conditions, particularly skin irritations or _____, can reflect systemic allergies or diseases. _____ or _____ may arise from many causes, such as a food allergy; itching or pruritus also can be the result of allergies. _____ is an acute form of dermatitis often caused by allergies.
ecchymosis (*pl.,* **ecchymoses**) [ĕk-ĭ-MŌ-sĭs (ĕk-ĭ-MŌ-sēz)] **petechiae** (*sing.,* **petechia**) [pē-TĒ-kē-ē, pē-TĔK-ē-ē (pē-TĒ-kē-ă, pē-TĔK-ē-ă)] **purpura** [PŬR-pū-ră] **rosacea** [rō-ZĀ-shē-ă]	_____ is a bluish-purple skin mark that may result from a skin injury that can cause blood to leak out of blood vessels. _____ are tiny, pin-point ecchymoses. _____ is a condition with extensive hemorrhages into the skin covering a wide area. It starts out with red areas, which turn purplish, and then brown, in a couple of weeks. _____ is a vascular disorder that appears as red blotches on the skin, particularly around the nose and cheeks.
furuncle [FYŪ-rŭng-kl] **carbuncle** [KĂR-bŭng-kl] **abscess** [ĂB-sĕs] **gangrene** [GĂNG-grēn]	Some diseases, infections, or inflammations cause skin conditions, such as a _____, a localized, pus-producing infection originating in a hair fol-licle; a _____, a pus-producing infection that starts in subcutaneous tissue and is usually accompanied by fever and an ill feeling; _____, a localized infection usually accompanied by pus and inflammation; and _____, *necrosis* (death) of tissue due to loss of blood supply.

STUDY TIP

Purpura may occur when the platelet count of the blood is low *(thrombocytopenia)*. It also may occur when the blood vessel wall is particularly fragile or has been damaged or if the skin is thin.

PRONOUNCE and DEFINE	Pronounce the following words aloud and write their meaning in the space provided.
gangrene	[GĂNG-grēn]
furuncle	[FYŪ-rŭng-kl]
roseola	[rō-ZĒ-Ō-lă]
pruritus	[prū-RĪ-tŭs]
eczema	[ĔK-sĕ-mă, ĔG-zĕ-mă]

SPELL and DEFINE	Identify if the following terms are spelled correctly. Correct the words that are spelled incorrectly. Write the definition for each word.	
	Spelling	Definition
kandidiasis		
pioderma		
rubela		
urticaria		
petekea		

UNDERSTAND Identify the term from the definition provided.

1. Blotchy red patches on the skin: _____
2. Another term for hives: _____
3. Another term for chickenpox: _____
4. Term for German measles: _____
5. A pus-producing infection originating in a hair follicle: _____

APPLY Read the following scenario and answer the question.

Lara Heber presents to the physician's office with the following symptoms:

- Purplish skin patch on left upper arm
- Ringworm
- Severe itching
- Inflammation of the skin with pus
- Infected hair follicle

Write the medical terms for the above symptoms.

_____
_____
_____
_____

STUDY TIP

Form a study group to learn medical terminology. Create games that will help to learn the spelling and meaning of the words.

Symptoms, Abnormalities, and Conditions II

Viral skin disease can cause skin disorders. This section includes more terms associated with diseases that manifest on or in the skin.

Pathological	PRACTICE II
	Provide the missing term(s) to complete the following sentences.
herpes [HĔR-pēz]	Some viruses cause skin problems. In some cases, these viruses are sexually transmitted infections (STIs) (such as some types of _____ and genital warts). (Sexually transmitted infections are discussed with the reproductive systems, covered in Chapters 16 and 17.)
herpes simplex virus type 1 [SĬM-plĕx] **herpes simplex virus type 2** **herpes zoster** [ZŎS-tĕr] **cold sore** **fever blister** **genital herpes** **shingles** [SHĬN-glz] **wart** [wŏrt] **verruca** (*pl.*, **verrucae**) [vĕ-RŪ-kă (vĕ-RŪ-kē)] **plantar wart** [PLĂN-tăr]	_____, _____, and _____ are all viral diseases caused by herpes viruses. Herpes 1, also called a _____ or _____, usually appears around the mouth. Herpes 2, also known as _____, affects the genital area. Herpes zoster, or _____, is an inflammation that affects the nerves on one side of the body and results in skin blisters. It can be extremely painful. A virus also may cause a _____ or _____. A _____ appears on the soles of the feet.
cellulitis [sĕl-yū-LĪ-tĭs]	_____ is inflammation of the dermis and subcutaneous portion of the skin.

PRONOUNCE and DEFINE	Pronounce the following terms aloud and write their meaning in the space provided.
herpes zoster	[HĔR-pēz ZŎS-tĕr]
plantar wart	[PLĂN-tăr wŏrt]
shingles	[SHĬN-glz]
cellulitis	[sĕl-yū-LĪ-tĭs]
wart	[wŏrt]

SPELL and DEFINE	Identify if the following terms are spelled correctly. Correct the words that are spelled incorrectly. Write the definition for each word.

	Spelling	Definition
shinglz		
herpes zoster		
herpes simplex		
veruka		
selyulitis		

1. Wart on sole of foot: _____
2. Herpes simplex type 2: _____
3. Inflammation of dermis and subcutaneous portion of skin: _____
4. Flesh-colored growth: _____
5. Herpes simplex type 1: _____

Did you know

Burns

When burning occurs, the faster the treatment starts, the better the outcome. Here are some tips for the following types of burns:

- **Heat burns.** It is important to smother any flames immediately. So if your clothing is on fire, stop, drop, and roll to smother the flames.
- **Liquid scald burns.** Run cool water over the burn for 10 to 20 minutes. Do not use ice.
- **Chemical burns.** Immediately call the Poison Control Center or 911 to find out how to treat burns from a chemical.
- **Electrical burns.** If the situation is safe, remove the person from the electrical source of the burn. If the person is not breathing, call 911 and begin CPR (discussed in Chapter 12).

Burns are classified by a system called the **"rule of nines,"** *illustrated in Figure 5-10.*

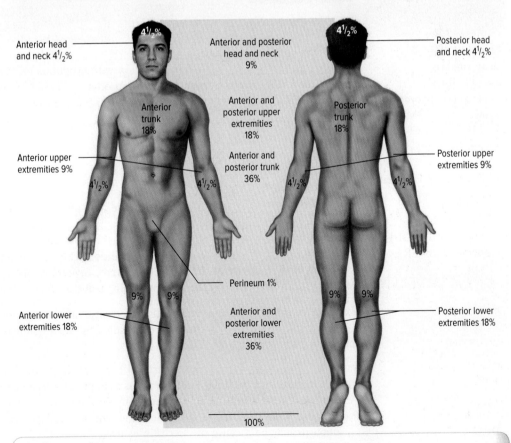

Figure 5-10 Rule of nines

Symptoms, Abnormalities, and Conditions III

Skin disorders can affect the skin and nails. This section includes terms associated with conditions of or affecting the skin or nails. Figure 5-11 shows a young person's forehead with acne.

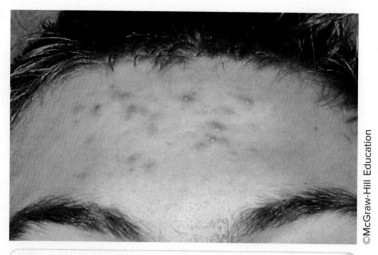

Figure 5-11 Acne

©McGraw-Hill Education

Pathological	**PRACTICE III**
	Provide the missing term(s) to complete the following sentences.
acne [ĂK-nē] **acne vulgaris** [vŭl-GĀR-ĭs] **comedo** (*pl.,* **comedos, comedones**) [KŌM-ē-dō, kō-MĒ-dō (KŌM-ē-dōz, kō-mē-DŌ-nĕz)] **blackheads** **whiteheads** [WHĪT-hĕd]	Other skin conditions include _____(also called _____), a skin condition with eruptions on the face and upper back. Acne usually starts around puberty and often is caused by overproduction of sebum. It usually includes several types of skin eruptions, such as _____ or _____, _____, pustules, and nodules.
scleroderma [sklēr-ō-DĚR-mă] **psoriasis** [sō-RĪ-ă-sĭs] **seborrhea** [sĕb-ō-RĒ-ă]	_____ is a chronic disease with abnormal thickening of the skin caused by the formation of new collagen. _____, a recurrent skin condition with scaly lesions on the trunk, arms, hands, legs, and scalp, is often associated with stress. _____, a condition with excessive production of sebum, is a result of overactivity of the sebaceous glands. *Seborrheic dermatitis* (also called *dandruff*), scaly eruptions on the face and scalp, is due to the overproduction of seborrhea.
burn	Exposure of the skin to heat, chemicals, electricity, radiation, or other irritants may cause a _____. Burns are classified by the amount or level of skin involvement and body surface area (BSA):
first-degree burns	1. _____ are superficial burns of the epidermis without blistering but with redness and swelling. Sunburn is an example of a first-degree burn. There is mild to moderate pain and the skin is intact but is often swollen and reddened, and it radiates heat. Cold compresses will relieve the pain and reduce the swelling. Continual sunburns may be a cause of later skin cancer.

second-degree burns	2. _____ affect the epidermis and dermis and involve blistering. The wound is sensitive to touch and very painful.
third-degree burns	3. _____ involve complete destruction of the skin, sometimes reaching into the muscle and bone and causing extensive scarring.
pediculosis [pĕ-DĬK-yū-LŌ-sĭs] **scabies** [SKĀ-bēz]	Some skin conditions are caused by insects. _____ is an inflammation with lice, often on the head *(pediculosis capitis)* or the genital area *(pediculosis pubis)*. _____, a contagious skin eruption that often occurs between fingers, on other areas of the trunk, or on the male genitalia, is caused by mites.
onychia [ō-NĬK-ē-ă] **onychitis** [ŏn-ĭ-KĪ-tĭs] **paronychia** [păr-ŏ-NĬK-ē-ă] **onychopathy** [ŏn-ĭ-KŎP-ă-thē]	Inflammations of the nail can be caused by infection, irritation, or fungi. _____ or _____ is a nail inflammation. _____ is an inflammation in the nail fold, the flap of skin overlapping the edges of the nail. Both of these inflammations often occur spontaneously in debilitated people. They also may result from a slight trauma. A general term for disease of the nails is _____.

PRONOUNCE and DEFINE	Pronounce the following terms aloud and write their meaning in the space provided.
comedo	[KŌM-ē-dō, kō-MĒ-dō]
scleroderma	[sklēr-ō-DĔR-mă]
seborrhea	[sĕb-ō-RĒ-ă]
pediculosis	[pĕ-DĬK-yū-LŌ-sĭs]
scabies	[SKĀ-bēz]

SPELL and DEFINE	Identify if the following terms are spelled correctly. Correct the words that are spelled incorrectly. Write the definition for each word.	
	Spelling	**Definition**
onikea		
paronikea		
pedikyulosis		
soriasis		
acne vulgaris		

UNDERSTAND   Identify the term from the definition provided.

1. Open hair follicle filled with bacteria and sebum: _____
2. Thickening of skin caused by an increase of collagen formation: _____
3. Disease of nail: _____
4. Lice infestation: _____
5. Skin eruption caused by a mite: _____

A concerned mother of an elementary child brings a note to you identifying that pediculosis has been identified at the school. Explain to the parent what this is.

_____

_____

Symptoms, Abnormalities, and Conditions IV

This section includes terms associated with abnormal growths on the skin and abnormal hair loss. Figure 5-12(c) shows malignant **melanoma** or skin cancer.

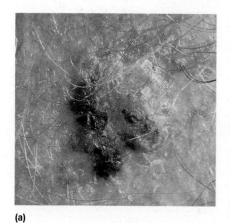
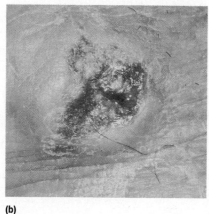
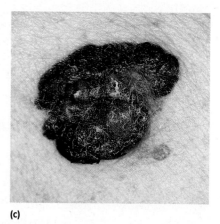

(a)   (b)   (c)

(a) ©Biophoto Associates/Science Source; (b) ©Clinical Photography, Central Manchester University Hospitals NHS Foundation Trust, UK/ Science Source; (c) ©James Stevenson/Science Source

Figure 5-12 Skin cancer: (a) squamous cell carcinoma, (b) basal cell carcinoma, (c) malignant melanoma

PRACTICE IV

Provide the missing term(s) to complete the following sentences.

Pathological	
neoplasms [NĒ-ō-plăzmz] **callus** [KĂL-ŭs] **corn** [kōrn] **keratosis** [kĕr-ă-TŌ-sĭs]	Some abnormal growths or _____ are benign. The most common benign neoplasms are a _____, a hard, thickened area of skin; a _____, hardening or thickening of skin on a toe; and _____, overgrowth of horny tissue on skin.
basal cell carcinoma [BĀ-săl sĕl kăr-sĭn-Ō-mă] **squamous cell carcinoma** [SKWĀ-mŭs sĕl kăr-sĭn-Ō-mă] **Kaposi sarcoma** [KĂ-pō-sē săr-KŌ-mă] **malignant melanoma** [mĕl-ă-NŌ-mă]	Some neoplasms are malignant. For example, _____ is cancer of the basal layer of the epidermis; _____ affects the squamous epithelium. _____ is often associated with AIDS. The incidence of _____ is rapidly increasing. This increase is thought to be due to the depletion of the Earth's ozone layer, which protects the skin from harmful UV rays. Many protective products, such as sunscreen, are widely available. One of the odd results of widespread sunscreen use is that skin cancers have increased in people who use them. This is because people who use the sunscreens actually feel that they can stay in the sun for much longer periods. The only effective skin cancer prevention is to avoid exposure to the sun as much as possible.
alopecia areata [ăl-ō-PĒ-shē-ă ā-rē-Ă-tă]	In most instances, hair loss is hereditary or due to a side effect of medication. However, hair loss can be a pathological condition, as in _____, a condition in which hair falls out in patches.

PRONOUNCE and DEFINE	Pronounce the following terms aloud and write their meaning in the space provided.
callus	[KĂL-ŭs]
Kaposi sarcoma	[KĂ-pō-sē săr-KŌ-mă]
keratosis	[kĕr-ă-TŌ-sĭs]
squamous cell carcinoma	[SKWĀ-mŭs sĕl kăr-sĭn-Ō-mă]
alopecia areata	[ăl-ō-PĒ-shē-ă ā-rē-Ă-tă]

SPELL and DEFINE	Identify if the following terms are spelled correctly. Correct the words that are spelled incorrectly. Write the definition for each word.	
	Spelling	Definition
kneoplasm		
urticaria		
purpora		
varicella		
rosola		

UNDERSTAND   Add the missing suffix to each term.

1. Nail inflammation: onych _____
2. Skin condition: dermat _____
3. Black tumor: melan _____
4. Hair disease: tricho _____
5. Horny tissue: kerat _____

LO 5.5 Surgical Terms

The following section includes terms associated with surgery of the integumentary system.

Surgical	PRACTICE — Provide the missing term(s) to complete the following sentences.
plastic surgery	Skin surgery includes the repair of various conditions. Sutures, stitches, or staples hold skin together while healing takes place. Various types of _____ may involve reconstructing areas of the skin, as after severe burns or radiation. Other types of skin surgery result in the removal of a part of a growth to test for the presence of cancer. Growths also are removed to keep a cancer from spreading.
skin graft autograft [ĂW-tō-grăft] allograft [ĂL-ō-grăft] homograft [HŌ-mō-grăft] heterograft [HĔT-ĕr-ō-grăft] xenograft [ZĔN-ō-grăft]	Plastic surgery is a general term for a variety of surgeries to correct defects resulting from injuries or birth defects or to enhance someone's idea of how he or she should look. Surgical correction of disfiguring physical defects is also known as *cosmesis*. Plastic surgery may involve the use of a _____. An _____ uses skin from one's own body. An _____ or _____ uses donor skin from another person. A _____ or _____ uses donor skin from one species to another (such as animal—for example, a pig—to human). A *dermatome* is an implement used to remove layers of skin for grafts.

continued on next page

Surgical	**PRACTICE**
	Provide the missing term(s) to complete the following sentences.
cryosurgery [KRĪ-ō-SĔR-jĕr-ē] **dermabrasion** [dĕr-mă-BRĀ-zhŭn] **debridement** [dā-brēd-MŎN] **curettage** [kyū-rĕ-TĂZH]	Plastic surgery also may use various methods to remove unwanted growths or scrape tissue or discolorations. _____ involves the removal of tissue by applying cold liquid nitrogen. _____ involves the use of brushes and emery papers to remove wrinkles, scars, and tattoos. _____ and _____ are the removal of dead tissue from a wound by scraping.
cauterized [KĂW-tĕr-īzd] **fulguration** [fŭl-gŭ-RĀ-shŭn]	Some surgical procedures of the skin involve the use of electricity or lasers to stop bleeding, remove tissue, or excise tissues for examination. Wounds may be _____, or burned, to coagulate an area that is bleeding. _____ is the use of electric sparks to destroy tissue.
biopsy [BĪ-ŏp-sē] **Mohs' surgery** [mōz]	A _____ is a cutting of tissue for microscopic examination. A *needle biopsy* is the removal of tissue by aspirating it through a needle. A *punch biopsy* is the use of a cylindrical instrument to remove a small piece of tissue (Figure 5-13). A *shave biopsy* is the removal of a layer of skin using a surgical blade. _____ is the removal of thin layers of malignant growth until a nonmalignant area is reached.

PRONOUNCE and DEFINE	Pronounce the following terms aloud and write their meaning in the space provided.
autograft	[ĂW-tō-grăft]
allograft	[ĂL-ō-grăft]
xenograft	[ZĔN-ō-grăft]
dermabrasion	[dĕr-mă-BRĀ-zhŭn]
curettage	[kyū-rĕ-TĂZH]

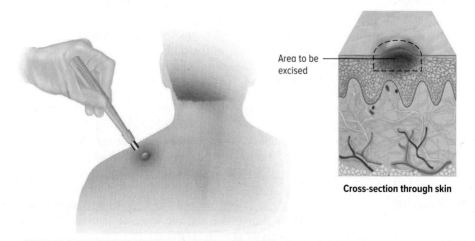

Area to be excised

Cross-section through skin

Figure 5-13 Punch biopsy instrument and procedure

SPELL and DEFINE	Identify if the following terms are spelled correctly. Correct the words that are spelled incorrectly. Write the definition for each word	
	Spelling	Definition
kawteriz		
fulgurashun		
biopse		
dabredmon		
criosurgerie		

UNDERSTAND Break apart the following combining terms. Identify the meaning of each part.

1. autograft _____
2. dermabrasion _____
3. homograft _____
4. cryosurgery _____
5. xenograft _____

APPLY Read the following scenario and respond accordingly.

Mr. David Horvath wants to know the difference between the various types of skin grafts. Explain the different types of skin grafts to him.

_____

_____

LO 5.6 Pharmacological Terms

Treatment of skin disorders involves the use of various medications. A wide variety of topical preparations can relieve symptoms and even kill agents that cause disease. Other treatments involve heat, light, and radiation. Figure 5-14 shows age-related changes of the skin. This section includes terms associated with the medications used to treat disorders of the integumentary system.

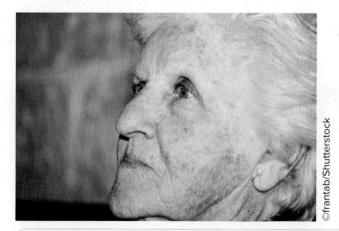

Figure 5-14 Age-related skin changes—note darkened spots

©frantab/Shutterstock

Pharmacological	**PRACTICE**
	Provide the missing term(s) to complete the following sentences.
chemotherapy [KĒ-mō-THĂR-ă-pē] **radiation therapy**	Cancer of the skin is sometimes successfully treated by _____ and/or _____. Chemotherapy uses chemicals to treat the malignant cells systematically. Radiation therapy uses high-energy radiation to bombard malignant cells, to destroy them.
ultraviolet light [ŭl-tră-VĪ-ō-lĕt]	The sun is beneficial in healing certain skin problems. Some lesions are treated with _____, which imitates some of the sun's rays. On the other hand, sunlight also may be the cause of many skin problems, such as certain carcinomas.
antihistamines [ĂN-tē-HĬS-tă-mēnz] **antibiotics** [ĂN-tē-bī-ŎT-ĭks] **antiseptics** [ĂN-tē-SĔP-tĭks] **antibacterials** [ĂN-tē-băk-TĒR-ē-ălz] **antifungals** [ĂN-tē-FŬNG-ălz]	_____ are medications used to control allergic skin reactions. They do so by blocking the effects of *histamines,* chemicals present in tissues that heighten allergic reactions. Other skin conditions are controlled by different medications. For example, _____ kill or slow the growth of microorganisms on the skin. _____ perform the same function. _____ kill or slow the growth of bacteria. _____ kill or slow the growth of fungal infections.
anti-inflammatory **corticosteroids** [KŌR-tĭ-kō-STĒR-oydz] **antipruritics** [ĂN-tē-prū-RĬT-ĭks] **anesthetic** [ăn-ĕs-THĔT-ĭk] **topical anesthetic**	_____ agents, particularly _____, reduce inflammation whereas _____ control itching. Some skin conditions are painful because of nerve conduction near the skin surface. An _____ and, especially in the case of surface pain, a _____ can relieve some of the pain associated with such conditions.
emollients [ē-MŎL-ē-ĕnts] **astringents** [ăs-TRĬN-jĕnts] **keratolytics** [KĔR-ă-tō-LĬT-ĭks] **alpha-hydroxy acids** [ĂL-fă-hī-DRŎK-sē ĂS-ĭdz]	Some skin conditions result in either oversecretion of oils or extreme dryness. _____ are agents that soothe or soften skin by moistening it or adding oils to it. _____ temporarily lessen the formation of oily material on the surface of the skin. These types of agents are often present in over-the-counter products. Other vitamin-based products to control skin aging (often containing vitamins A and C) also are often available over the counter. _____ remove warts and corns from the skin surface. _____ are fruit acids added to cosmetics to improve the skin's appearance.

PRONOUNCE and DEFINE	Pronounce the following terms aloud and write their meaning in the space provided.
corticosteroid	[KŌR-tĭ-kō-STĒR-oyd]
antipruritic	[ĂN-tē-prū-RĬT-ĭk]
emollient	[ē-MŎL-ē-ĕnt]
keratolytic	[KĔR-ă-tō-LĬT-ĭk]
antibiotic	[ĂN-tē-bī-ŎT-ĭk]

SPELL and DEFINE	Identify if the following terms are spelled correctly. Correct the words that are spelled incorrectly. Write the definition for each word.	
	Spelling	**Definition**
anesthetik		
antiseptik		
antehistamen		
kemotharape		
astrinjent		

UNDERSTAND	Complete the following sentences by filling in the blanks with the correct term.

1. Chemotherapy is used to treat _____.
2. Antibiotics are used to treat _____.
3. This class of medications would be used to treat allergic reactions: _____.
4. Astringents control _____.
5. Emollients may contain _____.

LO 5.7 Abbreviations

This section identifies abbreviations commonly used with the integumentary system.

ABBREVIATION REVIEW

Abbreviation	Definition
BSA	body surface area
bx, BX, Bx	biopsy
Derm	dermatology
HIV	human immunodeficiency virus/disease
HSV	herpes simplex virus
I&D	incision and drainage
ID	infectious disease
oint	ointment
PPD	purified protein derivative—used in skin test for tuberculosis
staph	staphylococcus
STI	sexually transmitted infections
strep	streptococcus
TB	tuberculosis

For each of the following words, identify its abbreviation.

1. Biopsy: _____
2. Tuberculosis: _____
3. Herpes simplex virus: _____
4. Incise and drain: _____

Read the following scenario and rewrite using appropriate medical terms.

"Please refer Mr. Jones to an ID for suspected strep or staph infection. He has been applying antibiotic oint without improvement for one month."

_____

_____

_____

_____

CHAPTER SUMMARY

	Learning Outcome	Summary
5.1	Identify parts of the skin and body membranes and discuss the function of each part.	The integumentary system includes the skin or integument, the hair, the nails, the sweat glands (also called the *sudoriferous glands*), and the oil-producing glands (also called the *sebaceous glands*). This system covers and protects the body, helps regulate the body's temperature, excretes some of the body's waste materials, and includes the body's sensors for pain and sensation.
5.2	Identify the major word parts used in building words that relate to the skin and body membranes.	Word building requires knowledge of the combining form and meaning.
5.3	Discuss common diagnostic tests, laboratory tests, and clinical procedures used in testing and treating disorders of the skin and body membranes.	Diagnostic, procedural, and laboratory findings assist the health care provider in diagnosing medical conditions. Often used in combination, these tests lead to a final diagnosis and assist in treatment planning.
5.4	Define the major pathological conditions of the skin and body membranes.	Pathological conditions of the skin and body membranes include lesions, diseases, and cancers.
5.5	Define surgical terms related to the skin and body membranes.	Skin surgery includes the repair of various conditions. Sutures, stitches, or staples hold skin together while healing takes place. Plastic surgery may involve reconstructing areas of the skin, as after severe burns or radiation. Other types of skin surgery result in the removal of a part of a growth to test for the presence of cancer. Growths also are removed to keep a cancer from spreading.
5.6	Explain common pharmacological agents used in treating disorders of the skin and body membranes.	Treatment of skin disorders involves the use of various medications. A wide variety of topical preparations can relieve symptoms and even kill agents that cause disease. Other treatments involve heat, light, and radiation.
5.7	Identify common abbreviations associated with the skin and body membranes.	Abbreviations are used to describe diseases, conditions, procedures, and treatments associated with the skin and body membranes.

Label the following on the accompanying figure.

- Free edge of nail
- Nail groove
- Lunula
- Nail body
- Cuticle

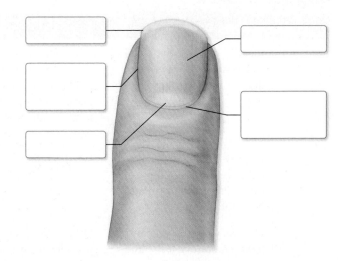

Correct the spelling and write the definition for each term. Say each term aloud.

1. integumentery: _____
2. onikotome: _____
3. adapose: _____
4. sebaceous: _____
5. collogen: _____

6. stratum corneum: _____
7. follical: _____
8. melanosite: _____
9. alopecia: _____
10. epadermis: _____

Complete the following sentences by filling in the blanks.

1. The thin layer of skin around the edge of a nail is called a(n) _____.
2. Hair follicles are found in the _____ (layer of the skin).
3. The outer layer of skin is the _____.
4. The top sublayer of the dermis is called _____.
5. Small sweat glands found all over the body are called _____ glands.
6. The subcutaneous layer consists of _____ tissue.
7. A pinkish nail is a sign of a(n) _____ nail.
8. The area where keratin and other cells mix with air under the nail is called the _____.
9. Sebaceous glands secrete _____.
10. Sweat glands are a(n) _____ gland.
11. Most adult hair loss is caused by _____ or a(n) _____.
12. Scabies is caused by _____.
13. Herpes simplex virus type 1 usually occurs around the area of the _____.
14. Herpes simplex virus type 2 usually occurs on the _____.
15. Warts are caused by a(n) _____.

Word Building: Break each of the following terms into word parts and write their meaning.

1. dermatoplasty, dermoplasty: _____

_____

2. mycodermatitis: _____

_____

3. trichoid: _____

_____

4. steatosis: _____

_____

5. adipocyte: _____

_____

6. onychomycosis: _____

_____

7. lipoma, steatoma, adipoma: _____

_____

8. xeroderma: _____

_____

9. melanosis: _____

_____

10. mycosis: _____

_____

Rewrite the following documentation using appropriate medical terms and abbreviations.
Mr. Smith is a 62-year-old male who reports a recent onset of baldness. Upon examination of the scalp, there are no open areas or pus. A smooth, slightly elevated area was noted by the left ear. Further examination revealed a bruise on the left arm and an open area on the forearm that was filled with pus. Another raised area on the arm was cut open and drained, and a sample was sent for testing.

Reviewing the Terms
Pronounce each of the following terms. Write the definitions on a separate sheet of paper. This review will take you through all the words you learned in this chapter. If you have difficulty with any words, make a flash card for later study. Refer to the English-Spanish and Spanish-English glossaries in the eBook.

abscess [ĂB-sĕs]
acne [ĂK-nē]
acne vulgaris [vŭl-GĀR-ĭs]
adip/o [ĂD-ĭ-pō]
adipose [ĂD-ĭ-pōs]
albinism [ĂL-bĭ-nĭzm]
allograft [ĂL-ō-grăft]
alopecia [ăl-ō-PĒ-shē-ă]
alopecia areata [ā-rē-Ă-tă]
alpha-hydroxy [ĂL-fă-hī-DRŎK-sē] **acid**
anesthetic [ăn-ĕs-THĔT-ĭk]
antibacterial [ĂN-tē-băk-TĒR-ē-ăl]

antibiotic [ĂN-tē-bī-ŎT-ĭk]
antifungal [ĂN-tē-FŬNG-ăl]
antihistamine [ĂN-tē-HĬS-tă-mēn]
anti-inflammatory [ĂN-tē-ĭn-FLĂM-ă-tō-rē]
antipruritic [ĂN-tē-prū-RĬT-ĭk]
antiseptic [ĂN-tē-SĔP-tĭk]
astringent [ăs-TRĬN-jĕnt]
autograft [ĂW-tō-grăft]
basal cell carcinoma [BĀ-săl sĕl kăr-sĭn-Ō-mă]
biopsy [BĪ-ŏp-sē]
birthmark
blackhead

bulla (*pl.*, **bullae**) [BŬL-ă (BŬL-ē)]
burn [bern]
callus [KĂL-ŭs]
candidiasis [kăn-dĭ-DĪ-ă-sĭs]
carbuncle [KĂR-bŭng-kl]
cauterize [KĂW-tĕr-īz]
cellulitis [sĕl-yū-LĪ-tĭs]
ceruminous [sĕ-RŪ-mĭn-ŭs] glands
chemotherapy [KĒ-mō-THĀR-ă-pē]
cherry angioma [ăn-jē-Ō-mă]
chloasma [klō-ĂZ-mă]
cicatrix [SĬK-ă-trĭks]
cold sore
collagen [KŎL-lă-jĕn]
comedo (*pl.*, **comedos, comedones**) [KŌM-ē-dō, kō-MĒ-dō
(KŌM-ē-dōz, kō-mē-DŌ-nĕz)]
corn [kōrn]
corticosteroid [KŌR-tĭ-kō-STĒR-oyd]
crust
cryosurgery [KRĪ-ō-SĔR-jĕr-ē]
curettage [kyū-rĕ-TĂZH]
cuticle [KYŪ-tĭ-kl]
cyst [sĭst]
debridement [dā-brēd-MŎN]
decubitus (*pl.*, **decubiti**) [dĕ-KYŪ-bĭ-tŭs (dĕ-KYŪ-bĭ-tī)] *or*
decubitus ulcer
depigmentation [dē-pĭg-mĕn-TĀ-shŭn]
derm/o [DĔR-mo]
dermabrasion [dĕr-mă-BRĀ-zhŭn]
dermat/o [DĔR-mă-tō]
dermatitis [dĕr-mă-TĪ-tĭs]
dermatology [dĕr-mă-TŎL-ō-jē]
dermis [DĔR-mĭs]
diaphoresis [DĪ-ă-fō-RĒ-sĭs]
discoid lupus erythematosus [DĬS-koyd LŪ-pŭs
ĕr-ĭ-thĕm-ă-TŌ-sŭs]
ecchymosis (*pl.*, **ecchymoses**) [ĕk-ĭ-MŌ-sĭs (ĕk-ĭ-MŌ-sēz)]
eccrine [ĔK-rĭn] glands
eczema [ĔK-sĕ-mă, ĔG-zĕ-mă]
emollient [ē-MŎL-ē-ĕnt]
epidermis [ĕp-ĭ-DĔR-mĭs]
erosion [ē-RŌ-zhŭn]
excoriation [ĕks-KŌ-rē-Ā-shŭn]
exocrine [ĔK-sō-krĭn] glands
exudate [ĔKS-yū-dāt]
fever blister
first-degree burn
fissure [FĬSH-ŭr]
fulguration [fŭl-gŭ-RĀ-shŭn]
furuncle [FYŪ-rŭng-kl]
gangrene [GĂNG-grēn]
genital herpes [HĔR-pēz]

hair follicle [FŎL-ĭ-kl]
hair root
hair shaft
herpes [HĔR-pēz]
herpes simplex virus type 1 [HĔR-pēz SĬM-plĕx]
herpes simplex virus type 2
herpes zoster [ZŎS-tĕr]
heterograft [HĔT-ĕr-ō-grăft]
hidr/o [hi-DRŌ *or* HĪ-drō]
hives
homograft [HŌ-mō-grăft]
hypodermis [hī-pō-DĔR-mĭs]
ichthy/o [ĭk-thē-ō]
impetigo [ĭm-pĕ-TĪ-gō]
integument [ĭn-TĔG-yū-mĕnt]
intradermal [ĬN-tră-DĔR-măl]
Kaposi sarcoma [KĂ-pō-sē săr-KŌ-mă]
keloid [KĒ-loyd]
kerat/o [kĕr-ă-TŌ]
keratin [KĔR-ă-tĭn]
keratolytic [KĔR-ă-tō-LĬT-ĭk]
keratosis [kĕr-ă-TŌ-sĭs]
lesion (*pl.*, **lesions**) [LĒ-zhŭn (LĒ-zhŭnz)]
lip/o [lĭp-ō]
lunula (*pl.*, **lunulae**) [LŪ-nū-lă (LŪ-nū-lē)]
macule [MĂK-yūl]
malignant melanoma [mĕl-ă-NŌ-mă]
Mantoux [măn-TŪ] test
melan/o [mĕl-ă-NŌ]
melanin [MĔL-ă-nĭn]
melanocyte [MĔL-ă-nō-sīt]
Mohs' [mōz] surgery
myc/o [mī-KŌ]
nail [nāl]
neoplasm [NĒ-ō-plăzm]
nevus (*pl.*, **nevi**) [NĒ-vŭs (NĒ-vī)]
nodule [NŎD-yūl]
onych/o [Ŏn-ĭ-kō]
onychia [ō-NĬK-ē-ă]
onychitis [ŏn-ĭ-KĪ-tĭs]
onychopathy [ŏn-ĭ-KŎP-ă-thē]
papule [PĂP-yūl]
paronychia [păr-ō-NĬK-ē-ă]
patch [pach]
patch test
pediculated [pĕ-DĬK-yū-lā-tĕd] polyp
pediculosis [pĕ-DĬK-yū-LŌ-sĭs]
petechiae (*pl.*, **petechiae**) [pē-TĒ-kē-ă, pē-TĔK-ē-ă
(pē-TĒ-kē-ē)]
pil/o [pī-lō]
pilonidal [pī-lō-NĪ-dăl] cyst
plantar [PLĂN-tăr] wart

plaque [plăk]
plastic surgery
polyp [PŎL-ĭp]
pore
pressure ulcer
pruritus [prū-RĪ-tŭs]
psoriasis [sō-RĪ-ă-sĭs]
purified protein derivative (PPD)
purpura [PŬR-pū-ră]
pustule [PŬS-tūl]
pyoderma [pī-ō-DĔR-mă]
radiation therapy
ringworm [RING-werm]
rosacea [rō-ZĀ-shē-ă]
roseola [rō-ZĒ-ō-lă]
rubella [rū-BĔL-ă]
rubeola [rū-BĒ-ō-lă]
scabies [SKĀ-bēz]
scale
scleroderma [sklĕr-ō-DĔR-mă]
scratch test
seb/o [sĕb-ō]
sebaceous [sĕ-BĀ-shŭs] cyst
sebaceous glands
seborrhea [sĕb-ō-RĒ-ă]
sebum [SĒ-bŭm]
second-degree burn
sessile [SĔS-ĭl] polyp
shingles [SHĬN-glz]
skin graft
squamous cell carcinoma [SKWĀ-mŭs sĕl kăr-sĭn-Ō-mă]

squamous epithelium [ĕp-ĭ-THĒ-lē-ŭm]
steat/o [stē-ă-TŌ]
stratified squamous epithelium [STRĂT-i-fīd]
stratum (pl., strata) [STRĂT-ŭm (STRĂ-tă)]
stratum corneum [KŌR-nē-ŭm]
stratum germinativum [jĕr-mĭ-NĀT-ĭ-vŭm]
striae [STRĪ-ē]
subcutaneous [sŭb-kyū-TĀ-nē-ŭs] layer
sweat glands [swĕt]
telangiectasia [tĕl-ĂN-jē-ĕk-TĀ-zē-ă]
third-degree burn
tine [tīn] test, TB tine
tinea [TĬN-ē-ă]
topical anesthetic
trich/o [trĭ-kō]
tumor [TŪ-mŏr]
ulcer [ŬL-sĕr]
ultraviolet light [ŭl-tră-VĪ-ō-lĕt]
urticaria [ŬR-tĭ-KĀR-ē-ă]
varicella [văr-ĭ-SĔL-ă]
vascular [VĂS-kyū-lăr] lesion
verruca (pl., verrucae) [vĕ-RŪ-kă (vĕ-RŪ-kē)]
vesicle [VĔS-ĭ-kl]
vitiligo [vĭt-ĭ-LĪ-gō]
wart [wōrt]
wheal [hwēl]
whitehead [WHĪT-hĕd]
xanth/o [zăn-THŌ]
xenograft [ZĔN-ō-grăft]
xer/o [zēr-ō]

The Musculoskeletal System

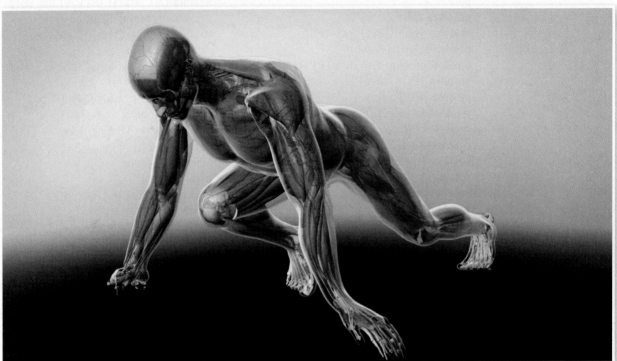

Learning Outcomes

After studying this chapter, you will be able to:

6.1   Identify the parts of the musculoskeletal system and discuss the function of each part.

6.2   Define combining forms used in building words that relate to the musculoskeletal system.

6.3   Identify common diagnostic tests, laboratory tests, and clinical procedures used in testing and treating disorders of the musculoskeletal system.

6.4   Define the major pathological conditions of the musculoskeletal system.

6.5   Define surgical terms related to the musculoskeletal system.

6.6   Discuss common pharmacological agents used in treating disorders of the musculoskeletal system.

6.7   Identify common abbreviations associated with the musculoskeletal system.

LO 6.1 Structure and Function of the Musculoskeletal System

The musculoskeletal system forms the framework that holds the body together, enables it to move, and protects and supports all the internal organs. This system includes bones, joints, and muscles. Figure 6-1 shows the musculoskeletal system.

This section provides an introduction to the basic musculoskeletal system combining terms and their meanings. Review this information prior to moving to the practices.

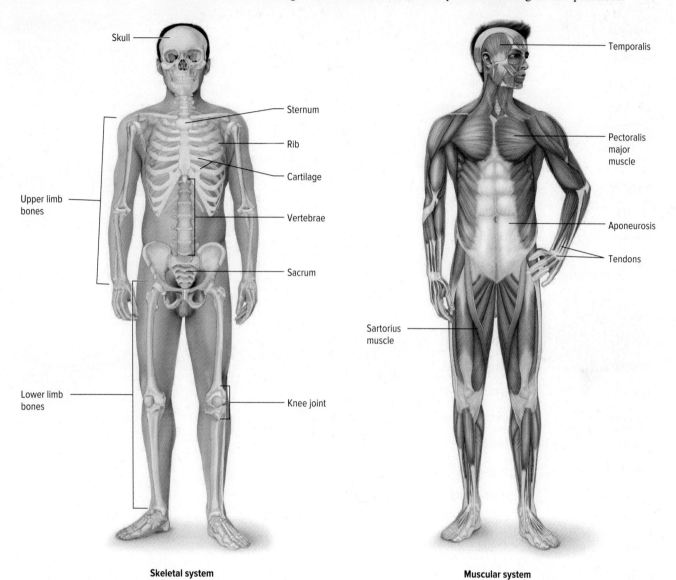

Figure 6-1 Bones and muscles

Combining Form	Meaning
ankyl/o	bent, crooked
arthr/o	joint
brachi/o	arm
burs/o	bursa

continued on next page

Combining Form	Meaning
calcane/o	heel
calci/o	calcium
carp/o	wrist
cephal/o	head
cervic/o	neck
chondr/o	cartilage
condyl/o	knob, knuckle
cost/o	rib
crani/o	skull
dactyl/o	fingers, toes
fasci/o	fascia
femor/o	femur
fibr/o	fiber
humer/o	humerus
ili/o	ilium
ischi/o	ischium
kyph/o	hump, bent
lamin/o	lamina
leiomy/o	smooth muscle
lumb/o	lumbar
maxill/o	upper jaw
metacarp/o	metacarpal
my/o	muscle
myel/o	spinal cord, bone marrow
oste/o	bone
patell/o	knee
ped/i, ped/o	foot
pelv/o	pelvis
phalang/o	finger or toe bone
pod/o	foot
pub/o	pubes
rachi/o	spine
radi/o	forearm bone

Combining Form	Meaning
rhabd/o	rod-shaped
rhabdomy/o	striated muscle
scapul/o	scapula
scoli/o	curved
spondyl/o	vertebra
stern/o	sternum
synov/o	synovial membrane
tars/o	tarsus
ten/o, tend/o, tendin/o	tendon
thorac/o	thorax
tibi/o	tibia
uln/o	ulna
vertebr/o	vertebra

Structure and Function

PRACTICE

Provide the missing term(s) to complete the following sentences.

musculoskeletal system [MŬS-kyū-lō-SKĔL-ē-tăl]
bones [bōnz]
joints [joynts]
muscles [MŬS-ĕlz]

The _____ forms the framework that holds the body together, enables it to move, and protects and supports all the internal organs. This system includes _____, _____, and _____.

osseous tissue [ŎS-ē-ŭs]
osteocytes [ŎS-tē-ō-sīts]
cartilage [KĂR-tĭ-lăj]

Bones are made of _____ and include a rich network of blood vessels and nerves. The cells of bone, called _____, are part of a dense network of connective tissue. The cells themselves are surrounded by calcium salts. During fetal development, bones are softer and flexible and are composed of _____ until the hardening process begins.

osteoblasts [ŎS-tē-ō-blăsts]
osteoclasts [ŎS-tē-ō-klăsts]
ossification [ŎS-ĭ-fĭ-KĀ-shŭn]
calcium [KĂL-sē-ŭm]
phosphorus [FŎS-fōr-ŭs]
vitamin D

Bone-forming cells are called _____. As bone tissue develops, some of it dies and is reabsorbed by _____. Later, if a bone breaks, osteoblasts will add new mineral matter to repair the break and the osteoclasts will remove any bone debris, thereby smoothing over the break. The hardening process and development of the osteocytes is called _____. This process is largely dependent on _____, _____, and _____.

skeleton [SKĔL-ē-tŏn]

The _____ of the body is made up of bones and joints. A mature adult has 206 bones that work together with joints and muscles to move the various parts of the body.

Fill in the term and pronounce the term aloud.

1. The cells of bones are called _____.
2. _____ are bone-forming cells.
3. _____ is the hardening process and osteocyte development.
4. The combining form for tibia is _____.
5. The combining form for wrist is _____.

SPELL and DEFINE

Identify if the following terms are spelled correctly. Correct the words that are spelled incorrectly. Write the definition for each word.

	Spelling	Definition
musculoskeletal		
osteochast		
osteofication		
phosferus		
cartilage		

UNDERSTAND

Identify the term from the definition provided.

1. Bone-forming cell: _____
2. Ten/o is the combining form for: _____
3. This cell reabsorbs dead bone cells: _____

APPLY

Read the following scenario and answer the question.

You are the nurse explaining to the client, Ms. Liz Hillesheim, how dietary intake impacts her bones. Ms. Hillesheim asks, "What should my diet include for strong bones?" How will you respond?

_____
_____
_____

Did you know ?

Calcium

Calcium is important for the formation of bones. It is recommended that you pay attention to your daily calcium intake throughout your life because lack of calcium is a factor in certain diseases, such as osteoporosis.

©C Squared Studios/Getty Images

Types of Bones and Bone Marrow

The bones function to provide shape, support, and a framework for the body. There are 206 bones in the skeletal system. Bones are classified according to their shape. Figure 6-2 shows the parts of a long bone. Figure 6-3 shows bone categories by shape. Figure 6-4 is a radiograph showing **epiphyseal plates.**

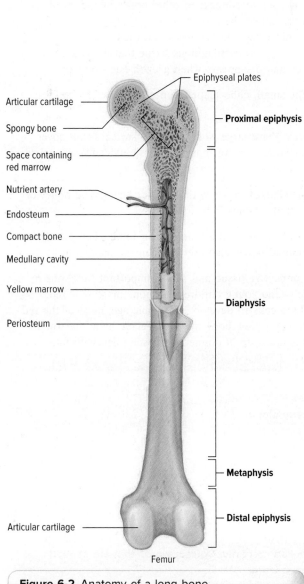

Articular cartilage
Spongy bone
Space containing red marrow
Nutrient artery
Endosteum
Compact bone
Medullary cavity
Yellow marrow
Periosteum
Articular cartilage
Femur

Epiphyseal plates
Proximal epiphysis
Diaphysis
Metaphysis
Distal epiphysis

Figure 6-2 Anatomy of a long bone

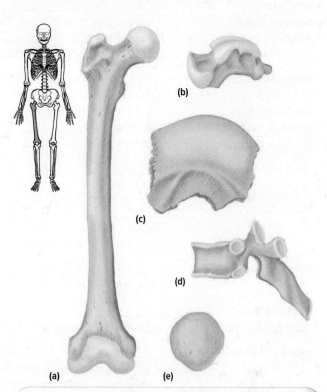

(a) (b) (c) (d) (e)

Figure 6-3 Bone categories classified by shape: (a) long, (b) short, (c) flat, (d) irregular, (e) sesamoid

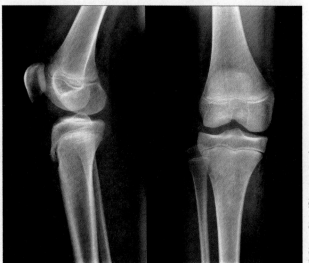

©ChooChin/Shutterstock

Figure 6-4 Epiphyseal plates

PRACTICE

Provide the missing term(s) to complete the following sentences.

There are many types of bones. The five most common categories include:

long bones **compact bone** **diaphysis** (*pl.*, **diaphyses**) [dī-ĂF-ĭ-sĭs (dī-ĂF-ĭ-sēz)]	1. The _____ form the extremities of the body. The legs and arms include this type of bone. The longest portion of a long bone is called the shaft. The outer portion is _____, solid bone that does not bend easily. This shaft is also called the _____.
epiphysis (*pl.*, **epiphyses**) [ĕ-PĬF-ĭ-sĭs (ĕ-PĬF-ĭ-sēz)] **epiphyseal plate** [ĕp-ĭ-FĬZ-ē-ăl plāt]	Each end of the shaft has an area shaped to connect to other bones by means of ligaments and muscle. These ends are called the proximal _____ and the distal epiphysis. As long bones grow, the diaphysis and the two epiphyses develop. The _____ is cartilaginous tissue that is replaced during growth years but eventually calcifies and disappears when growth has stopped.
short bones	2. _____ are the small, cube-shaped bones of the wrists, ankles, and toes.
flat bones	3. _____ generally have large, somewhat flat surfaces that cover organs or that provide a surface for large areas of muscle. The shoulder blades, pelvis, and skull include flat bones.
irregular bones	4. _____ are specialized bones with specific shapes. The bones of the ears, vertebrae, and face are irregular bones.
sesamoid bones [SĔS-ă-moyd bōnz]	5. _____ are bones formed in a tendon near joints. The patella (kneecap) is a sesamoid bone. Sesamoid bones also are found in the hands and feet.
marrow [MĂR-ō]	_____ is soft connective tissue and serves important functions in the production of blood cells. In infants and young children, all bone marrow is red, allowing much opportunity for red blood cells to develop. As people age, most of the red bone marrow decreases and is replaced by yellow bone marrow. Yellow bone marrow is found in most other adult bones and is made up of connective tissue filled with fat.

WRITE and PRONOUNCE

Fill in the term and pronounce the term aloud.

1. The patella is this type of bone: _____.
2. This is the end of a bone shaft: _____.
3. This is the middle section of a long bone: _____.
4. This closes when growth stops: _____.
5. This serves to produce blood cells: _____.

SPELL and DEFINE

Identify if the following terms are spelled correctly. Correct words that are spelled incorrectly. Write the definition for each word.

	Spelling	Definition
epiphisis		
diaphyses		
seasamoid		
osteofication		

Identify the term from the definition provided.

1. The toes are an example of what kind of bone? _____
2. The kneecap is an example of what kind of bone? _____

APPLY **Read the following scenario and answer the question.**

Dan Lange is a 17-year-old male who is 5′6″ tall. He asks you if you think he is going to get any taller. How will you answer him?

_____

_____

STUDY TIP

Find an unlabeled picture of the human skeleton and label the bones. This will help you to remember their location and correct spelling.

Bones of the Head

Cranial bones form the skull, which serves to protect the brain and the structures inside of the skull. Figure 6-5 shows the bones of the head. Figure 6-6 illustrates the sinuses.

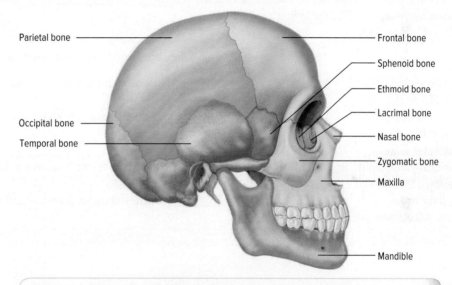

Parietal bone — Frontal bone — Sphenoid bone — Ethmoid bone — Lacrimal bone — Nasal bone — Zygomatic bone — Maxilla — Occipital bone — Temporal bone — Mandible

Figure 6-5 Right lateral view of the skull

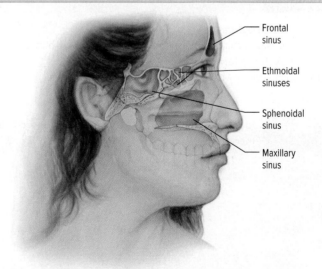

Frontal sinus — Ethmoidal sinuses — Sphenoidal sinus — Maxillary sinus

Figure 6-6 The sinuses

	Provide the missing term(s) to complete the following sentences.
sutures [SŪ-chŭrz] fontanelles [FŎN-tă-nĕlz]	The skull or cranial bones join at points called _____. The skull of a newborn is not completely joined and has soft spots, called _____.
frontal bone [FRŬN-tăl bōn] ethmoid bone [ĔTH-mŏyd bōn] parietal bone [pă-RĪ-ĕ-tăl bōn] temporal bone [TĔM-pŏ-răl bōn]	The skull contains the _____ (the forehead and roof of the eye sockets), the _____ (the nasal cavity and the orbits of the eyes), the _____ (top and upper parts of the sides of the skull), and the _____ (lower part of the skull and the lower sides, including the openings for the ears).
occipital bone [ŏk-SĬP-ĭ-tăl bōn] foramen magnum [fō-RĀ-mĕn MĂG-nŭm]	The back and base of the skull are covered by the _____. An opening in the occipital bone, the _____, is the structure through which the spinal cord passes.
	The head also has *facial bones,* each with a specific function, which include:
nasal bones [NĀ-zăl bōnz] lacrimal bones [LĂK-rĭ-măl bōnz] mandibular bone [măn-DĬB-yū-lăr bōn] mandible [MĂN-dĭ-bl] maxillary bones [MĂK-sĭ-lăr-ē bōnz]	1. _____ form the bridge of the nose. 2. _____ hold the lacrimal gland and the canals for the tear ducts. 3. The _____ or _____ is the lower jawbone and contains the sockets for the lower teeth. The mandible is the only movable bone in the face. 4. _____ form the upper jawbone and contain the sockets for the upper teeth.

WRITE and PRONOUNCE

Fill in the term and pronounce the term aloud.

1. This bone forms the nasal cavity: _____.
2. The spinal cord passes through this opening of the occipital bone: _____.
3. The sides of the skull are formed by the _____ bones.
4. The bone that forms the lower back portion of the skull is the _____.

SPELL and DEFINE

Identify if the following terms are spelled correctly. Correct the words that are spelled incorrectly. Write the definition for each word.

	Spelling	Definition
maxillary		
perital		
suchurz		
fontanelles		
lakrimail		

1. Removal of part of the skull: _____
2. Form the bridge of the nose: _____
3. The point where the cranial bones join: _____

APPLY   Read the following scenario and respond accordingly.

Kelly Brown experienced a head injury. Explain to her family the function of the cranial bones.

_____

_____

Spinal Column

The spinal or vertebral column extends from the skull to the pelvis. It serves to support and stabilize the body. Figure 6-7 shows the spinal column and Figure 6-8 shows the cervical vertebrae.

STUDY TIP

Here is an easy way to remember divisions of vertebrae in the spinal column: We eat breakfast at 7 (7 in cervical region), lunch at 12 (12 in the thoracic region), and dinner at 5 (5 in the lumbar region).

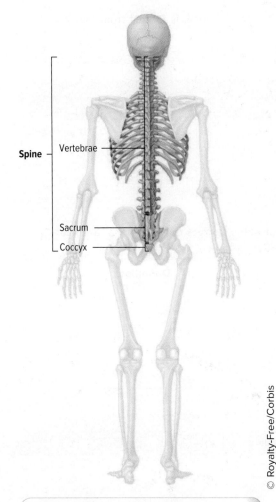

Spine

Vertebrae

Sacrum

Coccyx

© Royalty-Free/Corbis

Figure 6-7 The spinal column

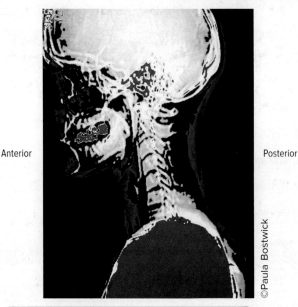

Anterior   Posterior

©Paula Bostwick

Figure 6-8 X-ray of the cervical vertebrae

PRACTICE

Provide the correct term(s) to complete the following sentences.

spinal column

vertebral column

vertebrae (*sing.*, **vertebra**)
[VĔR-tĕ-brē (VĔR-tĕ-bră)]

The _____ (also called the _____)
consists of five sets of _____.

disk [dĭsk]

Each vertebra is a bone segment with a thick _____ that separates the vertebrae. The disks cushion the vertebrae and help in movement and flexibility of the spinal column.

The five divisions of vertebrae include:

cervical vertebrae
[SĔR-vĭ-kl VĔR-tĕ-brē]

thoracic vertebrae
[thō-RĂS-ĭk VĔR-tĕ-brē]

lumbar vertebrae
[LŬM-băr VĔR-tĕ-brē]

sacrum [SĀ-krŭm]

coccyx [KŎK-sĭks]

1. The _____ are the seven vertebrae located in the neck.

2. The _____ are the 12 vertebrae that connect to the ribs.

3. The _____ are the five bones of the middle back.

4. The _____ is the curved bone of the lower back and consists of five separate bones at birth that fuse together in early childhood.

5. The _____, also called the tailbone, is formed from four bones fused together.

WRITE and PRONOUNCE

Fill in the term and pronounce the term aloud.

1. The tailbone: _____
2. Vertebrae in neck: _____
3. Separates vertebrae: _____
4. Vertebrae that connect ribs: _____
5. Vertebrae in middle back: _____

SPELL and DEFINE

Identify if the following terms are spelled correctly. Correct the words that are spelled incorrectly. Write the definition for each word.

	Spelling	Definition
koksiks		
lacrimeal		
sakrum		
vertebral		
thoracic		

UNDERSTAND

Identify the term from the definition provided.

1. Repair of the vertebra: _____
2. Removal of a disk: _____
3. An x-ray of the disks: _____
4. The lumbar vertebra consist of how many bones? _____
5. This is formed by four bones being fused together. _____

Mike Roth comes into his physician's office stating he fell on ice a week ago. He states he is having pain in his neck when he turns his head. He also states his lower back hurts. Document this using medical terms.

_____

_____

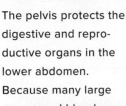

STUDY TIP

The pelvis protects the digestive and reproductive organs in the lower abdomen. Because many large nerves and blood vessels pass through it to supply the legs, injury to the pelvis can be life threatening.

Bones of the Chest and Pelvis

There are two weight-transferring transverse sections of bones. The upper is the group formed by the clavicle and scapula, which transfers the weight of the upper body to distribute it evenly to the spine. Any additional weight carried by one arm, such as a person holding a child, will be distributed evenly to the spine. The second weight-transferring transverse section is formed by the pelvic girdle. Figure 6-9 shows the rib cage.

The bones of the pelvis serve to support and protect the body. The pelvic girdle transfers the weight of the body from one leg to the other during running, walking, or any movement. Figure 6-10 shows the pelvis.

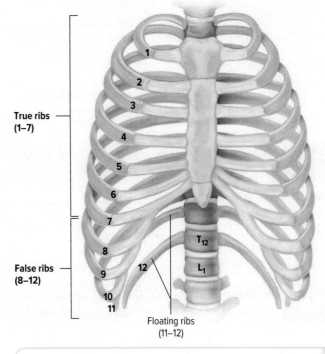

Figure 6-9 Rib cage

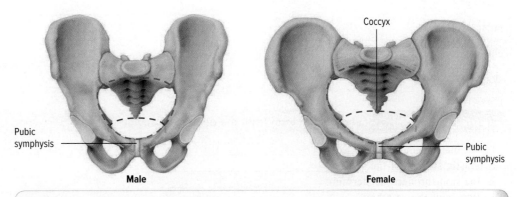

Figure 6-10 Male and female pelvis

Structure and Function	**PRACTICE**
	Provide the missing term(s) to complete the following sentences.
thorax [THŌ-răks] **clavicle** [KLĂV-ĭ-kl] **scapula** [SKĂP-yū-lă]	At the top of the _____ (chest cavity) are the _____ (anterior collarbone) and _____ (posterior shoulder bone).
sternum [STĔR-nŭm] **ribs** **true ribs**	Next is the _____ (breastbone), which extends down the middle of the chest. Extending out from the sternum are the 12 pairs of _____. The first seven pairs of ribs, the _____, are joined both to the vertebral column and to the sternum by costal cartilage.
pelvic girdle [PĔL-vĭk GER-dl] **ilium** [ĬL-ē-ŭm] **ischium** [ĬS-kē-ŭm] **pubis** [PYŪ-bĭs]	Below the thoracic cavity is the pelvic area. The _____ is a large bone that forms the hips and supports the trunk of the body. It is composed of three fused bones, including the _____, _____, and _____ (the anteroinferior portion of the hip bone). It is also the point of attachment for the legs.
pelvic cavity [PĔL-vĭk KAV-ĭ-tē] **pubic symphysis** [PYŪ-bĭk SĬM-fĭ-sĭs]	Inside the pelvic girdle is the _____. In the pelvic cavity are located the female reproductive organs, the sigmoid colon, the bladder, and the rectum. The area where the two pubic bones join is called the _____.
pelvis [PĔL-vĭs]	The major bone at the base of the trunk is the _____.

WRITE and PRONOUNCE	**Fill in the term and pronounce the term aloud.**

1. Between the neck and the abdomen is the _____.
2. The collarbone: _____
3. The shoulder blade: _____
4. Large bone that forms hips: _____
5. The bone at the base of the trunk: _____

SPELL and DEFINE	**Identify if the following terms are spelled correctly. Correct the words that are spelled incorrectly. Write the definition for each word.**

	Spelling	Definition
sternum		
ischeum		
pubic symphysis		
clavicle		
skapyula		

UNDERSTAND	**Identify the term from the definition provided.**

1. An incision into the thorax: _____
2. Plastic surgery of the skull: _____
3. Incision through the sternum: _____
4. Repair of the vertebra: _____
5. Removal of a disk: _____

Mr. Colin Stringer was in a motor vehicle accident. He is complaining of severe pain in his lower back and the area around his hips. Document this using medical terms.

_____

_____

_____

_____

Bones of the Extremities

The bones of the arms, hands, and legs allow the body to move. Muscles attach to these bones to aid in body movement. Figure 6-11 shows the bones of the arm and hand. Figure 6-12 shows the bones of the leg and foot.

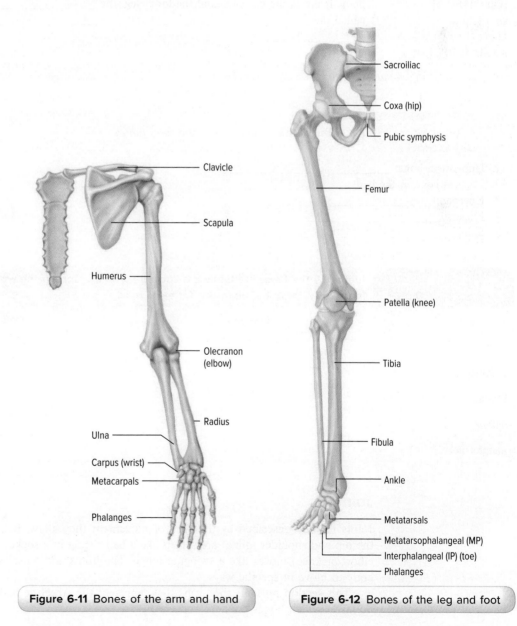

Figure 6-11 Bones of the arm and hand

Figure 6-12 Bones of the leg and foot

The Musculoskeletal System   **147**

PRACTICE

Provide the missing term(s) to complete the following sentences.

Terms	Practice
humerus [HYŪ-mĕr-ŭs] ulna [ŬL-nă] radius [RĀ-dē-ŭs] carpal bones [KĂR-păl bōnz]	The upper arm bone, the _____, attaches to the scapula and clavicle. The two lower arm bones are the _____ and the _____, which attach to the eight _____ of the wrist.
metacarpals [MĔT-ă-KĂR-pălz] phalanges [fă-LĂN-jēz]	The _____ are the five bones of the palm that radiate out to the finger bones, or the _____.
femur [FĒ-mŭr] tibia [TĬB-ē-ă] shin [shĭn] fibula [FĬB-yū-lă] patella [pă-TĔL-ă]	The _____ is the thigh bone. The femur is the longest bone in the body. It meets the two bones of the lower leg, the _____ (also called the _____) and _____, at the kneecap, or _____.

WRITE and PRONOUNCE

Fill in the term and pronounce the term aloud.

1. Upper arm bone: _____
2. Longest bone in the body: _____
3. Kneecap: _____
4. Fingers: _____
5. Shin: _____

SPELL and DEFINE

Identify if the following terms are spelled correctly. Correct the words that are spelled incorrectly. Write the definition for each word.

	Spelling	Definition
phemur		
phalanges		
fibula		
patela		
metakarpel		

Joints

Joints may be described by the type of movement they allow. Ball-and-socket joints (e.g., the hip and shoulder joints) are set up like a ball sitting in a socket. A hinge joint (e.g., the elbow or knee) moves like a swinging hinge. The joints and muscles allow the parts of the body to move in specific ways.

This section presents the terms that represent the structure and function of joints, the points at which bones connect.

Structure and Function	**PRACTICE** Provide the missing term(s) to complete the following sentences.
articulations [ăr-tĭk-yū-LĀ-shŭn]	Joints are also called _____, points where bones connect.
ligaments [LĬG-ă-mĕnts] **tendons** [TĔN-dŏnz]	Bones are connected to other bones with _____, bands of fibrous tissue. _____ are bands of fibrous tissue that connect muscles to bones. Movement takes place at the joints using the muscles, ligaments, and tendons.
synovial joints [sĭ-NŌ-vē-ăl joynts] **synovial membrane** [sĭ-NŌ-vē-ăl MĔM-brān] **synovial fluid** [sĭ-NŌ-vē-ăl FLŪ-ĭd] **bursa** (*pl.,* **bursae**) [BŬR-să (BŬR-sē)]	_____ are covered with a _____, which secretes _____, a joint lubricant that helps the joint move easily. The hip joint is an example of a synovial joint. Some spaces between tendons and joints have a _____, a sac lined with a synovial membrane. Bursae help the hands and feet to move by decreasing friction.

WRITE and PRONOUNCE

Fill in the term and pronounce the term aloud.

1. Attaches bone to bone: _____
2. Connects muscle to bone: _____
3. Space between tendons and joints: _____
4. A joint lubricant: _____
5. Shin: _____

SPELL and DEFINE

Identify if the following terms are spelled correctly. Correct the words that are spelled incorrectly. Write the definition for each word.

	Spelling	Definition
bursea		
sinoveal		
tendon		
artikulashunz		
patella		

STUDY TIP

We do not have to think about breathing, digesting, or urinating; our body does it on its own (involuntarily).

Muscles

Muscles contract and extend to provide body movement. During movement, a muscle contracts and extends the movable bone to which it is attached to move the bone in a specific direction. Different muscles have different functions. For example, the deltoid muscles are used to extend the arms, the biceps of the arm flex the forearms, and the masticatory muscles close and open the jaw for chewing. Figure 6-13 shows the three types of muscles. Figure 6-14 shows the origin and insertion of the biceps and triceps muscles.

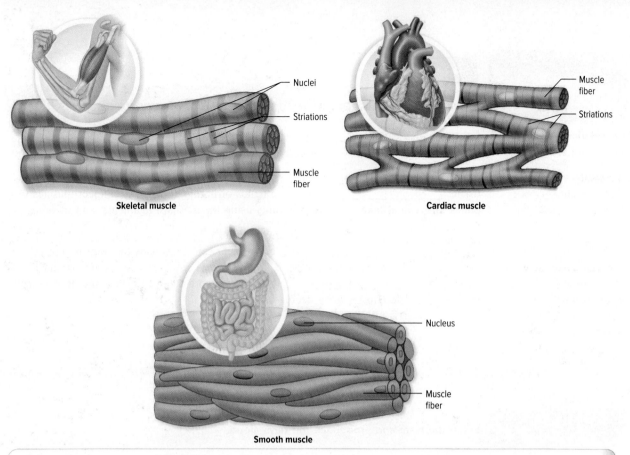

Figure 6-13 Three types of muscle

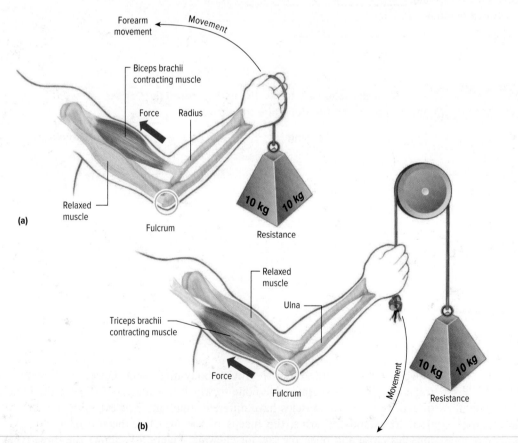

Figure 6-14 Origin and insertion of the biceps and triceps muscles: (a) muscle contracts with a force greater than resistance and shortens, (b) muscle contracts with a force less than resistance and lengthens

Structure and Function	**PRACTICE**
	Provide the missing term(s) to complete the following sentences.
voluntary striated [strī-ĀT-ĕd]	The _____ or _____ muscles can be contracted at will. These muscles are called skeletal muscles as they are responsible for the movement of all skeletal bones.
involuntary muscles smooth muscles visceral [VĬS-ĕr-ăl] **cardiac muscle** [KĂR-dē-ăk]	The _____ (also called _____ or _____ muscles) control movement that is not controlled voluntarily, such as respiration, urination, and digestion. Involuntary muscles move the internal organs and systems, such as the digestive system and the blood. _____, which controls the contractions of the heart, is the only involuntary muscle that is also striated.
fascia [FĂSH-ē-ă]	Most muscles are covered by _____, a band of connective tissue that supports and covers the muscle.

WRITE and PRONOUNCE	**Fill in the term and pronounce the term aloud.**

1. Voluntary muscles: _____
2. Smooth muscles: _____
3. Fibrous tissue that encloses muscles: _____

SPELL and DEFINE	**Identify if the following terms are spelled correctly. Correct the words that are spelled incorrectly. Write the definition for each word.**

	Spelling	Definition
verseal		
strieted		
fascia		

Did you know

Body Movement

Bones, joints, and muscles allow parts of the body to move in certain directions. To determine if movement can be done correctly, medical practitioners in a variety of fields look at the range of motion of the parts of the body. Also, position of the body involves placement in certain positions.

- **Flexion**—the bending of a limb.
- **Extension**—the straightening of a limb.
- **Rotation**—the circular movement of a part, such as the neck.
- **Abduction**—movement away from the body.
- **Adduction**—movement toward the body.
- **Supination**—a turning up, as of the hand.
- **Pronation**—a turning down, as of the hand.
- **Eversion**—moving the sole of the foot outward.
- **Inversion**—moving the sole of the foot inward.
- **Dorsiflexion**—a bending up, as of the ankle.
- **Plantar flexion**—a bending down, as of the ankle.

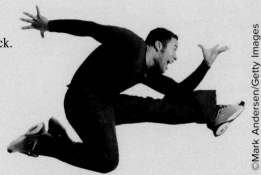

©Mark Andersen/Getty Images

STUDY TIP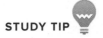

Think about abduction as something being taken away. With adduction, we are putting back.

LO 6.2 Word Building in the Musculoskeletal System

Word Building	PRACTICE
	Provide the missing combining form to complete the following sentences.
ankyl-osis [ĂNG-kĭ-LŌ-sĭs]	Fixation of a joint in a bent position, usually resulting from a disease, is _____ osis.
arthro-gram [ĂR-thrŏ-grăm]	_____ gram is an x-ray of a joint.
cranio-tomy [krā-nē-ŎT-ŏ-mē]	An incision into the skull is a _____ tomy.
brachio-cephalic [BRĀ-kē-ŏ-sĕ-FĂL-ĭk]	_____ cephalic: related to both the arm and the head.
burs-itis [bŭr-SĪ-tĭs]	Inflammation of a bursa is _____ itis.
cervico-dynia [SĔR-vĭ-kō-DĬN-ē-ă]	_____ dynia is neck pain.
chondro-plasty [KŎN-drŏ-plăs-tē]	Surgical repair of cartilage is _____ plasty.
fibr-oma [fī-BRŌ-mă]	_____ oma is a benign tumor in fibrous tissue.
humero-scapular [HYŪ-mĕr-ō-SKĂP-yū-lăr]	_____ scapular relates to both the humerus and the scapula.
ilio-femoral [ĬL-ē-ō-FĔM-ō-răl]	Relating to the ilium and the femur is _____ femoral.
ischio-dynia [ĬS-kē-ō-DĬN-ē-ă]	_____ dynia is pain in the ischium.
maxillo-facial [măk-SĬL-ō-FĀ-shăl]	_____ facial pertains to the jaws and face.
metacarp-ectomy [MĔT-ă-kăr-PĔK-tō-mē]	Excision of a metacarpal is a _____ ectomy.
myelo-cyst [MĪ-ĕ-lō-sĭst]	A cyst that develops in bone marrow is a _____ cyst.
osteo-arthritis [ŎS-tē-ō-ăr-THRĪ-tĭs]	Arthritis characterized by erosion of cartilage and bone as well as joint pain is _____ arthritis.
patell-ectomy [PĂT-ĕ-LĔK-tō-mē]	_____ ectomy is excision of the patella.
sterno-dynia [stĕr-nō-DĬN-ē-ă]	_____ dynia is sternum pain.
synov-itis [sĭn-ō-VĪ-tĭs]	Inflammation of a synovial joint is _____ itis.
vertebro-arterial [VĔR-tĕ-brō-ăr-TĒR-ē-ăl]	_____ arterial relates to a vertebral artery or to a vertebra and an artery.

Fill in the term and pronounce each term aloud.

1. Excision of the patella: _____
2. A cyst in the bone marrow: _____
3. Pain in the ischium: _____
4. Surgical repair of the cartilage: _____
5. Inflammation of a bursa: _____

SPELL and DEFINE

Identify if the following terms are spelled correctly. Correct the words that are spelled incorrectly. Write the definition for each word.

	Spelling	Definition
bursitis		
scapulodynia		
phalangectomy		
tendonitis		

UNDERSTAND

Identify the term from the definition provided.

1. Joint pain due to cartilage erosion: _____
2. Removal of a bursa: _____
3. Removal of a disk: _____
4. Bone-forming cell: _____
5. X-ray of joint: _____
6. Repair of cervical vertebrae: _____

APPLY

Read the following scenario and respond accordingly.

Mr. Ted Whaley fell while shoveling snow. He is now having pain in his left knee. When he fell, the muscles tore away from the bone and the tissue that connects bone to bone was pulled away. His primary physician is referring him to Dr. Ziesel, a bone doctor. Rewrite this scenario using correct medical terminology.

_____

_____

_____

_____

LO 6.3 Diagnostic, Procedural, and Laboratory Terms

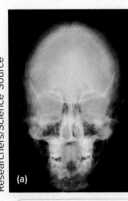 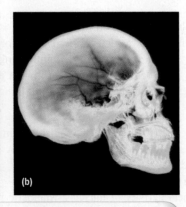

Diagnostic, procedural, and laboratory findings assist in the diagnosis of medical conditions. Often used in combination, these tests lead to a final diagnosis and assist in treatment planning. Figure 6-15 shows radiographs of the skull. Figure 6-16 shows a finger goniometer, an instrument used to measure the range of motion of finger joints. Figure 6-17 is a view of a torn meniscus in the knee.

(a): ©LunaGrafix/Photo Researchers/Science Source; (b): ©David Roberts/SPL/Photo Researchers/Science Source

Figure 6-15 Radiographs of the skull: (a) anterior view, (b) right lateral view

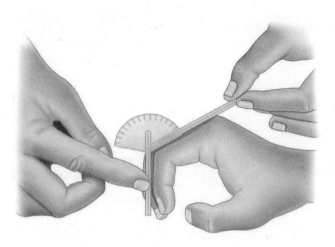

Figure 6-16 Finger goniometer

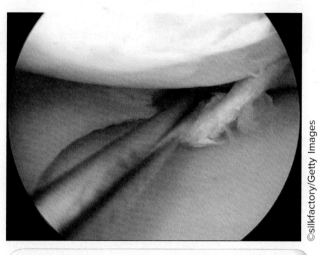

©silkfactory/Getty Images

Figure 6-17 Arthroscopic view of torn meniscus in the knee

Diagnostic	PRACTICE
	Provide the missing term(s) to complete the following sentences.
orthopedists [ōr-thō-PĒ-dĭsts] **orthopedic surgeon** [ōr-thō-PĒ-dĭk] **osteopaths** [ŎS-tē-ō-păths] **rheumatologists** [rū-mă-TŎL-ō-jĭsts] **podiatrists** [pō-DĪ-ă-trĭsts] **chiropractors** [kī-rō-PRĂK-tōrz]	The musculoskeletal system is often the site of pain caused by conditions in the system itself or by symptoms of other systemic conditions. Specialists in the musculoskeletal system include _____ or _____, physicians who treat disorders of the musculoskeletal system; _____, physicians who combine manipulative procedures with conventional treatment; _____, physicians who treat disorders of the joints specifically, and of the musculoskeletal system generally; _____, medical specialists who treat disorders of the foot; and _____, health care professionals who manipulate the spine to treat certain ailments.
arthrography [ăr-THRŎG-ră-fē] **arthroscopy** [ăr-THRŎS-kō-pē]	Diagnosing bone and muscle ailments often involves taking x-rays, scans, or radiographs or performing internal examinations to determine if an abnormality is present. _____ is the examination of joints using radiography (x-rays). _____ is the internal examination of a joint using a lighted instrument capable of directly viewing, cutting, irrigating, obtaining biopsy material, and more, through a small incision.
diskography [dĭs-KŎG-ră-fē] **myelography** [MĪ-ĕ-LŎG-ră-fē] **electromyogram** [ē-lĕk-trō-MĪ-ō-grăm] **bone scan**	_____ is the examination of disks by injecting a contrast medium into the spine and using radiography. Computed tomography (CT) scans can reveal joint, bone, or connective tissue disease. _____ is the use of radiography of the spinal cord to identify spinal cord conditions. An _____ is a graphic image of the electrical activity of muscles. Magnetic resonance imaging (MRI) may be used to detect disorders of the musculoskeletal system, especially of soft tissue. A _____ is used to detect tumors.

rheumatoid factor test serum creatine phosphokinase (CPK) [KRĒ-ă-tēn fŏs-fō-KĪ-nās] serum calcium [SĒR-ŭm KĂL-sĭ-ŭm] serum phosphorus [SĒR-ŭm FŎS-fōr-ŭs] uric acid test [YŪR-ĭk]	Laboratory tests measure the levels of substances found in some musculoskeletal disorders. Rheumatoid arthritis may be confirmed by a _____. High levels of _____ appear in some disorders such as a skeletal injury. The measurement of _____ and _____ in the blood indicates the body's incorporation of those substances in the bones. A _____ can detect gout.
goniometer [gō-nē-ŎM-ĕ-tĕr] densitometer [dĕn-sĭ-TŎM-ĕ-tĕr]	Tests for range of motion (ROM) in certain joints can indicate movement or joint disorders. A _____ is used to measure motion in the joints. A _____ uses light and x-ray images to measure bone density for osteoporosis, a disease that can lead to bone fractures and that is most common in postmenopausal women.

WRITE and PRONOUNCE

Fill in the term and pronounce each term aloud.

1. Radiograph of a joint: _____
2. Radiographic image of the spinal cord: _____
3. Examination of a joint with an instrument: _____
4. Physician who treats disorders of the joints: _____
5. Radiographic image of a disk: _____

SPELL and DEFINE

Identify if the following terms are spelled correctly. Correct the words that are spelled incorrectly. Write the definition for each word.

	Spelling	Definition
goniometre		
desitometer		
myelography		
arthrografe		
electramyelogram		

UNDERSTAND

Break down the following words into their component parts.

1. arthroscopy: _____
2. osteopath: _____
3. podiatrist: _____
4. goniometer: _____
5. myelography: _____

APPLY

Read the following scenario and rewrite using medical terms.

The patient is here today to see the bone doctor for surgery after having seen a health care professional that manipulated her spine due to low back, leg, and foot pain. The foot doctor is making the referral.

_____

_____

Pathological Terms

Pathological conditions can occur throughout the musculoskeletal system. These conditions may be present at birth or occur throughout the lifespan. Figure 6-18 shows two types of spina bifida.

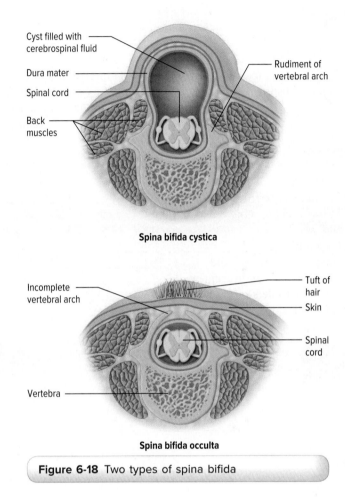

Cyst filled with
cerebrospinal fluid

Dura mater

Spinal cord

Back
muscles

Rudiment of
vertebral arch

Spina bifida cystica

Incomplete
vertebral arch

Vertebra

Tuft of
hair

Skin

Spinal
cord

Spina bifida occulta

Figure 6-18 Two types of spina bifida

Pathological	**PRACTICE** Provide the correct term(s) to complete the following sentences.
spina bifida [SPĪ-nă BĬF-ĭ-dă]	Musculoskeletal disorders arise from congenital conditions, injury, degenerative disease, or other systemic disorders. With birth defects, such as _____, there is an opening in the spinal cord that may produce paralysis.
herniated disk [HĔR-nē-ā-tĕd] **sciatica** [sī-ĂT-ĭ-kă] **rickets** [RĬK-ĕts]	A _____, in which the center of the disk is compressed and presses on nerves in the neural canal, can lead to _____, pain radiating down the leg from the lower back. Some diseases, such as _____, which causes deformities in the legs, may result from a vitamin D deficiency.

talipes calcaneus [TĂL-ĭ-pēz kăl-KĀ-nē-ŭs] **talipes valgus** [TĂL-ĭ-pēz VĂL-gŭs] **talipes varus** [TĂL-ĭ-pēz VĀ-rŭs] **calcar** [KĂL-kăr] **spur** [spŭr]	Foot deformities may occur in or involve the ankle joint. _____ is a deformity of the heel due to weakened calf muscles; _____ is excessive eversion of the foot; and _____ is excessive inversion of the foot. A _____ or _____ is a bony projection growing out of a bone.

WRITE and PRONOUNCE

Fill in the term and pronounce each term aloud.

1. A foot deformity characterized by eversion: _____
2. Pain in the lower back that radiates down the leg: _____
3. A bony projection growing out of a bone: _____
4. A disease caused by vitamin D deficiency: _____
5. A heel deformity that is a result of a weakened calf muscle: _____

SPELL and DEFINE

Identify if the following terms are spelled correctly. Correct the words that are spelled incorrectly. Write the definition for each word.

	Spelling	Definition
rickets		
calcar		
spina bifida		
talipez kalkaneus		
siaticka		

UNDERSTAND

Build Your Medical Vocabulary: Match the word on the left with the proper definition on the right.

1. _____ herniated disk
2. _____ talipes varus
3. _____ talipes valgus
4. _____ rickets
5. _____ congenital defect

a. characterized by excessive eversion of the foot
b. lack of vitamin D
c. protrusion of a disk into the neural canal
d. characterized by excessive inversion of the foot
e. spina bifida

APPLY

Read the following scenario and respond accordingly.

The nurse is teaching a client diagnosed with rickets. Explain what rickets is in terms the client can understand.

_____

_____

STUDY TIP

The opposite of valgus (outward) is varus (inward).

Symptoms, Abnormalities, and Conditions

Fractures

One of the most common problems with bones is that they can break, or fracture. There are many types of fractures; for example, an *avulsion fracture* is caused when a ligament is pulled, and an *intracapsular fracture* occurs within the capsule of a joint. Figure 6-19 shows the different types of fractures that can occur.

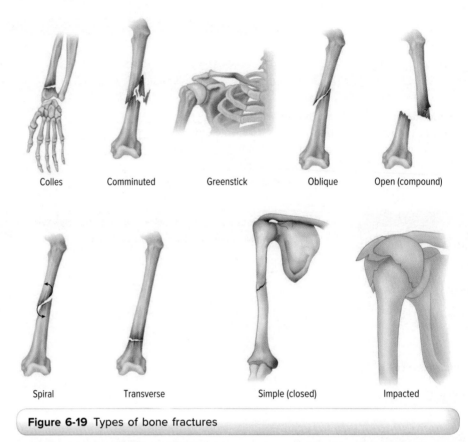

Colles   Comminuted   Greenstick   Oblique   Open (compound)

Spiral   Transverse   Simple (closed)   Impacted

Figure 6-19 Types of bone fractures

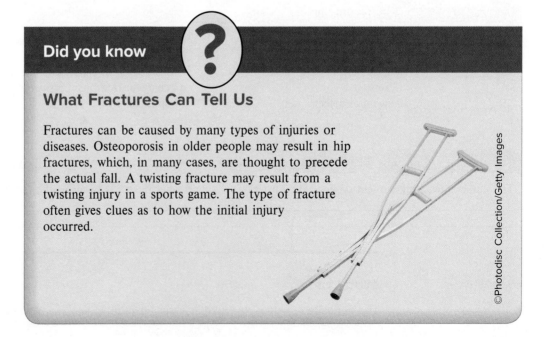

Did you know ?

What Fractures Can Tell Us

Fractures can be caused by many types of injuries or diseases. Osteoporosis in older people may result in hip fractures, which, in many cases, are thought to precede the actual fall. A twisting fracture may result from a twisting injury in a sports game. The type of fracture often gives clues as to how the initial injury occurred.

©Photodisc Collection/Getty Images

Joints

Disorders of the joints can occur due to everyday use of the joint or may be related to an injury. Figure 6-20 shows the damage caused by osteoporosis. Figure 6-21 is a nuclear scan that compares a healthy knee to an arthritic knee.

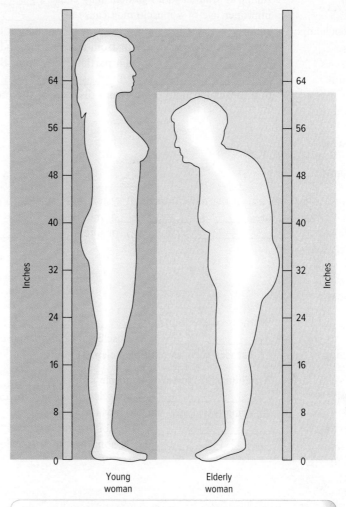

Young woman   Elderly woman

Figure 6-20 Damage caused by osteoporosis

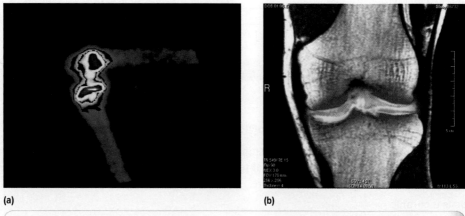

(a)   (b)

(a): ©CNRI/Science Source;
(b): ©Alfred Pasieka/Science Source

Figure 6-21 Nuclear scan showing (a) healthy knee and (b) knee with arthritis

Pathological	Provide the correct term(s) to complete the following sentences.
sprain [sprān] **strain** [strān] **tendinitis** *or* **tendonitis** [těn-dǐn-ĪT-ĭs] **dislocation** [dis-lō-KĀ-shŭn] **subluxation** [sŭb-lŭk-SĀ-shŭn] **osteoporosis** [ŎS-tē-ō-pō-RŌ-sǐs] **contracture** [kŏn-TRĂK-chūr]	Injury or trauma to a ligament may cause a _____. Overuse or improper use of a muscle may cause a _____. Overworking a joint may cause _____, an inflammation of a tendon. _____ may result from an injury or from a strenuous, sudden movement. A _____ is a partial dislocation. Bones may lose their density (_____). _____, extreme resistance to stretching of a muscle, usually results from diseases of the muscle fibers or from an injury.
ostealgia [ŏs-tē-ĂL-jē-ă] **osteodynia** [ŏs-tē-ō-DĬN-ē-ă] **myalgia** [mī-ĂL-jē-ă] **myodynia** [MĪ-ō-DĬN-ē-ă] **arthralgia** [ăr-THRĂL-jē-ă]	Pain in the musculoskeletal system may appear in the bones (_____ or _____), muscles (_____ or _____), or joints (_____).
ankylosis [ĂNG-kǐ-LŌ-sǐs] **spastic** [SPĂS-tǐk] **spasms** [spăzmz]	Stiffness of the joints (_____) may be an indicator of several diseases. _____ muscles have abnormal contractions (_____) in diseases such as multiple sclerosis.
hypertrophy [hī-PĔR-trō-fē] **flaccid** [FLĂK-sǐd *or* FLĂS-ĭd] **hypotonia** [HĪ-pō-TŌ-nē-ă] **rigor** [RĬG-ōr] **rigidity** [ri-JID-i-tē] **dystonia** [dǐs-TŌ-nē-ă]	An abnormal increase in muscle size is _____. _____ muscles are flabby in tone. _____ is abnormally reduced muscle tension and _____ (also called _____) is abnormal muscle stiffness, as seen in lockjaw. _____ is abnormal tone (tension) in a muscle.
tetany [TĔT-ă-nē] **tremor** [TRĔM-ōr] **atrophy** [ĂT-rō-fē] **muscular dystrophy** [MŬS-kyū-lăr DĬS-trō-fē] **myositis** [mī-ō-SĪ-tǐs]	A painfully long muscle contraction is _____. Shaking (_____) appears in a number of diseases such as Parkinson's disease. Some muscles _____ (shrink) as a result of disuse or specific diseases such as _____, a progressive, degenerative disorder affecting skeletal muscles. A muscle inflammation is _____.

STUDY TIP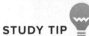

Osteoarthritis is a chronic degenerative disease. Rheumatoid arthritis is a chronic inflammatory process.

Bones and Spinal Cord

The bones and spinal cord also can be affected by diseases and disorders. This section presents additional terms relating to musculoskeletal pathology. Figure 6-22 shows two types of spinal curvature.

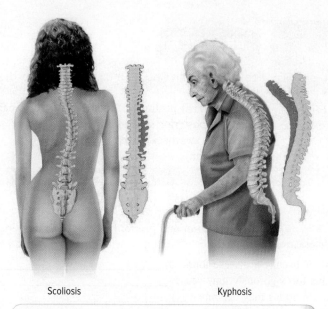

Scoliosis   Kyphosis

Figure 6-22 Two types of spinal curvatures

Pathological	PRACTICE
	Provide the missing term(s) to complete the following sentences.
bony necrosis [nĕ-KRŌ-sĭs] **bursitis** [bŭr-SĪ-tĭs] **bunion** [BŬN-yŭn]	Some bone tissue dies (_____), often as a result of loss of blood supply. The bursa may become inflamed, causing _____. Inflammation of the bursa on the side of the big toe causes a _____.
arthritis [ăr-THRĪ-tĭs] **osteoarthritis** [ŎS-tē-ō-ăr-THRĪ-tĭs] **degenerative arthritis** [dē-JEN-er-ă-tĭv ăr-THRĪ-tĭs] **rheumatoid arthritis** [RŪ-mă-tŏyd ăr-THRĪ-tĭs] **gouty arthritis** [GŎWT-ē ăr-THRĪ-tĭs] **gout** [gŏwt] **podagra** [pō-DĂG-ră] **crepitation** [krĕp-ĭ-TĀ-shŭn] **crepitus** [KRĔP-ĭ-tŭs] **osteomyelitis** [ŎS-tē-ō-mī-ĕ-LĪ-tĭs]	A common inflammation of the joints is _____. Arthritis is a name for many different joint diseases, such as _____ or _____ (arthritis characterized by erosion of joint cartilage); _____ (a systemic disease affecting connecting tissue); and _____ or _____ (a disease characterized by joint _____, pain in the big toe, and other joint pains). Certain types of arthritis may cause _____ (also called _____), noise made when affected surfaces rub together. Infections in the bone may cause _____.
	Various tumors may develop in the muscle, bone, bone marrow, and joints. Types of musculoskeletal tumors include:
myeloma [mī-ĕ-LŌ-mă] **myoma** [mī-Ō-mă] **osteoma** [ŏs-tē-Ō-mă] **osteosarcoma** [ŎS-tē-ō-săr-KŌ-mă]	1. Bone marrow tumor, _____. 2. Benign muscle tumor, _____. 3. Benign bone tumor, _____. 4. Malignant bone tumor, _____.

continued on next page

Pathological

kyphosis [kī-FŌ-sĭs]
lordosis [lōr-DŌ-sĭs]
scoliosis [skō-lē-Ō-sĭs]

Provide the missing term(s) to complete the following sentences.

Some abnormal posture conditions may cause pain. These include _____ (abnormal posterior spinal curvature), _____ (anterior spinal curvature resulting in swayback), and _____ (abnormal lateral curvature of the spinal column).

WRITE and PRONOUNCE

Fill in the term and pronounce each term aloud.

1. Osteoporosis is usually a disease found in _____ women.
2. Playing tennis too vigorously may cause _____ of the elbow.
3. Underworked muscles may become _____.
4. A muscle tumor is a(n) _____.
5. A slipped disk is called _____.

SPELL and DEFINE

Identify if the following terms are spelled correctly. Correct the words that are spelled incorrectly. Write the definition for each word.

	Spelling	Definition
kiphosis		
osteomyelitis		
flacksid		
arthralagia		
siattica		

UNDERSTAND

Build Your Medical Vocabulary: Match the word on the left with the proper definition on the right.

1. _____ myo-
2. _____ myelo-
3. _____ rhabdo-
4. _____ osteo-
5. _____ arthro-
6. _____ chiro-

a. bone
b. hand
c. rod-shaped
d. joint
e. bone marrow
f. muscle

APPLY

Read the following scenario and respond accordingly.

Read the following scenario and rewrite it using correct medical terminology.

The nurse is taking a health history of 76-year-old Nicole Young. Nicole states that when she was younger, she injured the ligament in her left ankle multiple times while playing basketball. Later in life, she reports she twisted the same ankle and was diagnosed with an inflamed tendon. She states that while riding her bicycle last year, she fell and partially dislocated her right shoulder. Lastly, she tells the nurse that last year she was told she had decreased bone density and was subject to fractures.

_____

_____

_____

_____

LO 6.5 Surgical Terms

Orthopedic surgery may involve repairing, grafting, replacing, excising, or reconstructing parts of the musculoskeletal system. Surgeons also make incisions to take biopsies. Almost any major part of the musculoskeletal system can now be surgically replaced. This section presents terms relating to surgery and the musculoskeletal system.

STUDY TIP

Make sure you have learned all of the terms before completing the exercises.

Surgical	PRACTICE
	Provide the missing term(s) to complete the following sentences.
amputation [ĂM-pyū-TĀ-shŭn] **prosthetic devices** [prŏs-THĔT-ĭk] **bone grafting** **orthosis** [ŏr-THŌ-sĭs] **orthotic** [ŏr-THŎT-ĭk]	In some situations (as with loss of circulation in diabetes, cancer of a limb, or severe infection), _____ of a limb may be necessary. _____ now routinely replace knees and hips when injury or degenerative disease has worn down joints. _____ can be used to repair a defect. An _____ or _____ may be used to provide support and prevent movement during treatment.
casting **splinting** **traction** [TRĂK-shŭn] **external fixation devices** **internal fixation device**	Fractures are treated by _____, _____, surgical manipulation, or placement in _____. Casts and splints are considered _____, which are devices that surround a fractured body part to hold the bones in place while healing. These may be used in combination with an _____, such as a pin placed internally to hold bones together. Pins for internal fixation are usually metal or hard plastic. A pin may be placed permanently or it may be removed after the bone has healed.
osteotomy [ŏs-tē-ŎT-ō-mē]	_____ is an incision into a bone.
tenotomy [tĕ-NŎT-ō-mē] **myoplasty** [MĪ-ō-plăs-tē]	_____ is the cutting into a tendon to repair a muscle. _____ is muscle repair.
arthroplasty [ĂR-thrō-plăs-tē] **arthrocentesis** [ĂR-thrō-sĕn-TĒ-sĭs] **synovectomy** [sĭn-ō-VĔK-tō-mē]	_____ is joint repair. _____ is a puncture into a joint. A _____ is the removal of part or all of the synovial membrane of a joint.
arthrodesis [ăr-THRŎD-ĕ-sĭs *or* ăr-thrō-DĒ-sĭs] **spondylosyndesis** [SPŎN-dĭ-lō-sĭn-DĒ-sĭs] **bursectomy** [bŭr-SĔK-tō-mē] **bunionectomy** [bŭn-yŭn-ĔK-tō-mē]	_____ and _____ are two types of joint fusion. A _____ is the removal of an affected bursa. A _____ is the removal of a bunion. This operation is usually performed on the big toe. Other types of toe repair may correct such things as *hammer toe,* where one or more toes are permanently flexed to one side.
laminectomy [LĂM-ĭ-NĔK-tō-mē]	Some musculoskeletal surgery is done by arthroscopy. _____, or removal of part of a vertebra, may alleviate the pain of a herniated disc.

1. Repair of the bone is _____.
2. _____ is cutting into a tendon to repair a muscle.
3. A joint repair is called _____.
4. Removal of part of the vertebrae is a _____.
5. Removal of a bunion is a _____.

SPELL and DEFINE   Identify if the following terms are spelled correctly. Correct the words that are spelled incorrectly. Write the definition for each word.

	Spelling	Definition
osteotome		
arthosentesis		
myelplasty		
tenotome		
osteoplastie		

UNDERSTAND   Form two surgical words for each of the following word roots by adding suffixes learned in previous chapters.

1. osteo: _____ and _____
2. arthro: _____ and _____
3. myo: _____ and _____
4. spondylo: _____ and _____
5. cranio: _____ and _____

APPLY   Read the following scenario and answer the questions.

Kathy Brode, a 56-year-old female, suffered an injury while running. The physician prescribed rest and medication first, to be followed by a gradual program of physical therapy. Kathy missed about six weeks of work and seemed fine until she started to run again. At that time, Kathy twisted her knee, leaving her writhing in pain. It was the same knee on which fluid had accumulated during the previous week. X-rays showed no fractures. Later, after examination by a specialist, arthroscopic surgery was recommended. Kathy had to go through another rehabilitative program (rest, medication, and physical therapy) after the surgery.

1. A program of physical therapy was prescribed for Kathy. Which one of her tests was most important in determining whether she could exercise? Why? _____
   _____

2. Is physical therapy always appropriate for a musculoskeletal injury? _____

LO 6.6 Pharmacological Terms

Most medications for treatment of the musculoskeletal system treat symptoms, not causes. The following medications all relieve or relax the area of pain by either numbing the area or reducing the inflammation. This section includes terms associated with the medications used to treat skin disorders.

Pharmacological	PRACTICE
	Provide the missing term(s) to complete the following sentences.
muscle relaxant	An agent that relieves muscle stiffness is a _____.
nonsteroidal anti-inflammatory drug (NSAID) [nŏn-STĔR-oy-dăl]	An agent that reduces inflammation without the use of steroids is a _____.
narcotic [năr-KŎT-ĭk]	An agent that relieves pain by affecting the body in ways that are similar to opium is a _____.
analgesic [ăn-ăl-JĒ-zĭk]	An agent that relieves pain is an _____.
anti-inflammatory (corticosteroid) [KŎR-tĭ-kō-STĔR-oyd]	An agent that reduces inflammation is _____.

WRITE and PRONOUNCE

Fill in the term and pronounce each term aloud.

1. This medication addresses muscle stiffness: _____.
2. Opium is this type of medication: _____.
3. This medication relieves pain: _____.
4. Inflammation is reduced by: _____.

UNDERSTAND

Identify which type of medication could be used to treat the following conditions.

1. bursitis: _____
2. myalgia: _____
3. bone infection: _____
4. arthritis: _____
5. arthralgia: _____

LO 6.7 Abbreviations

The following are abbreviations associated with the musculoskeletal sytsem.

Abbreviation	ABBREVIATION REVIEW
	Definition
AKA	above the knee amputee
AROM	active range of motion
BKA	below the knee amputee
C1, C2, and so on	first, second, and so on, cervical vertebrae
CPK	creatine phosphokinase
CTS	carpel tunnel syndrome

continued on next page

Abbreviation	Definition
D.O.	Doctor of Osteopathy
EMG	electromyogram
Fx	fracture
NSAID	nonsteroidal anti-inflammatory drug
PROM	passive range of motion
ROM	range of motion
TMJ	temporomandibular joint

UNDERSTAND   Identify the abbreviation for the following terms

1. Active range of motion: _____
2. Creatine phosphokinase: _____
3. Carpel tunnel syndrome: _____
4. Fracture: _____

APPLY   Read the following scenario and rewrite using appropriate medical terms

Mrs. Smith has a history of a Fx left leg; CTS; right AKA. She presents today with limited AROM in her left arm and pain with PROM in her left leg.

_____

_____

Chapter Review

CHAPTER SUMMARY

	Learning Outcome	Summary
6.1	Identify the parts of the musculoskeletal system and discuss the function of each part.	The musculoskeletal system forms the framework that holds the body together, enables it to move, and protects and supports all the internal organs.
6.2	Define combining forms used in building words that relate to the musculoskeletal system.	Word building requires knowledge of the combining form and meaning.
6.3	Identify common diagnostic tests, laboratory tests, and clinical procedures used in testing and treating disorders of the musculoskeletal system.	Diagnostic, procedural, and laboratory findings assist the health care provider in diagnosing medical conditions. Often used in combination, these tests lead to a final diagnosis and assist in treatment planning.
6.4	Define the major pathological conditions of the musculoskeletal system.	Pathological conditions can occur throughout the musculoskeletal system. These conditions may be present at birth or occur throughout the lifespan.
6.5	Define surgical terms related to the musculoskeletal system.	Orthopedic surgery may involve repair, grafting, replacement, excision, or reconstruction of parts of the musculoskeletal system. Surgeons also make incisions to take biopsies.
6.6	Discuss the common pharmacological agents used in treating disorders of the musculoskeletal system.	Most medications used to treat disorders of the musculoskeletal system treat symptoms, not the causes. Often, treatment includes medications to relieve or relax the painful area by either numbing the area or reducing the inflammation.
6.7	Identify abbreviations commonly associated with the musculoskeletal system.	Abbreviations are frequently used to describe location, disease, or care provided.

Label this figure with these terms:

1. vertebrae
2. coccyx
3. sacrum
4. spine

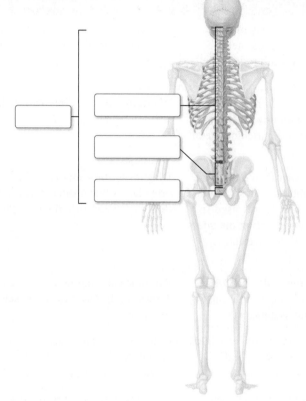

Label this figure with these terms:

1. carpus
2. olecranon
3. humerus
4. phalanges
5. metacarpals

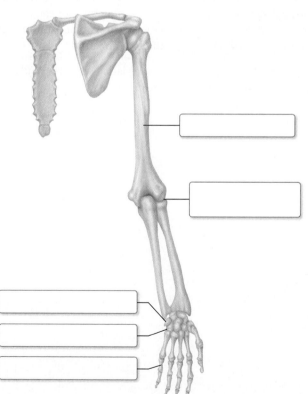

Correct the spelling and write the definition. Say each term aloud.

	Spelling	Definition
1. spazmz		
2. kaltar		
3. rumatolojist		
4. fashea		
5. mielografe		
6. diafhysis		
7. osteoklasts		
8. kokkix		
9. falanjez		
10. iskeum		

IMPLEMENT

Match the definition in the second column to the terms in the first.

1. _____ amputation   a. Replacement device
2. _____ prosthesis   b. Molding
3. _____ orthosis, orthotic   c. Muscle repair
4. _____ traction   d. Bone cutting
5. _____ casting   e. Limb removal
6. _____ splinting   f. Bone repair
7. _____ myoplasty   g. External supporting or immobilizing device
8. _____ osteoplasty   h. Wrapping to immobilize
9. _____ osteotomy   i. Pulling to straighten
10. _____ arthroplasty   j. Joint repair

Complete the words using the combining forms learned in this chapter.

1. Joint pain: _____ dynia
2. Plastic surgery of the skull: _____ plasty
3. Of the upper jaw and its teeth: _____ dental
4. Operation on the instep of the foot: _____ tomy
5. Examination of joints using x-ray: _____ graphy
6. Production of fibrous tissue: _____ plasia
7. Inflammation of the foot: _____ itis
8. Instrument for measuring spine curvature: _____ meter
9. Incision through the sternum: _____ tomy
10. A hernia in the femur: _____ cele

Fill in the Blanks: Complete the sentences by filling in the blanks.

1. The extremities of the body include mostly _____ bones.
2. A mature adult has a total of _____ bones.
3. Soft connective tissue with high nutrient content in the center of some bones is called _____.
4. An infant's skull generally has soft spots known as _____.
5. Disks in the spinal column have a soft, fibrous mass in the middle called the _____.
6. A deformity of the heel due to weakened calf muscles is called _____.
7. Ribs that attach to both the vertebral column and the sternum are called _____.
8. Another name for kneecap is _____.
9. The largest tarsal is called the _____ or heel.
10. The only muscle that is both striated and involuntary is the _____ muscle.

DECONSTRUCT

Janet Connolly (age 48) reports pain in her left upper leg. She states she has pain with and without movement. The left leg is rotated outward and there is pain when the ankle is bent upward. Rewrite the information using medical terms and any appropriate abbreviations.

_____

_____

Reviewing the Terms
Pronounce each of the following terms. Write the definitions on a separate sheet of paper. This review will take you through all the words you learned in this chapter. If you have difficulty with any words, make a flash card for later study. Refer to the English-Spanish and Spanish-English glossaries in the eBook.

acetabul/o [ăs-ě-TĂB-yū-lō]
acetabulum [ăs-ě-TĂB-yū-lŭm]
acromi/o [ă-KRŌ-mē-ō]
acromion [ă-KRŌ-mē-ŏn]
amphiarthrosis (*pl.*, **amphiarthoses**) [ĂM-fĭ-ăr-THRŌ-sĭs (ĂM-fĭ-ăr-THRŌ-sēz)]
amputation [ĂM-pyū-TĀ-shŭn]
analgesic [ăn-ăl-JĒ-zĭk]
ankle [ĂNG-kl]
ankyl/o [ĂNG-kĭ-LŌ]
ankylosis [ĂNG-kĭ-LŌ-sĭs]
anti-inflammatory (corticosteroid) [KŎR-tĭ-kō-STĔR-oyd])
arthr/o [ĂR-thrō]
arthralgia [ăr-THRĂL-jē-ă]
arthritis [ăr-THRĪ-tĭs]
arthrocentesis [ĂR-thrō-sĕn-TĒ-sĭs]
arthrodesis [ăr-THRŎD-ě-sĭs *or* ăr-thrō-DĒ-sĭs]
arthrography [ăr-THRŎG-ră-fē]
arthroplasty [ĂR-thrō-plăs-tē]
arthroscopy [ăr-THRŎS-kō-pē]
articular [ăr-TĬK-yū-lăr] **cartilage**
articulation [ăr-tĭk-yū-LĀ-shŭn]
atlas [ĂT-lăs]
atrophy [ĂT-rō-fē]

axis [ĂK-sĭs]
bone
bone grafting
bone head
bone scan
bony necrosis [nĕ-KRŌ-sĭs]
brachi/o [BRĀ-kē-ō]
bunion [BŬN-yŭn]
bunionectomy [bŭn-yŭn-ĔK-tō-mē]
burs/o [BŬR-sō]
bursa (*pl.*, **bursae**) [BŬR-să (BŬR-sē)]
bursectomy [bŭr-SĔK-tō-mē]
bursitis [bŭr-SĪ-tĭs]
calcane/o [kăl-KĀ-nē-ō]
calcaneus [kăl-KĀ-nē-ŭs]
calcar [KĂL-kăr]
calci/o [KĂL-sē-ō]
calcium [KĂL-sē-ŭm]
cancellous [KĂN-sě-lŭs] **bone**
cardiac [KĂR-dē-ăk] **muscle**
carp/o [KĂR-pō]
carpal [KĂR-păl] **tunnel syndrome**
carpus [KĂR-pŭs], **carpal** [KĂR-păl] **bones**
cartilage [KĂR-tĭ-lăj]

cartilaginous [kăr-tĭ-LĂJ-ĭ-nŭs] disk
casting
cephal/o [SĔF-ă-lō]
cervic/o [SĔR-vĭ-kō]
cervical [SĔR-vĭ-kl] vertebrae
chiropractor [kī-rō-PRĂK-tōr]
chondr/o [KŎN-drō]
chondromalacia [KŎN-drō-mă-LĀ-shē-ă]
clavicle [KLĂV-ĭ-kl]
closed fracture
coccyx [KŎK-sĭks]
Colles' [kōlz] fracture
comminuted [KŎM-ĭ-nū-tĕd] fracture
compact bone
complex fracture
complicated fracture
compound fracture
compression fracture
condyl/o [KŎN-di-lō]
condyle [KŎN-dīl]
contracture [kŏn-TRĂK-chūr]
cost/o [KŎS-tō]
crani/o [KRĀ-nē-ō]
crepitation [krĕp-ĭ-TĀ-shŭn], crepitus [KRĔP-ĭ-tŭs]
crest
dactyl/o [DĂK-tĭ-lō]
degenerative arthritis [dē-JEN-er-ă-tĭv ăr-THRĪ-tĭs]
densitometer [dĕn-sĭ-TŎM-ĕ-tĕr]
diaphysis [dī-ĂF-ĭ-sĭs]
diarthroses (sing., diarthrosis)
[dī-ăr-THRŌ-sēz (dī-ăr-THRŌ-sĭs)]
disk [dĭsk]
diskography [dĭs-KŎG-ră-fē]
dislocation [dis-lō-KĀ-shŭn]
dorsal vertebrae
dystonia [dĭs-TŌ-nē-ă]
elbow [ĔL-bō]
electromyogram [ē-lĕk-trō-MĪ-ō-grăm]
endosteum [ĕn-DŎS-tē-ŭm]
epiphyseal [ĕp-ĭ-FĬZ-ē-ăl] plate
epiphysitis [ĕ-pĭf-ĭ-SĪ-tĭs]
ethmoid [ĔTH-moyd] bone
exostosis [ĕks-ŏs-TŌ-sĭs]
external fixation device
fasci/o [FĂSH-ē-ō]
fascia (pl., fasciae) [FĂSH-ē-ă (FĂSH-ē-ē)]
femor/o [FĔM-ō-rō]

femur [FĒ-mūr]
fibr/o [FĬ-brō]
fibula [FĬB-yū-lă]
fissure [FĬSH-ŭr]
flaccid [FLĂK-sĭd or FLĂS-ĭd]
flat bones
fontanelle [FŎN-tă-nĕl]
foramen [fō-RĀ-mĕn]
foramen magnum [MĂG-nŭm]
fossa (pl., fossae) [FŎS-ă (FŎS-ē)]
fracture [FRĂK-chŭr]
frontal [FRŬN-t ăl] bone
frontal sinuses
goniometer [gō-nē-ŎM-ĕ-tĕr]
gouty arthritis, gout [GŎWT-ē, gŏwt]
greenstick fracture
hairline fracture
heel [hēl]
herniated [HĔR-nē-ă-tĕd] disk
humer/o [HYŪ-mĕr-ō]
humerus [HYŪ-mĕr-ŭs]
hypertrophy [hī-PĔR-trō-fē]
hypotonia [HĪ-pō-TŌ-nē-ă]
ili/o [ĬL-ē-ō]
ilium [ĬL-ē-ŭm]
impacted fracture
incomplete fracture
insertion
internal fixation device
intervertebral [ĭn-tĕr-VĔR-tĕ-brăl] disk
involuntary muscles
irregular bones
ischi/o [ĬS-kē-ō]
ischium [ĬS-kē-ŭm]
joint [joynt]
kyph/o [kī-FŌ]
kyphosis [kī-FŌ-sĭs]
lacrimal [LĂK-rĭ-măl] bone
lamin/o [LĂM-ĭ-nō]
lamina (pl., laminae) [LĂM-ĭ-nă (LĂM-ĭ-nē)]
laminectomy [LĂM-ĭ-NĔK-tō-mē]
leiomy/o [LĪ-ō-mī-Ō]
leiomyoma [LĪ-ō-mī-Ō-mă]
leiomyosarcoma [LĪ-ō-MĪ-ō-săr-KŌ-mă]
ligament [LĬG-ă-mĕnt]
long bone
lordosis [lōr-DŌ-sĭs]

lumb/o [LŬM-bō]
lumbar [LŬM-băr] vertebrae
malleolus (pl., malleoli) [mă-LĒ-ō-lŭs (mă-LĒ-ō-lī)]
mandible [MĂN-dĭ-bl]
mandibular [măn-DĬB-yū-lăr] bone
marrow [MĂR-ō]
mastoid [MĂS-toyd] process
maxill/o [măk-SĬL-ō]
maxillary [MĂK-sĭ-lăr-ē] bone
maxillary sinus
medullary [MĔD-ū-lăr-ē] cavity
metacarp/o [MĔT-ă-KĂR-pō]
metacarpal [MĔT-ă-KĂR-păl]
metaphysis [mĕ-TĂF-ĭ-sĭs]
metatarsal [MĔT-ă-TĂR-săl] bones
muscle [MŬS-ĕl]
muscle relaxant
muscular dystrophy [MŬS-kyū-lăr DĬS-trō-fē]
musculoskeletal [MŬS-kyū-lō-SKĔL-ĕ-tăl] system
my/o [MĪ-ō]
myalgia [mī-ĂL-jē-ă]
myel/o [MĪ-ĕ-lō]
myelography [MĪ-ĕ-LŎG-ră-fē]
myeloma [mī-ĕ-LŌ-mă]
myodynia [MĪ-ō-DĬN-ē-ă]
myoma [mī-Ō-mă]
myoplasty [MĪ-ō-plăs-tē]
myositis [mī-ō-SĪ-tĭs]
narcotic [năr-KŎT-ĭk]
nasal [NĀ-zăl] bones
nasal cavity
nonsteroidal [nŏn-STĔR-oy-dăl] anti-inflammatory drug (NSAID)
occipital [ŏk-SĬP-ĭ-tăl] bone
olecranon [ō-LĔK-ră-nŏn or Ō-lē-KRĀ-nŏn]
open fracture
origin
orthopedic [ōr-thō-PĒ-dĭk] surgeon
orthopedist [ōr-thō-PĒ-dĭst]
orthosis [ōr-THŌ-sĭs], orthotic [ōr-THŎT-ĭk]
osseous [ŎS-ē-ŭs] tissue
ossification [ŎS-ĭ-fĭ-KĀ-shŭn]
oste/o [ŎS-tē-ō]
ostealgia [ŏs-tē-ĂL-jē-ă]
osteoarthritis [ŎS-tē-ō-ăr-THRĪ-tĭs]
osteoblast [ŎS-tē-ō-blăst]

osteoclasis [ŎS-tē-ŎK-lă-sĭs]
osteoclast [ŎS-tē-ō-klăst]
osteocyte [ŎS-tē-ō-sīt]
osteodynia [ŏs-tē-ō-DĬN-ē-ă]
osteoma [ŏs-tē-Ō-mă]
osteomyelitis [ŎS-tē-ō-mī-ĕ-LĪ-tĭs]
osteopath [ŎS-tē-ō-păth]
osteoplasty [ŎS-tē-ō-plăs-tē]
osteoporosis [ŎS-tē-ō-pō-RŌ-sĭs]
osteosarcoma [ŎS-tē-ō-săr-KŌ-mă]
osteotomy [ŏs-tē-ŎT-ō-mē]
palatine [PĂL-ă-tīn] bone
parietal [pă-RĪ-ĕ-tăl] bone
patell/o [pă-TĔL-ō]
patella [pă-TĔL-ă]
pathological fracture
ped/i, ped/o [PĒ-dē, pē-dō]
pelv/i [PĔL-vĭ]
pelvic [PĔL-vĭk] cavity
pelvic girdle
pelvis [PĔL-vĭs]
periosteum [pĕr-ē-ŎS-tē-ŭm]
phalang/o [fă-Lăn-jō]
phalanges (sing., phalanx) [fă-LĂN-jēz (FĂ-lăngks)]
phantom limb, phantom pain
phosphorus [FŎS-fōr-ŭs]
physical therapy
pod/o [pō-DŌ]
podagra [pō-DĂG-ră]
podiatrist [pō-DĪ-ă-trĭst]
process [PRŌ-sĕs, PRŎS-ĕs]
prosthetic [prŏs-THĔT-ĭk] device
pub/o [PYŪ-bō]
pubic symphysis [PYŪ-bĭk SĬM-fĭ-sĭs]
pubis [PYŪ-bĭs]
rachi/o [rā-kē-ō]
radi/o [RĀ-dē-ō]
radius [RĀ-dē-ŭs]
reduction
rhabd/o [RĂB-dō]
rhabdomy/o [RĂB-dō-mī-ō]
rhabdomyoma [RĂB-dō-mī-Ō-mă]
rhabdomyosarcoma [RĂB-dō-mī-ō-săr-KŌ-mă]
rheumatoid [RŪ-mă-toyd] arthritis
rheumatoid factor test
rheumatologist [rū-mă-TŎL-ō-jĭst]

rib

rickets [RĬK-ĕts]

rigidity

rigor [RĬG-ōr]

sacrum [SĀ-krŭm]

scapul/o [SKĂP-yū-lō]

scapula [SKĂP-yū-lă]

sciatica [sī-ĂT-ĭ-kă]

scoli/o [skō-lē-Ō]

scoliosis [skō-lē-Ō-sĭs]

sella turcica [SĔL-ă TŬR-sĭ-kă]

sequestrum [sē-KWĔS-trŭm]

serum calcium [SĔR-ŭm KĂL-sĭ-ŭm]

serum creatine phosphokinase (CPK) [KRĒ-ă-tēn fŏs-fō-KĬ-nās]

serum phosphorus [FŎS-fōr-ŭs]

sesamoid [SĔS-ă-moyd] bone

shin [shĭn]

short bones

simple fracture

sinus [SĪ-nŭs]

skeleton [SKĔL-ĕ-tŏn]

smooth muscles

spasm [spăzm]

spastic [SPĂS-tĭk]

sphenoid [SFĒ-noyd] bone

sphenoid sinus

spina bifida [SPĪ-nă BĬF-ĭ-dă]

spinal column

spinal curvature

spinous [SPĪ-nŭs] process

splinting

spondyl/o [SPŎN-dĭ-lō]

spondylolisthesis [SPŎN-dĭ-lō-lĭs-THĒ-sĭs]

spondylosis [spŏn-dĭ-LŌ-sĭs]

spondylosyndesis [SPŎN-dĭ-lō-sĭn-DĒ-sĭs]

spongy bone

sprain [sprān]

spur [spŭr]

stern/o [STĔR-nō]

sternum [STĔR-nŭm]

strain [strān]

striated [strī-ĀT-ĕd] muscles

styloid [STĪ-loyd] process

subluxation [sŭb-lŭk-SĀ-shŭn]

sulcus (pl., sulci) [SŬL-kŭs (SŬL-sī)]

suture [SŪ-chŭr]

symphysis [SĬM-fĭ-sĭs]

synarthrosis [SĬN-ăr-THRŌ-sĭs]

synov/o [sĭ-NŌ-vō]

synovectomy [sĭn-ō-VĔK-tō-mē]

synovial [sĭ-NŌ-vē-ăl] fluid

synovial joint

synovial membrane

talipes calcaneus [TĂL-ĭ-pēz kăl-KĀ-nē-ŭs]

talipes valgus [VĂL-gŭs]

talipes varus [VĀ-rŭs]

tars/o [TĂR-sō]

tarsus [TĂR-sŭs], tarsal [TĂR-săl] bones

temporal [TĔM-pō-răl] bone

temporomandibular [TĔM-pō-rō-măn-DĬB-yū-lăr] joint (TMJ)

ten/o, tend/o, tendin/o [TĔN-ō, TĔN-dō, tĕn-dĭn-ō]

tendinitis (tendonitis) [tĕn-dĭn-ĪT-ĭs]

tendon [TĔN-dŏn]

tenotomy [tĕ-NŎT-ō-mē]

tetany [TĔT-nē]

thorac/o [THŌR-ă-kō]

thoracic [thō-RĂS-ĭk] vertebrae

thorax [THŌ-răks]

tibi/o [TĬB-ē-ō]

tibia [TĬB-ē-ă]

Tinel's [tĭ-NĔLZ] sign

traction [TRĂK-shŭn]

transverse [trănz-VĔRS] process

tremor [TRĔM-ōr]

trochanter [trō-KĂN-tĕr]

true ribs

tubercle [TŪ-bĕr-kl]

tuberosity [TŪ-bĕr-ŎS-ĭ-tē]

uln/o [ŬL-nō]

ulna [ŬL-nă]

uric [YŪR-ĭk] acid test

vertebr/o [VĔR-tĕ-brō]

vertebra (pl., vertebrae) [VĔR-tĕ-bră (VĔR-tĕ-brē)]

vertebral body

vertebral column

visceral [VĬS-ĕr-ăl] muscles

vitamin D

voluntary muscles

vomer [VŌ-mĕr]

zygomatic [ZĪ-gō-MĂT-ĭk] bone

The Nervous System

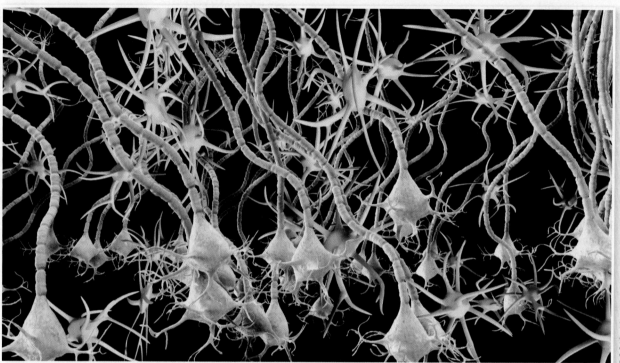

Learning Outcomes

After studying this chapter, you will be able to:

7.1 Identify the parts of the nervous system and discuss the function of each part.

7.2 Recall the major word parts used in building words that relate to the nervous system.

7.3 Identify the common diagnostic tests, laboratory tests, and clinical procedures used in testing and treating disorders of the nervous system.

7.4 Define the major pathological conditions of the nervous system.

7.5 Explain the meaning of surgical terms related to the nervous system.

7.6 Recognize common pharmacological agents used in treating disorders of the nervous system.

7.7 Identify common abbreviations associated with the nervous system.

LO 7.1 Structure and Function of the Nervous System

The nervous system directs the function of all the human body systems. Every activity, whether voluntary or involuntary, is controlled by some of the more than 100 billion nerve cells throughout the body. The nervous system is divided into two subsystems: the *central nervous system* and the *peripheral nervous system*. Figure 7-1 shows a nerve cell. Figure 7-2 illustrates the network of nerves in the body.

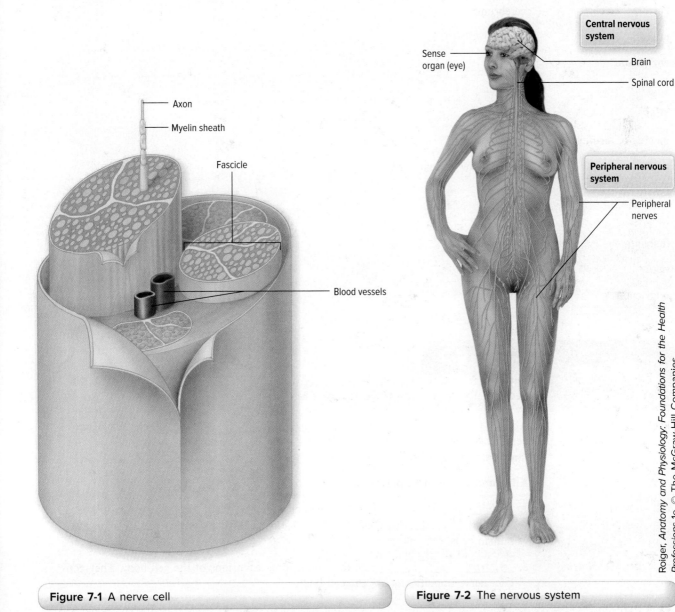

Figure 7-1 A nerve cell

Figure 7-2 The nervous system

Roiger, *Anatomy and Physiology: Foundations for the Health Professions 1e*, © The McGraw-Hill Companies

Building Your Nervous System Vocabulary

This section provides an introduction to the basic nervous system combining terms and their meanings. Review this information prior to moving to the practices.

Combining Form	Meaning
cephal/o	head
cerebell/o	cerebellum
cerebr/o, cerebr/i	cerebrum
crani/o	cranium
encephal/o	brain
gangli/o	ganglion
gli/o	neuroglia
mening/o, meningi/o	meninges
myel/o	bone marrow, spinal cord
neur/o, neur/i	nerve
spin/o	spine
thalam/o	thalamus
vag/o	vagus nerve
ventricul/o	ventricle

Structure and Function	PRACTICE
	Provide the missing term(s) to complete the following sentences.
nerve cell neuron [NŪR-ŏn]	A _____ or _____ is the basic element of the nervous system. Neurons are highly specialized types of cells and vary greatly in function, shape, and size.
	All neurons have three parts:
cell body	1. The _____ has branches or fibers that reach out to send or receive impulses. The cell body contains all the biological structures that are common to all human cells.
dendrites [DĔN-drīts]	2. _____ are thin, branching extensions of the cell body. They conduct nerve impulses *toward* the cell body.
axon [ĂK-son] myelin sheath [MĪ-ĕ-lĭn shēth]	3. The _____ conducts nerve impulses *away from* the cell body. It is generally a single branch covered by fatty tissue called the _____. This protective sheath prevents the nerve from transmitting impulses in the wrong direction.

terminal end **fibers** **synapse** [SĬN-ăps] **neurotransmitter** [NŪR-ō-trăns-MĬT-ĕr]	Outside the myelin sheath is a membranous covering called the neurilemma. At the end of the axon, there are _____ through which the impulse passes when leaving the neuron. The nerve impulse then jumps from one neuron to the next over a space called a _____. The nerve impulse is stimulated to jump over the synapse by a _____ and by various substances produced by, and located in, tiny sacs at the end of the terminal end fibers.
excitability [ĕk-SĪ-tă-BĬL-ĭ-tē] **stimulus** [STĬM-yū-lŭs] **conductivity** [kŏn-dŭk-TĬV-ĭ-tē]	All neurons also have two basic properties: _____, the ability to respond to a _____ (anything that arouses a response), and _____, the ability to transmit a signal.
	The three types of neurons are:
efferent (motor) neurons [ĔF-ĕr-ĕnt NŪR-ŏnz] **afferent (sensory)** **neurons** [ĂF-ĕr-ĕnt NŪR-ŏnz] **interneurons** [ĬN-tĕr-NŪR-ŏnz]	1. _____, which convey information to the muscles and glands from the central nervous system. 2. _____, which carry information from sensory receptors to the central nervous system. 3. _____, which carry and process sensory information.
	Some nerves contain combinations of at least two types of neurons.
nerves [nĕrvz] **acetylcholine** [ăs-ĕ-tĭl-KŌ-lēn] **norepinephrine** [nŏr-ĕp-ĭ-NĔF-rĭn] **nerve impulse** **receptors** [rē-SĔP-tĕrz]	Neurons are microscopic entities that form bundles called _____, the bearers of electrical messages to the organs and muscles of the body. The body's cells contain stored electrical energy that is released when the cells receive outside stimuli or when internal chemicals (e.g., _____ or _____) stimulate the cells. The released energy passes through the nerve cell, causing a _____, which is received or transmitted by tissues or organs called _____. These impulses are then transmitted to other receptors throughout the body.
	Certain neuroglia, along with the almost solid walls of the brain's capillaries, form what is known as the *blood–brain barrier,* a barrier that permits a few chemical substances to reach the brain's neurons but blocks most.

PRONOUNCE and DEFINE	Pronounce the following terms aloud and write their meaning in the space provided.
afferent	[ĂF-ĕr-ĕnt]
nerve	[nĕrv]
efferent	[ĔF-ĕr-ĕnt]
norepinephrine	[nŏr-ĕp-ĭ-NĔF-rĭn]
acetylcholine	[ăs-ĕ-tĭl-KŌ-lēn]

SPELL and DEFINE	Identify if the following terms are spelled correctly. Correct the words that are spelled incorrectly. Write the definition for each word.	
	Spelling	**Definition**
neuroglia		
norepinefrine		
sinapse		
myelin sheath		
internurons		

UNDERSTAND	Build Your Medical Vocabulary: Match the word on the left with its function on the right.

1. _____ afferent
2. _____ efferent
3. _____ nerves
4. _____ axon
5. _____ excitability
6. _____ conductivity

a. Sends electrical messages
b. Ability to respond to a stimulus
c. Carry information from sensory receptors to central nervous system
d. Carries impulse away from body
e. Ability to transmit a signal
f. Carry information to muscles and glands

APPLY	Read the following scenario and respond accordingly.

You are teaching a class about afferent and efferent neurons. Describe to the students the differences between these two types of neurons.

_____

_____

_____

_____

The Central Nervous System and the Brain

The central nervous system (CNS) consists of the brain and spinal cord. Within the brain, there are different areas with very distinct functions. It is the role of the CNS to receive an impulse, process the information, and respond with an appropriate action. Figure 7-3 shows the human brain. Figure 7-4 illustrates what parts of the brain control certain activities.

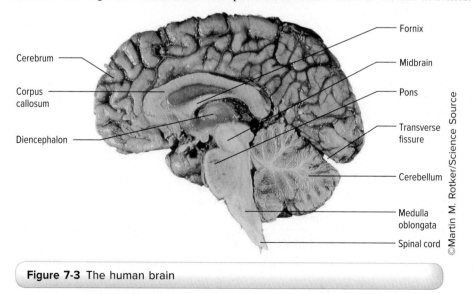

Figure 7-3 The human brain

©Martin M. Rotker/Science Source

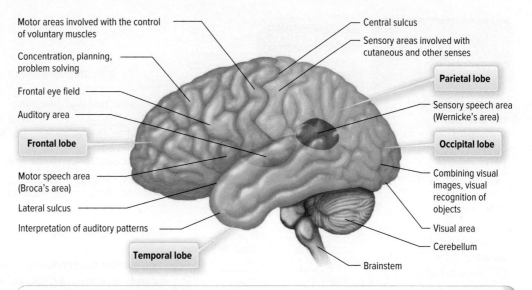

Motor areas involved with the control of voluntary muscles

Concentration, planning, problem solving

Frontal eye field

Auditory area

Frontal lobe

Motor speech area (Broca's area)

Lateral sulcus

Interpretation of auditory patterns

Temporal lobe

Central sulcus

Sensory areas involved with cutaneous and other senses

Parietal lobe

Sensory speech area (Wernicke's area)

Occipital lobe

Combining visual images, visual recognition of objects

Visual area

Cerebellum

Brainstem

Figure 7-4 Centers of control in the brain

Structure and Function	PRACTICE
	Provide the missing term(s) to complete the following sentences.
central nervous system	The _____ (CNS) consists of the brain and spinal cord. The word *central* is the key to understanding the purpose of this subsystem. It is the center of control, receiving and interpreting all stimuli and sending nerve impulses to instruct muscles and glands to take or respond to certain actions. Designated actions throughout the body include both voluntary and involuntary movement, sight, hearing, thinking, secretion of hormones, memory, and responses to outside stimuli.
brain [brān]	The human adult _____ weighs about 3 pounds, is 85% water, has the consistency of gelatin, contains more than 100 billion neurons, and is responsible for controlling the body's many functions and interactions with the outside world.
	The brain has four major divisions:
brainstem **midbrain** **pons** [pŏnz] **medulla oblongata** [mĕ-DŪL-ă ŏb-lŏng-GĂ-tă]	1. The _____ is made up of the _____ (involved with visual reflexes), the _____ (controls certain respiratory functions), and the _____ (contains centers that regulate heart and lung functions, swallowing, vomiting, coughing, and sneezing).
cerebellum [sĕr-ĕ-BĔL-ŭm]	2. The _____ is the area that coordinates musculoskeletal movement to maintain posture, balance, and muscle tone.
cerebrum [SĔR-ĕ-brŭm, sĕ-RĒ-brŭm] **cerebral cortex** [SĔR-ĕ-brăl KŌR-tĕks]	3. Above the cerebellum lies the _____, the third major brain structure. The cerebrum is the largest area of the brain, taking up about 85% of its mass. The cerebrum has two hemispheres, with an outer portion called the _____. The inner portion is divided into two hemispheres, one on the left and one on the right.

continued on next page

Structure and Function	**PRACTICE** Provide the missing term(s) to complete the following sentences.
fissures [FĬSH-ŭrz] **convolutions** [kŏn-vō-LŪ-shŭnz]	The cerebral cortex (area of conscious decision making) has many _____ and _____ and is composed of gray matter, the substance in the brain composed mainly of nerve cells and dendrites.
basal ganglia [BĀ-săl GĂNG-glē-ă] **frontal lobe** [FRŬN-tăl lōb] **parietal lobe** [pă-RĪ-ĕ-tăl lōb] **temporal lobe** [TĔM-pŏ-răl lōb] **occipital lobe** [ŏk-SĬP-ĭ-tăl lōb]	Below the cerebral cortex is white matter, the substance in the brain composed mainly of nerve fibers, and masses of gray matter called the _____ (involved with musculoskeletal movement). The left and right hemispheres of the cerebrum are each divided into four parts or lobes: a. The _____ controls voluntary motor movements, emotional expression, and moral behavior. b. The _____ controls and interprets the senses and taste. c. The _____ controls memory, equilibrium, emotion, and hearing. d. The _____ controls vision and various forms of expression.
corpus callosum [KŌR-pŭs kă-LŌ-sŭm]	The two hemispheres of the cerebrum are connected by the _____, a bridge of nerve fibers that relays information between the two hemispheres.
diencephalon [dī-ĕn-SĔF-ă-lŏn] **thalamus** [THĂL-ă-mŭs] **hypothalamus** [HĪ-pō-THĂL-ă-mŭs] **epithalamus** [ĔP-ĭ-THĂL-ă-mŭs] **ventral thalamus**	The _____ is the deep portion of the brain containing the _____, _____, _____, and _____. These parts of the diencephalon serve as relay centers for sensations. They also integrate with the autonomic nervous system in the control of heart rate, blood pressure, temperature regulation, water and electrolyte balance, digestive functions, behavioral responses, and glandular activities.
cranium [KRĀ-nē-ŭm] **cerebrospinal fluid (CSF)** [SĔR-ĕ-brō-spī-năl FLŪ-ĭd] **ventricles** [VĔN-trĭ-klz]	The brain sits inside the _____, a strong bony structure that protects it. The area between the brain and the cranium is filled with _____, a watery substance that contains various compounds and flows throughout the brain and around the spinal cord. This watery fluid cradles and cushions the brain. The fluid acts as a shock absorber in the event of head trauma. _____, or cavities in the brain, also contain this fluid. The meninges also protect the brain.

PRONOUNCE and DEFINE	Pronounce the following terms aloud and write their definitions in the space provided.
diencephalon	[dī-ĕn-SĔF-ă-lŏn]
fissures	[FĬSH-ŭrz]
sulci	[SŬL-sī]
convolutions	[kŏn-vō-LŪ-shŭnz]
gyri	[JĪ-rī]
pons	[pŏnz]

SPELL and DEFINE	Identify if the following terms are spelled correctly. Correct the words that are spelled incorrectly. Write the definition for each word.	
	Spelling	**Definition**
cereberum		
corpus callosum		
thaleamus		
ventriclaes		
epithralmus		

UNDERSTAND Complete the following:

1. The frontal lobe is responsible for _____.
2. Visual recognition occurs in the _____.
3. The temporal lobe is responsible for _____.
4. The thalamus is responsible for _____.
5. Emotions are controlled by the _____.
6. The parietal lobe is responsible for _____.

APPLY Read the following scenario and answer the questions.

Mr. Robert Jones experienced a head injury. He is having difficulty reading and he seems to be distracted easily. What part of his brain was most likely affected? What other symptoms might Mr. Jones experience?

_____
_____
_____
_____

STUDY TIP

The brain is protected by the meninges, which consist of three layers: dura mater, arachnoid, and pia mater.

Spinal Cord and Meninges

The spinal cord extends down from the occipital bone to the space between the first and second lumbar vertebrae. The function of the spinal cord is to conduct sensory impulses to the brain, conduct motor impulses from the brain, and coordinate certain reflexes. The meninges are membranes that cover the brain and spinal cord. Figure 7-5 shows the shape and parts of the spinal cord. Figure 7-6 illustrates the detailed structure of the spinal cord.

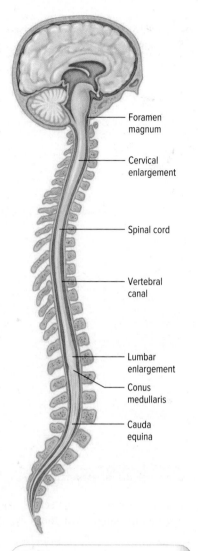

Figure 7-5 Shape and parts of the spinal cord

Foramen magnum

Cervical enlargement

Spinal cord

Vertebral canal

Lumbar enlargement

Conus medullaris

Cauda equina

STUDY TIP

Severe spinal cord injuries usually result in some type of paralysis. Research is underway to grow replacement cells for injured nerves. It is expected that some types of paralysis will be cured in the future.

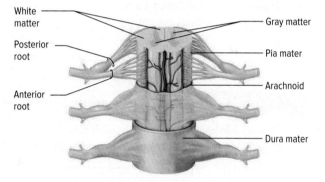

Figure 7-6 Detailed spinal cord structure

White matter

Posterior root

Anterior root

Gray matter

Pia mater

Arachnoid

Dura mater

PRACTICE

Structure and Function	Provide the missing term(s) to complete the following sentences.
spinal cord	The _____ extends from the medulla oblongata of the brain to the area around the second lumbar vertebra in the lower back. The spinal cord is contained within the vertebral column. The space that contains the spinal column is called the vertebral canal. The spinal cord is protected by the bony structure of the vertebral column, by the cerebrospinal fluid that surrounds it, and by the spinal meninges.
meninges [mĕ-NĬN-jēz]	The _____ are three layers of connective tissue membranes that cover the brain and spinal cord.
dura mater [DŪ-ră MĀ-tĕr]	The outer layer, the _____ (from Latin, "hard mother"), is a tough, fibrous membrane that covers the entire length of the spinal cord and contains channels for blood to enter brain tissue.

arachnoid [ă-RĂK-noyd] **subdural space** [sŭb-DŪR-ăl spās]	The middle layer, the _____, is a weblike structure that runs across the space (called the _____) containing cerebrospinal fluid.
pia mater [PĪ-ă MĀ-tĕr, PĒ-ă MĀ-tĕr]	The _____ (Latin, "tender mother"), the innermost layer of meninges, is a thin membrane containing many blood vessels that nourish the spinal cord.
epidural space [ĕp-ĭ-DŪ-răl spās]	The space between the pia mater and the bones of the spinal cord is called the _____. It contains blood vessels and some fat. It is the space into which anesthetics may be injected to dull pain (as during childbirth and some pelvic operations) or contrast material for certain diagnostic procedures.

PRONOUNCE and DEFINE	Pronounce the following terms aloud and write their meaning in the space provided.
pia mater	[PĪ-ă, PĒ-ă; MĀ-tĕr, MĂ-tĕr]
meninges	[mĕ-NĬN-jēz]
arachnoid	[ă-RĂK-noyd]
epidural	[ĕp-ĭ-DŪ-răl]
subdural	[sŭb-DŪR-ăl]

SPELL and DEFINE	Identify if the following terms are spelled correctly. Correct the words that are spelled incorrectly. Write the definition for each word.

	Spelling	Definition
arachnoid		
duremeter		
piamater		
subdural space		
epidural space		

UNDERSTAND	Build Your Medical Vocabulary: Match the word(s) on the left with the definition on the right.

1. _____ meninges
2. _____ pia mater
3. _____ archnoid space
4. _____ epidural space
5. _____ subdural space

a. Inner layer of meninges
b. Middle layer of meninges
c. Space between dura mater and pia mater
d. Protects the brain and spinal cord
e. Space between pia mater and spinal cord bones

Mr. John Smith was in a motor vehicle accident and has experienced a spinal cord injury. If Mr. Smith's spinal cord was severed, what symptoms do you think might occur?

_____

_____

_____

Peripheral Nervous System

The peripheral nervous system (PNS) includes a network of nerves that branch off of the brain and spinal cord. The PNS, which includes the cranial and spinal nerves, is divided into two subsystems: the somatic nervous system and the autonomic nervous system. Table 7-1 lists the cranial nerves and their functions. Table 7-2 lists the major spinal nerve divisions and their functions. Figure 7-7 shows the spinal cord regions and nerves.

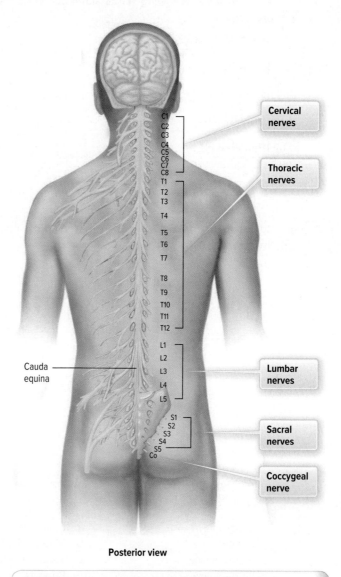

Posterior view

Figure 7-7 Spinal cord regions and nerves

TABLE 7-1   The 12 Pairs of Cranial Nerves and Their Functions

Pair of Cranial Nerves	Primary Type of Nerve	Function
I olfactory	sensory	involved in sense of smell
II optic	sensory	involved in sense of vision
III oculomotor	motor	involved in movement of eyes, controlling both the exterior and interior parts
IV trochlear	motor	involved in muscles that move the eyes
V trigeminal	sensory and motor	involved in eyes, tear glands, scalp, forehead, teeth, gums, lips, and muscles of the mouth
VI abducens	motor	involved with muscle conditioning
VII facial	sensory and motor	involved with taste, facial expressions, tear glands, and salivary glands
VIII vestibulocochlear	sensory	involved in equilibrium and hearing
IX glossopharyngeal	sensory and motor	involved in pharynx, tonsils, tongue, and carotid arteries; stimulates salivary glands
X vagus	sensory and motor	involved in speech, swallowing, heart muscles, smooth muscles, and certain glands
XI accessory (cranial and spinal)	motor	involved in muscles of the soft palate, pharynx, larynx, neck, and back
XII hypoglossal	motor	involved in muscles that move the tongue

TABLE 7-2   Major Spinal Nerve Divisions and Their Functions

Region of Spinal Cord	Location	Functions of Nerves
cervical	neck	involved in muscles of the back of the head and neck and in the diaphragm
brachial	lower neck, axilla	involved in the muscles and skin of the neck, shoulder, arm, and hand
lumbar	posterior abdominal wall	involved in abdominal skin and muscles
sacral	posterior pelvic wall	involved in the muscles of the buttocks, thighs, feet, legs, and voluntary sphincters
coccygeal	coccyx and surrounding area	skin in coccyx region

STUDY TIP

The parasympathetic nervous system is responsible for the "rest and digest" functions of the body. The sympathetic nervous system responds to stress and initiates our "fight or flight" response.

Structure and Function	**PRACTICE**
	Provide the missing term(s) to complete the following sentences.
cranial nerves [KRĀ-nē-ăl nĕrvz] **spinal nerves**	The peripheral nerve system includes 12 pairs of _____ that carry impulses to and from the brain and 31 pairs of _____ that carry messages to and from the spinal cord and the torso and extremities of the body.
	The 31 pairs of spinal nerves are grouped according to the segments of the spinal cord out of which they extend. The peripheral nerves are further divided into two subsystems—the somatic and autonomic nervous systems—according to their function.
somatic nervous system [sō-MĂT-ĭk]	Nerves of the _____ receive and process sensory input from the skin, muscles, tendons, joints, eyes, tongue, nose, and ears. They also excite the voluntary contraction of skeletal muscles.
autonomic nervous system [ăw-tō-NŎM-ĭk]	Nerves of the _____ carry impulses from the central nervous system to glands, various smooth (involuntary) muscles, cardiac muscle, and various membranes. The autonomic nervous system stimulates organs, glands, and senses by stimulating secretions of various substances.
sympathetic nervous system [sĭm-pă-THĔT-ĭk] **parasympathetic nervous system** [păr-ă-sĭm-pă-THĔT-ĭk]	The autonomic nervous system is further divided into the _____ and the _____. In general, the two systems play opposite roles. The sympathetic system operates when the body is awakening, increasing activity, or under stress. It helps to activate responses necessary to react to sudden changes in activity level or to dangerous or abnormal situations. These nerves control the "fight or flight" reaction to stress. This means it tells the body when to fight back or to flee in dangerous situations. The parasympathetic system, on the other hand, operates to keep the body in homeostasis, or balance, under normal conditions, as in the "rest and digest" activity of the body.

SPELL and DEFINE	Identify if the following terms are spelled correctly. Correct the words that are spelled incorrectly. Write the definition for each word.

	Spelling	Definition
perismpathatic		
autonamitic		
somatic		
sympathetic		
cranial		

Build Your Medical Vocabulary: Match the word on the left with its function on the right.

1. _____ Somatic nervous system
2. _____ Autonomic nervous system
3. _____ Sympathetic nervous system
4. _____ Parasympathetic nervous system
5. _____ Cranial nerve

a. Promotes homeostasis
b. Carries impulses to and from the brain
c. Excites voluntary contraction of skeletal muscles
d. Stimulates secretions
e. Fight or flight

APPLY **Read the following scenario and answer the question.**

Mrs. Gina Jones comes to the physician's office and states that every time she gets into a stressful situation, she notices her heart rate increases, her respiratory rate increases, and she begins to sweat. She is concerned that she has a psychological disorder and needs some medication. As the nurse, how will you respond to Mrs. Jones?

_____
_____
_____

LO 7.2 Word Building in the Nervous System

Word Building	PRACTICE
	Provide the correct combining form to complete each of the following sentences.
encephal-itis [ĕn-sĕf-ă-LĪ-tĭs]	Inflammation of the brain is _____ itis.
vag-otomy [vă-GŎT-ō-mē]	Surgical severing of the vagus nerve is _____ otomy.
cerebell-itis [sĕr-ĕ-bĕl-Ī-tĭs]	Inflammation of the cerebellum is _____ itis.
gangli-form [GANG-glē-fōrm]	Having the shape of a ganglion is _____ form.
ventricul-itis [ven-trik-ū-LĪ-tĭs]	Inflammation of the ventricles of the brain is _____ itis.
neur-itis [nū-RĪ-tĭs]	_____ itis is inflammation of a nerve.
cranio-facial [KRĀ-nē-ō-FĀ-shăl]	Relating to the face and the cranium is _____ facial.
myelo-malacia [MĪ-ĕ-lō-ma-LĀ-shē-ă]	Softening of the spinal cord is _____ malacia.
glio-matosis [glī-ō-mă-TŌ-sĭs]	_____ matosis is abnormal growth of neuroglia in the brain or spinal column.
thalamo-tomy [thal-ă-MOT-ō-mē]	_____ tomy is an incision into the thalamus to destroy a portion causing or transmitting sensations of pain.
ceph-algia [se-FAL-jē-ă]	Pain in the head is _____ algia.
meningo-cele [mĕ-NĬNG-gō-sēl]	A _____ cele is a protrusion of the spinal meninges above the surface of the skin.

PRONOUNCE and DEFINE	Pronounce the following terms aloud and write their meaning in the space provided.
gliomatosis	[glī-ō-mă-TŌ-sĭs]
ventriculitis	[ven-trik-ū-LĪ-tĭs]
gangliform	[GANG-glē-fōrm]
craniofacial	[KRĀ-nē-ō-FĀ-shăl]
encephalitis	[ĕn-sĕf-ă-LĪ-tĭs]

SPELL and DEFINE	Identify if the following terms are spelled correctly. Correct the words that are spelled incorrectly. Write the definition for each word.	
	Spelling	Definition
meninxes		
thalomus		
ganoglia		
gyri		
synapse		

UNDERSTAND — Fill in the blanks.

1. The brain and spinal cord are protected by three layers of meninges. Name the three layers in order from inside the skull to the brain and describe the structure of each.
   a. _____
   b. _____
   c. _____
2. Neuron structures that conduct nerve impulses away from the cell body are called _____.
3. The spinal cord connects to the brain at the _____.
4. The part of the brain with two hemispheres is called the _____.
5. The part of the brainstem that controls certain respiratory functions is called the _____.
6. The deep portion of the brain is called the _____.
7. The bony structure protecting the brain is the _____.
8. Ventricles hold _____.

APPLY — Read the following scenario and answer the questions.

In the past few months, Jose Gutierrez has been having trouble buttoning his shirts and remembering things. He also has developed a limp. Dr. Chin orders some tests. Mr. Gutierrez has no history of cerebrovascular accident (CVA) or stroke but is experiencing numbness in his fingers and has some difficulty walking. Dr. Stanley will test for CVA, but because Mr. Gutierrez has a history of normal blood pressure, he suspects another disorder.

1. Mr. Gutierrez has some new problems. According to his symptoms, what areas of his body might have been affected by some disorder? _____
2. What nerves might affect Mr. Gutierrez's walking? _____

STUDY TIP

If you missed any of the answers in this set of exercises, go back and rewrite them until all have been completed correctly.

LO 7.3 Diagnostic, Procedural, and Laboratory Terms

Diagnostic, procedure, and laboratory findings assist the physician in diagnosing medical conditions. Often used in combination, these tests lead to a final diagnosis and assist in treatment planning. Figure 7-8 shows an electroencephalogram (EEG). Figure 7-9 depicts a brain scan showing the effects of cocaine (blue) on the normal brain (yellow).

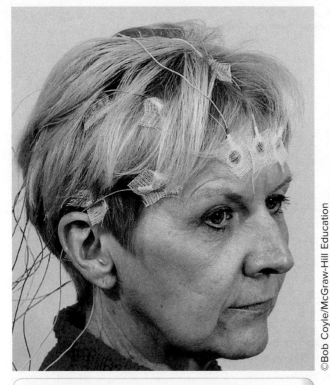

©Bob Coyle/McGraw-Hill Education

Figure 7-8 An electroencephalogram (EEG)

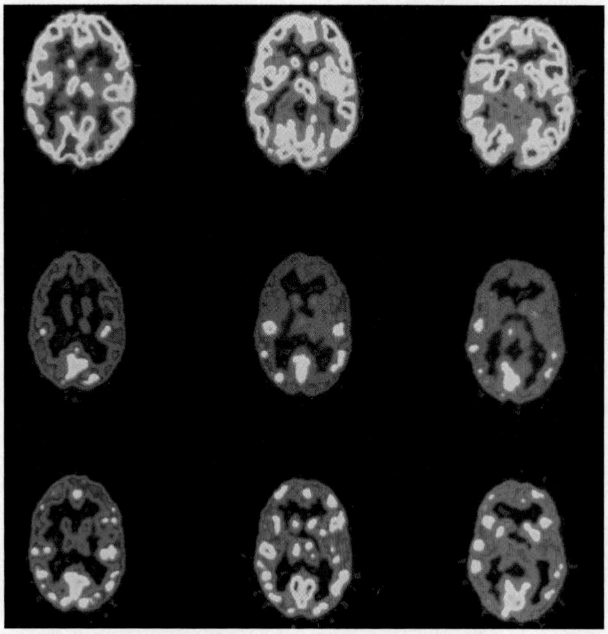

©Brookhaven National Laboratory/Getty Images

Figure 7-9 A brain scan showing the effects of cocaine

Diagnostic	**PRACTICE**
	Provide the missing term(s) to complete the following sentences.
electroencephalogram (EEG) [ē-LĔK-trō-ĕn-SĔF-ă-lō-grăm]	Many of the diagnostic tests used to examine the nervous system include electrodiagnostic procedures. An _____ is a record of the electrical impulses of the brain. This record can detect abnormalities that signal certain neurological conditions.
nerve conduction velocity	Peripheral nervous system diseases can sometimes be detected by shocking the peripheral nerves and timing the conductivity of the shock. This procedure is called _____.
polysomnography (PSG) [PŎL-ē-sŏm-NŎG-ră-fē]	_____ is a recording of electrical and movement patterns during sleep to diagnose sleep disorders, such as *sleep apnea,* a dangerous breathing disorder.
	Various types of imaging are used to visualize the structures of the brain and spinal cord. *Magnetic resonance imaging (MRI)* is the use of magnetic fields and radio waves to visualize structures. *Magnetic resonance angiography (MRA)* is the imaging of blood vessels to detect various abnormalities. *Intracranial MRA* is the visualizing of the head to check for aneurysms and other abnormalities. *Extracranial MRA* is the imaging of the neck to check the carotid artery for abnormalities.

continued on next page

Diagnostic	PRACTICE
	Provide the missing term(s) to complete the following sentences.
SPECT (single-photon emission computed tomography) brain scan **PET (positron emission tomography) scan** [pĕt (PŎZ-Ĭ-trŏn ē-MĬ-shŭn tō-MŎG-ră-fē)]	_____ is a procedure that produces brain images using radioactive isotopes. _____ is a procedure that produces brain images using radioactive isotopes and tomography. It gives highly accurate images of the brain structures and physiology and can provide diagnoses of various brain disorders.
computerized (axial) tomography (CT or CAT) scan [(ĂKS-ē-ăl) tō-MŎG-ră-fē]	_____ uses tomography to show cross-sectional radiographic images.
myelogram [MĪ-ĕ-lō-grăm] **cerebral angiogram** [SĔR-ĕ-brăl AN-jē-ō-gram]	X-rays are used to diagnose specific malformations or disorders. A _____ is an x-ray of the spinal cord after a contrast medium is injected. A _____ is an x-ray of the brain's blood vessels after a contrast medium is injected.
encephalogram [ĕn-SĔF-ă-lō-grăm]	*Encephalography* is the radiographic study of the ventricles of the brain. The record made by this study is called an _____.
transcranial sonogram [trănz-KRĀ-nē-ăl SŎN-ō-grăm]	Sound waves are used to create brain images in a _____ for diagnosing and managing head and stroke trauma. Ultrasound also is used in *echoencephalography,* encephalography using ultrasound waves.
reflex [RĒ-flĕks] **Babinski reflex** [bă-BĬN-skē]	A _____ is an involuntary muscular contraction in response to a stimulus. Reflex testing can aid in the diagnosis of certain nervous system disorders. The _____ is a reflex on the plantar surface of the foot.
lumbar (spinal) puncture [LŬM-băr PŬNK-choor]	Cerebrospinal fluid that has been withdrawn from between two lumbar vertebrae during a _____ can be studied for the presence of various substances, which may indicate certain diseases.

STUDY TIP

The Babinski reflex occurs when the great toe flexes toward the top of the foot and the other toes fan out when the sole of the foot has been stroked. This is normal in very young children, but in clients older than age two, it indicates damage to the nerve pathways.

STUDY TIP

Clients with a suspected concussion should be watched to make sure there is no change in their level of consciousness. This change could lead to an unconscious state (coma).

PRONOUNCE and DEFINE	Pronounce the following terms aloud and write their meaning in the space provided.
electroencephalogram	[ē-LĔK-trō-ĕn-SĔF-ă-lō-grăm]
myelogram	[MĪ-ĕ-lō-grăm]
encephalogram	[ĕn-SĔF-ă-lō-grăm]
reflex	[RĒ-flĕks]
Babinski	[bă-BĬN-skē]

SPELL and DEFINE	Identify if the following terms are spelled correctly, Correct the words that are spelled incorrectly. Write the definition for each word.	
	Spelling	Definition
babenskez		
reflecks		
mylogram		
polysomnography		
transcranial sonagram		

UNDERSTAND Circle the correct answer.

1. A myelogram is an x-ray of the **spinal cord/neck.**
2. Reflexes are **voluntary/involuntary** muscular contractions.
3. An encephalogram is a record of a study of the **spinal cord/brain ventricles.**
4. A lumbar puncture removes **blood/cerebral spinal fluid.**
5. PET is an extremely accurate **imaging/laboratory** system.
6. Reflexes are caused by **electrical waves/stimulation.**

APPLY   Read the following scenario and answer the questions.

Dr. Stanley orders an electroencephalogram of Mr. Gutierrez's brain. He also orders some additional blood tests. Dr. Stanley performs a number of reflex tests. The abnormalities he finds confirm his initial suspicion of Parkinson disease. He prescribes several medications and schedules a visit for Mr. Gutierrez in three weeks to discuss his progress. He asks Mr. Gutierrez to keep a daily log of his walking ability, any vision changes, his speech, and tremors for the three weeks until his appointment.

1. Why does Dr. Stanley want Mr. Gutierrez to keep a log? _____

_____

2. What might Mr. Gutierrez's abnormal reflex tests indicate? _____

_____

LO 7.4 Pathological Terms

Trauma and Congenital Disorders

Trauma and congenital disorders can affect the nervous system. Some conditions, depending on severity, may affect a person throughout his or her lifespan.

Pathological	PRACTICE
	Provide the missing term(s) to complete the following sentences.
	Some neurological disorders are caused by **trauma.** Although bones, cerebrospinal fluid, and the meninges protect the nervous system from most types of external trauma, they cannot protect against everything. The blood–brain barrier protects the brain from most infectious diseases.
concussion [kŏn-KŬSH-ŭn] **coma** [KŌ-mă]	A _____ is an injury to the brain from an impact with an object. Cerebral concussions usually clear within 24 hours. Concussions may be followed by nausea, disorientation, dizziness, and/or vomiting. A severe concussion can lead to _____, an abnormally deep sleep with little or no response to stimuli. Coma also can result from other causes, such as stroke.
brain contusion [kŏn-TŪ-zhŭn]	A more serious trauma than concussion is a _____, a bruising of the surface of the brain without penetration into the brain. Brain contusions can result in extreme disorientation, listlessness, and even death.
	Traumatic injury, as during a car accident, also may cause the brain to hit the skull and then to rebound to the other side of the skull. This is called a *closed head trauma* because there is no penetration of the skull. *Shaken baby syndrome* is a severe form of closed head trauma in which a young child experiences head trauma (as a result of falling, being shaken, or other trauma), causing the brain to hit the sides of the skull and creating potentially fatal damage.
	A *subdural hematoma* (between the dura mater and the arachnoid or at the base of the dura mater) is a tumorlike collection of blood often caused by trauma.
	Injuries that result in penetration of the brain through the skull are usually extremely serious and often fatal. Depending on the degree of penetration and the place penetrated, permanent brain damage may result.
	Congenital disorders of the brain or spinal cord can be devastating and have an impact on the activities of daily living.
spina bifida [SPĪ-nă BĬF-ĭ-dă] **meningocele** [mĕ-NĬNG-gō-sēl] **meningomyelocele** [mĕ-nĭng-gō-MĪ-ĕ-lō-sēl]	_____ is a defect in the spinal column (Figure 7-10). *Spina bifida occulta* is a covered lesion of the vertebra that is generally visible only by x-ray. This is the least severe form of spina bifida. *Spina bifida cystica* is a more severe form of the condition, usually with a _____ (protrusion of the spinal meninges above the surface of the skin) or a _____ (protrusion of the meninges and spinal cord).
Tay-Sachs disease [TĀ-săks]	_____ is a hereditary disease found primarily in the descendants of Eastern European Jews. It is a genetic disease characterized by an enzyme deficiency that causes deterioration in the central nervous system's cells.
hydrocephalus [hī-drō-SĔF-ă-lŭs]	_____ is an overproduction of fluid in the brain. It usually occurs at birth (although it can occur in adults with infections or tumors) and is treated with a shunt placed from the ventricle of the brain to the peritoneal space to relieve pressure by draining fluid.

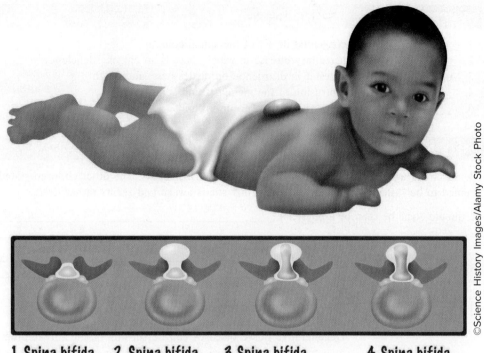

1. Spina bifida occulta 2. Spina bifida with meningocele 3. Spina bifida with meningomyelocele 4. Spina bifida with myeloschisis

Figure 7-10 Types of spina bifida

PRONOUNCE and DEFINE	Pronounce the following terms aloud and write their meaning in the space provided.
spina bifida	[SPĪ-nă BĬF-ĭ-dă]
Tay-Sachs	[TĀ-săks]
hydrocephalus	[hī-drō-SĚF-ă-lŭs]
concussion	[kŏn-KŬSH-ŭn]
contusion	[kŏn-TŪ-zhŭn]

SPELL and DEFINE	Identify if the following terms are spelled correctly. Correct the words that are spelled incorrectly. Write the definition for each word.	
	Spelling	**Definition**
Taysacks		
hydrocefales		
meningomyelocele		
encefalgram		
contuson		

Fill in the blanks.

1. _____ is a congenital defect of the spinal column.
2. _____ is a hereditary disease in which there is an enzyme deficiency.
3. A _____ can result in disorientation, listlessness, and death.
4. _____ is a protrusion of the meninges and spinal cord.
5. _____ is treated with a shunt to drain fluid.

Read the following scenario and answer the questions.

Josie Martin, age 9 years, fell off the 14-foot slide during recess. The other children stated that after the fall, she seemed to be "asleep" for a moment. Currently she is awake and seems rather tired.

1. Should Josie be seen by a physician? _____

_____

2. Why should there be a concern regarding this fall? _____

_____

Degenerative Nerve Diseases

Degenerative nerve diseases can be serious or life threatening. Some degenerative diseases may be genetic in cause or occur with the aging process, and some are due to lifestyle choices. Oftentimes, there is no cure; the goal is to address symptoms, decrease pain, and keep the client mobile. The following table includes terms associated with degenerative diseases and the nervous system.

Pathological	PRACTICE Provide the missing term(s) to complete the following sentences.
dementia [dē-MĔN-shē-ă] **Alzheimer disease** [ĂLTS-hī-mĕr] **amnesia** [ăm-NĒ-zē-ă] **apraxia** [ă-PRĂK-sē-ă] **agnosia** [ăg-NŌ-zē-ă]	Degenerative diseases of the central nervous system can affect almost any part of the body. Deterioration in mental capacity is found in _____ and _____, a progressive degeneration of neurons in the brain, eventually leading to death. Some symptoms that worsen as Alzheimer disease progresses are _____ (loss of memory), _____ (inability to properly use familiar objects), and _____ (inability to receive and understand outside stimuli).
amyotrophic lateral sclerosis (ALS) [ă-mī-ō-TRŌ-fĭk LĂT-ĕr-ăl sklĕ-RŌ-sĭs] **Lou Gehrig disease** [GĔR-ĭg]	_____ is a degenerative disease of the motor neurons leading to loss of muscular control and death. It is also known as _____.
Huntington chorea [kōr-Ē-ă]	Several other degenerative diseases are not necessarily fatal. _____ is a hereditary disease with uncontrollable jerking movements and progressive loss of neural control.
multiple sclerosis (MS) [MŬL-tĭ-pŭl sklĕ-RŌ-sĭs] **demyelination** [dē-MĪ-ĕ-lĭ-NĀ-shŭn] **gait** [gāt] **paresthesia** [pār-ĕs-THĒ-zē-ă]	_____ is the destruction of the myelin sheath, a process called _____, leading to muscle weakness, unsteady _____ (walking), _____ (odd sensations, such as tingling, stinging, etc.), extreme fatigue, and some paralysis. In certain cases, it can lead to death.

myasthenia gravis [mī-ăs-THĒ-nē-ă GRĂV-ĭs]	_____, a disease with muscle weakness, can be treated to avoid the overproduction of antibodies that block neurotransmitters from sending proper nerve impulses to skeletal muscles.
Parkinson disease [PAR-kin-sŏn] dopamine [DŌ-pă-mēn]	_____, a degeneration of nerves in the brain, causes tremors, weakness of muscles, and difficulty in walking. It is treated with drugs that increase the levels of _____ in the brain. Treatment helps relieve symptoms but does not cure the disease.

PRONOUNCE and DEFINE	Pronounce the following terms aloud and write their meaning in the space provided.
multiple sclerosis (MS)	[MŬL-tĭ-pŭl sklĕ-RŌ-sĭs]
demyelination	[dē-MĪ-ĕ-lĭ-NĀ-shŭn]
gait	[gāt]
paresthesia	[pār-ĕs-THĒ-zē-ă]
chorea	[kōr-Ē-ă]

SPELL and DEFINE	Identify if the following terms are spelled correctly. Correct the words that are spelled incorrectly. Write the definition for each word.	
	Spelling	Definition
dopamine		
demylinashun		
giate		
paresthesia		
myasthenia graves		

UNDERSTAND	Build Your Medical Vocabulary: Match the degenerative disorder on the left with its symptom on the right.

1. _____ Alzheimer disease
2. _____ amnesia
3. _____ agnosia
4. _____ amyotrophic lateral sclerosis
5. _____ apraxia

a. Loss of memory
b. Disease of motor neurons
c. Inability to use familiar objects
d. Deterioration in mental capacity
e. Inability to receive and understand outside stimuli

APPLY	Read the following scenario and answer the question.

Mrs. Amy Shine is 49 years old. She has tested positive for Huntington chorea. She asks the nurse what symptoms will occur and what she needs to do to avoid progression of the disease. How should the nurse respond?

_____

_____

_____

_____

Did you know

Huntington Chorea or Huntington Disease (HD)

Huntington chorea is characterized by jerking, uncontrollable movement of the limbs, trunk, and face (chorea); progressive loss of mental abilities; and the development of psychiatric problems. The disease progresses without remission over 10 to 25 years and patients ultimately are unable to care for themselves. Huntington disease (HD) usually appears between the ages of 30 and 50 but can develop in younger and older people.

HD is a familial disease, passed from parent to child through a mutation in the normal gene. Each child of an HD parent has a 50–50 chance of inheriting the HD gene. If a child does not inherit the HD gene, he or she will not develop the disease and cannot pass it on. A person who inherits the HD gene will sooner or later develop the disease. Whether one child inherits the gene has no bearing on whether others will or will not inherit the gene.

Nondegenerative Nerve Disorders

Severe neurological disorders cause paralysis, convulsions, and other symptoms but are not necessarily degenerative or congenital. This section identifies terms associated with nondegenerative disorders of the nervous system.

Pathological	PRACTICE
	Provide the missing term(s) to complete the following sentences.
palsy [PĂWL-zē] **cerebral palsy** [SĔR-ĕ-brăl PĂWL-zē] **Bell's palsy** [bĕlz PĂWL-zē] **ataxia** [ă-TĂK-sē-ă]	_____ is partial or complete paralysis. _____ includes lack of motor coordination from cerebral damage during gestation or birth. _____ is paralysis of one side of the face. It usually disappears after treatment. _____ is lack of voluntary muscle coordination resulting from disorders of the cerebellum, pons, or spinal cord.
epilepsy [ĔP-ĭ-LĔP-sē] **aura** [ĂW-ră] **absence seizures** [AB-sens SĒ-zhŭrz] **petit mal seizures** [PĔ-tē măhl SĒ-zhŭrz] **tonic-clonic seizures** [TŎN-ĭk-KLŎN-nĭk SĒ-zhŭrz] **grand mal seizures** [grand măhl SĒ-zhŭrz]	_____ is chronic, recurrent seizure activity. This disease has been known since ancient times, when victims were thought to be under the influence of outside forces. Now it is understood that this disease occurs because of abnormal conditions in the brain that cause sudden excessive electrical activity. The seizures caused by this activity can be preceded by an _____, a collection of symptoms felt just before the actual seizure. Seizures may be mild or intense. _____ or _____ are mild and usually include only a momentary disorientation with the environment. _____ or _____ are much more severe and include loss of consciousness, convulsions, and twitching of limbs.

Tourette syndrome [tū-RĔT SĬN-drōm] tics [tĭks]	_____ is a neurological disorder that causes uncontrollable, involuntary sounds and _____ (twitching). Some drugs are helpful in controlling symptoms and allowing sufferers to lead normal lives.

PRONOUNCE and DEFINE	Pronounce the following terms aloud and write their meaning in the space provided.
epilepsy	[ĔP-ĭ-LĔP-sē]
aura	[ĂW-ră]
Tourette	[tū-RĔT]
palsy	[PĂWL-zē]
tics	[tĭks]

SPELL and DEFINE	Identify if the following terms are spelled correctly. Correct the words that are spelled incorrectly. Write the definition for each word.	
	Spelling	**Definition**
tonick klonec		
cerebral palsy		
seezur		
petite mal		
ataxea		

UNDERSTAND	Mark the following statements as true or false.

1. If the client with Tourette syndrome focuses, symptoms will subside. **True** **False**
2. Absence seizures and petit mal seizures are the same. **True** **False**
3. Ataxia may be exhibited as being clumsy while walking. **True** **False**
4. Tics crawl on the skin. **True** **False**
5. During a petit mal seizure the client will exhibit a brief disorientation. **True** **False**

APPLY	Read the following scenario and answer the questions.

Mrs. April Johnson is experiencing a seizure.

1. What should the health care provider observe during the seizure?

_____
_____
_____

2. Why is it important for the health care provider to be able to describe what was observed?

_____
_____
_____

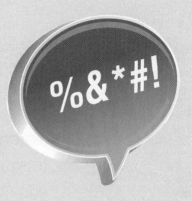
Infections and Inflammations

Infections and inflammations of the nervous system can be very serious, even deadly in some cases. Some of the symptoms of nervous system infections and inflammations may be exhibited as pain and even skin conditions. This section includes major infections and inflammations affecting the nervous system.

Pathological	PRACTICE
	Provide the missing term(s) to complete the following sentences.
shingles [SHĬNG-glz], **meningitis** [mĕ-nĭn-JĪ-tĭs]	Infectious diseases of the nervous system include _____ and _____. Shingles is a viral disease caused by the herpes zoster virus. Its symptoms include pain in the peripheral nerves and blisters on the skin.
pyrogenic meningitis [pī-rō-JĔN-ĭk mĕ-nĭn-JĪ-tĭs] **bacterial meningitis** [bac-TĒR-ē-ăl mĕ-nĭn-JĪ-tĭs] **viral meningitis** [VĪ-răl mĕ-nĭn-JĪ-tĭs]	Several types of meningitis, inflammation of the meninges, can be infectious. _____ (also called _____) is caused by bacteria and includes such symptoms as fever, headache, and stiff neck. It is usually treated with antibiotics. In some severe cases, it can be fatal. _____ is caused by viruses and, although it has the same symptoms as pyrogenic meningitis, it is usually allowed to run its course. Medication can be given for some of the more uncomfortable symptoms (fever, headache).
neuritis [nū-RĪ-tĭs] **myelitis** [mī-ĕ-LĪ-tĭs] **encephalitis** [ĕn-sĕf-ă-LĪ-tĭs] **cerebellitis** [sĕr-ĕ-bĕl-Ī-tĭs] **gangliitis** [găng-glē-Ī-tĭs] **radiculitis** [ră-dĭk-yū-LĪ-tĭs] **sciatica** [sī-ĂT-ĭ-kă]	Inflammation can also occur in the nerves (_____), the spinal cord (_____), the brain (_____), the cerebellum (_____), the ganglion (_____), or the spinal nerve roots (_____). Some specific nerve inflammations, such as _____, cause pain in the area served by the nerve. This is a common cause of lower back and leg pain.

PRONOUNCE and DEFINE	Pronounce the following terms aloud and write their meaning in the space provided.
neuritis	[nū-RĪ-tĭs]
myelitis	[mī-ĕ-LĪ-tĭs]
encephalitis	[ĕn-sĕf-ă-LĪ-tĭs]
cerebellitis	[sĕr-ĕ-bĕl-Ī-tĭs]
gangliitis	[găng-glē-Ī-tĭs]

SPELL and DEFINE	Identify if the following terms are spelled correctly. Correct the words that are spelled incorrectly. Write the definition for each word.	
	Spelling	Definition
progyenic meningitis		
meningitis		
shenglez		
sciatica		
radiculitis		

UNDERSTAND	Break the following terms into its component parts and define each component.
meningitis	
cerebellitis	
myelitis	
gangliitis	
ataxia	
myelomalacia	

APPLY	Read the following scenario and answer the questions.

The physician tells Jaime Shew's family that she has viral meningitis. He states that Jamie's symptoms should subside in a few days.

1. What is viral meningitis?

_____

_____

_____

2. What symptoms is Jaime most likely exhibiting?

_____

_____

_____

3. How is viral meningitis usually treated?

_____

_____

_____

Abnormal Growths

STUDY TIP

Don't forget to update your flash cards.

About one-third of all brain tumors are growths that spread from cancers in other parts of the body (lungs, breasts, skin, etc.). The remaining tumors can be benign or malignant. In either case, the pressure and the distortion of the brain caused by the tumor may result in many other neurological symptoms. This section presents abnormal growths relating to the nervous system.

Pathological	PRACTICE
	Provide the missing term(s) to complete the following sentences.
glioma [glī-Ō-mă] **meningioma** [mĕ-NĬN-jē-Ō-mă] **astrocytoma** [ĂS-trō-sī-TŌ-mă] **oligodendroglioma** [ŎL-ĭ-gō-DĔN-drō-glī-Ō-mă] **glioblastoma multiforme** [GLĪ-ō-blăs-TŌ-mă MŬL-tĭ-fŏrm]	_____ (tumors that arise from neuroglia) and _____ (tumors that arise from the meninges) can be either benign or malignant. Both may be removed surgically. _____, _____, and _____ are all types of gliomas, with the latter being the most malignant. Tumors can be treated surgically if they have not infiltrated or affected certain essential areas of the brain. Radiation and medication may be used to try to reduce tumor growth.
ganglion [GĂNG-glē-ŏn]	Some nontumorous growths can cause pain from pressure on nerves. A _____ is any group of nerve cells bunched together to form a growth or cyst, usually arising from a wrist tendon.

PRONOUNCE and DEFINE	Pronounce the following terms aloud and write their meaning in the space provided.
oligodendroglioma	[ŎL-ĭ-gō-DĔN-drō-glī-Ō-mă]
glioblastoma multiforme	[GLĪ-ō-blăs-TŌ-mă MŬL-tĭ-fŏrm]
glioma	[glī-Ō-mă]
meningioma	[mĕ-NĬN-jē-Ō-mă]
astrocytoma	[ĂS-trō-sī-TŌ-mă]

SPELL and DEFINE	Identify if the following terms are spelled correctly. Correct the words that are spelled incorrectly. Write the definition for each word.	
	Spelling	**Definition**
gleeoblastoma multaiform		
ganglion		
meninioma		
astrositomia		

UNDERSTAND	Break the following terms into its component parts and define each component.
meningioma	
glioblastoma	
oligodendroglioma	
astrocytoma	

APPLY	Answer the following question.

Discuss why the size of tumors within the nervous system is important.

_____

_____

_____

_____

Vascular Disorders

Vascular disorders in the nervous system can cause significant changes in a person's lifestyle. Depending on the severity, vascular disorders can be deadly. This section presents vascular disorders that can affect the nervous system.

Pathological	PRACTICE
	Provide the missing term(s) to complete the following sentences.
cerebrovascular accident (CVA) [SĔR-ĕ-brō-VĂS-kyū-lăr] **stroke** [strōk] **cerebral infarction** [SĔR-ĕ-brăl ĭn-FĂRK-shŭn] **thrombus** [THRŎM-bŭs] **occlusion** [ō-KLŪ-zhŭn] **thrombotic stroke** [thrŏm-BŎT-ĭk strōk]	Vascular problems, such as *arteriosclerosis,* may cause a _____, a disruption in the normal blood supply to the brain. Various types of _____ (_____) result from this disruption. A _____ (stationary blood clot) may cause _____ (blocking of a blood vessel), which in turn may cause a _____.
transient ischemic attacks (TIAs) [ĭs-KĒ-mĭk] **embolic stroke** [ĕm-BŎL-ĭk strōk] **embolus** [ĔM-bō-lŭs]	As the blockage grows, the person may experience milder symptoms before a major stroke. These short incidents are known as _____. They may be symptomless or may cause brief disorientation and speech and motor difficulty. An _____ is caused by an _____, a clot that travels from somewhere in the body to the cerebral arteries and blocks a small vessel, causing a sudden stroke.
hemorrhagic stroke [hĕm-ō-RĂJ-ĭk strōk] **aneurysm** [ĂN-yū-rĭzm]	A _____ is caused by blood escaping from a damaged cerebral artery. It may be caused by sudden trauma or an _____, bursting of the wall of an artery after abnormal widening or weakening.

continued on next page

Pathological	**PRACTICE**
	Provide the missing term(s) to complete the following sentences.
dysphasia [dĭs-FĀ-zē-ă] **aphasia** [ă-FĀ-zē-ă]	Strokes can be mild and result in complete recovery, or they can range from mild to severe, with symptoms that remain permanently. Common symptoms are thought disorders, _____ (speech difficulty), _____ (loss of speech), loss of muscular control, some paralysis, and disorientation. (Note that dysphasia is different from *dysphagia,* difficulty in swallowing, discussed in Chapter 14.)
fainting [FĀNT-ĭng] **syncope** [SĬN-kŏ-pē] **somnolence** [SŎM-nō-lĕns] **narcolepsy** [NĂR-kō-lĕp-sē]	Some states of consciousness are changed by lack of oxygen or brain abnormalities that affect the flow of blood and oxygen to the brain. _____ or _____ is caused by lack of oxygen to the brain. _____ (extreme sleepiness) and _____ (uncontrollable, sudden lapses into deep sleep) are altered states of consciousness.

PRONOUNCE and DEFINE	Pronounce the following terms aloud and write their meaning in the space provided.
somnolence	[SŎM-nō-lĕns]
narcolepsy	[NĂR-kō-lĕp-sē]
aneurysm	[ĂN-yū-rĭzm]
embolus	[ĔM-bō-lŭs]
cerebrovascular	[SĔR-ĕ-brō-VĂS-kyū-lăr]

SPELL and DEFINE	Identify if the following terms are spelled correctly. Correct the words that are spelled incorrectly. Write the definition for each word.	
	Spelling	**Definition**
afaszea		
desfaszea		
anurism		
thrombic strok		
syncope		

UNDERSTAND	Complete each sentence by filling in the blanks with the correct term.

1. Uncontrollable, sudden lapse into a deep sleep is called _____.
2. Extreme sleepiness is known as _____.
3. The medical term for speech difficulty is _____.
4. A stationary blood clot is called a(n) _____.
5. A blood clot that moves is called a(n) _____.

From the Perspective Of . . .

Who: Registered Nurse

Other Aliases: Office Nurse, Clinical Care Coordinator, Lead Nurse, RN, Charge Nurse, Hospice Nurse, Clinical Administrator

Job Duties: Obtaining vital signs; assessing patient status; gathering health histories, allergies, and medications. The registered nurse assists the physician with procedures and provides care for the patient after treatment and educates the patient on side effects and disease/conditions. Often, the RN is a lead administrator in many cases and is able to provide other services available to the patient, including specialty care.

That is why medical terminology is important to me.

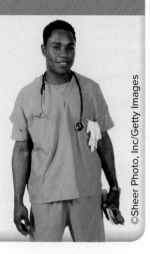
©Sheer Photo, Inc/Getty Images

LO 7.5 Surgical Terms

Surgery is performed on the nervous system to treat a variety of diseases and disorders. Surgery on the nervous system is always high risk due to the potential for permanent injury. This section presents terms relating to surgery and the nervous system.

Surgical	PRACTICE Provide the missing term(s) to complete the following sentences.
neurosurgeons [nūr-ō-SĔR-jŭnz]	_____ are the specialists who perform surgery on the brain and spinal cord. Neurosurgery is considered high risk because the potential for permanent injury is great. When some brain diseases, such as epilepsy, do not respond well to drugs, they may, in extreme cases, require surgery.
lobectomy [lō-BĔK-tō-mē] **lobotomy** [lō-BŎT-ō-mē]	A _____ is removal of a portion of the brain to treat epilepsy and other disorders, such as brain cancer. A _____, severing of nerves in the frontal lobe of the brain, was once considered a primary method for treating mental illness. Now it is rarely used. Laser surgery to destroy damaged parts of the brain is also used to treat some neurological disorders.
craniectomy [krā-nē-ĔK-tō-mē] **craniotomy** [krā-nē-ŎT-ō-mē] **stereotaxy** [stĕr-ē-ō-TĂK-sē] **stereotactic surgery** [stĕr-ē-ō-TĂK-tĭk SER-jer-ē]	When it is necessary to operate directly on the brain (as in the case of a tumor), a _____, removal of part of the skull, or a _____, incision into the skull, may be performed. _____ or _____ is the destruction of deep-seated brain structures using three-dimensional coordinates to locate the structures.
neuroplasty [NŪR-ō-PLĂS-tē] **neurectomy** [nū-RĔK-tō-mē] **neurotomy** [nū-RŎT-ō-mē] **neurorrhaphy** [nūr-ŌR-ă-fē] **vagotomy** [vā-GŎT-ō-mē]	_____ is the surgical repair of a nerve. _____ is the surgical removal of a nerve. A _____ is the dissection of a nerve. A _____ is the suturing of a severed nerve. A _____ is the severing of the vagus nerve to relieve pain.

PRONOUNCE and DEFINE	Pronounce the following terms aloud and write their meaning in the space provided.
neuroplasty	[NŪR-ō-PLĂS-tē]
neurectomy	[nū-RĔK-tō-mē]
neurotomy	[nū-RŎT-ō-mē]
neurorrhaphy	[nūr-ŌR-ă-fē]
vagotomy	[vă-GŎT-ō-mē]

SPELL and DEFINE	Identify if the following terms are spelled correctly. Correct the words that are spelled incorrectly. Write the definition for each word.	
	Spelling	Definition
nurwrecktome		
nuroplastie		
stereotakie		
lobaotomie		
stereotactic		

UNDERSTAND	Complete each sentence by filling in the blanks with the correct term.

1. Cutting the vagus nerve for pain relief is called _____.
2. The incision into the frontal lobe is called a(n) _____.
3. The removal of a portion of the brain is called a(n) _____.
4. Suturing of a severed nerve is _____.
5. Removal of a nerve is _____.
6. Repair of a nerve is _____.
7. Vagotomy is severing the _____ nerve.
8. "A specialist that performs neurological surgery is a _____".

APPLY	Read the following scenario and answer the questions.

Mr. Randy Allen was injured in a car accident 3 years ago. At that time, he experienced some nerve damage in his leg. A neurosurgeon was called in to see if she could repair enough of the leg nerves to allow Mr. Allen to walk. She operated, and the results were mixed. Mr. Allen experienced improvement with his walking after undergoing physical therapy.

1. The damaged leg nerves could actually be a result of an injury elsewhere in the body. What particular nerves or areas might the neurosurgeon examine before determining exactly where to operate?

_____

_____

2. Why was physical therapy ordered for Mr. Allen?

_____

_____

LO 7.6 Pharmacological Terms

Medications may be used to treat neurological disorders and diseases. Many neurological medications may treat more than one neurological disorder.

STUDY TIP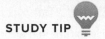

Have a friend quiz you over the terms and their correct spelling.

Pharmacological

PRACTICE

Provide the missing term(s) to complete the following sentences.

analgesics
[ăn-ăl-JĒ-zĭks]
anticonvulsants
[ĂN-tē-kŏn-VŬL-sănts]
narcotics
[năr-KŎT-ĭks]
sedatives [SĔD-ă-tĭvz]
hypnotics [hĭp-NŎT-ĭks]
anesthetics
[ăn-ĕs-THĔT-ĭks]

The nervous system can be the site of severe pain. _____ relieve pain. Other problems of the nervous system may be associated with diseases such as epilepsy. _____ are often used to treat epilepsy and other disorders to lessen or prevent convulsions. _____ relieve pain by inducing a stuporous or euphoric state. _____ and _____ relax the nerves and sometimes induce sleep. _____ block feelings or sensation and are used in surgery. They can be given *locally* (to numb sensation to one section of the body) or *generally* (to numb sensation to the entire body).

PRONOUNCE and DEFINE

Pronounce the following terms aloud and write their meaning in the space provided.

analgesics	[ăn-ăl-JĒ-zĭks]
anticonvulsant	[ĂN-tē-kŏn-VŬL-sănt]
hypnotic	[hĭp-NŎT-ĭk]
sedatives	[SĔD-ă-tĭvz]
anesthetics	[ăn-ĕs-THĔT-ĭks]

SPELL and DEFINE

Identify if the following terms are spelled correctly. Correct the words that are spelled incorrectly. Write the definition for each word.

	Spelling	Definition
narkotic		
sedative		
anethetick		
hipnotik		
analgesic		

UNDERSTAND

Complete each sentence by filling in the blanks with the correct term.

1. An agent that induces sleep is called a(n) _____.
2. An agent that relieves nervousness is called a(n) _____.
3. An agent that causes loss of feeling is called a(n) _____.
4. A drug prescribed for epilepsy is probably a(n) _____.
5. Pain is relieved with a(n) _____ without mind altering effects (or without inducing a euphoric state).
6. A pain reliever that induces a euphoric state is a(n) _____.

Read the following scenario and answer the question.

Pain management is a delicate art. Physicians have to consider the addictive nature and strong side effects of many painkillers while making the patient comfortable enough to recover. Many physicians and medical ethicists have endorsed the unlimited use of pain medication for those with terminal diseases. Pain management is an important medical practice because pain itself can be so debilitating. What might explain the reluctance of some practitioners to allow unlimited painkillers?

_____

_____

LO 7.7 Abbreviations

ABBREVIATION REVIEW

Abbreviation	Definition
ALS	amyotrophic lateral sclerosis
CNS	central nervous system
CSF	cerebrospinal fluid
CVA	cerebrovascular accident
EEG	electroencephalogram
ICP	intracranial pressure
MRA	magnetic resonance angiography
MRI	magnetic resonance imaging
PNS	peripheral nervous system
SCI	spinal cord injury
TENS	transcutaneous electrical nerve stimulation
TIA	transient ischemic attack

UNDERSTAND | Identify the abbreviation for the following terms.

1. electroencephalogram: _____
2. amyotrophic lateral sclerosis: _____
3. magnetic resonance angiography: _____
4. spinal cord injury: _____
5. cerebrospinal fluid: _____

APPLY | Read the following scenario and rewrite using appropriate medical terms.

Mr. Jones presents to the emergency department after a motor vehicle accident. Experienced TIA last week; may now have a CVA. Will evaluate for SCI and get MRI, MRA, and EEG. Concerned ICP is elevated. May have a CSF leak.

_____

_____

_____

Chapter Review

CHAPTER SUMMARY

	Learning Outcome	Summary
7.1	Identify the parts of the nervous system and discuss the function of each part.	The nervous system directs the function of all the human body systems. The nervous system is divided into two subsystems: the *central nervous system* and the *peripheral nervous system*.
7.2	Recall the major word parts used in building words that relate to the nervous system.	Word building requires knowledge of the combining form and meaning.
7.3	Identify the common diagnostic tests, laboratory tests, and clinical procedures used in testing and treating disorders of the nervous system.	Diagnostic, procedural, and laboratory findings assist the health care provider in diagnosing medical conditions. Often used in combination, these tests lead to a final diagnosis and assist in treatment planning.
7.4	Define the major pathological conditions of the nervous system.	Pathological conditions of the nervous system can include trauma and congenital disorders, degenerative and nondegenerative conditions such as paralysis and convulsions, infections, inflammations, vascular disorders, tumors, and growths.
7.5	Explain the meaning of surgical terms related to the nervous system.	Surgery is performed on the nervous system to treat a variety of diseases and disorders. Surgery on the nervous system is always high risk due to the potential for permanent injury.
7.6	Recognize common pharmacological agents used in treating disorders of the nervous system.	Medications may be used to treat neurological disorders and diseases. Many neurological medications may treat more than one neurological disorder.
7.7	Identify common abbreviations associated with the nervous system.	Abbreviations are commonly used to describe disease, diagnostic procedures, and treatments of the nervous system.

1. Label the parts of the brain.

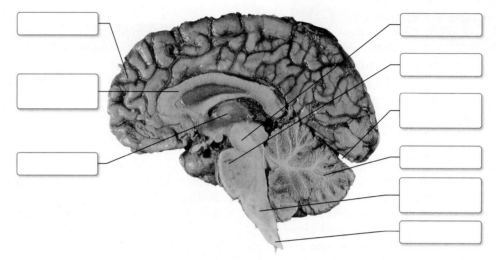

©Martin M. Rotker/Science Source

2. Label the following parts of the spine.

a. Lumbar nerves
b. Sacral nerves
c. Cervical nerves
d. Thoracic nerves
e. Coccygeal nerves

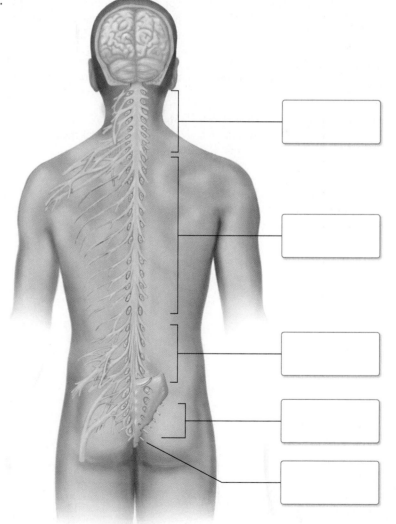

Posterior view

Pronounce the following terms aloud.

anesthetic	[ăn-ĕs-THĔT-ĭk]
acetylcholine	[ăs-ĕ-tĭl-KŌ-lēn]
convolutions	[kŏn-vō-LŪ-shŭnz]
efferent	[ĔF-ĕr-ĕnt]
neurorrhaphy	[nūr-ŌR-ă-fē]
encephalogram	[ĕn-SĔF-ă-lō-grăm]
Alzheimer	[ĂLTS-hī-mĕr]
ventricle	[VĔN-trĭ-kl]
dopamine	[DŌ-pă-mēn]

Identify if all of the following terms are spelled correctly.

axion	nuroplastie	paristhesha
neurietisu	thalamus	occlusion
microalagia	radiculitis	norepinephrine
dincfalone		

Match the definition in the right-hand column to the correct word in the left-hand column.

1. _____ neuroglia		a. Gray matter
2. _____ meninges		b. Weblike meningeal layer
3. _____ neuron		c. Internal chemical
4. _____ acetylcholine		d. Cell that does not transmit impulses
5. _____ excitability		e. Fissures
6. _____ ventricle		f. Area between pia mater and spinal bones
7. _____ basal ganglia		g. Responsiveness to stimuli
8. _____ sulci		h. Protective membranes
9. _____ arachnoid		i. Cell that transmits impulses
10. _____ epidural space		j. Cavity for fluid

Find at least two nervous system combining forms in each word. Write the combining forms and their definitions in the space provided.

1. encephalomyelitis: _____
2. craniomeningocele: _____
3. glioneuroma: _____
4. cerebromeningitis: _____
5. spinoneural: _____
6. neuroencephalomyelopathy: _____

Add the combining form that completes the word.

1. Acting upon the vagus nerve: _____ tropic
2. Tumor consisting of ganglionic neurons: ganglio _____ oma
3. Myxoma containing glial cells: _____ myxoma
4. Relating to nerves and meninges: neuro _____ eal

Break the word apart and define the combining form that relates to the nervous system.

1. parencephalia: _____
2. angioneurectomy: _____
3. cephalomegaly: _____
4. myelitis: _____
5. meningocyte: _____
6. neurocyte: _____
7. craniomalacia: _____
8. vagotropic: _____
9. glioblast: _____
10. cerebrosclerosis: _____

DECONSTRUCT

Steven Phillps has complained of a headache for the last month. He states that he is not sleeping well and the headache is almost constant. After checking Steven's reflexes, including the Babinski, the physician states he wants to order the following tests: electroencephalogram, PET scan, CT scan, and polysomnography.

Explain to Steven why each of the tests would be ordered.

_____

_____

_____

Reviewing the Terms

Pronounce each of the following terms. Write the definitions on a separate sheet of paper. This review will take you through all the words you learned in this chapter. If you have difficulty with any words, make a flash card for later study. Refer to the English-Spanish and Spanish-English glossaries in the eBook.

absence seizure [SĔ-zhŭr]

acetylcholine [ăs-ĕ-tĭl-KŌ-lēn]

afferent [ĂF-ĕr-ĕnt] **(sensory) neuron**

agnosia [ăg-NŌ-zē-ă]

Alzheimer [ĂLTS-hī-mĕr] **disease**

amnesia [ăm-NĒ-zē-ă]

amyotrophic lateral sclerosis (ALS) [ă-mī-ō-TRŌ-fĭk LĂT-ĕr-ăl sklĕ-RŌ-sĭs]

analgesic [ăn-ăl-JĒ-zĭk]

anesthetic [ăn-ĕs-THĔT-ĭk]

aneurysm [ĂN-yū-rĭzm]

anticonvulsant [ĂN-tē-kŏn-VŬL-sănt]

aphasia [ă-FĀ-zē-ă]

apraxia [ă-PRĂK-sē-ă]

arachnoid [ă-RĂK-noyd]

astrocytoma [ĂS-trō-sī-TŌ-mă]

ataxia [ă-TĂK-sē-ă]

aura [ĂW-ră]

autonomic [ăw-tō-NŎM-ĭk] **nervous system**

axon [ĂK-sōn]

Babinski [bă-BĬN-skē] **reflex**

bacterial meningitis [bac-TĒR-ē-ăl mĕ-nĭn-JĪ-tĭs]

basal ganglia [BĀ-săl GĂNG-glē-ă]

Bell's palsy [PĂWL-zē]

brain [brān]

brain contusion [kŏn-TŪ-zhŭn]

brainstem

cell body

central nervous system

cerebell/o [sĕr-ĕ-BĔL-ō]

cerebellitis [sĕr-ĕ-bĕl-Ī-tĭs]

cerebellum [sĕr-ĕ-BĔL-ŭm]

cerebr/o, cerebr/i [SĔR-ĕ-brō, SĔR-ĕ-bri]

cerebral angiogram

cerebral cortex [SĔR-ĕ-brăl KOR-tĕks]

cerebral infarction [SĔR-ĕ-brăl ĭn-FĂRK-shŭn]

cerebral palsy [PĂWL-zē]

cerebrospinal [SĔR-ĕ-brō-spī-năl] fluid (CSF)

cerebrovascular [SĔR-ĕ-brō-VĂS-kyū-lăr] accident (CVA)

cerebrum [SĔR-ĕ-brŭm, sĕ-RĒ-brŭm]

coma [KŌ-mă]

computerized (axial) tomography
[(ĂKS-ē-ăl) tō-MŎG-ră-fē] (CT or CAT) scan

concussion [kŏn-KŬSH-ŭn]

conductivity [kŏn-dŭk-TĬV-ĭ-tē]

convolutions [kŏn-vō-LŪ-shŭnz]

corpus callosum [KOR-pŭs kă-LŌ-sŭm]

crani/o [KRĀ-nē-ō]

cranial [KRĀ-nē-ăl] nerves

craniectomy [krā-nē-ĔK-tō-mē]

craniotomy [krā-nē-ŎT-ō-mē]

cranium [KRĀ-nē-ŭm]

dementia [dē-MĔN-shē-ă]

demyelination [dē-MĪ-ĕ-lĭ-NĀ-shŭn]

dendrite [DĔN-drīt]

diencephalon [dī-ĕn-SĔF-ă-lŏn]

dopamine [DŌ-pă-mēn]

dura mater [DŪ-ră MĀ-tĕr]

dysphasia [dĭs-FĀ-zē-ă]

efferent [ĔF-ĕr-ĕnt] (motor) neuron

electroencephalogram [ē-LĔK-trō-ĕn-SĔF-ă-lō-grăm]
(EEG)

embolic [ĕm-BŎL-ĭk] stroke

embolus [ĔM-bō-lŭs]

encephal/o [ĕn-SĔF-ă-Lō]

encephalitis [ĕn-sĕf-ă-LĪ-tĭs]

encephalogram [ĕn-SĔF-ă-lō-grăm]

epidural [ĕp-ĭ-DŪ-răl] space

epilepsy [ĔP-ĭ-LĔP-sē]

epithalamus [ĔP-ĭ-THĂL-ă-mŭs]

evoked potentials [ē-VŌKT pō-TĔN-shălz]

excitability [ĕk-SĪ-tă-BĬL-ĭ-tē]

fainting

fissure [FĬSH-ŭr]

frontal lobe [FRŬN-tăl lōb]

gait [gāt]

gangli/o [GĂNG-glē-ō]

gangliitis [găng-glē-Ī-tĭs]

ganglion (pl., ganglia, ganglions) [GĂNG-glē-ŏn
(-a, -ons)]

gli/o [GLĪ-ō]

glioblastoma multiforme [GLĪ-ō-blăs-TŌ-mă
MŬL-tĭ-fŏrm]

glioma [glī-Ō-mă]

grand mal [măhl] seizure

gyrus (pl., gyri) [JĪ-rŭs (JĪ-rī)]

hemorrhagic [hĕm-ō-RĂJ-ĭk] stroke

Huntington chorea [kōr-Ē-ă]

hydrocephalus [hī-drō-SĔF-ă-lŭs]

hypnotic [hĭp-NŎT-ĭk]

hypothalamus [HĪ-pō-THĂL-ă-mŭs]

interneuron [ĬN-tĕr-NŪR-ŏn]

lobectomy [lō-BĔK-tō-mē]

lobotomy [lō-BŎT-ō-mē]

Lou Gehrig [GĔR-ĭg] disease

lumbar [LŬM-băr] (spinal) puncture

medulla oblongata [mĕ-DŪL-ă ŏb-lŏng-GĂ-tă]

mening/o, meningi/o [mĕ-NĬNG-gō, mĕ-NĬN-jē-ō]

meninges (sing., meninx) [mĕ-NĬN-jēz (MĔ-nĭngks)]

meningioma [mĕ-NĬN-jē-Ō-mă]

meningitis [mĕ-nĭn-JĪ-tĭs]

meningocele [mĕ-NĬNG-gō-sēl]

meningomyelocele [mĕ-nĭng-gō-MĪ-ĕ-lō-sēl]

microglia [mī-KRŎG-lē-ă]

midbrain

multiple sclerosis (MS) [MŬL-tĭ-pŭl sklĕ-RŌ-sĭs]

myasthenia gravis [mī-ăs-THĒ-nē-ă GRĂV-ĭs]

myel/o [mī-ĕ-Lŏ]

myelin sheath [MĪ-ĕ-lĭn shēth]

myelitis [mī-ĕ-LĪ-tĭs]

myelogram [MĪ-ĕ-lŏ-grăm]

narcolepsy [NĂR-kō-lĕp-sē]

narcotic [năr-KŎT-ĭk]

nerve [nĕrv]

nerve cell

nerve conduction velocity

nerve impulse

neur/o, neur/i [NŪ-rō, NŪ-ri]

neurectomy [nū-RĔK-tō-mē]

neuritis [nū-RĪ-tĭs]

neuroglia [nū-RŎG-lē-ă]

neuroglial [nū-RŎG-lē-ăl] cell

neuron [NŪR-ŏn]

neuroplasty [NŪR-ō-PLĂS-tē]

neurorrhaphy [nūr-ŌR-ă-fē]

neurosurgeon [nūr-ō-SĔR-jŭn]

neurotomy [nū-RŎT-ō-mē]

neurotransmitters [NŬR-ō-trăns-MĬT-ĕrz]

norepinephrine [nŏr-ĕp-ĭ-NĔF-rĭn]

occipital lobe [ŏk-SĬP-ĭ-tăl lōb]

occlusion [ō-KLŪ-zhŭn]

oligodendroglia [ŎL-ĭ-gō-dĕn-DRŎG-lē-ă]

oligodendroglioma [ŎL-ĭ-gō-DĔN-drŏ-glī-Ō-mă]

parasympathetic [pār-ă-sĭm-pă-THĔT-ĭk] nervous system

paresthesia [pār-ĕs-THĒ-zē-ă]

parietal lobe [pă-RĪ-ĕ-tăl lōb]

Parkinson [PAR-kin-sŏn] disease

peripheral [pĕ-RĬF-ĕ-răl] nervous system

PET (positron emission tomography) [PŎZ-ĭ-trŏn ē-MĬ-shŭn tō-MŎG-ră-fē] scan

petit mal [PĔ-tē măhl] seizure

pia mater [PĪ-ă MĂ-tĕr, PĒ-ă MĀ-tĕr]

polysomnography [PŎL-ē-sŏm-NŎG-ră-fē] (PSG)

pons [pŏnz]

pyrogenic [pī-rō-JĔN-ĭk] meningitis

radiculitis [ră-dĭk-yū-LĪ-tĭs]

receptor [rē-SĔP-tĕr]

reflex [RĒ-flĕks]

sciatica [sī-ĂT-ĭ-kă]

sedative [SĔD-ă-tĭv]

shingles [SHĬNG-glz]

somatic [sō-MĂT-ĭk] nervous system

somnolence [SŎM-nō-lĕns]

SPECT (single-photon emission computed tomography) brain scan

spin/o [SPĪ-nō]

spina bifida [SPĪ-nă BĬF-ĭ-dă]

spinal cord

spinal nerves

spine [spīn]

stereotaxy [stĕr-ē-ō-TĂK-sē], stereotactic [stĕr-ē-ō-TĂK-tĭk] surgery

stroke [strōk]

subdural [sŭb-DŪR-ăl] space

sulcus (pl., sulci) [SŬL-kŭs (SŬL-sī)]

sympathetic [sĭm-pă-THĔT-ĭk] nervous system

synapse [SĬN-ăps]

syncope [SĬN-kŏ-pē]

Tay-Sachs [T-săks] disease

temporal lobe [TĔM-pŏ-răl lōb]

terminal end fibers

thalam/o [THĂL-ă-mō]

thalamus [THĂL-ă-mŭs]

thrombotic [thrŏm-BŎT-ĭk] stroke

thrombus [THRŎM-bŭs]

tics [tĭks]

tonic-clonic [TŎN-ĭk-KLŎN-nĭk] seizure

Tourette [tū-RĔT] syndrome

transcranial sonogram [trănz-KRĀ-nē-ăl SŎN-ō-grăm]

transient ischemic [ĭs-KĒ-mĭk] attack (TIA)

vag/o [VĀ-gŏ]

vagotomy [vă-GŎT-ō-mē]

vagus nerve [VĀ-gŭs nĕrv]

ventral thalamus

ventricle [VĔN-trĭ-kl]

ventricul/o [ven-TRĬK-ū-lō]

viral meningitis [VĪ-răl mĕ-nĭn-JĪ-tĭs]

The Sensory System

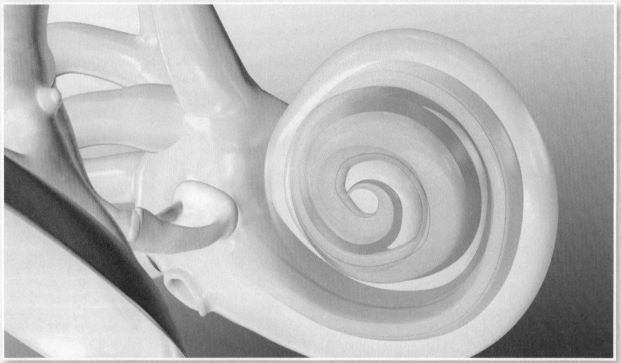

Learning Outcomes

After studying this chapter, you will be able to:

8.1 Identify the parts of the sensory system and discuss the function of each part.

8.2 Define combining forms used in building words that relate to the sensory system.

8.3 Recall the common diagnostic tests, laboratory tests, and clinical procedures used in treating disorders of the sensory system.

8.4 Define the major pathological conditions of the sensory system.

8.5 Define surgical terms related to the sensory system.

8.6 Recognize common pharmacological agents used in treating disorders of the sensory system.

8.7 Identify common abbreviations associated with the sensory system.

Structure and Function of the Sensory System

The sensory system includes any organ or part involved in the perceiving and receiving of stimuli from the outside world and from within our bodies. Aristotle, a Greek philosopher who lived more than 2,000 years ago, identified the five senses: sight, touch, hearing, smell, and taste. These senses are popularly thought of as the sensory system even though most of the senses are based on stimulation of nerves in the nervous system. The specialized nerve endings of each of the senses are neurons with specialized dendrites that respond to only one sensation. When stimulated, the electrochemical signal progresses to the brain for interpretation as with any afferent signal of the nervous system.

Sensory organs are also known as sensory receptors. These contain specialized receptor cells that are able to receive stimuli. They are designed to receive only certain stimuli (such as sound in the ear and light waves in the eye). Sensory receptor cells send impulses to the afferent (conductive) nerves in the central nervous system to interpret the stimuli. Figure 8-1 illustrates the organs of the sensory system.

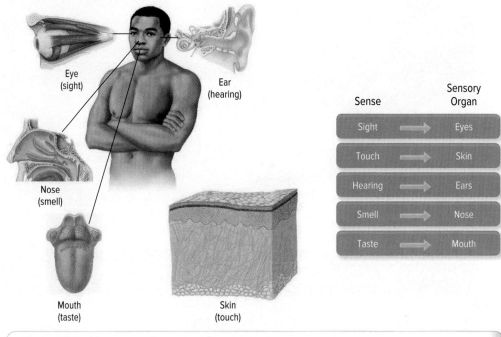

Figure 8-1 The organs of the sensory system

Building Your Sensory System Vocabulary

This section provides an introduction to basic sensory system combining terms and their meanings. Review this information prior to moving to the practices.

Combining Form	Meaning
audi/o, audit/o	hearing
aur/o, auricul/o	hearing
blephar/o	eyelid
cerumin/o	wax
cochle/o	cochlea

Combining Form	Meaning
conjunctiv/o	conjunctiva
cor/o, core/o	pupil
corne/o	cornea
cycl/o	ciliary body
glauc/o	gray or silver
ir/o, irid/o	iris
kerat/o	cornea
lacrim/o	tears
mastoid/o	mastoid process
myring/o	eardrum, middle ear
nas/o	nose
ocul/o	eye
ophthalm/o	eye
opt/o, optic/o	eye
ossicul/o	ossicle
phac/o, phak/o	lens
presby/o	old
pupill/o	pupil
retin/o	retina
salping/o	tube
scler/o	white of the eye
scot/o	darkness
tympan/o	eardrum, middle ear
uve/o	uvea

Sight—the Eye

The eyes are organs that detect light and stimulate sensory receptors. The eyes contain about 70% of all the receptors in the human body. Figure 8-2 shows an eye and Figure 8-3 illustrates the parts of an eye.

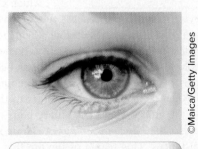

©Maica/Getty Images

Figure 8-2 An eye

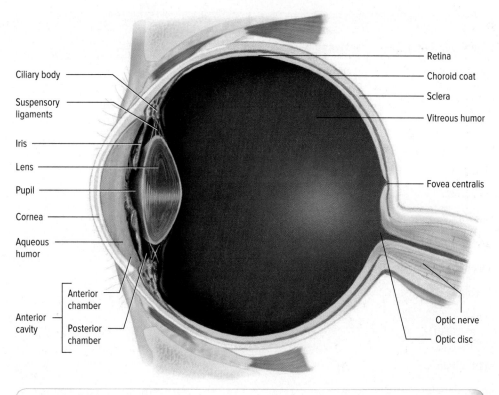

Ciliary body

Suspensory
ligaments

Iris

Lens

Pupil

Cornea

Aqueous
humor

Anterior
chamber

Anterior
cavity

Posterior
chamber

Retina

Choroid coat

Sclera

Vitreous humor

Fovea centralis

Optic nerve

Optic disc

Figure 8-3 Details of the eye

Structure and Function	PRACTICE
	Provide the missing term(s) to complete the following sentences.
sclera [SKLĒR-ă] **cornea** [KŌR-nē-ă] **refraction** [rē-FRĂK-shŭn] **eyelid** [Ī-lĭd] **conjunctiva** (*pl.,* **conjunctivae**) [kŏn-jŭnk-TĬ-vă (kŏn-jŭnk-TĬ-vē)]	Each eye is made up of three layers: the sclera, the choroids, and the retinal layer. The outer layer is a smooth, firm, white posterior section called the _____. It is made of a thick, tough membrane. The sclera supports the eyeball. The _____ is the transparent, anterior section, which is the first place where light is bent, or refracted, as it enters the eye. This section has a greater curvature to capture and direct light into the eye. The sclera has blood vessels that nourish the cornea (which has no blood supply). The cornea is transparent, has no blood vessels, and bends (or refracts) light rays in a process called _____. The outer layer is covered by the _____. The anterior surface of the eye and the posterior surface of the eyelid are lined with a mucous membrane (the _____).
choroid [KŌ-royd] **ciliary body** [SĬL-ē-ăr-ē BOD-ē] **pupil** [PYŪ-pĭl] **lens** [lĕnz] **iris** [Ī-rĭs] **uvea** [YŪ-vē-ă]	The _____ or middle layer, is a vascular layer of blood vessels, consisting of a thin posterior membrane. Anteriorly, this is continuous with the _____, which contains the ciliary muscles, used for focusing the eyes. Vision is the process that begins when light is refracted as it hits the cornea and again when it hits the retina. Light passes through the _____, the black circular center of the eye, then passes through the _____, a colorless, flexible transparent body behind the _____, the colored part of the eye that expands and contracts in response to light, thereby opening and closing the pupil. From there it goes to the lens, which is suspended by ligaments that extend to the ciliary body. The ciliary body contracts to change the shape of the lens in a process called *accommodation*. Accommodation allows the eye to focus on objects at varying distances. This region of the eye that includes the iris, ciliary body, and choroid is known as the _____.

retina [RĔT-ĭ-nă] **rods** [rŏdz] **cones** [kōnz] **optic nerve**	The interior layer of the eye is called the *retinal layer*. It contains the _____, a light-sensitive membrane that can decode the light waves and send the information on to the brain, which interprets what we see. The retina itself has many layers. The thick layer of nervous tissue is called neuroretina, which consists of specialized nerve receptor cells called _____, sensors of black and white shades, and _____, sensors of color and the brightest light. There are three types of cones, one each for red, green, and blue. There are approximately 125 million rods and 7 million cones in each eye, along with other nerve cells, that convert the light images received to nerve impulses that are then transmitted through the _____ to the appropriate lobes of the brain.
	The region where the retina connects to the optic nerve, where there are no rods or cones to receive images, is called the *optic disk* or *blind spot*. Light causes a chemical change in the rods and cones that allows them to convert the images to nerve impulses. The thin layer of the retina is made of pigmented epithelial tissue, which, along with the choroid, absorbs stray light that is not absorbed by the neuroretina and prevents reflections from the back of the retina.
eyebrows [Ī-brŏwz] **eyelashes** [Ī-lăsh-ĕz] **lacrimal glands** [LĂK-rĭ-măl glandz] **tears** [tērz]	Several other structures are important to the eye. The eyelids close to protect the eyes or to allow rest and sleep. The _____ and _____ help keep foreign particles from entering the eye. The _____ secrete moisture into the lacrimal ducts or tear ducts. The resulting _____ moisten the eyes, wash foreign particles off the eye, and distribute water and nutrients to parts of the eye. Tears may flow heavily as a reaction to allergies, infections, or emotional upset.

PRONOUNCE and DEFINE	Pronounce the following words aloud and write their meaning in the space provided.
uvea	[YŪ-vē-ă]
lacrimal glands	[LĂK-rĭ-măl glandz]
conjunctiva	[kŏn-jŭnk-TĬ-vă]
sclera	[SKLĒR-ă]
iris	[Ī-rĭs]

SPELL and DEFINE	Identify if the following terms are spelled correctly. Correct the words that are spelled incorrectly. Write the definition for each word.	
	Spelling	**Definition**
korneea		
ilshez		
lakrimeal glands		
lenz		
pyupill		

UNDERSTAND	Identify the term from the definition provided.

1. Colored part of eye: _____
2. Transparent body behind iris: _____
3. Refraction occurs here: _____
4. Transmits information to the brain related to light waves: _____
5. Nerve that transmits impulses from eye to brain: _____

Explain to a sixth-grade health class how sight occurs.

_____

_____

Did you know ❓

Eye Color

Newborns with light skin are almost always born with blue eyes, even though their eyes may later turn brown or green. Eye color is determined by heredity. It takes several months for the melanocytes to be distributed to the anterior portion of the eye. Babies with darker skin normally have a higher concentration of melanocytes to begin with, and their eyes at birth are almost always dark. Albinos are born with no melanocytes in their bodies and they are, therefore, much more sensitive to light and have no pigment in the irises of their eyes.

©PeopleImages/Getty Images

©wavebreakmedia/Shutterstock

Hearing and Equilibrium—the Ear

The ear is an organ of hearing and equilibrium (balance). There are three major divisions of the ear: external, middle, and inner. Figure 8-4 shows an ear and Figure 8-5 illustrates the parts of an ear.

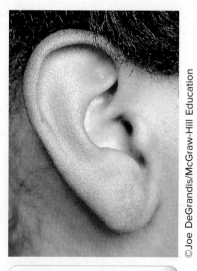

©Joe DeGrandis/McGraw-Hill Education

Figure 8-4 An ear

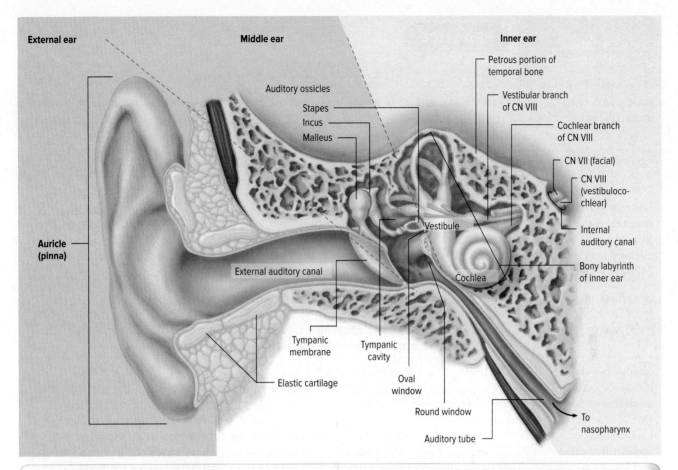

External ear

Middle ear

Inner ear

Petrous portion of temporal bone

Vestibular branch of CN VIII

Auditory ossicles

Stapes

Incus

Malleus

Cochlear branch of CN VIII

CN VII (facial)

CN VIII (vestibuloco-chlear)

Internal auditory canal

Vestibule

Auricle (pinna)

Bony labyrinth of inner ear

External auditory canal

Cochlea

Tympanic membrane

Tympanic cavity

Oval window

Elastic cartilage

Round window

To nasopharynx

Auditory tube

Figure 8-5 Details of the ear

Did you know ?

Ears

Driving down a mountain sometimes causes you to feel and hear a popping sound. The eustachian tubes react quickly to equalize the pressure caused by exposure to a high altitude when the eardrum membrane is stretched. The eardrum "pops" back into place when pressure is equalized.

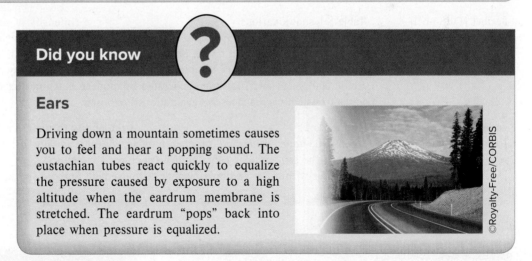

©Royalty-Free/CORBIS

Structure and Function	PRACTICE
	Provide the missing term(s) to complete the following sentences.
ear [ēr]	The three major divisions of the _____ are the *external ear*, the *middle ear*, and the *inner ear*.

continued on next page

Structure and Function	PRACTICE
	Provide the missing term(s) to complete the following sentences.
auricle [ĂW-rĭ-kl] **pinna** [PĬN-ă]	The external ear begins on the outside of the head with a funnel-like structure called the _____ or _____. This structure leads through part of the skull known as the *temporal bone* (which itself has a bony projection called the *mastoid process*) to an S-shaped tube called the *external auditory meatus.* The external auditory meatus contains glands that secrete *cerumen,* or earwax, a brownish-yellow, waxy substance.
eardrum [ĒR-drŭm] **tympanic membrane** [tĭm-PĂN-ĭk] **auditory ossicles** [ĂW-dĭ-tōr-ē ŎS-ĭ-klz]	The middle ear includes the *tympanic cavity,* in which sits the _____ (_____) and the _____, three small, specially shaped bones. The eardrum is an oval, semitransparent membrane with skin on its outer surface and a mucous membrane on the inside. Sound waves change the pressure on the eardrum, which moves back and forth, thereby producing vibrations.
eustachian tube [yū-STĀ-shŭn, yū-STĀ-kē-ăn]	The middle ear is connected to the pharynx through the _____ (*auditory tube*). This tube helps equalize air pressure on both sides of the eardrum, which is essential to hearing. The eustachian tube is connected to the nasal cavity. This explains why children are more susceptible to ear infections following a head cold.
osseous labyrinth [ŎS-sē-ŭs LĂB-ĭ-rĭnth] **membranous labyrinth** [MĔM-bră-nus LĂB-ĭ-rĭnth] **semicircular canals** **cochlea** [KOK-lē-ă]	The inner ear is a system of two tubes: the _____ and the _____. The osseous labyrinth is a bony canal in the temporal bone. The labyrinths include three _____, structures important to equilibrium, and a _____, a snail-shaped structure important to hearing. The cochlea has a membrane that has hairlike receptor cells located on the membrane's surface. The hairs move back and forth in response to sound waves and eventually send messages via neurotransmitters through the eighth cranial nerve and to the brain for interpretation.
decibel [DĔS-ĭ-bĕl]	Table 8-1 shows various _____ (intensity of sound) levels that can be heard by a normal human ear. The scale of decibels (dB) gives the intensity of sound in progressions multiplied by 10. So 10 dB is 10 times greater than the lowest perceptible decibel, 20 dB is 100 times as great as 10 dB, and so on. The easy availability of electronic equipment and the sound generated by modern machines have raised the decibel levels to which each successive generation is exposed.
equilibrium [ē-kwĭ-LĬB-rē-ŭm] **vestibule** [VĔS-tĭ-būl]	The sense of _____ is the ability to maintain steady balance either when still, *static equilibrium,* or when moving, *dynamic equilibrium.* The bony chamber between the semicircular canal and the cochlea is called the _____. Structures within the vestibule respond to movement and aid in maintaining balance.

PRONOUNCE and DEFINE	Pronounce the following terms aloud and write their meaning in the space provided.
equilibrium	[ē-kwĭ-LĬB-rē-ŭm]
pinna	[PĬN-ă]
auricle	[ĂW-rĭ-kl]
eustachian tube	[yū-STĀ-shŭn *or* yū-STĀ-kē-ăn tūb]
vestibule	[VĔS-tĭ-būl]

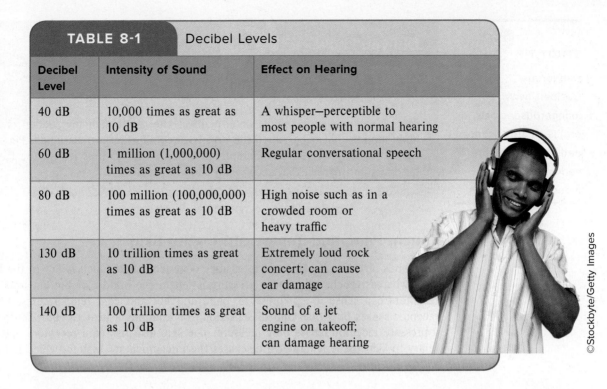

TABLE 8-1	Decibel Levels	
Decibel Level	Intensity of Sound	Effect on Hearing
40 dB	10,000 times as great as 10 dB	A whisper—perceptible to most people with normal hearing
60 dB	1 million (1,000,000) times as great as 10 dB	Regular conversational speech
80 dB	100 million (100,000,000) times as great as 10 dB	High noise such as in a crowded room or heavy traffic
130 dB	10 trillion times as great as 10 dB	Extremely loud rock concert; can cause ear damage
140 dB	100 trillion times as great as 10 dB	Sound of a jet engine on takeoff; can damage hearing

©Stockbyte/Getty Images

SPELL and DEFINE	Identify if the following terms are spelled correctly. Correct the words that are spelled incorrectly. Write the definition for each word.	
	Spelling	Definition
youstashun tube		
ekwllibreum		
awerikl		
pina		
desibel		

UNDERSTAND Identify the term from the definition provided.

1. Also known as pinna: _____
2. Produces vibrations: _____
3. Assists with balance: _____
4. Organ of hearing: _____
5. Snail-shaped structure within inner ear: _____

APPLY Read the following scenario and respond accordingly.

Bob Noel works in a factory. During his visit to the physician, he states that his employer is asking him to wear ear plugs. Explain to Mr. Noel why wearing ear plugs is important.

_____

_____

_____

Did you know

Motion Sickness

Motion sickness in a vehicle or airplane is the result of many sudden changes in body motion that occur when the organs of equilibrium are disrupted. People experience motion sickness at different rates. Some medications relieve the feelings of dizziness and nausea that accompany motion sickness.

Touch, Pain, and Temperature—the Skin

The skin's layers sense different intensities of touch. Light touch is felt in the top layer of skin, whereas touch with harder pressure is felt in the middle or bottom layer. The skin's receptors can sense touch, pressure, pain, and hot and cold temperatures. Each type of receptor senses only one kind of sensation; for example, a heat receptor senses only heat; a pressure receptor senses only pressure. The skin also has pain receptors that senses any injury to skin tissue. Chapter 5 discusses the integumentary system, which is incorporated within the skin.

Smell and Taste

The sense of smell is the ability to perceive a scent due to the olfactory nerves. The sense of taste occurs when the taste buds on the tongue's surface send messages to the brain. The loss of the sense of smell or taste can have a major impact on our everyday life.

Structure and Function	PRACTICE
	Provide the missing term(s) to complete the following sentences.
olfactory organs [ŏl-FĂK-tō-rē ŌR-gănz]	The sense of smell, or *olfactory stimulation,* is activated by *olfactory receptors* located at the top of the nasal cavity. The olfactory receptors are neurons covered with cilia that send small messages to the brain. The receptors are located within the _____, yellowish-brown masses along the top of the nasal cavity. For the sense of smell to sense an object, the object must be dissolved in a liquid in the olfactory organs. The sense of smell is closely related to the sense of taste.
taste buds **papillae** (*sing.,* **pappila**) [pă-PĬL-ē (pă-PĬL-ă)] **taste cells**	_____ are organs that sense the taste of food. Most taste buds are on the surface of the tongue in small raised structures called _____, but some also line the roof of the mouth and the walls of the pharynx. Each taste bud contains receptor cells, called _____. Nerve fibers wrapped around the taste cells transmit impulses to the brain. The taste buds are activated when the item being tasted dissolves in the watery fluid surrounding the taste buds. The salivary glands secrete this fluid. There are at least four types of taste buds to match the primary taste sensations—sweet, sour, salty, and bitter. Different sections of the tongue contain concentrations of receptors for each of the taste sensations. There are also receptors that sense the texture, odor, and temperature of food. In the case of food that is too hot, too spicy, or too cold, some pain receptors are activated. The combination of the primary taste sensations and the aroma of food will be interpreted in the brain as the specific flavor of food. This explains why someone with a head cold does not have a good appetite.

PRONOUNCE and DEFINE	Pronounce the word aloud and write the meaning.
olfactory	[ōl-FĂK-tō-rē]
papillae	[pă-PĬL-ē]

APPLY	Answer the following question.

You have lost your sense of smell. What impact might this have on your everyday life?

_____

_____

_____

_____

Did you know

Skin

One of the remarkable advances in genetic engineering is the ability to grow replacement skin. The new skin is grown from cells of skin from various parts of the body and can be used to replace burned or injured areas. If the skin is working once it is put in place, it will continue to grow and function like normal skin—helping to regulate body temperature, preventing foreign material from entering the body, and protecting inner organs from bruises.

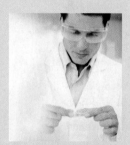

©Palo Alto/Eric Audras/ Getty Images

LO 8.2 Word Building in the Sensory System

Word Building	PRACTICE
	Provide the correct combining form for each of the following sentences.
myring-itis [mĭr-ĭn-JĬ-tĭs]	_____ itis is inflammation of the tympanic membrane.
cyclo-dialysis [sī-klō-dī-ĂL-ĭ-sĭs]	Method of relieving intraocular pressure in glaucoma is _____ dialysis.
conjunctivo-plasty [kŏn-JŬNK-tĭ-vō-plas-tē]	_____ plasty is plastic surgery on the conjunctiva.
phac-oma [fa-KŌ-mă]	_____ oma is a tumor of the lens.
scler-ectasia [sklēr-ĕk-TĀ-zē-ă]	Bulging of the sclera is _____ ectasia.
audio-meter [aw-dē-OM-ĕ-ter]	Instrument for measuring hearing is an _____ meter.

continued on next page

Word Building	**PRACTICE**
	Provide the correct combining form for each of the following sentences.
irido-ptosis [ĬR-ĭ-dŏp-TŌ-sĭs]	_____ ptosis is prolapse of the iris.
ossicul-ectomy [ŎS-ĭ-kū-LEK-tō-mē]	_____ ectomy is removal of one of the ossicles of the middle ear.
uve-itis [ū-vē-Ī-tĭs]	Inflammation of the uvea is _____ itis.
blephar-itis [blĕf-ă-RĪ-tĭs]	_____ itis is inflammation of the eyelid.
lacrimo-tomy [lăk-rĭ-MOT-ō-mē]	Incision into the lacrimal duct is _____ tomy.
opto-meter [ŏp-TŎM-ĕ-ter]	Instrument for determining eye refraction is an _____ meter.
corneo-scleral [KŌR-nē-ō-SKLĒR-ăl]	_____ scleral pertains to the cornea and sclera.
tympano-plasty [TĬM-pă-nō-plas-tē]	Repair of a damaged middle ear is _____ plasty.
mastoid-itis [măs-toy-DĪ-tĭs]	_____ itis is inflammation of the mastoid process.
coreo-plasty [KŌR-ē-ō-plas-tē]	Surgical correction of the size and shape of a pupil is _____ plasty.
kerato-conus [KER-ă-tō-KŌ-nŭs]	_____ conus is abnormal protrusion of the cornea.
pupillo-meter [PŪ-pĭ-LŎM-ĕ-ter]	Instrument for measuring the diameter of the pupil is a _____ meter.
dacryo-lith [DĂK-rē-ō-lith]	A calculus in the tear duct is a _____ lith.
ophthalmo-scope [ŏf-THĂL-mō-skōp]	Instrument for studying the interior of the eyeball is an _____ scope.
auriculo-cranial [ăw-RĬK-ū-lō-KRĀ-nē-ăl]	_____ cranial pertains to the auricle of the ear and the cranium.
retin-itis [rĕt-ĭ-NĪ-tĭs]	Inflammation of the retina is _____ itis.
cerumino-lytic [sĕ-ROO-mĭ-nō-LIT-ĭk]	Agent for softening earwax is a _____ lytic.
oculo-dynia [OK-ū-lō-DIN-ē-ă]	_____ dynia is pain in the eyeball.
scoto-meter [skō-TŎM-ĕ-ter]	Instrument for evaluating a _scotoma,_ or blind spot, is a _____ meter.
cochleo-vestibular [KOK-lē-ō-ves-TIB-ū-lăr]	Pertaining to the cochlea and the vestibule of the ear is _____ vestibular.
naso-sinusitis [NĀ-zō-sī-nŭ-SĪ-tĭs]	_____ sinusitis is inflammation of the nasal and sinus cavities.

PRONOUNCE and DEFINE	Pronounce the following terms aloud and write their meaning in the space provided.
blepharitis	[blĕf-ă-RĪ-tĭs]
uveitis	[ū-vē-Ī-tĭs]
ophthalmoscope	[ŏf-THĂL-mō-skōp]
nasosinusitis	[NĀ-zō-sī-nŭ-SĪ-tĭs]
ceruminolytic	[sĕ-ROO-mĭ-nō-LIT-ĭk]

SPELL and DEFINE	Identify if the following terms are spelled correctly. Correct the words that are spelled incorrectly. Write the definition for each word.	
	Spelling	Definition
wretinitis		
pupilimeter		
lakrimiotome		
oddiometr		
erdiptoeses		

UNDERSTAND	Find the Roots. From the following list of combining forms and from the list of suffixes in previous chapters, write the word that matches the definition (not all will be used).

a. audi/o   b. blephar/o   c. core/o   d. dacryocyst/o   e. irid/o

f. kerat/o   g. opt/o   h. ot/o   i. retin/o   j. scler/o

1. _____ Inflammation of the ear
2. _____ Instrument for determining eye refraction
3. _____ Study of the ear
4. _____ Inflammation of the cornea
5. _____ Instrument to examine the cornea
6. _____ Disease of the iris
7. _____ Pain in the tear sac
8. _____ Repair of the pupil

APPLY	Read the following scenario and answer the question.

You are reviewing the medical record of Kelly Post, a 68-year-old woman who just left the physician's office. The physician documented the following conditions:

- oculodynia
- mastoiditis
- conjunctivitis

What conditions does Ms. Post have?

_____
_____
_____
_____

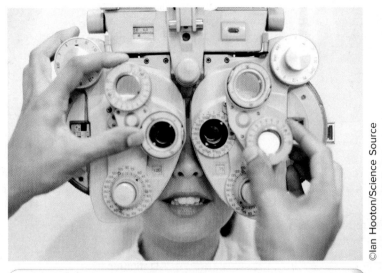

Figure 8-6 An optometrist using equipment to examine the eyes

©Ian Hooton/Science Source

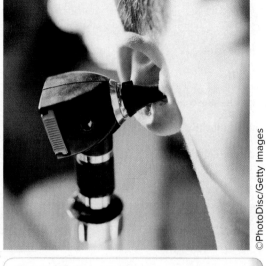

Figure 8-7 An otoscope

©PhotoDisc/Getty Images

LO 8.3 Diagnostic, Procedural, and Laboratory Terms

Diagnostic, procedural, and laboratory testing assists in the diagnosis and treatment of the sensory conditions. Diagnosis of the sensory system usually includes testing of the sense in question and examination of the sensory structures. Loss of a sense can cause serious problems for an individual. In some cases, senses can be partially or totally restored through the use of prosthetic devices, transplants, or medication. In other cases, patients must adapt to the loss of a sense. Figure 8-6 shows an optometrist with equipment. Figure 8-7 shows an otoscope being used to examine the ear.

Diagnostic	PRACTICE
	Provide the missing term(s) to complete the following sentences.

	Diagnosing the Eye
ophthalmologist [ŏf-thăl-MŎL-ō-jĭst] **optometrist** [ŏp-TŎM-ĕ-trĭst]	An _____ (medical doctor who specializes in treatment and surgeries of the eye) and an _____ (a trained nonmedical specialist who can examine patients for vision problems and prescribe lenses) both perform routine eye examinations. The most common diagnostic test of the eye is the visual acuity test, which measures the ability to see objects clearly at measured distances. The most common chart is the *Snellen Chart*. Perfect vision measures 20/20 on such a test. The first number, 20, is the distance (typically 20 feet) from which the person being tested reads a chart with black letters of different sizes. The second number is the distance from which the person being tested can read the size of the letters in relation to someone with normal vision. If the test shows that the subject can read only the letters on the 400 line, then the vision would be measured as 20/400. The 400 line means that someone with normal vision would be able to see from 400 feet away what the person being tested can see without corrective lenses at only 20 feet. A reading that shows less than 20/20 (e.g., 20/13) means that a person can read something at 20 feet that most people with 20/20 vision would be able to read at only 13 feet.

tonometry [tō-NŎM-ĕ-trē] **ophthalmoscopy** [ŏf-thăl-MŎS-kō-pē] **optician** [ŏp-TĬSH-ŭn]	The next step in a routine eye examination is to examine peripheral vision, the area one is able to see to the side with the eyes looking straight ahead. This is usually done by telling a patient to follow a finger placed in front of the eyes while facing straight ahead. (In diagnosing some diseases, peripheral vision is tested in an examination called a *visual field examination*.) Depending on the patient's age, most routine eye examinations also include _____, a measurement of pressure within the eye (a test for glaucoma), and _____ (visual examination of the interior of the eye). If the patient needs corrective lenses, an _____ (trained technician who makes and fits corrective lenses) can fill the prescription written by an ophthalmologist or an optometrist. Most optometrists and some ophthalmologists also fill prescriptions for lenses.
	For further diagnosis of the eye, a *slit lamp ocular device* is used to view the interior of the eye magnified through a microscope. *Fluorescein angiography* is the injection of a contrast medium into the blood vessels to observe the movement of blood throughout the eye. This test is for people with diabetes and other diseases that may manifest lesions on various parts of the eye.

Diagnosing the Ear

otologist [ō-TŎL-ō-jĭst] **audiologist** [ăw-dē-ŎL-ō-jĭst] **otorhinolaryngologists** [Ō-tō-rī-nō-lăr-ĭng-GŎL-ō-jĭsts] **otoscopy** [ō-TŎS-kō-pē] **audiometry** [ăw-dē-ŎM-ĕ-trē] **audiogram** [ĂW-dē-ō-grăm]	Hearing tests are routinely given to young children to see if they have any hearing deficit. Later, hearing is checked when a person notices hearing loss or when that person's friends and family suspect it. An _____ is an ear specialist and an _____ is a nonmedical hearing specialist. _____ are specialists who practice *otorhinolaryngology,* the medical specialty covering the ear, nose, and throat. They all perform thorough examinations that include _____, visual examination of the ear using an *otoscope,* a lighted viewing device. Such an examination also might include _____, the measurement of various acoustic frequencies to determine what frequencies the patient can or cannot hear. The device used is an *audiometer* and the results of the test are plotted on a graph, an _____. The inside of the ear may be tested using a *pneumatic otoscope,* an otoscope that allows air to be blown into the ear to view the movement of the eardrum. A *tuning fork* compares the conduction of sound in one ear or between the two ears. The *Rinne test* and the *Weber test* are two tuning fork tests.

Diagnosing Other Senses

	The nose is usually observed as part of a general examination or, more specifically, a respiratory examination. Loss of the sense of smell is often the result of a disease process or of aging. The tongue and other parts of the mouth and the skin also are observed during a general examination. Loss of taste or touch also may be part of a disease process or of aging.

UNDERSTAND

Know Your Senses. For each of the following diagnostic tests or devices, write A for eye, B for ear, or C for both eye and ear.

1. audiogram: _____
2. tuning fork: _____
3. otoscope: _____
4. Snellen chart: _____

5. Rinne test: _____
6. tonometer: _____
7. visual acuity: _____
8. ophthalmoscope: _____

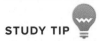
LO 8.4 Pathological Terms

Eye Disorders

Lost or damaged senses are illnesses in themselves. The disruption of losing or damaging a sense organ can lead to other related illnesses. Much of the pathology of the sensory system results from age-related disorders or just age-related wear and tear on the sensory organs. Figures 8-8 and 8-9 illustrate some common eye disorders.

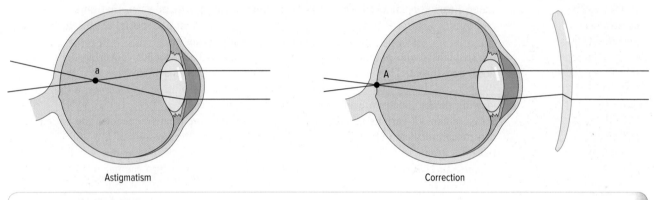

Figure 8-8 Astigmatism and correction

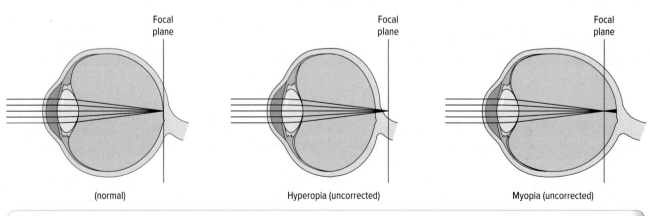

Figure 8-9 Hyperopia and myopia

PRACTICE

Provide the missing term(s) to complete the following sentences.

	Eye Disorders
contact lenses	The most common eye disorders involve defects in the curvature of the cornea and/or lens or defects in the refractive ability of the eye due to an abnormally short or long eyeball. Such disorders are usually managed with corrective lenses. Corrective lenses may be placed in frames to be worn on the face or may be in the form of _____, which are placed directly over the cornea of the eye and centered on the pupil. Contact lenses come in a variety of types, including disposable, hard, soft, and long-term wear. The degree of correction of the lenses depends on the results of a visual acuity examination.
astigmatism [ă-STĬG-mă-tĭzm] **hyperopia** [hī-pĕr-Ō-pē-ă] **farsightedness** **myopia** [mī-Ō-pē-ă] **nearsightedness** **presbyopia** [prĕz-bē-Ō-pē-ă]	An eye examination may reveal an _____, distortion of sight because light rays do not come to a single focus on the retina. It also may reveal _____ (_____) or _____ (_____). All three are errors of refraction, the bending of light that causes light rays to fall at one point on the retina. Hyperopia is the focusing of light rays behind the retina and myopia is the focusing of light rays in front of the retina. _____ is the loss of close reading vision due to lessened ability to focus and accommodate. It is a common disorder after age 40 and another type of refractive disorder.
strabismus [stră-BĬZ-mŭs] **esotropia** [ĕs-ō-TRŌ-pē-ă] **exotropia** [ĕk-sō-TRŌ-pē-ă] **asthenopia** [ăs-thĕ-NŌ-pē-ă] **eyestrain** **diplopia** [dĭ-PLŌ-pē-ă] **photophobia** [fō-tō-FŌ-bē-ă]	_____ is eye misalignment (sometimes called "cross-eyed"). Two types of strabismus are _____, deviation of one eye inward, and _____, deviation of one eye outward. _____, or _____, is a condition in which the eyes tire easily because of weakness of the ocular or ciliary muscles. Symptoms may include pain in or around the eyes, headache, dimness of vision, dizziness, and light nausea. _____ is double vision. _____ is extreme sensitivity to light, sometimes as a result of a disease.
cataracts [CĂT-ă-răkts]	_____ are cloudiness of the lens of the eye. They are usually a result of the aging process but can be congenital or the result of a disease process or injury. Also, some types of medication may hasten the lens clouding. Cataracts may be repaired with an intraocular lens implant.
glaucoma [glăw-KŌ-mă] **blindness**	_____ is any disease caused by increased intraocular pressure of the aqueous humor. The pressure misaligns the lens and cornea and causes damage to the ciliary body. It can be treated in most cases by the use of special eye medications or surgical procedures (including laser treatments) to relieve the pressure. If not treatable, it can lead to _____, loss of vision.
macular degeneration [MĂK-yū-lăr dē-jen-er-Ā-shŭn]	There are many other causes of blindness, such as congenital defects, trauma to the eyes, and _____. Macular degeneration is the breakdown of macular tissue, which leads to loss of central vision, the vision we use for reading, driving, and watching television. Some specific conditions within the eye may affect vision. One such condition is *papilledema*, or *edema* of the optic disk. Diseases of other body systems can affect the senses. *Diabetic retinopathy* is a complication of diabetes mellitus that can result in vision loss.
	The retina can tear or become detached and need surgical repair. Many of these conditions and other situations can lead to a form of partial blindness known as *legal blindness*. Legal blindness is a range of sight set by states. For example, someone whose vision can be corrected only to 20/400 may be considered legally blind.

continued on next page

PRACTICE

Provide the missing term(s) to complete the following sentences.

exophthalmos or exophthalmus
[ĕk-sŏf-THĂL-mos, ĕk-sŏf-THĂL-mŭs]
lacrimation
[lăk-rĭ-MĀ-shŭn]
nystagmus
[nĭs-STĂG-mŭs]

The eyeball can protrude abnormally, as in _____ or _____, usually caused by hyperthyroidism. _____ is excessive tearing and _____ is excessive eyeball movement.

blepharospasm [BLĔF-ă-rō-spăzm]
blepharitis [BLĔF-ă-RĪ-tĭs]
conjunctivitis [kŏn-jŭnk-tĭ-VĪ-tĭs]
pinkeye
blepharoptosis [BLĔF-ă-RŎP-tō-sĭs]
chalazion [kă-LĀ-zē-ŏn]
trichiasis [trĭ-KĪ-ă-sĭs]
sty, stye [stī]

Inflammations and conditions of the eyelid include _____, involuntary eyelid movement causing excessive blinking; _____, inflammation of the eyelid; _____ or _____, a highly infectious inflammation of the conjunctiva; and _____, paralysis of the eyelid causing drooping. A _____ is a nodular inflammation that usually forms on the eyelid. _____ is abnormal growth of eyelashes in a direction that causes them to rub on the eye. A _____ is an infection of a sebaceous gland in the eyelid.

iritis [ī-RĪ-tĭs]
keratitis [kĕr-ă-TĪ-tĭs]
retinitis [rĕt-ĭ-NĪ-tĭs]
scleritis [sklĕ-RĪ-tĭs]

Inflammation of other parts of the eye include _____, inflammation of the iris; _____, inflammation of the cornea; _____, inflammation of the retina; and _____, inflammation of the sclera.

PRONOUNCE and DEFINE

Pronounce the following terms aloud and write their meaning in the space provided.

astigmatism	[ă-STĬG-mă-tĭzm]
hyperopia	[hī-pĕr-Ō-pē-ă]
blepharoptosis	[BLĔF-ă-RŎP-tō-sĭs]
chalazion	[kă-LĀ-zē-ŏn]
keratitis	[kĕr-ă-TĪ-tĭs]

SPELL and DEFINE

Identify if the following terms are spelled correctly. Correct the words that are spelled incorrectly. Write the definition for each word.

	Spelling	Definition
blefaroptosis		
konjunktivitis		
eksofthalmous		
lakrimashun		
sti		

Fill in the blanks with the correct terms.

1. An inflammation of the conjunctiva: _____
2. Excessive blinking: _____
3. Inflammation of the eyelid: _____
4. Abnormal growth in the direction of the eyelashes: _____
5. Excessive eyeball movement: _____

APPLY **Read the following scenario and respond accordingly.**

You are the nurse gathering information on a new client, Julie Halbritter. Ms. Halbritter reports the following symptoms:

• Reddened lump on her eyelid
• Reddened, inflamed left eye with excessive tearing and blinking

Using correct medical terminology, write Ms. Halbritter's symptoms.

_____
_____
_____
_____

Ear Disorders

The sense of hearing can be diminished or lost in a number of situations. Hearing loss can impact nearly every aspect of an individual's life.

PRACTICE

Pathological	Provide the missing term(s) to complete the following sentences.
deafness **otosclerosis** [ō-tō-sklĕ-RŌ-sĭs] **tinnitus** [tĭ-NĪ-tŭs, TĬ-nĭ-tŭs] **otalgia** [ō-TĂL-jē-ă] **otorrhagia** [ō-tō-RĀ-jē-ă] **otorrhea** [ō-tō-RĒ-ă] **vertigo** [VĔR-tĭ-gō, vĕr-TĪ-gō]	_____ is either partial or total hearing loss. *Conductive hearing loss* is caused by lessening of vibrations of the ear. *Sensorineural hearing loss* (also known as nerve deafness) is caused by lesions or dysfunction of those parts of the ear necessary to hearing. *Cerumen impaction,* abnormal wax buildup, can diminish hearing. _____ is the hardening of bone within the ear. _____ is a constant ringing or buzzing in the ear. _____ or *earache* can interfere with hearing. _____, bleeding in the ear, and _____, purulent matter draining from the ear, also can impair hearing, usually temporarily. The sense of equilibrium is disturbed in _____, dizziness.
otitis media [ō-TĪ-tĭs MĒ-dē-ă] **otitis externa** [ō-TĪ-tĭs ĕks-TĔR-nă]	Various ear inflammations can diminish hearing or cause pain. _____ is inflammation of the middle ear. *Suppurative otitis media* is bacterial in nature and is often found in children. *Serous otitis media* is fluid contained in the middle ear, preventing free movement of the tympanic membrane. _____, also known as *swimmer's ear,* is a fungal infection of the external ear canal, often occurring in hot weather.
Ménière's disease [mĕn-YERZ di-ZĒZ]	_____ is elevated fluid pressure within the cochlea, causing disturbances of the equilibrium and vertigo.

PRONOUNCE and DEFINE	Pronounce the following terms aloud and write their meaning in the space provided.
otorrhagia	[ō-tō-RĀ-jē-ă]
otorrhea	[ō-tō-RĒ-ă]
vertigo	[VĔR-tĭ-gō, vĕr-TĪ-gō]
Ménière's disease	[mĕn-YERZ di-ZĒZ]
otosclerosis	[ō-tō-sklĕ-RŌ-sĭs]

SPELL and DEFINE	Identify if the following terms are spelled correctly. Correct the words that are spelled incorrectly. Write the definition for each word.	
	Spelling	**Definition**
otorajea		
otorea		
tinitus		
otidus medea		
vertego		

UNDERSTAND	Sense the Diseases. For each of the diseases listed, write A for eye, B for ear, or C for nose to indicate the organ associated with that disease.

1. conjunctivitis: _____
2. cataract: _____
3. labyrinthitis: _____
4. otitis media: _____
5. presbyopia: _____

6. allergic rhinitis: _____
7. macular degeneration: _____
8. nasosinusitis: _____
9. Ménière's disease: _____
10. tinnitus: _____

LO 8.5 Surgical Terms

Surgery may be performed on the sensory system. Sensory deficits may be restored; removal of cancerous tumors and cosmetic changes may occur through surgical intervention. This section presents terms for surgery in the sensory system.

Surgical	PRACTICE
	Provide the missing term(s) to complete the following sentences.
keratoplasty [KĔR-ă-tō-plăs-tē]	Some of the sense organs require surgery at various times. Corneal transplants or _____ may give or restore sight. Implantation of new sound wave devices may give or restore hearing. The eye, ear, and nose are also the sites of plastic surgery to correct congenital defects or the signs of aging. Microscopic laser surgery or microsurgery often is used to operate on the small, delicate sensory organs. Vision correction surgery is becoming quite common as advances in laser surgery make this possible.
blepharoplasty [BLĔF-ă-rō-plăst-ē] otoplasty [Ō-tō-plăs-tē] tympanoplasty [TĬM-pă-nō-plăs-tē]	Plastic surgery is used in _____, eyelid repair; _____, surgical repair of the outer ear; and _____, eardrum repair. In some cases, removal of part of a sensory organ becomes necessary to treat a disorder or because a part has become damaged or cancerous.

enucleation [ē-nū-klē-Ā-shŭn] **iridectomy** [ĭr-ĭ-DĔK-tō-mē] **iridotomy** [ĭr-ĭ-DŎT-ō-mē]	*Cataract extraction* is the removal of a cloudy lens from the eye. It is usually followed by an *intraocular lens (IOL) implant,* during which an artificial lens is implanted to replace the natural lens that was removed. It is unusual for patients to be unable to tolerate the implant. When they do, however, special glasses are prescribed that allow the patient some, usually limited, sight. _____ is the removal of an eyeball. _____ is removal of part of the iris. An _____ is an incision into the iris to allow aqueous humor to flow from the posterior to the anterior chambers. Correction of nearsightedness is also available with a laser procedure that changes the curvature of the cornea by making spokelike incisions around it. A retina can tear or become detached due to a trauma.
stapedectomy [stā-pĕ-DĔK-tō-mē] **myringotomy** [mĭr-ĭng-GŎT-ō-mē]	In the ear, hearing can sometimes be aided by a _____, removal of the stapes to correct otosclerosis and insertion of tissue to substitute for a damaged stapes. A _____ is the insertion of a small, polyethylene (PE or pressure-equalizing) tube to help drain fluid, thereby relieving some of the symptoms of otitis media. This operation is done frequently on infants and children with recurring ear infections.

PRONOUNCE and DEFINE	Pronounce the following terms aloud and write their meaning in the space provided.
stapedectomy	[stā-pĕ-DĔK-tō-mē]
myringotomy	[mĭr-ĭng-GŎT-ō-mē]
enucleation	[ē-nū-klē-Ā-shŭn]
iridectomy	[ĭr-ĭ-DĔK-tō-mē]
blepharoplasty	[BLĔF-ă-rō-plăst-ē]

SPELL and DEFINE	Identify if the following terms are spelled correctly. Correct the words that are spelled incorrectly. Write the definition for each word.	
	Spelling	**Definition**
stapedktome		
miringgotome		
enukleashun		
tympanoplasty		
keratoplasty		

UNDERSTAND	Fill in the blanks with the correct terms.

1. A patient sustaining a third-degree burn to the pinna would likely require _____.
2. A stapedectomy would be performed to correct _____.
3. Cryoretinopexy would be performed to correct a _____ retina.
4. A corneal _____ may restore sight.
5. A child with chronic otitis media may need a _____.

During the assessment, the physician asks the medical assistant to schedule surgery to correct Mr. Smith's droopy eyelids that are obstructing his vision. What procedure would the medical assistant schedule?

_____

_____

_____

_____

LO 8.6   Pharmacological Terms

Pharmacological agents may be used to treat sensory system symptoms, diseases, and conditions or may be used to assist in identifying conditions. Medications may be used for a short or an extended time.

Pharmacological	PRACTICE
	Provide the missing term(s) to complete the following sentences.
	Eyes and ears can both be treated with the instillation of drops.
	Antibiotic ophthalmic solution is an antibacterial agent used to treat eye infections, such as conjunctivitis.
mydriatic [mī-drē-ĂT-ĭk] **miotic** [mī-ŎT-ĭk]	A _____ solution dilates the pupil during an eye examination. A _____ solution causes the pupil to contract. Antiglaucoma medications, ophthalmic decongestants, and moisturizers also may be used.
	The eye and the ear can both be irrigated and flushed with water or solution to remove foreign objects. Ear irrigation (lavage) is the irrigation of the ear canal to remove excessive cerumen buildup. Wax emulsifiers remove cerumen. Antibiotics, antihistamines, anti-inflammatories, and decongestants are used to relieve ear infections, allergies, inflammations, and congestion. Antiemetics may be used to decrease nausea related to ear disorders.

UNDERSTAND   **Fill in the blanks with the correct terms.**

1. What medication might be prescribed for conjunctivitis? _____
2. During an eye exam, what agent helps to open part of the eye for better viewing? _____
3. What type of medication might be prescribed for otitis media? _____
4. What type of medication might be prescribed for allergies? _____

LO 8.7 Abbreviations

ABBREVIATION REVIEW

Abbreviation	Definition
ASL	American Sign Language
dB	decibel
IOL	intraocular lens
IOP	intraocular pressure

APPLY   **Answer the question.**

How would you explain to the patient what the difference is between IOP and IOL?

_____

_____

_____

Chapter Review

	Learning Outcome	Summary
8.1	Identify the parts of the sensory system and discuss the function of each part.	The sensory system includes any organ or part involved in the perceiving and receiving of stimuli from the outside world and from within our bodies. The senses include vision, hearing, touch, pain, temperature, smell, and taste.
8.2	Define combining forms used in building words that relate to the sensory system.	Word building requires knowledge of the combining form and meaning.
8.3	Recall the common diagnostic tests, laboratory tests, and clinical procedures used in testing and treating disorders of the sensory system.	Diagnostic, procedural, and laboratory findings assist the health care provider in diagnosing medical conditions. Often used in combination, these tests lead to a final diagnosis and assist in treatment planning.
8.4	Define the major pathological conditions of the sensory system.	Lost or damaged senses are illnesses in themselves. The disruption of losing or damaging a sense organ can lead to related illnesses. Much of the pathology of the sensory system results from age-related disorders or just age-related wear and tear on the sensory organs.
8.5	Define surgical terms related to the sensory system.	Surgery may be performed on the sensory system. Sensory deficits may be restored; removal of cancerous tumors and cosmetic changes may occur through surgical intervention.
8.6	Recognize common pharmacological agents used in treating disorders of the sensory system.	Pharmacological agents may be used to treat conditions or may be used to assist in identifying conditions. Medications may be used for a short or extended timeframe.
8.7	Identify common abbreviations associated with the sensory system.	Abbreviations are used to describe diseases, conditions, and treatments within the sensory system.

RECALL

Identify the organs of the sensory system.

a. sight: _____
b. smell: _____
c. taste: _____
d. touch: _____
e. hearing: _____

Write the correct spelling in the blank space to the right of any misspelled words. Pronounce the word aloud. Write the definition of each word.

	Spelling	Definition
koroyd		
sileare		
chochlea		
miotik		
midreatik		
miopea		
glawkoma		
otoskope		
pupile		
diplopea		

IMPLEMENT

Match each term in the left column with its definition in the right column.

1. _____ iris
2. _____ sclera
3. _____ pupil
4. _____ decibel
5. _____ eustachian
6. _____ lacrimal gland
7. _____ cones
8. _____ stapes
9. _____ tympanic membrane
10. _____ auricle
11. _____ cerumen

a. Tough, white, outer coating of eyeball
b. Dark opening of the eye, surrounded by the iris
c. Earwax
d. Moisten eyes and produce tears
e. Eardrum
f. Intensity of sound
g. Stirrup
h. Auditory tube
i. Pinna
j. Receptor that perceives color and bright light
k. Colored portion of the eye

Complete the sentences by filling in the blanks with the correct terms.

1. _____ and _____ are receptor cells that sense light and color.
2. _____ receptors perceive light rays.
3. _____ is the focusing on distant objects.
4. The _____ houses the taste buds.
5. A sty is caused by _____.
6. Farsightedness caused by the focusing of light rays behind the retina is _____.
7. _____ is an inflammation of the tympanic membrane.
8. A chalazion is a nodular inflammation typically occurring in the _____.
9. Labyrinthitis occurs in the labyrinth of the _____.
10. _____ is sensitivity to light.

Find the Roots: From the following list of combining forms and from the list of suffixes in Chapter 3, write the word that matches the definition (not all roots may be used).

1. audi/o	2. blephar/o	3. core/o	4. dacryocyst/o	5. irid/o
6. kerat/o	7. opt/o	8. ot/o	9. retin/o	10. scler/o

a. _____ Softening of the sclera

b. _____ Inflammation of the sclera and cornea

c. _____ Inflammation of the eyelid

d. _____ Pertaining to the retina

e. _____ Paralysis of the iris

f. _____ Earache

g. _____ Study of hearing (disorders)

h. _____ Inflammation of the eyelid

i. _____ Discharge from the ear

j. _____ Instrument to measure hearing

DECONSTRUCT

Mr. Stevenson's grandson came for a few days' visit with his mother. The 2-year-old has had fairly frequent ear infections. During the stay, the child woke up screaming and clutching his ear. A local 24-hour clinic diagnosed severe otitis media and prescribed medication. When the boy returned home, his pediatrician performed a myringotomy. Ten months later, the child has gone without any ear inflammations and is back for a return visit with his grandparents. On the second day of the visit, however, the boy started rubbing his eyes and complained of itching. His mother noticed a reddish area around the edge of his eyelid.

1. Is the child's otitis media infectious?
2. What is a myringotomy?
3. What was the likely cause of the child's itchy eyelids?
4. Is it surprising that Mr. Stevenson, who played with his grandson frequently, developed the same condition 5 days later? Why or why not? _____

Reviewing the Terms

Pronounce each of the following terms. Write the definitions on a separate sheet of paper. This review will take you through all the words you learned in this chapter. If you have difficulty with any words, make a flash card for later study. Refer to the English-Spanish and Spanish-English glossaries in the eBook.

aphakia [ă-FĀ-kē-ă]

asthenopia [ăs-thě-NŌ-pē-ă]

astigmatism [ă-STĬG-mă-tĭzm]

audi/o, audit/o [ĂW-dē-ō, ĂW-dĭ-tō]

audiogram [ĂW-dē-ō-grăm]

audiologist [ăw-dē-ŎL-ō-jĭst]

audiometry [ăw-dē-ŎM-ě-trē]

auditory ossicles [ĂW-dĭ-tōr-ē ŎS-ĭ-klz]

aur/o, auricul/o [ĂW-rō, aw-RIK-ū-lō]

auricle [ĂW-rĭ-kl]

blephar/o [BLĚF-ă-rō]

blepharitis [BLĚF-ă-RĪ-tĭs]

blepharochalasis [BLĚF-ă-rō-KĂL-ă-sĭs]

blepharoplasty [BLĚF-ă-rō-plăst-ē]

blepharoptosis [BLĚF-ă-RŎP-tō-sĭs]

blepharospasm [BLĚF-ă-rō-spăzm]

blindness

cataracts [CĂT-ă-răkts]

cerumin/o [sě-ROO-mĭ-nō]

chalazion [kă-LĀ-zē-ŏn]

cholesteatoma [kō-lěs-tē-ă-TŌ-mă]

choroid [KŌ-royd]

ciliary [SĬL-ē-ăr-ē] body

cochle/o [KOK-lē-o]

cochlea (pl., cochleae) [KOK-lē-ă (KOK-lē-ē)]

cones [kōnz]

conjunctiv/o [kŏn-jŭnk-TĬ-vō]

conjunctiva (pl., conjunctivae) [kŏn-jŭnk-TĬ-vă (kŏn-jŭnk-TĬ-vē)]

conjunctivitis [kŏn-jŭnk-tĭ-VĬ-tĭs]

contact lenses

cor/o, core/o, corne/o [KŌR-ō, KŌR-ē-ō, KŌR-nē-ō]

cornea [KŌR-nē-ă]

cryoretinopexy [KRĪ-ō-RĚT-ĭ-nō-PĔK-sē]

cycl/o [SĪ-klō]

deafness

decibel [DĚS-ĭ-bĕl]

diplopia [dĭ-PLŌ-pē-ă]

ear [ēr]

eardrum [ĒR-drŭm]

enucleation [ē-nū-klē-Ā-shŭn]

equilibrium [ē-kwĭ-LĬB-rē-ŭm]

esotropia [ĕs-ō-TRŌ-pē-ă]

eustachian [yū-STĀ-shŭn, yū-STĀ-kē-ăn] tube

exophthalmos, exophthalmus [ĕk-sŏf-THĂL-mos, ĕk-sŏf-THĂL-mŭs]

exotropia [ĕk-sō-TRŌ-pē-ă]

eye [ī]

eyebrow [Ī-brŏw]

eyelashes [Ī-lăsh-ĕz]

eyelid [Ī-lĭd]

eyestrain [Ī-strān]

farsightedness

glaucoma [glăw-KŌ-mă]

hearing

hyperopia [hī-pĕr-Ō-pē-ă]

ir/o, irid/o [Ī-rō, ĬR-ĭ-dō]

iridectomy [ĬR-ĭ-DĔK-tō-mē]

iridotomy [ĭr-ĭ-DŎT-ō-mē]

iris [Ī-rĭs]

iritis [ĭ-RĪ-tĭs]

kerat/o [KĚR-ă-tō]

keratitis [kĕr-ă-TĪ-tĭs]

keratoplasty [KĚR-ă-tō-plăs-tē]

labyrinthitis [LĂB-ĭ-rĭn-THĪ-tĭs]

lacrim/o [LĂK-rĭ-mō]

lacrimal [LĂK-rĭ-măl] glands

lacrimation [lăk-rĭ-MĀ-shŭn]

lens [lĕnz]

macula [MĂK-yū-lă]

macula lutea [lū-TĒ-ă]

macular [MĂK-yū-lăr] degeneration

malleus [MĂL-ē-ŭs]

mastoid/o [măs-TOY-dō]

mastoiditis [măs-toy-DĪ-tĭs]

membranous labyrinth [MĚM-bră-nŭs LĂB-ĭ-rĭnth]

Ménière's disease [mĕn-YERZ di-ZĒZ]

miotic [mī-ŎT-ĭk]

mydriatic [mī-drē-ĂT-ĭk]

myopia [mī-Ō-pē-ă]

myring/o [mĭ-RĬNG-gō]

myringitis [mĭr-ĭn-JĪ-tĭs]

myringotomy [mĭr-ĭng-GŎT-ō-mē]

nas/o [NĀ-zō]

nearsightedness

neuroretina [nūr-ō-RĚT-ĭ-nă]

nyctalopia [nĭk-tă-LŌ-pē-ă]

nystagmus [nĭs-STĂG-mŭs]

ocul/o [Ŏk-ū-lō]

olfactory [ōl-FĂK-tō-rē] organs

ophthalm/o [ŏf-THĂL-mō]

ophthalmologist [ŏf-thăl-MŎL-ō-jĭst]

ophthalmoscopy [ŏf-thăl-MŎS-kō-pē]

opt/o, optic(o) [Ŏp-tō, ŎP-tĭ-kō]

optic nerve

optician [ŏp-TĬSH-ŭn]

optometrist [ŏp-TŎM-ĕ-trĭst]

organ of Corti [KŌR-tē]

osseous labyrinth [ŎS-sē-ŭs LĂB-ĭ-rĭnth]

ossicul/o [ŏ-SĬK-ū-lō]

otalgia [ō-TĂL-jē-ă]

otitis externa [ō-TĪ-tĭs ĕks-TĔR-nă]

otitis media [MĒ-dē-ă]

otoliths [Ō-tō-lĭths]

otologist [ō-TŎL-ō-jĭst]

otoplasty [Ō-tō-plăs-tē]

otorhinolaryngologist [Ō-tō-RĪ-nō-lăr-ĭng-GŎL-ō-jĭst]

otorrhagia [ō-tō-RĀ-jē-ă]

otorrhea [ō-tō-RĒ-ă]

otosclerosis [ō-tō-sklĕ-RŌ-sĭs]

otoscopy [ō-TŎS-kō-pē]

papillae [pă-PĬL-ē]

paracusis [PĂR-ă-KŪ-sĭs]

perilymph [PĔR-ĭ-lĭmf]

phac/o, phak/o [FĀ-kō]

phacoemulsification [FAK-ō-ē-mŭl-sĭ-fĭ-KĀ-shŭn]

photophobia [fō-tō-FŌ-bē-ă]

pinkeye

pinna [PĬN-ă]

presbyacusis [prĕz-bē-ă-KŪ-sĭs]

presbyopia [prĕz-bē-Ō-pē-ă]

pseudophakia [sū-dō-FĀ-kē-ă]

pupil [PYŪ-pĭl]

pupill/o [pyū-pĭ-lō]

refraction [rē-FRĂK-shŭn]

retin/o [RĔT-ĭ-nō]

retina [RĔT-ĭ-nă]

retinitis [rĕt-ĭ-NĪ-tĭs]

retinitis pigmentosa [pĭg-mĕn-TŌ-să]

rods [rŏdz]

scler/o [SKLĒR-ō]

sclera (pl., sclerae) [SKLĒR-ă (SKLĒR-ē)]

scleritis [sklĕ-RĪ-tĭs]

scot/o [skō-tō]

scotoma [skō-TŌ-mă]

semicircular canals

sensory receptors

sensory system

sight

smell

stapedectomy [stā-pĕ-DĔK-tō-mē]

stapes (pl., stapes, stapedes) [STĀ-pēz (STĀ-pĕ-dēz)]

strabismus [stră-BĬZ-mŭs]

sty, stye [stī]

taste [tāst]

taste buds

taste cells

tears [tērz]

tinnitus [tĭ-NĪ-tŭs, TĬ-nĭ-tŭs]

tonometry [tō-NŎM-ĕ-trē]

touch

trabeculectomy [tră-BĔK-yū-LĔK-tō-mē]

trichiasis [trĭ-KĪ-ă-sĭs]

tympan/o [TĬM-pă-nō]

tympanic [tĭm-PĂN-ĭk] membrane

tympanitis [tĭm-pă-NĪ-tĭs]

tympanoplasty [TĬM-pă-nō-plăs-tē]

uve/o [YŪ-vē-o]

uvea [YŪ-vē-ă]

vertigo [VĔR-tĭ-gō, vĕr-TĪ-gō]

vestibule [VĔS-tĭ-būl]

The Endocrine System

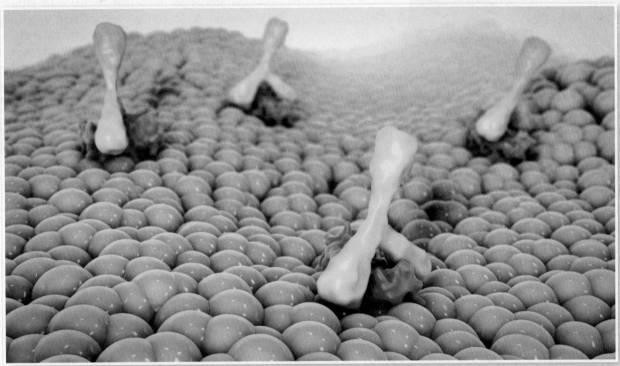

Learning Outcomes

After studying this chapter, you will be able to:

9.1 Recall the parts of the endocrine system and discuss the function of each part.

9.2 Define combining forms used in building words that relate to the endocrine system.

9.3 Recall the common diagnostic tests, laboratory tests, and clinical procedures used to test and treat disorders of the endocrine system.

9.4 Define the major pathological conditions of the endocrine system.

9.5 Define surgical terms related to the endocrine system.

9.6 Recognize common pharmacological agents used in treating disorders of the endocrine system.

9.7 Identify common abbreviations associated with the endocrine system.

LO 9.1 Structure and Function of the Endocrine System

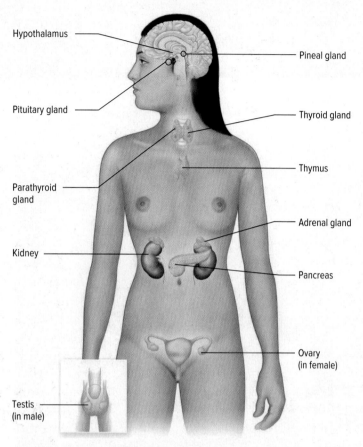

Hypothalamus

Pineal gland

Pituitary gland

Thyroid gland

Thymus

Parathyroid gland

Adrenal gland

Kidney

Pancreas

Ovary (in female)

Testis (in male)

Figure 9-1 Endocrine glands

The endocrine system is a group of glands that act as the body's master regulator. It helps to maintain homeostasis by regulating the production of chemicals that affect most functions of the body. It secretes hormones that aid the nervous system in reacting to stress and is an important regulator of growth and development. Hormones are secreted by glands and carried in the bloodstream to various parts of the body. Each type of hormone is transported differently throughout the body because of its chemical properties. Hormone release is triggered by various factors including age and substances that increase or decrease the levels of hormone released.

Figure 9-1 shows the endocrine system and Figure 9-2 shows the bodily functions affected by the endocrine system. Table 9-1 outlines the endocrine glands, their secretions, and their functions.

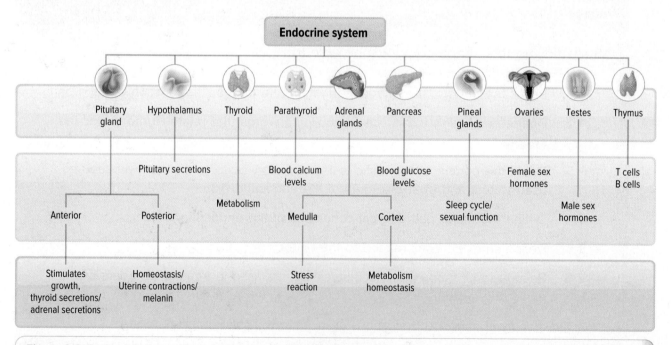

Figure 9-2 Bodily functions affected by the endocrine system

TABLE 9-1	Endocrine Glands, Their Secretions, and Their Functions	
Endocrine Gland or Tissue	**Hormone**	**Function**
hypothalamus	pituitary-regulating hormones	either stimulates or inhibits pituitary secretions
neurohypophysis (pituitary gland—posterior)	antidiuretic hormone (ADH), vasopressin oxytocin melanocyte-stimulating hormone (MSH)	increases water reabsorption stimulates uterine contractions and lactation stimulates the production of melanin
adenohypophysis (pituitary gland—anterior)	growth hormone (GH), somatotrophic hormone (STH) thyroid-stimulating hormone (TSH) adrenocorticotropic hormone (ACTH) follicle-stimulating hormone (FSH), luteinizing hormone (LH) prolactin	stimulates bone and muscle growth; regulates some metabolic functions, such as the rate at which cells utilize carbohydrates and fats stimulates thyroid gland to secrete hormones stimulates secretion of adrenal cortex hormones stimulates development of ova and production of female hormones stimulates breast development and milk production
thyroid	thyroxine (T4), triiodothyronine (T3) calcitonin	regulates metabolism; stimulates growth lowers blood calcium as necessary to maintain homeostasis
parathyroid	parathormone, parathyroid hormone (PTH)	increases blood calcium as necessary to maintain homeostasis
adrenal medulla	epinephrine (adrenaline), norepinephrine (noradrenaline)	works with the sympathetic nervous system to react to stress
adrenal cortex	glucocorticoids (cortisol, corticosteroids, corticosterone), mineralocorticoids (aldosterone), gonadocorticoids (androgens)	affects metabolism and growth; aids in electrolyte and fluid balances
pancreas (in islets of Langerhans)	insulin, glucagons	maintains homeostasis in blood glucose concentration
pineal gland	melatonin	affects sexual functions and wake–sleep cycles
ovaries	estrogen (estradiol, the most powerful estrogen), progesterone	promotes development of female sex characteristics, menstrual cycle, reproductive functions
testes	androgen, testosterone	promotes development of male sex characteristics, sperm production
thymus gland	thymosin, thymic humoral factor (THF), factor thymic serum (FTS)	aids in development of T cells and some B cells; function not well understood

Building Your Endocrine Vocabulary

This section provides an introduction to the endocrine system combining terms and their meanings. Review this information prior to moving to the practice.

Combining Form	Meaning
aden/o	gland
adren/o, adrenal/o	adrenal glands
gluc/o	glucose
glyc/o	glycogen
gonad/o	sex glands
pancreat/o	pancreas
parathyroid/o	parathyroid
thyr/o, thyroid/o	thyroid gland

Structure and Function	PRACTICE
	Provide the missing term(s) to complete the following sentences.
glands [glăndz] hormones [HŌR-mōnz] target cells receptors [rē-SĔP-tĕrz]	The endocrine system is made up of various _____ and other tissue that secrete _____, specialized chemicals, into the bloodstream. The hormones are effective only in specific _____, cells that have _____ that recognize a compatible hormone. A group of such cells forms target tissue. Minute amounts of hormones can initiate a strong reaction in some target cells.
exocrine glands [ĔK-sō-krĭn glăndz] endocrine glands [ĔN-dō-krĭn glăndz] ductless glands	Unlike _____, which secrete substances into ducts directed toward a specific location, _____ or tissue secretes hormones into the bloodstream. They are also known as _____. Some endocrine glands are also exocrine glands. For example, as an endocrine gland, the pancreas secretes insulin, and as an exocrine gland, it releases digestive juices through ducts to the small intestine.

PRONOUNCE and DEFINE	Pronounce the following terms aloud and write their meaning in the space provided.
hormones	[HŌR-mōnz]
receptors	[rē-SĔP-tĕrz]
exocrine	[ĔK-sō-krĭn]
endocrine	[ĔN-dō-krĭn]

Identify if the following terms are spelled correctly. Correct the words that are spelled incorrectly. Write the definition for each word.

	Spelling	Definition
ductless glands		
indokrin glands		
xsokin gland		
target cells		
resepterz		

UNDERSTAND Match the term on the left to its function on the right.

1. _____ exocrine
2. _____ endocrine
3. _____ target cells
4. _____ receptor
5. _____ hormone
6. _____ gland

a. Secretes hormones
b. Recognize hormones
c. Secretes into ducts
d. Substance secreted by glands
e. Ductless gland
f. Receptors that match specific hormones

APPLY Read the following scenario and answer the question.

You must give an overview of the endocrine system to Elizabeth Boone's fifth-grade class. How will you explain it?

_____

_____

_____

Hypothalamus, Pineal Gland, and Pituitary Gland

The hypothalamus either stimulates or inhibits pituitary secretions. The pineal gland affects sexual functions and wake–sleep cycles. The anterior and posterior pituitary glands affect vital functions of the body, including growth and metabolism. Figure 9-3 shows the hypothalamus and pituitary glands.

Structure and Function

PRACTICE

Provide the missing term(s) to complete the following sentences.

Hypothalamus

hypothalamus
[HĪ-pō-THĂL-ă-mŭs]
releasing factor
inhibiting factor

The _____ is a part of the nervous system that serves as an endocrine gland because it analyzes the body's condition and directs the release of hormones that regulate pituitary hormones. The hormones released by the hypothalamus have either a _____ (allowing the secretion of other hormones to take place) or an _____ (preventing the secretion of other hormones). The hypothalamus regulates the body's temperature, blood pressure, heartbeat, metabolism of fats and carbohydrates, and sugar levels in the blood. The hypothalamus is located in the brain superior to the pituitary gland.

Pineal Gland

pineal gland
[PĬN-ē-ăl glănd]
melatonin [měl-ă-TŌN-ĭn]

The _____ is located superior and posterior to the pituitary gland. It releases _____, a hormone that is believed to affect sleep and the functioning of the gonads.

continued on next page

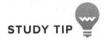
The hypothalamus and pituitary are located in close proximity. This provides a direct link to the nervous system.

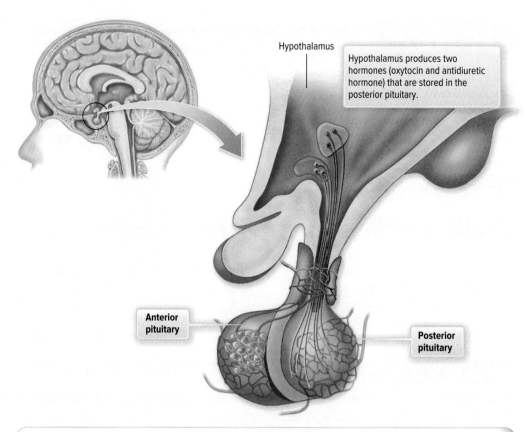

Hypothalamus

Hypothalamus produces two hormones (oxytocin and antidiuretic hormone) that are stored in the posterior pituitary.

Anterior pituitary

Posterior pituitary

Figure 9-3 The hypothalamus and pituitary glands

Structure and Function	PRACTICE
	Provide the missing term(s) to complete the following sentences.

Pituitary Gland

pituitary gland [pĭ-TŪ-ĭ-tār-ē glănd] hypophysis [hī-PŎF-ĭ-sĭs] adenohypophysis [ĂD-ĕ-nō-hī-PŎF-ĭ-sĭs] neurohypophysis [NŪR-ō-hī-PŎF-ĭ-sĭs]	The _____, also called the _____, is located at the base of the brain. The pituitary is the body's master gland in regulating or aiding in the secretion of essential hormones. The pituitary consists of an *anterior lobe* (_____) and a *posterior lobe* (_____).

PRONOUNCE and DEFINE	Pronounce the following terms aloud and write their meaning in the space provided.
hypothalamus	[HĪ-pō-THĂL-ă-mŭs]
adenohypophysis	[ĂD-ĕ-nō-hī-PŎF-ĭ-sĭs]
neurohypophysis	[NŪR-ō-hī-PŎF-ĭ-sĭs]
pineal	[PĬN-ē-ăl]
melatonin	[mĕl-ă-TŌN-ĭn]

UNDERSTAND Match the term on the left to its description on the right.

1. _____ adenohypophysis   a. Affects sleep patterns
2. _____ hypothalamus   b. Regulates pituitary hormones
3. _____ melatonin   c. Secretes melatonin
4. _____ pituitary gland   d. Anterior lobe of pituitary gland
5. _____ pineal gland   e. Essential for metabolic functions

APPLY Read the following scenario and answer the questions.

Marcy Capell experienced a head injury that affected the hypothalamus.

1. How might this injury affect the body?

_____
_____
_____

2. What glands might have been impacted by this injury that could result in system-wide complications?

_____
_____
_____

Did you know

Biological Rhythms

All living things have biological cycles determined by nature. Humans are considered to have three basic biological rhythms or biorhythms: *ultradian, infradian,* and *circadian.* Ultradian rhythms are those cycles (heartbeat, respiration) that are shorter than 24 hours. Infradian rhythms are those cycles (menstrual, ovulation) that are longer than 24 hours. Circadian rhythms occur in the 24-hour sleep–wake periods. Most of these cycles are affected by two things: factors outside the body and factors inside the body. Factors outside the body can include almost any environmental changes, such as light and dark, weather, physical activity, and stress. Factors inside the body are affected mostly by hormones released from the endocrine system. People with circadian rhythm disorders (such as insomnia) are sometimes treated with hormone supplements. In addition, some health care practitioners believe that understanding and regulating the body's biorhythms may be a key to maintaining health. There are many Internet sites that promote personal software for mapping your own biorhythms. Many of these are not based on scientific understanding of body rhythms.

Thyroid Gland, Parathyroid Glands, Thymus Gland, and Adrenal Glands

The thyroid gland affects metabolism and calcium levels within the body. Though the thymus gland is not well understood, it does aid in the development of T and B cells. Metabolism, growth, fluid, and electrolyte balance are affected by the hormones of the adrenal glands. Figure 9-4 shows the thyroid gland and Figure 9-5 the parathyroid glands. Figure 9-6 shows the adrenal glands.

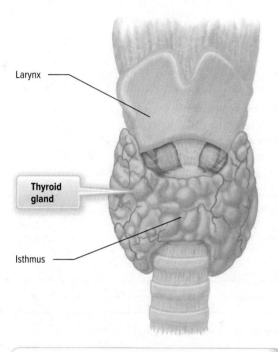

Figure 9-4 Thyroid gland

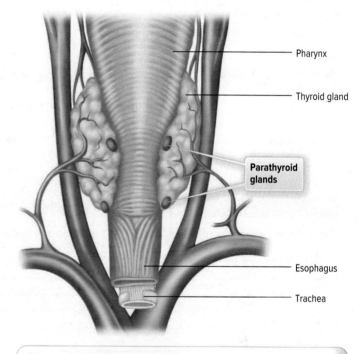

Figure 9-5 Parathyroid glands

STUDY TIP

If the thyroid glands are removed, the parathyroids also are removed.

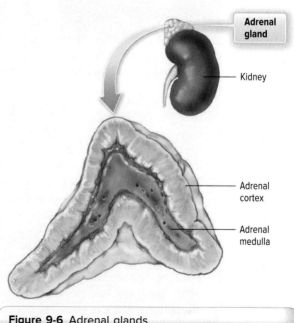

Figure 9-6 Adrenal glands

<table>
<tr><td></td><td>**PRACTICE**

Provide the missing term(s) to complete the following sentences.</td></tr>
</table>

Thyroid Gland

thyroid gland [THĪ-royd glănd] **isthmus** [ĬS-mŭs] **Adam's apple**	The _____ consists of a left lobe and a right lobe. The lobes sit on either side of the trachea. The two lobes are connected by the _____, a narrow strip of tissue on the ventral surface of the trachea. Above the thyroid gland sits the thyroid cartilage, a large piece of cartilage that covers the larynx and produces the protrusion on the neck known as the _____.
metabolism [mĕ-TĂB-ō-lĭzm] **thyroxine** [thī-RŎK-sēn, -sĭn] T_4 **triiodothyronine** [trī-Ī-ō-dō-THĪ-rō-nēn] T_3 **calcitonin** [kăl-sĕ-TŌ-nĭn]	Thyroid secretions control _____ (the chemical changes in cells that provide energy for vital processes and activities and through which new material is assimilated) and blood calcium concentrations. Two of the hormones secreted, _____, or *tetraiodothyronine* (_____), and _____ (_____), are produced in the thyroid gland using iodine from blood that circulates through the gland. These compounds circulate throughout the bloodstream helping to stimulate and control various bodily functions, such as regulating the metabolizing of carbohydrates, lipids, and proteins.

_____ is secreted from the outside surface of thyroid cells. It is a hormone that helps lower blood calcium concentration. |

Parathyroid Glands

parathyroid glands [păr-ă-THĪ-royd glăndz]	The _____ are four oval-shaped glands located on the dorsal side of the thyroid. The parathyroids help regulate calcium and phosphate levels, two elements necessary to maintain homeostasis.

Thymus Gland

thymus gland [THĪ-mŭs glănd]	The _____ is considered an endocrine gland because it secretes a hormone and is ductless; however, it is also part of the immune system. (Chapter 13 discusses the immune system.)

Adrenal Glands

adrenal glands [ă-DRĒ-năl glăndz] **suprarenal glands** [SŪ-pră-RĒ-năl glăndz] **adrenal cortex** [ă-DRĒ-năl KŎR-tĕks] **adrenal medulla** [ă-DRĒ-năl mĕ-DŪL-ă] **electrolytes** [ē-LĔK-trō-līts] **sympathomimetic** [SĬM-pă-thō-mĭ-MĔT-ĭk] **catecholamines** [kăt-ĕ-KŌL-ă-mēnz]	The _____ (or _____) are a pair of glands. Each of the glands sits atop a kidney. Each gland consists of two parts: the _____ (the outer portion) and the _____ (the inner portion). The adrenal glands regulate _____ (essential mineral salts that conduct electricity and are decomposed by it) in the body. The mineral salts affect metabolism and blood pressure. The adrenal glands are also _____, imitative of the sympathetic nervous system, as in response to stress. The adrenal medulla secretes a class of hormones, _____ (*epinephrine* and *norepinephrine*), in response to stress.

PRONOUNCE and DEFINE	Pronounce the following terms aloud and write their meaning in the space provided.
parathyroid	[păr-ă-THĪ-royd]
adrenal	[ă-DRĒ-năl]
sympathomimetic	[SĬM-pă-thō-mǐ-MĚT-ĭk]
calcitonin	[kăl-sĕ-TŌ-nǐn]
catecholamines	[kăt-ĕ-KŌL-ă-mēnz]

SPELL and DEFINE	Identify if the following terms are spelled correctly. Correct the words that are spelled incorrectly. Write the definition for each word.	
	Spelling	Definition
elekrolite		
ismus		
triiodothyronine		
thirocksen		
metabolism		

UNDERSTAND Fill In the blanks.

1. If the thyroid is removed, the _____ are also removed.
2. The _____ gland is ductless.
3. _____ stimulates growth.
4. _____ is the outer portion of the adrenal gland.
5. _____ produces chemical changes to provide energy.

APPLY Read the following scenario and answer the questions.

Angie Herting had a thyroidectomy.

1. What is the function of the thyroid gland?

_____

_____

2. How might a removal of the thyroid affect Angie's body?

_____

_____

Pancreas, Ovaries, and Testes

The pancreas secretes enzymes to maintain a normal blood glucose level. Estrogen and progesterone are secreted by the ovaries. The testes secrete testosterone, which is responsible for sperm production. Figure 9-7 shows the structure of the pancreas.

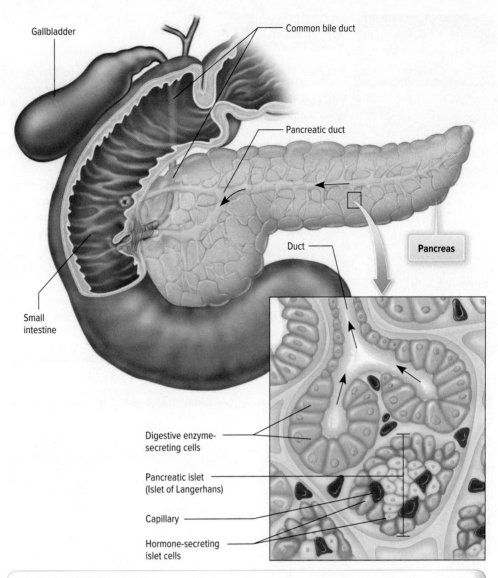

Figure 9-7 The pancreas

continued on next page

Structure and Function

pancreas
[PĂN-krē-ăs]
islets of Langerhans
[Ī-lets LĂN-gĕr-hănz]
insulin [ĬN-sū-lĭn]
glucagon [GLŪ-kă-gŏn]
beta cells [BĀ-tă sĕlz]
alpha cells [ĂL-fă sĕlz]
glycogen [GLĪ-kō-jĕn]

PRACTICE

Provide the missing term(s) to complete the following sentences.

The _____ helps in maintaining a proper level of blood glucose. Within the pancreas, the _____, specialized hormone-producing cells, secrete _____ to lower blood sugar when blood sugar levels are high and _____ to raise blood sugar levels when they are low. Insulin is produced by _____ in the islets of Langerhans, and glucagon is produced by _____ in the islets. When insulin is released in response to high blood sugar levels, it stimulates the glucose to be sent to the body's cells for energy as needed and to be converted to a starchy substance, _____, that is stored for later use in the liver and muscle. When glucagon is released in response to low blood sugar levels, it stimulates stored glycogen to be transformed into glucose again.

PRACTICE

Provide the missing term(s) to complete the following sentences.

	The pancreas is both an endocrine and an exocrine gland. The islets of Langerhans serve endocrine functions and the remaining cells, its exocrine ones (as discussed in the digestive system section in Chapter 14).

Ovaries

ovaries [Ō-văr-ēz]	The _____ are in the female pelvic region, one at the top of each fallopian tube. (Chapter 17 describes the female reproductive system.) The ovaries produce the immature egg cell, which, when fertilized, becomes the fetus. The ovaries also produce the female sex hormones *estrogen* and *progesterone*.

Testes

testes [TĔS-tēz] testicles [TĔS-tĭ-klz] androgens [ĂN-drō-jĕnz]	The two _____ (or _____) are located in the scrotum, a sac on the outside of the male body. The testes produce spermatozoa, which fertilize ova. The testes also produce male sex hormones called _____. The major androgen is *testosterone*. (Chapter 16 describes the male reproductive system.)

PRONOUNCE and DEFINE

Pronounce the following terms aloud and write their meaning in the space provided.

ovaries	[Ō-văr-ēz]
testes	[TĔS-tēz]
pancreas	[PĂN-krē-ăs]
alpha	[ĂL-fă]
glycogen	[GLĬ-kō-jĕn]

SPELL and DEFINE

Identify if the following terms are spelled correctly. Correct the words that are spelled incorrectly. Write the definition for each word.

	Spelling	Definition
islands of Longerhans		
glicojen		
testes		
androgen		
beta cells		

UNDERSTAND

Fill in the blanks.

1. _____ cell that produces insulin.
2. _____ produces glucagon.
3. The _____ are located at the top of the fallopian tubes.
4. The female and male sex hormones are _____, _____, and _____.
5. _____ is stored in the liver and muscles.

Mark Haas's blood sugar is elevated.

1. What gland is responsible for blood sugar levels?

_____

_____

_____

2. If the blood sugar is elevated, what should occur in the body?

_____

_____

_____

3. What happens in the body if Mr. Haas's blood sugar is low?

_____

_____

_____

LO 9.2 Word Building in the Endocrine System

The combining forms that relate specifically to the endocrine system include the following:

Word Building	PRACTICE — Provide the correct combining form to complete each of the following sentences.
pancreat-itis [păn-krē-ă-TĪ-tĭs]	_____ itis is inflammation of the pancreas.
glyco-lysis [glī-KŎL-ĭ-sĭs]	Conversion of glycogen to glucose is _____ lysis.
adeno-pathy [ad-ĕ-NOP-ă-thē]	_____ pathy is glandular or lymph node disease.
gonado-tropin [GŌ-nad-ō-TRŌ-pĭn]	_____ tropin is a hormone that aids in growth of gonads.
gluco-genesis [gloo-kō-JEN-ĕ-sĭs]	Production of glucose is _____ genesis.
adreno-megaly [ă-DRĒ-nō-MEG-ă-lē]	Enlargement of the adrenal glands is _____ megaly.
thyro-toxic [thī-rō-TOK-sik]	_____ toxic is having excessive amounts of thyroid hormones.
parathyroid-ectomy [PĂ-ră-thī-roy-DĔK-tō-mē]	_____ ectomy is excision of the parathyroid glands.

PRONOUNCE and DEFINE — Say the following words aloud and write the meaning in the space provided.	
pancreatitis	[PĂN-krē-ă-TĪ-tĭs]
glycolysis	[glī-KŎL-ĭ-sĭs]
adrenomegaly	[ă-DRĒ-nō-MEG-ă-lē]
parathyroidectomy	[PĂ-ră-thī-roy-DĔK-tō-mē]
gonadotropin	[GŌ-nad-ō-TRŌ-pĭn]

SPELL and DEFINE	Identify if the following terms are spelled correctly. Correct the words that are spelled incorrectly. Write the definition for each word.	
	Spelling	Definition
adenohypophysis		
adenal gland		
hypophisis		
suparenal gland		
sympathomimetic		

UNDERSTAND — Match each hormone with its function.

1. May affect sleep habits
2. Reacts to stress
3. Decreases urine output
4. Stimulates uterine contractions and lactation
5. Helps transport glucose to cells and decreases blood sugar
6. Stimulates breast development and lactation
7. Affects electrolyte and fluid balances
8. Regulates rate of cellular metabolism
9. Promotes growth and maintenance of male sex characteristics and sperm production
10. Aids in the development of the immune system

a. ADH
b. prolactin
c. insulin
d. aldosterone
e. oxytocin
f. thyroxine
g. testosterone
h. thymus
i. melatonin
j. epinephrine

APPLY — Complete the following:

Using the combining forms learned in this chapter, construct five words about the endocrine system that fit the definitions provided.

1. Inflammation of the thyroid: _____
2. Inflammation of the pancreas: _____
3. Production of glycogen: _____
4. Removal of the thyroid gland: _____
5. Removal of the adrenal gland: _____

From the Perspective Of . . .

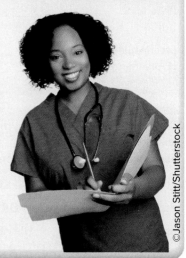

Who: Medical Coder/Biller

Other Aliases: CPC, Medical Secretary, Clinic Billing Specialist, Patient Account Representative, Medical Administrative Assistant

Job Duties: Assigning proper health care billing codes to diseases and procedures based on physician findings; submitting paperwork to insurance companies for processing; answering and resolving patient concerns with billing; operating office equipment (computer EMR system, fax, copier, postage).

A big part of the coder/biller's work includes dealing with difficult situations between insurance companies and patient satisfaction. Information, symptoms, and questions need to be spelled and recorded accurately for correct processing, as many bills are on a timeline for submission.

That is why medical terminology is important to me.

©Jason Stitt/Shutterstock

LO 9.3 Diagnostic, Procedural, and Laboratory Terms

Diagnostic, procedural, and laboratory findings assist in diagnosing the medical condition. Often used in combination, these tests lead to a final diagnosis and assist in treatment planning. Figure 9-8 shows a blood glucose test.

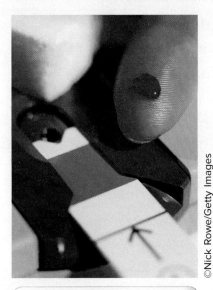

©Nick Rowe/Getty Images

Figure 9-8 Blood glucose test

Diagnostic	**PRACTICE** Provide the missing term(s) to complete the following sentences.
fasting blood sugar **glucose tolerance** **test (GTT)** **blood sugar** **blood glucose** **postprandial** **blood sugar** [pōst-PRĂN-dē-ăl] **urine sugar** **glycated hemoglobin** [GLĪ-kă-tĕd hē-mō-GLŌ-bĭn]	Endocrine functions affect homeostasis, the maintenance of fluid balance in the body. Levels of hormones, minerals, glucose, and other substances affect overall health. Blood and urine test results often can confirm a suspected diagnosis (usually based on symptoms such as sudden weight loss, fatigue, and abnormal thirst, as in the case of diabetes). Blood sugar levels vary depending on when the last meal was eaten. A _____ test and a _____ are both taken after a 12-hour fast. However, in the glucose tolerance test, the blood sugar test is repeated every 3 to 5 hours after the patient ingests a concentrated glucose solution. Patients can check _____ or _____ levels themselves to track fluctuations in blood sugar. A _____ (after eating) _____ is a test for blood sugar usually taken about 2 hours after a meal. A _____ is a test for ketones and/or sugar in urine, both of which may indicate diabetes. For people already diagnosed with diabetes, a _____ test or A1C tracks average blood sugar readings over the previous 2 to 3 months.
radioactive immunoassay **(RIA)** **thyroid function** **test or study** **radioactive iodine** **uptake** **thyroid scan**	Overall endocrine functioning is tested in a blood test. Many hormones and electrolytes are present in the blood. Endocrine function can be tested in the plasma by using a _____, a test that uses radioactive iodine to locate various substances in the plasma. Thyroid functioning can be tested using a _____, which is a blood test that measures the various hormones secreted by the thyroid. A _____ test is a measure of how quickly the thyroid gland absorbs ingested iodine. A _____ is a test for cancer or other abnormalities using radionuclide imaging.

PRONOUNCE and DEFINE	Pronounce the following terms aloud and write their meaning in the space provided.
postprandial	[pōst-PRĂN-dē-ăl]
glycated hemoglobin	[GLĪ-kā-tĕd hē-mō-GLŌ-bĭn]
testicles	[TĔS-tĭ-klz]
sympathomimetic	[SĬM-pă-thō-mĭ-MĔT-ĭk]
catecholamines	[kăt-ĕ-KŌL-ă-mēnz]

SPELL and DEFINE	Identify if the following terms are spelled correctly. Correct the words that are spelled incorrectly. Write the definition for each word.	
	Spelling	Definition
radioactive immunoassay		
glikated hemaglobin		
postprandeal blud sugar		
blud glucos		
thyroid scan		

UNDERSTAND	For each test, write D if it is a test for diabetes or T if it is a test for thyroid function.

1. Fasting blood sugar: _____
2. Radioactive iodine uptake: _____
3. Radioactive immunoassay: _____
4. Urine sugar: _____
5. Glucose tolerance test: _____

APPLY	Read the following scenario and answer the questions.

Diane Welp is a 45-year-old woman who has noticed some disturbing symptoms, such as unusual fatigue, excessive thirst, and excessive urination since her last checkup. She called her physician, Dr. John Colter, for an appointment. Dr. Colter examined her and sent her to a lab for several tests. Gail's tests came back with abnormally high blood sugar.

1. Dr. Colter ordered a urinalysis and blood tests. Why?

_____

_____

2. What organ is the likely origin of Gail's abnormally high blood sugar?

_____

_____

LO 9.4 Pathological Terms

Pituitary, Thyroid, Parathyroid, and Adrenal Disorders

Disorders of the pituitary, thyroid, parathyroid, and adrenal glands can affect many functions within the body. The Practice table introduces terms relating to disorders of the endocrine system. Figures 9-9, 9-10, and 9-11 show examples of thyroid disorders.

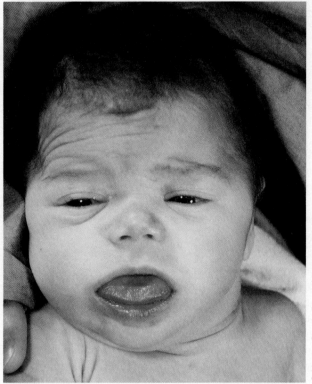

©Alamy Stock Photo/Alamy

Figure 9-9 Cretinism in an infant—note protruding tongue

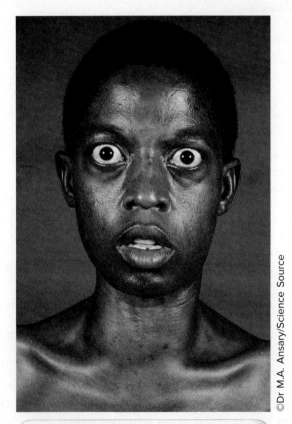

©Dr M.A. Ansary/Science Source

Figure 9-10 Graves disease—note the bulging eyes

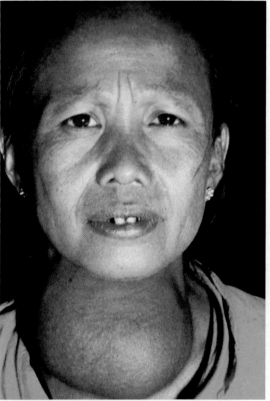

©Lester V. Bergman/Corbis/Getty Images

Figure 9-11 An iodine deficiency—note the goiter at the neck

Pathological	

Fill in the correct term(s) to complete the following sentences.

hypersecretion [HĪ-pĕr-sĕ-KRĒ-shŭn] **hyposecretion** [HĪ-pō-sĕ-KRĒ-shŭn]	Diseases of the endocrine system commonly involve lack of homeostasis. In other words, either too much or too little of a hormone or substance in the body creates an imbalance and, often, a disorder or disease. Most endocrine illnesses are the result of _____ (oversecretion) or _____ (undersecretion) of one or more hormones. Hypersecretion can be caused by excessive stimulating hormone; a bacterial, viral, or other illness in an endocrine gland; or a tumor. Hypersecretion is treated either with medication or by surgery. Hyposecretion can be due to a suppressed stimulating hormone or atrophy of a gland. Hyposecretion is usually treated with hormone supplements.

Pituitary Disorders

acromegaly [ăk-rō-MĔG-ă-lē] **gigantism** [JĪ-găn-tĭzm] **dwarfism** [DWŌRF-ĭzm]	Pituitary abnormalities include _____ (hypersecretion of growth hormone after puberty), which causes abnormal enlargement of features (such as the nose, ears, jaws, and fingers) after childhood. Hypersecretion of growth hormone from the pituitary gland may result in _____, which causes abnormal growth, even to more than 8 feet tall. Hyposecretion of the same growth hormone may result in dwarfism, which is stunted growth. Dwarfism caused by hyposecretion of growth hormone results in an extremely small person, but one with normally proportioned features. _____ with disproportionate features is usually caused by the congenital absence of the thyroid gland or by another genetic defect.
diabetes insipidus [dī-ă-BĒ-tēz ĭn-SĬP-ĭ-dŭs] **polyuria** [pŏl-ē-YŪ-rē-ă] **polydipsia** [pŏl-ē-DĬP-sē-ă] **syndrome of inappropriate ADH (SIADH)**	In addition to growth problems, hyposecretion of vasopressin or antidiuretic hormone causes _____, a disease with _____ (excessive amount of water excreted in the urine) and _____ (excessive and constant thirst). It can be treated with an antidiuretic medication. Hypersecretion of antidiuretic hormone causes _____, which results in excessive water retention.

Thyroid Disorders

hyperthyroidism [hī-pĕr-THĪ-royd-ĭzm] **Graves disease** [grāvz di-ZĒZ] **thyrotoxicosis** [THĪ-rō-tŏk-sĭ-KŌ-sĭs] **exophthalmos** [ĕk-sŏf-THĂL-mos] **goiter** [GOY-tĕr]	The thyroid gland may become overactive, causing _____, also known as _____ or _____. Symptoms of Graves disease are consistent with increased T_3 and T_4, which cause increased metabolic rate, weight loss, insomnia, and sweating. _____, bulging of the eyes, is a complication that can occur in some instances of Graves disease. A _____ also can be caused by hypersecretion from the thyroid gland, a tumor, or lack of iodine in the diet, causing the gland to expand and create a massive growth in the neck.
hypothyroidism [HĪ-pō-THĪ-royd-ĭzm] **myxedema** [mĭk-sĕ-DĒ-mă]	_____, underactivity of the thyroid gland, causes sluggishness and slow metabolism, often resulting in obesity. _____ is a specific type of hypothyroidism in adults with a range of symptoms, including puffiness in the extremities, slow muscular response, and excessively dry skin. As with other types of hypothyroidism, myxedema can be treated with synthetic hormones. Fetal hypothyroidism may result in a form of dwarfism (once called *cretinism;* now referred to as *congenital hypothyroidism*), which results in small physical stature as well as slow mental development. If caught early enough, at birth through newborn screening, it can be treated with a synthetic form of thyroxine.

Parathyroid Disorders

hyperparathyroidism [HĪ-pĕr-pă-ră-THĪ-royd-ĭzm] **hypoparathyroidism** [HĪ-pō-pă-ră-THĪ-royd-ĭzm] **tetany** [TĔT-ă-nē]	The parathyroid glands help control blood calcium levels, which contribute to bone growth and muscular health. _____ (overactivity of the parathyroid glands) is usually caused by a tumor in the parathyroid gland. It often results in many clinical symptoms, from bone loss to severe cases of kidney failure. _____ (underactivity of the parathyroid glands) results in low blood calcium levels, causing many symptoms such as bone loss and some muscle paralysis (_____). Medications and supplements that increase calcium absorption are available treatments that may be prescribed.

Adrenal Disorders

hyperadrenalism [HĪ-pĕr-ă-DRĒN-ă-lĭzm] **hypoadrenalism** [HĪ-pō-ă-DRĒN-ă-lĭzm] **hirsutism** [HĔR-sū-tĭzm] **virilism** [VĬR-ĭ-lĭzm] **Cushing syndrome** [KUSH-ĭng SIN-drōm]	The adrenal glands may be overactive (_____) or underactive (_____). Hyperadrenalism is usually caused by an adrenal tumor. It is usually cured by removal of the tumor. *Adrenogenital syndrome* results in symptoms of excessive androgens in both men and women, which, in turn, can result in _____, abnormal hair growth. _____ is also a condition with excessive androgen secretion. Virilism results in mature masculine features in children. Administration of steroids can keep the overactivity in balance. _____ results from an oversecretion of ACTH.
Addison disease [ĂD-ĭ-sŏn di-ZĒZ]	Hypoadrenalism also is known as _____. It may result in anemia, abnormal skin pigment, and general malaise. It can be controlled with cortisone.

PRONOUNCE and DEFINE	Pronounce the following terms aloud and write the meaning in the space provided.
polydipsia	[pŏl-ē-DĬP-sē-ă]
polyuria	[pŏl-ē-YŪ-rē-ă]
virilism	[VĬR-ĭ-lĭzm]
hirsutism	[HĔR-sū-tĭzm]
myxedema	[mĭk-sĕ-DĒ-mă]

SPELL and DEFINE	Identify if the following terms are spelled correctly. Correct the words that are spelled incorrectly. Write the definition for each word.	
	Spelling	**Definition**
poledpsea		
thirotoksikosis		
acromegaly		
dworfizm		
eksofthalmus		

Match the following conditions to the symptoms.

1. _____ Addison disease
2. _____ Cushing syndrome
3. _____ diabetes insipidus
4. _____ Graves disease
5. _____ SIADH
6. _____ myxedema

a. Hyposecretion of antidiuretic hormone
b. Excessive secretion of antidiuretic hormone
c. Overactive adrenal glands
d. Underactive thyroid gland
e. Underactive adrenal glands
f. Overactive thyroid gland

APPLY **Read the following scenario and answer the questions.**

Tammy Noel reports to the nurse that she has an enlarged area on her neck. She also states that she frequently urinates large amounts and is extremely thirsty.

1. What do you think is wrong with Tammy?

_____

_____

_____

2. As the medical assistant, document Tammy's symptoms using medical terminology.

_____

_____

_____

Pancreatic Disorders (Including Diabetes)

Pancreatic disorders frequently lead to diabetes. Diabetes can impact many other systems within the body. The following Practice table presents terms relating to disorders of the pancreas, including diabetes.

Did you know ?

Misleading Common Terms

In certain parts of the country, both types of diabetes are simply called *sugar,* as in the phrase "he has sugar." Sometimes common terms for diseases seem to misrepresent what the disease is. Diabetes is in fact an underproduction of or resistance to *insulin,* although in the past, many people thought it was caused by sugar alone.

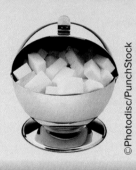

©Photodisc/PunchStock

Pathological	PRACTICE
	Provide the missing term(s) to complete the following sentences.
pancreatitis [PĂN-krē-ă-TĪ-tĭs] **hypoglycemia** [HĪ-pō-glī-SĒ-mē-ă] **diabetes mellitus** [dī-ă-BĒ-tēz MĔL-ĭ-tŭs, mĕ-LĪ-tŭs]	Sometimes, the pancreas may become inflamed, as in _____. Hyperinsulinism is the hypersecretion of insulin and may cause _____, a lowering of blood sugar levels that deprives the body of needed glucose. It can be controlled with dietary changes. Hyposecretion of insulin can cause _____, a widespread disease that affects about 4% of the U.S. population.

diabetes [dī-ă-BĒ-tēz] **type 1 diabetes** **(insulin-dependent** **diabetes mellitus or** **IDDM)** **type 2 diabetes** **(noninsulin-dependent** **diabetes mellitus or** **NIDDM)** **glucosuria** [glū-kō-SŪ-rē-ă] **glycosuria** [glī-kō-SŪ-rē-ă]	_____ occurs either as _____ or as _____. Type 1 diabetes usually occurs in childhood and is the result of underproduction of insulin by the beta cells. Glucose accumulates and overflows into the urine (_____, _____). Type 1 diabetes can be treated with controlled doses of insulin. Type 2 diabetes used to occur only in adulthood but now also occurs in younger people and even in teens and children. It usually occurs in overweight people whose responsiveness to insulin is abnormally low. This response is called _insulin resistance._
	Both types of diabetes can lead to _insulin shock,_ a condition where an overdosage of insulin causes symptoms such as tremors, tachycardia, hunger, dizziness, and cool moist skin. If left untreated, insulin shock can lead to _diabetic coma._
diabetic nephropathy [dī-ă-BĚT-ĭk nĕ-FRŎP-ă-thē] **diabetic neuropathy** [dī-ă-BĚT-ĭk nū-RŎP-ă-thē] **diabetic retinopathy** [dī-ă-BĚT-ĭk rĕt-ĭ-NŎP-ă-thē] **acidosis** [ăs-ĭ-DŌ-sĭs] **ketoacidosis** [KĒ-tō-ă-sĭ-DŌ-sĭs] **ketosis** [kē-TŌ-sĭs]	Complications of diabetes cover a wide range of ailments, from circulatory problems to infections to organ failure. _____ is a kidney disease resulting from serious diabetes. _____ is loss of sensation in the extremities. _____ is gradual visual loss leading to blindness. The body uses stored fat to replace glucose, thereby causing _____, _____, and _____, all of which are marked by the abnormal presence of ketone bodies in the blood and urine.
	Before the discovery of insulin as a compound that affects blood sugar levels, people with diabetes usually died of some of the many complications of the disease. Diabetes is still not curable—but it is controllable.

PRONOUNCE and DEFINE	**Pronounce the following terms aloud and write the meaning in the space provided.**
glucosuria	[glū-kō-SŪ-rē-ă]
glycosuria	[glī-kō-SŪ-rē-ă]
diabetic nephropathy	[dī-ă-BĚT-ĭk nĕ-FRŎP-ă-thē]
neuropathy	[nū-RŎP-ă-thē]
retinopathy	[rĕt-ĭ-NŎP-ă-thē]
acidosis	[ăs-ĭ-DŌ-sĭs]

SPELL and DEFINE	**Identify if the following terms are spelled correctly. Correct the words that are spelled incorrectly. Write the definition for each word.**	
	Spelling	**Definition**
keytoesis		
asidoesis		
glikosurea		
glucosuria		
pancreatitis		

UNDERSTAND | Write A for adrenal, PA for pancreas, PI for pituitary, and T for thyroid to indicate the gland from which each of the following diseases arise.

1. acromegaly: _____
2. diabetes mellitus: _____
3. exophthalmos: _____
4. gigantism: _____
5. goiter: _____
6. myxedema: _____
7. Cushing syndrome: _____
8. Graves disease: _____

APPLY | Read the following scenario and answer the questions.

Kelly Post has lost 12 pounds rapidly over the last couple of months, is feeling abnormally tired, and is unusually thirsty. Dr. Colter referred her to an endocrinologist. Kelly decides to wait until after the holidays to make her appointment with the endocrinologist. She thinks that she will watch what she eats and then go to the doctor when she is less busy. For a few days, she moderates her eating and feels a little better. However, on the big holiday weekend, Kelly goes to several parties, drinks, and overeats. When she wakes up in the morning, she feels dizzy, is in a cold sweat, and feels very hungry. Right away, she realizes that something is terribly wrong. Because it is a holiday weekend, she has a friend take her to the emergency room. Once there, her symptoms are worse. The emergency room doctor tests her blood sugar and finds it very low. After she has eaten something, he tests it again. Because Kelly is overweight, the doctor suspects that her body is not sensitive to insulin. Kelly is sent to Dr. Malpas, an endocrinologist, the very next day.

1. What disease does Dr. Colter think Kelly may have?

   _____

   _____

2. What test for blood glucose is taken after a meal? Explain how the test is run.

   _____

   _____

3. What type of diabetes does Kelly appear to have?

   _____

   _____

4. What might some recommendations be for Kelly's diet? What other lifestyle changes might the doctor suggest?

   _____

   _____

Did you know

Diabetes and Diet

For many years, doctors prescribed a high-protein, low-carbohydrate diet for diabetics. In recent years, increased understanding of how food is metabolized by the body has led to changes in diets prescribed for diabetics. Most newly diagnosed diabetics are given a varied diet by a physician or dietitian that is tailored to their specific needs—current weight, level of diabetes (mild, moderate, severe), and lifestyle. The American Dietetic Association and the American Diabetes Association provide the dietary information on which most diets for diabetics are based. A diabetic's personalized daily diet might include four fruit exchanges, three protein exchanges, three bread exchanges, and seven vegetable exchanges.

Many suppliers of processed food, particularly those foods aimed at the health-conscious consumer, now list exchanges as part of their nutrition labels, as shown here.

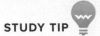

1/4 Carbohydrates   1/4 Protein   1/2 Vegetables

(fork & knife): ©C Squared Studios/Getty Images

STUDY TIP

Test Your Knowledge

1. Exophthalmos is associated with Graves disease. **True** or **False**?
2. The thyroid is connected by the parathyroids. **True** or **False**?
3. The adrenal glands are located in the mediastinum. **True** or **False**?

Cancers of the Endocrine System

Cancers occur commonly in the endocrine system. Many, such as thyroid cancer, can be treated by removing the affected gland and supplementing with a synthetic version of the necessary hormones that are consequently missing from the body. Some cancers, such as pancreatic cancer, are almost always fatal because no effective treatments are currently available.

LO 9.5 Surgical Terms

Certain endocrine glands that become diseased can be surgically removed. Synthetic versions of the hormones they produce are given to the patients to help their bodies perform the necessary endocrine functions once the glands are removed.

Surgical

adenectomy
[ă-dĕ-NĔK-tō-mē]
adrenalectomy
[ă-drē-năl-ĔK-tō-mē]
hypophysectomy
[hī-pŏf-ĭ-SĔK-tō-mē]
pancreatectomy
[PĂN-krē-ă-TĔK-tō-mē]
parathyroidectomy
[PĂ-ră-thī-roy-DĔK-tō-mē]
thymectomy
[thī-MĔK-tō-mē]
thyroidectomy
[thī-roy-DĔK-tō-mē]

PRACTICE

Provide the missing term(s) to complete the following sentences.

An _____ is the removal of any gland.

An _____ is the removal of an adrenal gland.

Removal of the pituitary gland is a _____.

The pancreas is removed in a _____.

Removal of the parathyroid gland is performed in a _____ and removal of the thymus gland is performed in a _____.

A _____ is the removal of the thyroid.

PRONOUNCE and DEFINE	Pronounce the following terms aloud and write the meaning in the space provided.
adenectomy	[ă-dĕ-NĔK-tō-mē]
adrenalectomy	[ă-drē-năl-ĔK-tō-mē]
hypophysectomy	[hī-pŏf-ĭ-SĔK-tō-mē]
pancreatectomy	[PĂN-krē-ă-TĔK-tō-mē]
parathyroidectomy	[PĂ-ră-thī-roy-DĔK-tō-mē]

SPELL and DEFINE	Identify if the following terms are spelled correctly. Correct the words that are spelled incorrectly. Write the definition for each word.	
	Spelling	**Definition**
thimektome		
hipofsectome		
adenektome		
thyroidectomy		
parathyroidectomy		

UNDERSTAND	Supply the missing root word to the suffix to complete the term.

1. Removal of a gland: _____ ectomy
2. Removal of the pituitary gland: _____ ectomy
3. Removal of an adrenal gland: _____ ectomy
4. Removal of the thymus gland: _____ ectomy
5. Removal of part of the pancreas: _____ ectomy
6. Removal of the thyroid gland: _____ ectomy

APPLY	Read the following scenario and answer the questions.

Phil Byrd has had an overactive thyroid since he was a child. Lately, Phil's hyperthyroidism has increased. Dr. Rothburg biopsies Phil's thyroid and tells Phil it would be best to remove it.

1. What did Dr. Rothburg probably find that necessitated thyroid removal?

_____

_____

2. What is the medical term for removal of the thyroid?

_____

_____

3. What is a complication of removing the thyroid?

_____

_____

LO 9.6 Pharmacological Terms

This section identifies terms associated with the medications used to treat endocrine system disorders.

Pharmacological

PRACTICE

Provide the missing term(s) to complete the following sentences.

hormone replacement therapy (HRT) **antihypoglycemic** [ĂN-tē-HĪ-pō-glī-SĒ-mĭk] **antihyperglycemic** [ĂN-tē-HĪ-pĕr-glī-SĒ-mĭk] **hypoglycemic** [HĪ-pō-glī-SĒ-mĭk] **human growth hormone** **steroids** [STĒR-oyd, STĒR-oyd]	Hormonal deficiencies are sometimes treated with _____. Common types of hormone therapy include synthetic thyroid, estrogen, and testosterone. Other medications include those that regulate levels of substances in the body, such as glucose levels in diabetics. An _____ raises blood sugar. An _____ or _____ lowers blood sugar. Instead of, or in addition to, using drugs to regulate blood sugar, many diabetics are now treated with medications that increase their sensitivity to their own insulin. _____ (somatotropin) occurs naturally in the body. In some cases of dwarfism, it is given to promote growth during childhood. _____ are used to control symptoms and treat many diseases occurring within and outside the endocrine system. Steroids also can be abused for muscle growth. Women who are in perimenopause or menopause itself must weigh the risks of HRT (increased risk of cancer and clots in some studies) with its benefits (alleviation of symptoms, prevention of heart disease, and osteoporosis).
radioactive iodine therapy	Many cancers of the endocrine system require surgical removal and/or chemotherapy or radiation. A thyroid tumor also may be treated with _____ to eradicate the tumor.

PRONOUNCE and DEFINE

Pronounce the following terms aloud and write the meaning in the space provided.

antihypoglycemic	[ĂN-tē-HĪ-pō-glī-SĒ-mĭk]
antihyperglycemic	[ĂN-tē-HĪ-pĕr-glī-SĒ-mĭk]
hypoglycemic	[HĪ-pō-glī-SĒ-mĭk]
steroids	[STĔR-oydz, STĒR-oydz]

SPELL and DEFINE

Identify if the following terms are spelled correctly. Correct the words that are spelled incorrectly. Write the definition for each word.

	Spelling	Definition
sterold		
hipogliseemick		
radioactive iodine therapy		
antihypoglycemic		

UNDERSTAND

Identify the medication needed to relieve the described symptoms associated with a hormonal disease.

1. This medication lowers blood glucose levels: _____
2. Treats hormonal deficiencies: _____
3. Treats low blood glucose: _____
4. Helps to control symptoms of menopause: _____
5. May be given to promote growth due to dwarfism: _____

Mr. Jim Grott has dwarfism. He asks his nurse about human growth hormone. How should the nurse respond?

_____
_____
_____

LO 9.7 Abbreviations

ABBREVIATION REVIEW

Abbreviation	Definition
ADH	antidiuretic hormone
DM	diabetes mellitus
GH	growth hormone
GTT	glucose tolerance test
HRT	hormone replacement therapy
IDDM	insulin-dependent diabetes mellitus
RIA	radioactive immunoassay
SIADH	syndrome of inappropriate antidiuretic hormone
t3, T3	triiodothyronine
t4	thyroxine

UNDERSTAND   Match the abbreviation to the definition.

1. _____ IDDM
2. _____ SIADH
3. _____ HRT
4. _____ T3
5. _____ GH

a. growth hormone
b. hormone replacement therapy
c. syndrome of inappropriate antidiuretic hormone
d. insulin-dependent diabetes mellitus
e. triiodothyronine

APPLY   Read the following scenario and respond accordingly.

Per physician notes, the patient has diabetes insipidus due to hypersecretion of ADH resulting in SIADH. No history of DM.

Explain to the patient what this means.

_____
_____
_____

CHAPTER SUMMARY

	Learning Outcome	Summary
9.1	Recall the parts of the endocrine system and discuss the function of each part.	The function of the endocrine system is to secrete hormones. The endocrine glands include the following: • hypothalamus • neurohypophysis (pituitary gland—posterior) • adenohypophysis (pituitary gland—anterior) • thyroid • parathyroid • adrenal medulla • adrenal cortex • pancreas (in islets of Langerhans) • pineal gland • ovaries • testes • thymus gland
9.2	Define combining forms used in building words that relate to the endocrine system.	Word building requires knowledge of the combining form and meaning.
9.3	Recall the common diagnostic tests, laboratory tests, and clinical procedures used to test and treat disorders of the endocrine system.	Diagnostic, procedural, and laboratory findings assist the health care provider to diagnose medical conditions. Often used in combination, these tests lead to a final diagnosis and assist in treatment planning.
9.4	Define the major pathological conditions of the endocrine system.	Diseases of the endocrine system commonly involve lack of homeostasis. In other words, either too much or too little of a hormone or substance in the body creates an imbalance and, often, a disorder or disease.
9.5	Define surgical terms related to the endocrine system.	Certain endocrine glands that become diseased can be surgically removed. Synthetic versions of the hormones they produce are given to the patients to help their bodies perform the necessary endocrine functions once the glands are removed.
9.6	Recognize common pharmacological agents used in treating disorders of the endocrine system.	Medications are used to treat a variety of endocrine disorders. Many of the medications must be taken for life.
9.7	Identify common abbreviations associated with the endocrine system.	Abbreviations are used to describe diseases, conditions, procedures, and treatments associated with the endocrine system.

Label the glands on the accompanying figure.

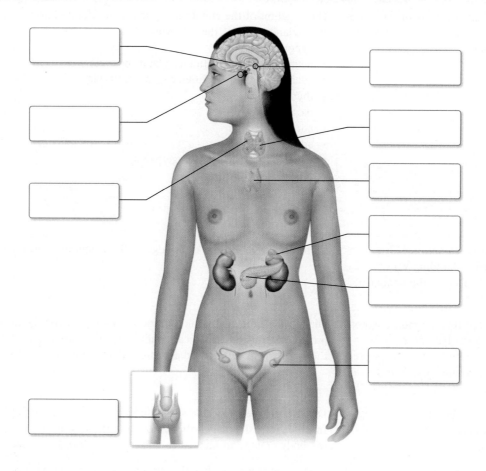

Pronounce the following terms aloud.

calcitonin	[kăl-sĕ-TŌ-nĭn]
catecholamines	[kăt-ĕ-KŌL-ă-mēnz]
exocrine	[ĔK-sō-krĭn]
exophthalmos	[ĕk-sŏf-THĂL-mŏs]
hypophysis	[hī-PŎF-ĭ-sĭs]
hyposecretion	[HĪ-pō-sĕ-KRĒ-shŭn]
thyrotoxicosis	[THĪ-rō-tŏk-sĭ-KŌ-sĭs]
thyroxine	[thī-RŎK-sēn, -sĭn]

Identify if the following terms are spelled correctly. Correct the words that are spelled incorrectly. Write the meaning.

1. adenohypophysis: _____
2. adenal: _____
3. hypophisis: _____
4. suparenal: _____
5. sympathomimetic: _____
6. pituatary: _____
7. lutinizing: _____
8. triiodothyronine: _____

IMPLEMENT

Write the definitions for the following terms.

1. adrenalectomy: _____
2. pancreatectomy: _____
3. adenoma: _____
4. gonadotropin: _____
5. thyromegaly: _____

Define the treatment for the following conditions.

1. Treatment for Graves disease: _____
2. Treatment for severe virilism: _____
3. Treatment for a cancerous gland: _____
4. Treatment for hyperparathyroidism: _____
5. Treatment for acromegaly: _____

In each word, find the combining form that relates to the endocrine system and provide its definition.

1. adenohypophysis: _____
2. neurohypophysis: _____
3. pancreatectomy: _____
4. thyroidectomy: _____
5. thymectomy: _____

DECONSTRUCT

Helene Fisher is a 52-year-old female who comes to the physician's office with the following complaint: bulging eyes, rapid heart rate, weight loss, increased hunger, and inability to sleep.

1. As the nurse, discuss the symptoms with the physician using medical terminology.

_____

_____

_____

2. Based on her symptoms, the nurse suspects what endocrine disorder?

_____

_____

_____

Reviewing the Terms

Define and pronounce each of the following terms. This review will take you through all the words you learned in this chapter. If you have difficulty with any words, make a flash card for later study. Refer to the English-Spanish and Spanish-English glossaries in the eBook.

acidosis [ăs-ĭ-DŌ-sĭs]

acromegaly [ăk-rō-MĔG-ă-lē]

Adam's apple

Addison [ĂD-ĭ-sŏn] disease

aden/o [ĂD-ě-nō]

adenectomy [ă-dě-NĔK-tō-mē]

adenohypophysis [ĂD-ě-nō-hī-PŎF-ĭ-sĭs]

adren/o, adrenal/o [ă-DRĒ-nō, ă-DRĒ-nă-lō]

adrenal cortex [ă-DRĒ-năl KŌR-těks]

adrenal gland

adrenal medulla [mě-DŪL-ă]

adrenalectomy [ă-drē-năl-ĔK-tō-mē]

adrenaline [ă-DRĔN-ă-lĭn]

aldosterone [ăl-DŎS-těr-ōn]

alpha [ĂL-fă] cells

androgen [ĂN-drō-jěn]

antihyperglycemic [ĂN-tē-HĪ-pěr-glī-SĒ-mĭk]

antihypoglycemic [ĂN-tē-HĪ-pō-glī-SĒ-mĭk]

beta [BĀ-tă] cells

blood sugar, blood glucose

calcitonin [kăl-sě-TŌ-nĭn]

catecholamines [kăt-ě-KŌL-ă-mēnz]

corticosteroid [KŌR-tĭ-kō-STĒR-oyd]

cortisol [KŌR-tĭ-sŏl]

Cushing [KUSH-ĭng] syndrome

diabetes [dī-ă-BĒ-tēz]

diabetes insipidus [ĭn-SĬP-ĭ-dŭs]

diabetes mellitus [MĔL-ĭ-tŭs, mě-LĪ-tŭs]

diabetic nephropathy [dī-ă-BĔT-ĭk ně-FRŎP-ă-thē]

diabetic neuropathy [nū-RŎP-ă-thē]

diabetic retinopathy [rět-ĭ-NŎP-ă-thē]

ductless gland

dwarfism [DWŌRF-ĭzm]

electrolyte [ē-LĔK-trō-līt]

endocrine [ĔN-dō-krĭn] gland

epinephrine [EP-i-NEF-rin]

exocrine [ĔK-sō-krĭn] gland

exophthalmos [ĕk-sŏf-THĂL-mos, ĕk-sŏf-THĂL-mŭs]

fasting blood sugar

gigantism [JĪ-găn-tĭzm]

gland [glănd]

gluc/o [GLŪ-kō]

glucagon [GLŪ-kă-gŏn]

glucose tolerance test (GTT)

glucosuria [glū-kō-SŪ-rē-ă]

glyc/o [GLĪ-kō]

glycated hemoglobin [GLĪ-kā-těd hē-mō-GLŌ-bĭn]

glycogen [GLĪ-kō-jěn]

glycosuria [glī-kō-SŪ-rē-ă]

goiter [GOY-těr]

gonad/o [gō-NĂD-ō]

Graves [grāvz] disease

hirsutism [HĔR-sū-tĭzm]

hormone [HŌR-mōn]

hormone replacement therapy (HRT)

human growth hormone

hyperadrenalism [HĪ-pěr-ă-DRĒN-ă-lĭzm]

hyperparathyroidism [HĪ-pěr-pă-ră-THĪ-royd-ĭzm]

hypersecretion [HĪ-pěr-sě-KRĒ-shŭn]

hyperthyroidism [hī-pěr-THĪ-royd-ĭzm]

hypoadrenalism [HĪ-pō-ă-DRĒN-ă-lĭzm]

hypoglycemia [HĪ-pō-glī-SĒ-mē-ă]

hypoglycemic [HĪ-pō-glī-SĒ-mĭk]

hypoparathyroidism [HĪ-pō-pă-ră-THĪ-royd-ĭzm]

hypophysectomy [hī-pŏf-ĭ-SĔK-tō-mē]

hypophysis [hī-PŎF-ĭ-sĭs]

hyposecretion [HĪ-pō-sě-KRĒ-shŭn]

hypothalamus [HĪ-pō-THĂL-ă-mŭs]

hypothyroidism [HĪ-pō-THĪ-royd-ĭzm]

inhibiting factor

insulin [ĬN-sū-lĭn]

islets [Ī-lets] of Langerhans [LĂN-gěr-hănz]

isthmus [ĬS-mŭs]

ketoacidosis [KĒ-tō-ă-sĭ-DŌ-sĭs]

ketosis [kē-TŌ-sĭs]

melatonin [mĕl-ă-TŌN-ĭn]

metabolism [mĕ-TĂB-ō-lĭzm]

myxedema [mĭk-sĕ-DĒ-mă]

neurohypophysis [NŪR-ō-hī-PŎF-ĭ-sĭs]

ovary [Ō-văr-ē]

pancreas [PĂN-krē-ăs]

pancreat/o [PĂN-krē-ă-tō]

pancreatectomy [PĂN-krē-ă-TĚK-tō-mē]

pancreatitis [PĂN-krē-ă-TĪ-tĭs]

parathormone [păr-ă-THŌR-mōn] (PTH)

parathyroid [păr-ă-THĪ-royd] gland

parathyroid/o [păr-ă-THĪ-royd-ō]

parathyroidectomy [PĂ-ră-thī-roy-DĚK-tō-mē]

pineal [PĬN-ē-ăl] gland

pituitary [pĭ-TŪ-ĭ-tār-ē] gland

polydipsia [pŏl-ē-DĬP-sē-ă]

polyuria [pŏl-ē-YŪ-rē-ă]

postprandial [pōst-PRĂN-dē-ăl] blood sugar

radioactive immunoassay (RIA)

radioactive iodine therapy

radioactive iodine uptake

receptor [rē-SĚP-tĕr]

releasing factor

steroid [STĚR-oyd, STĒR-oyd]

suprarenal [SŪ-pră-RĒ-năl] gland

sympathomimetic [SĬM-pă-thō-mĭ-MĚT-ĭk]

syndrome of inappropriate ADH (SIADH)

target cell

testicle [TĚS-tĭ-kl]

testis (pl., testes) [TĚS-tĭs (TĚS-tēz)]

tetany [TĚT-ă-nē]

thymectomy [thī-MĚK-tō-mē]

thymus [THĪ-mŭs] gland

thyr/o, thyroid/o [THĪ-rō, THĪ-roy-dō]

thyroid function test or study

thyroid [THĪ-rŏyd] gland

thyroid scan

thyroidectomy [thī-roy-DĚK-tō-mē]

thyrotoxicosis [THĪ-rō-tŏk-sĭ-KŌ-sĭs]

thyroxine [thī-RŎK-sēn, -sĭn] (T$_4$)

triiodothyronine [trī-Ī-ō-dō-THĪ-rō-nēn] (T$_3$)

type 1 diabetes (insulin-dependent diabetes mellitus or IDDM)

type 2 diabetes (noninsulin-dependent diabetes mellitus or NIDDM)

urine sugar

virilism [VĬR-ĭ-lĭzm]

The Blood System

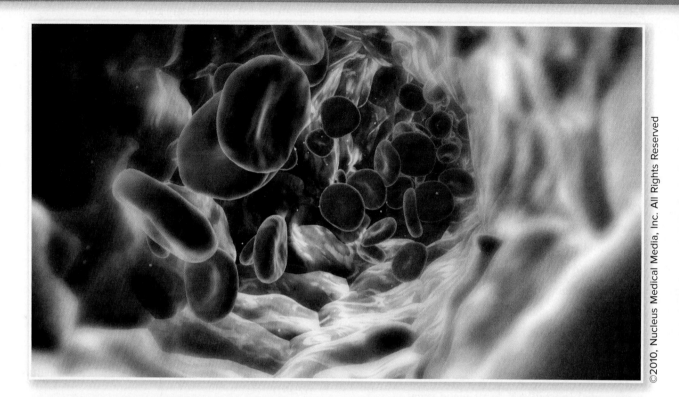

Learning Outcomes

After studying this chapter, you will be able to:

10.1 Identify the parts of the blood system and discuss the function of each part.

10.2 Recall the major word parts used in building words that relate to the blood system.

10.3 Identify the common diagnostic tests, laboratory tests, and clinical procedures used in testing and treating disorders of the blood system.

10.4 Define the major pathological conditions of the blood system.

10.5 Explain the meaning of surgical terms related to the blood system.

10.6 Recognize common pharmacological agents used in treating disorders of the blood system.

10.7 Identify common abbreviations associated with the blood system.

LO 10.1 Structure and Function of the Blood System

Blood is a complex mixture of cells, water, and various biochemical agents, such as proteins and sugars. It transports life-sustaining nutrients, oxygen, and hormones to all parts of the body. As a transport medium for waste products from cells of the body, it prevents toxic buildup. It helps maintain the stability of the fluid volume that exists within body tissues (a form of homeostasis, the maintaining of balance), and it helps regulate body temperature. Without blood, human life is not possible. An average adult has about 5 liters of blood circulating within the body. The volume of blood changes with body size, usually equaling about 8% of body weight. If a person loses blood, either through bleeding or by donating blood, most of the blood volume is replaced within 24 hours. If bleeding is extensive, blood transfusions may be necessary.

Figure 10-1a illustrates the blood system, with arteries shown in red and veins shown in blue. Figure 10-1b is a schematic showing the path of blood through the body.

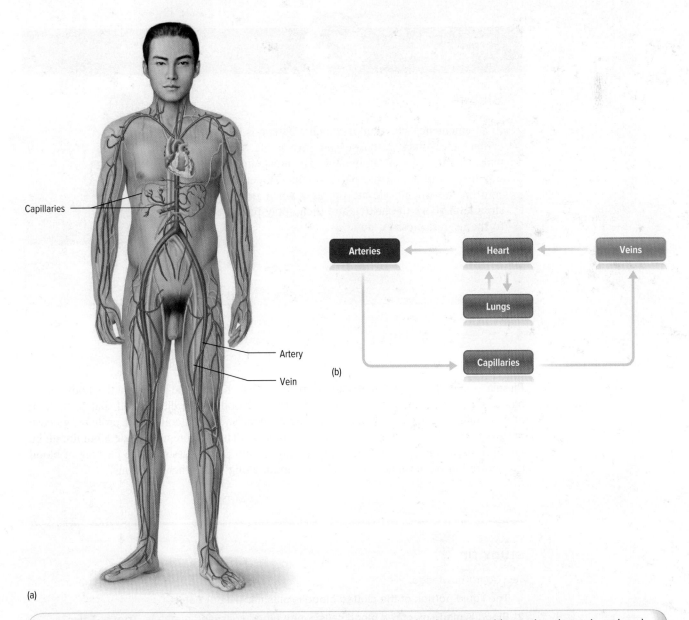

Figure 10-1 Blood circulation within the cardiovascular system: (a) the blood system, with arteries shown in red and veins shown in blue; (b) a schematic showing the path blood takes through the body.

Combining Form	Meaning
agglutin/o	clumping
eosino	rosy red
erythr/o	red
hemo, hemat/o	blood
leuk/o	white
phag/o	eating, devouring

Did you know

Blood

In an emergency situation, in which a person is hemorrhaging, a quick response can save a life. First, make sure the person can breathe. The most effective way to control hemorrhaging is to apply direct pressure on the wound, elevate the area when possible (to a level above the heart), and then apply pressure to the nearest pressure point.

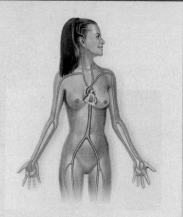

Plasma

Plasma is the clear liquid that makes up more than half of the blood in the body. When blood is separated, the plasma (about 55% of the blood) is the clear liquid that is made up of 92% water and 8% organic and inorganic chemicals. The 8% consists of proteins, glucose, nutrients, gases, electrolytes, and other substances. Plasma proteins include albumin, globulin, fibrinogen, and prothrombin. The proteins within plasma assist in the clotting of blood, transportation of substances through the blood, along with other functions.

STUDY TIP

Test Your Knowledge:

1. The liquid portion of the clotted blood is plasma. **True** or **False**?

2. Blood is made up of red blood cells, white blood cells, and platelets. **True** or **False**?

3. Heparin prevents blood from clotting. **True** or **False**?

Platelets

Platelets, or thrombocytes, are cells that circulate in the blood that are needed for blood clotting. Platelets also are used for wound healing. Produced in the bone marrow, platelets are the first to react to an injury to the body.

Structure and Function	PRACTICE
	Provide the missing term(s) to complete the following sentences.
albumin [ăl-BYŪ-mĭn] **globulin** [GLŎB-yū-lĭn] **fibrinogen** [fĭ-BRĬN-ō-jĕn] **prothrombin** [prō-THRŎM-bĭn]	The main groups of plasma proteins are _____ (which helps regulate water movement between blood and tissue), _____, _____, and _____. Plasma proteins cannot pass through capillaries and, in order to maintain a balance of fluids on both sides of the capillary walls, they create pressure that forces water into the bloodstream. Leakage of water out of the bloodstream can cause edema (swelling). An injury can upset the balance of water in the blood and, if too much water is lost, eventually can lead to shock.
gamma globulins [GĂ-mă GLŎB-yū-lĭnz] **electrophoresis** [ē-lĕk-trō-FŌR-ē-sĭs] **plasmapheresis** [PLĂZ-mă-fĕ-RĒ-sĭs]	Globulins have different functions, depending on their type. The *alpha* and *beta globulins,* which are joined in the liver, transport lipids and fat-soluble vitamins. _____ arise in the lymphatic tissue and function as part of the immune system. Globulins can be separated from each other when plasma is placed in a special solution and electrical currents attract the different proteins to move in the direction of the electricity through a process called _____. Blood also may be *centrifuged,* put in a device that separates blood elements by spinning. _____ is a process that uses centrifuging to take a patient's blood and return only red cells to that patient.
coagulation [kō-ăg-yū-LĀ-shŭn] **thromboplastin** [thrŏm-bō-PLĂS-tĭn] **fibrin clot** [FĬ-brĭn klot] **thrombin** [THRŎM-bĭn] **heparin** [HĔP-ă-rĭn]	Fibrinogen and prothrombin are essential for blood _____, the process of clotting. The clot is formed by platelets that rush to the site of an injury. They clump at the site and release a protein, _____, which combines with calcium and various clotting factors (I–V and VII–XIII) to form the _____. _____, an enzyme, helps in formation of the clot. The clot tightens while releasing serum, a clear liquid. Blood clotting at the site of a wound is essential. Without it, one would bleed to death. Blood clotting inside blood vessels, however, can cause major cardiovascular problems. Some elements of the blood, such as _____, prevent clots from forming during normal circulation.

PRONOUNCE and DEFINE	Pronounce the following terms aloud and write their meaning in the space provided.
coagulation	[kō-ăg-yū-LĀ-shŭn]
electrophoresis	[ē-lĕk-trō-FŌR-ē-sĭs]
gamma globulin	[GĂ-mă GLŎB-yū-lĭn]
prothrombin, fibrinogen	[prō-THRŎM-bĭn], [fĭ-BRĬN-ō-jĕn]

SPELL and DEFINE	Identify if the following terms are spelled correctly. Correct the words that are spelled incorrectly. Write the definition for each word.	
	Spelling	**Definition**
plazmaferesis		
albyumin		
thrombin		
thromboplatin		
coagulation		

UNDERSTAND — Identify the term from the definition provided.

1. Protein that aids in clotting: _____
2. Enzyme that aids in clot formation: _____
3. The process of clotting: _____
4. Clot-forming threads: _____

APPLY — Read the following scenario and respond accordingly.

Blake Greenhaw has a clotting disorder. Explain to Mr. Greenhaw how normal clotting occurs.

_____

_____

_____

_____

Did you know ?

Stem Cells

In recent years, researchers have found that stem cells can be used to combat some diseases. It is theorized that stem cells may be the ultimate cure for many chronic and devastating ailments. Because most usable stem cells must come from human embryos obtained from abortions or in vitro fertilization, their use has become controversial.

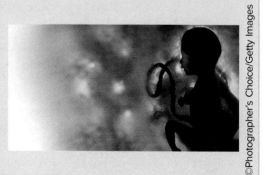

©Photographer's Choice/Getty Images

Blood Cells

Blood cells are composed of red and white cells. The red blood cells are responsible for carrying oxygen; the white blood cells fight infection.

Provide the missing term(s) to complete the following sentences.

erythrocytes
[ĕ-RĬTH-rō-sīts]
leukocytes [LŪ-kō-sīts]
thrombocytes
[THRŎM-bō-sīts]
hematocrit
[HĒ-mă-tō-krĭt,
HĔM-ă-tō-krĭt]
stem cells

The solid part of the blood that is suspended in the plasma consists of the red blood cells (RBCs), also called _____; white blood cells (WBCs), also called _____; and platelets, also referred to as _____. These cells, or the solids in the blood, make up about 45% of the blood. The measurement of the percentage of packed red blood cells is known as the _____. Most blood cells are formed as _____, or immature blood cells in the bone marrow. Stem cells mature in the bone marrow before entering the bloodstream and becoming *differentiated*, specialized in their purpose. The term *differential*, which you will see on written orders for blood tests, refers to the percentage of each type of white blood cell in the bloodstream.

STUDY TIP

Erythropoietin is used in the treatment of AIDS patients to encourage red blood cell production.

Erythrocytes (Red Blood Cells), Leukocytes, and Platelets

Table 10-1 identifies the types of white blood cells. Figure 10-2 shows erythrocytes. Figure 10-3 shows leukocytes. Figure 10-4 shows the development of elements of blood.

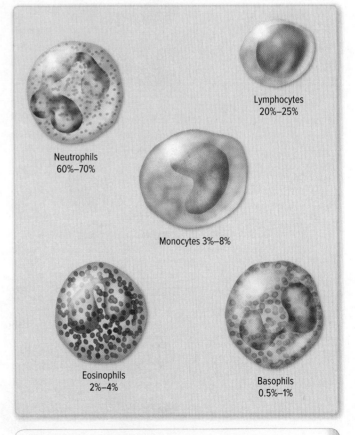

Figure 10-3 Leukocytes

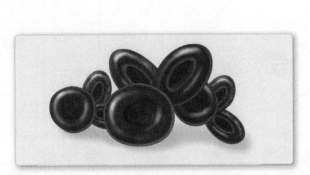

Figure 10-2 Erythrocytes

TABLE 10-1	Types of Leukocytes
Leukocytes	Function
Granulocytes	A type of white blood cell that is released during infections, allergic reactions, and asthma.
basophils	release heparin and histamine
eosinophils	remove unwanted particles
neutrophils	kill parasites and help control inflammation
Agranulocytes	White blood cells that work to coordinate the body's defense system against infectious agents.
lymphocytes	important to immune system
monocytes	destroy large unwanted particles

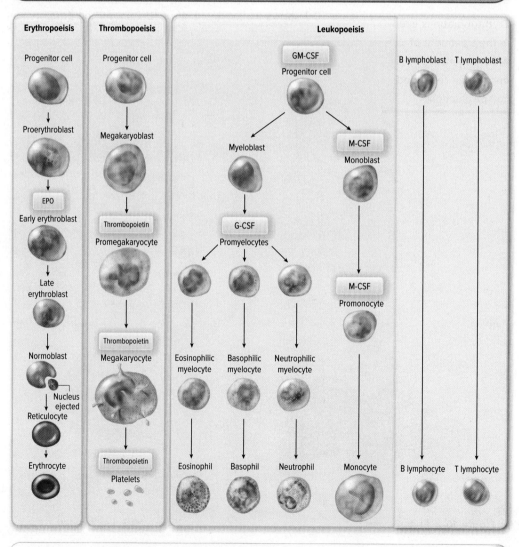

Figure 10-4 Development of blood elements

Provide the missing term(s) to complete the following sentences.

	Erythrocytes or Red Blood Cells
erythropoietin [ĕ-rĭth-rō-POY-ĕ-tĭn]	A hormone produced in the kidneys, _____ stimulates the production of red blood cells in the bone marrow. When stem cells mature into erythrocytes, they lose their nucleus and become biconcave.
hemoglobin [hē-mō-GLŌ-bĭn]	A protein within red blood cells, _____ aids in the transport of oxygen to the cells of the body. Oxygen molecules have the ability to bond with hemoglobin molecules. When a red blood cell has oxygen on board, it becomes bright red in color. Oxygen-poor red blood cells are a deep burgundy color.
heme [hēm] **globin** [GLŌ-bĭn] **red blood cell count**	About one-third of each red blood cell is made up of hemoglobin. Hemoglobin is composed of _____, a pigment containing iron, and _____, a protein. Erythrocytes live for about 120 days. Some are removed from circulation each day to maintain a steady concentration of red blood cells. *Macrophages* are cells formed from stem cells that consume damaged or aged cells. The average number of red blood cells in 1 cubic millimeter of blood is 4.6 to 6.4 million for adult males and 4.2 to 5.4 million for adult females. This measurement is known as the _____.
	Leukocytes
	Leukocytes, or white blood cells, protect against disease in various ways—for example, by destroying foreign substances. Leukocytes are transported in the bloodstream to the site of an infection. There are two main groups of leukocytes: granulocytes and agranulocytes.
granulocytes [GRĂN-yū-lō-sĭts]	The first group, _____, have a granular cytoplasm and have nuclei with several lobes when viewed under a microscope and when stain is used. There are three types of granulocytes:
neutrophils [NŪ-trō-fĭlz]	1. _____ are the most plentiful leukocytes (more than half of the white blood cells in the bloodstream). They do not stain distinctly with either an acidic or an alkaline dye. Their purpose is to remove small particles of unwanted material from the bloodstream.
eosinophils [ē-ō-SĬN-ō-fĭlz]	2. _____ make up only about 1% to 3% of the leukocytes in the bloodstream. Their granules stain bright red in the presence of an acidic red dye called eosin. Their purpose is to kill parasites and to help control inflammations and allergic reactions.
basophils [BĀ-sō-fĭlz] **histamine** [HĬS-tă-mēn]	3. _____ make up less than 1% of the leukocytes in the bloodstream. Their granules stain dark purple in the presence of alkaline dyes. They release heparin, an anticlotting factor, and _____, a substance involved in allergic reactions.
agranulocytes [ā-GRĂN-yū-lō-sĭts]	The second group of leukocytes, _____, have cytoplasm with no granules. Their single nucleus does not have the dark-staining elements of granulocytes. There are two types of agranulocytes:
monocytes [MŎN-ō-sĭts]	1. _____, the largest blood cells, make up about 3% to 9% of the leukocytes in the bloodstream. They destroy large particles of unwanted material (such as old red blood cells) in the bloodstream.
lymphocytes [LĬM-fō-sĭts]	2. _____ make up about 25% to 33% of the leukocytes in the bloodstream. They are essential to the immune system, as discussed in Chapter 13.

continued on next page

PRACTICE

Provide the missing term(s) to complete the following sentences.

Platelets

megakaryocytes [mĕg-ă-KĀR-ē-ō-sīts]	Platelets, or thrombocytes, are fragments that break off from large cells in red bone marrow called _____. Platelets live for about 10 days and help in blood clotting. Platelets adhere to damaged tissue and to one another and group together to control blood loss from a blood vessel.

PRONOUNCE and DEFINE

Pronounce the following terms aloud and write their meaning in the space provided.

lymphocyte	[LĬM-fō-sīt]
erythropoietin	[ĕ-rĭth-rō-POY-ĕ-tĭn]
granulocytes	[GRĂN-yū-lō-sīts]
basophils	[BĀ-sō-fĭlz]
histamine	[HĬS-tă-mēn]

SPELL and DEFINE

Identify if the following terms are spelled correctly. Correct the words that are spelled incorrectly. Write the definition for each word.

	Spelling	Definition
erithopoyetin		
hemoglobin		
basofilz		
granyulosits		
megakareosits		

UNDERSTAND

Identify the term from the definition.

1. Hormone that stimulates red blood cell production: _____
2. Substance involved in allergic reactions: _____
3. Cells that function to control inflammation and allergic reactions: _____
4. Large blood cell whose fragments produce platelets: _____

Blood Types

The following Practice introduces terms involved with transfusion and blood types. Table 10-2 lists the four blood types and their characteristics. Figure 10-5 describes the four blood types and Figure 10-6 lists the blood factors. Figure 10-7 describes the Rh factor and pregnancy.

TABLE 10–2		Blood Types	
Blood Type	**Antigen**	**Antibody**	**Transfusion Match**
A	A	anti-B	Can donate to blood types A and AB.
B	B	anti-A	Can donate to blood types B and AB.
AB	A and B	neither anti-A nor anti-B	Can donate to blood type AB only but can receive from all others. Universal receiver.
O	neither A nor B	both anti-A and anti-B	Can donate to all blood types. Universal donor.

ABO Blood Types

Erythrocytes	Antigen A	Antigen B	Antigens A and B	Neither antigen A nor B
	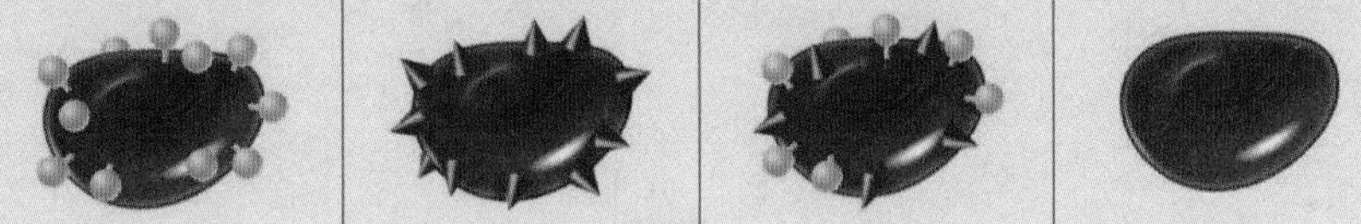			
Plasma	Anti-B antibodies	Anti-A antibodies	Neither anti-A nor anti-B antibodies	Both anti-A and anti-B antibodies
Blood type	**Type A** Erythrocytes with type A surface antigens and plasma with anti-B antibodies	**Type B** Erythrocytes with type B surface antigens and plasma with anti-A antibodies	**Type AB** Erythrocytes with both type A and type B surface antigens, and plasma with neither anti-A nor anti-B antibodies	**Type O** Erythrocytes with neither type A nor type B surface antigens, but plasma with both anti-A and anti-B antibodies

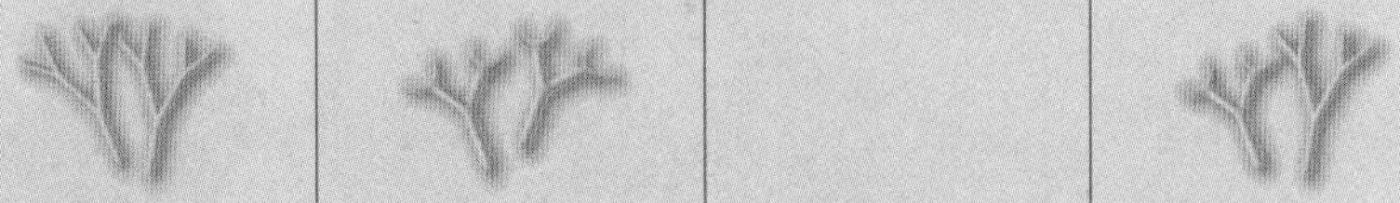

Figure 10-5 Blood types

Rh Blood Types

Erythrocytes	Antigen D	No antigen D
	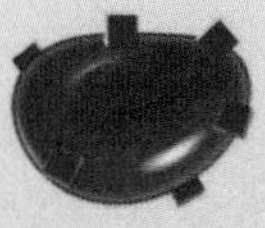	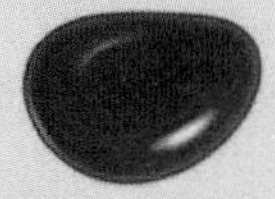
Plasma	No anti-D antibodies	Anti-D antibodies (after prior exposure) 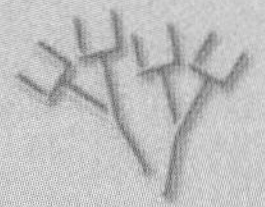
Blood type	**Rh positive** Erythrocytes with type D surface antigens and plasma with no anti-D antibodies	**Rh negative** Erythrocytes with no type D surface antigens and plasma with anti-D antibodies, only if there has been prior exposure to Rh-positive blood

Figure 10-6 Blood factors

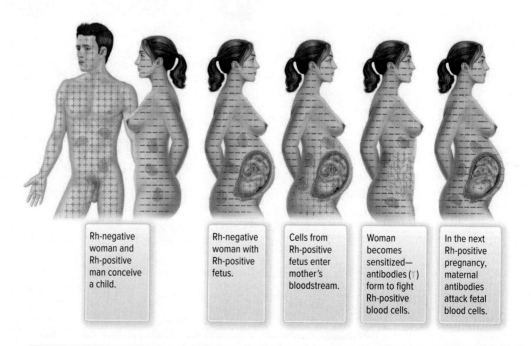

Rh-negative woman and Rh-positive man conceive a child.

Rh-negative woman with Rh-positive fetus.

Cells from Rh-positive fetus enter mother's bloodstream.

Woman becomes sensitized—antibodies (Y) form to fight Rh-positive blood cells.

In the next Rh-positive pregnancy, maternal antibodies attack fetal blood cells.

Figure 10-7 Rh factor and pregnancy

Did you know

Transfusions

Two early scientists attempted various experimental transfusions. Sir Christopher Wren (1632–1723), a famous English architect and scientist, did biological experiments in which he injected fluids into the veins of animals. This process is regarded as an early attempt at blood transfusions. During the same century, a French physician, Jean Baptiste Denis (1643–1704), tried unsuccessfully to transfuse sheep's blood into a human. Later, experiments with transfusing human blood succeeded somewhat, but the majority of people receiving transfusions died—until the advent of blood typing in the twentieth century. Once blood factors and typing became routine, transfusions were widely used in surgery. Later, it was found that some infections (hepatitis, AIDS) were transmitted by blood. Now, donated blood is carefully screened for infections.

©Liquidlibrary/PictureQuest

Structure and Function	PRACTICE
	Provide the missing term(s) to complete the following sentences.
transfusion [trăns-FYŪ-zhŭn] **blood types or groups**	When blood is needed for _____, the blood being donated is tested for type and put into one of four human _____. The donated blood must be tested because an incompatible blood type from a donor can cause adverse reactions. Blood typing is based on the antigens (substances that promote an immune response) and antibodies (special proteins) present in the blood. The most common type of blood in the population is O, followed by A, B, and AB in descending order.
agglutination [ă-glū-tĭ-NĀ-shŭn]	The danger in transfusing blood of a different type is that _____, or clumping of the antigens, stops the flow of blood, which can be fatal. People with type O blood have no antigens, so people with type O can donate to all other types and are, therefore, called *universal donors* from all blood types. AB blood are called *universal recipients* because they can receive blood from people with all the other types and not experience clotting.
Rh factor **Rh-positive** **Rh-negative** **agglutinogens** [ă-glū-TĬN-ō-jĕnz]	In addition to the four human blood types, there is a positive or negative element in the blood. _____ is a type of antigen first identified in rhesus monkeys. _____ blood contains this factor and _____ blood does not. The factor contains any of more than 30 types of _____, substances that cause agglutination, and can be fatal to anyone who receives blood with a factor different from the donor's blood.

APPLY	Read the following scenario and answer the question.

Michelle Davis is pregnant with her third child. Mrs. Davis's blood type is O negative. Her husband's blood type is B positive. How might this affect the fetus?

_____

_____

_____

_____

LO 10.2 Word Building in the Blood System

Word Building	PRACTICE
	Provide the correct combining form to complete the following sentences.
eosino-penia [Ē-ŏ-sĭn-ō-PĒ-nē-ă]	_____ penia is an abnormally low count of eosinophils.
leuko-blast [LŪ-kō-blăst]	An immature white blood cell is a _____ blast.
erythro-cyte [ĕ-RĬTH-rō-sīt]	A red blood cell is an _____ cyte.
thrombo-cyte [THRŎM-bō-sīt]	A cell involved in blood clotting is a _____ cyte.
agglutino-gens [ă-glū-TĬN-ō-jĕnz]	_____ gens cause the production of agglutinin.
phago-cyte [FĂG-ō-sīt]	A cell that consumes other substances, such as bacteria, is a _____ cyte.
hemo-dialysis [HĒ-mō-dī-ĂL-ĭ-sĭs]	_____ dialysis is external dialysis performed by separating solid substances and water from the blood.
cyto-plasm [SĪ-tō-plazm]	_____ plasm is the solution that fills the cell and that is enclosed by the cell membrane.

PRONOUNCE and DEFINE	Pronounce the following terms aloud and write their meaning in the space provided.
hemodialysis	[HĒ-mō-dī-ĂL-ĭ-sĭs]
thrombocyte	[THRŎM-bō-sīt]
erythrocyte	[ĕ-RĬTH-rō-sīt]
phagocyte	[FĂG-ō-sīt]
leukoblast	[LŪ-kō-blăst]

UNDERSTAND	After each of the following terms, indicate which component of blood is most closely related by writing a, b, or c in the space provided.

a. red blood cell
b. white blood cell
c. component of plasma

1. albumin _____
2. leukocyte _____
3. hemoglobin _____
4. eosinophils _____
5. neutrophils _____
6. fibrinogen _____
7. histamine _____
8. basophils _____

9. lymphocytes _____

10. monocyte _____

Find the Type: Write the correct blood type—A, B, AB, or O—in the space provided.

1. _____ Has A and B antigens
2. _____ Has neither A nor B antigens
3. _____ Has only B antigens
4. _____ Has only A antigens
5. _____ Has both anti-A and anti-B antibodies
6. _____ Has neither anti-A nor anti-B antibodies
7. _____ Has only anti-A antibodies
8. _____ Has only anti-B antibodies

LO 10.3 Diagnostic, Procedural, and Laboratory Terms

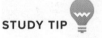

STUDY TIP

After answering,
go back and define
each term.

The following Practice defines some of the major diagnostic, procedural, and laboratory terms related to the blood system. Figure 10-8 shows a patient during venipuncture. Table 10-3 lists common blood analyses.

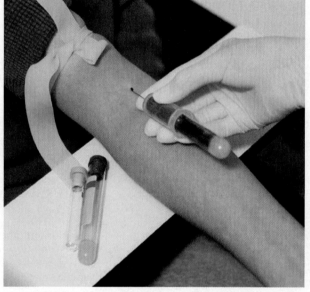

©Keith Brofsky/Getty Images

Figure 10-8 Venipuncture

TABLE 10-3	Common Blood Analyses	
Test or Procedure	**Purpose of Test**	**Common Diseases/Disorders That May Be Indicated**
complete blood count (CBC)	common screen for basic medical checkup	iron-deficiency anemia, bacterial or viral infection, internal bleeding, dehydration, aplastic anemia, impaired renal function, liver disease, circulatory disorders
blood chemistry	test of plasma for presence of most substances, such as glucose, cholesterol, uric acid, and electrolytes	diabetes, hyperlipidemia, gout, circulatory disorders, impaired renal function, liver diseases, general metabolic disorders

continued on next page

TABLE 10-3	Common Blood Analyses	
Test or Procedure	**Purpose of Test**	**Common Diseases/Disorders That May Be Indicated**
biochemistry panel	group of automated tests for various common diseases or disorders	same as blood chemistry
blood indices	measurement of size, volume, and content of red blood cells	classification of anemias
blood culture	test of a blood specimen in a culture in which microorganisms are observed; test for infections	septicemia, bacterial infections
erythrocyte sedimentation rate (ESR); sedimentation rate (SR)	test for rate at which red blood cells fall through plasma; indicator of inflammation and/or tissue injury	infections, joint inflammation, sickle cell anemia, liver and kidney disorders
white blood cell differential and red blood cell morphology	test for number of types of leukocytes and shape of red blood cells	infection, anemia, blood cells, poikilocytosis, anisocytosis
platelet count (PLT)	test for number of thrombocytes in a blood sample	hemorrhage, infections, malignancy, hypersplenism, aplastic anemia, thrombocytopenia
partial thromboplastin time (PTT)	test for coagulation defects	vitamin K deficiency, hepatic disease, hemophilia, hemorrhagic disorders
prothrombin time (PT)	test for coagulation defects	vitamin K deficiency, hepatic disease, hemorrhagic disorders, hemophilia
antiglobulin test	test for antibodies on red blood Coombs' test	Rh factor and anemia cells
white blood count (WBC)	number of white blood cells in a sample (usually done as part of a complete blood count [CBC])	bacterial or viral infection, aplastic anemia, leukemia, leukocytosis
red blood count (RBC)	number of red blood cells in a sample (usually done as part of a complete blood count [CBC])	polycythemia, dehydration, iron-deficiency anemia, blood loss, erythropoiesis
hemoglobin (HGB, Hgb)	level of hemoglobin in blood (usually done as part of a complete blood count [CBC])	polycythemia, dehydration, anemia, sickle cell anemia, recent hemorrhage
hematocrit (HCT, Hct)	measure of packed red blood cells in a sample (usually done as part of a complete blood count [CBC])	polycythemia, dehydration, blood loss, anemia

PRACTICE

Provide the missing term(s) to complete the following sentences.

phlebotomy
[flĕ-BŎT-ō-mē]
venipuncture
[VĔN-ĭ-pŭnk-chŭr,
VĒ-nĭ-pŭnk-chŭr]

_____ or _____, the withdrawal of blood for examination, is probably the most frequently used diagnostic tool in medicine. Various measurements provide a clue as to someone's general health and aid in diagnosing specific conditions.

Most of the blood tests described in Table 10-3 are performed in a laboratory. Names of tests may vary according to the region of the country or the practice of a particular doctor.

UNDERSTAND

Match the name of the test in the column on the left to its correct description in the column on the right.

1. _____ blood culture
2. _____ hematocrit
3. _____ sedimentation rate
4. _____ white blood count
5. _____ antiglobulin test
6. _____ biochemistry panel
7. _____ prothrombin time
8. _____ complete blood count

a. Clotting factors test
b. Antibodies on red blood cells
c. Rate at which red blood cells fall
d. Group of automated tests
e. Most common blood test
f. Growing microorganisms in a culture
g. Number of white blood cells
h. Measure of packed red blood cells

LO 10.4 Pathological Terms

Many diseases and disorders have some effect on the blood, but they are really diseases of other body systems. For example, diabetes is a disorder of the endocrine system, but its diagnosis includes an analysis of blood glucose levels.

Pathological

PRACTICE

Provide the missing term(s) to complete the following sentences.

dyscrasia
[dĭs-KRĀ-zē-ă]

Actual diseases of the blood are characterized by changes in the supply or characteristics of blood cells, presence of microorganisms affecting the blood, or presence or lack of certain substances in the blood. _____ is a general term for any disease of the blood with abnormal material present.

anemia
[ă-NĒ-mē-ă]

_____ is a general term for a condition in which the red blood cells do not transport enough oxygen to the tissues due to a deficiency in number or quality of red blood cells. The most common types of anemia include:

- *Iron-deficiency anemia,* a lack of enough iron in the blood that affects the production of hemoglobin.
- *Aplastic anemia,* a failure of the bone marrow to produce enough red blood cells.
- *Pernicious anemia,* a condition in which the shape and number of the red blood cells change due to a lack of sufficient vitamin B_{12}.

continued on next page

Pathological	PRACTICE

Provide the missing term(s) to complete the following sentences.

sickle cell anemia
[SĬ-kl sĕl ă-NĒ-mē-ă]

- _____, a hereditary condition (usually in persons of African American ancestry) characterized by sickle-shaped red blood cells and a breakdown in red blood cell membranes.
- *Hemolytic anemia,* a disorder characterized by destruction of red blood cells.
- *Posthemorrhagic anemia,* a disorder resulting from a sudden, dramatic loss of blood.

thalassemia
[thăl-ă-SĒ-mē-ă]

- _____, an inherited disorder (usually in people of Mediterranean origin) resulting in an inability to produce sufficient hemoglobin (the most severe form of which is *Cooley anemia*).

von Willebrand disease
[vŏn WĬL-lĕ-brănd di-zēz]
hemophilia
[hē-mō-FĬL-ē-ă]
thrombocytopenia
[THRŎM-bō-sī-tō-PĒ-nē-ă]
purpura [PŬR-pū-ră]

_____ is a hemorrhagic disorder in which there is a greater tendency to bleed due to the lack of a clotting factor called *factor VIII.* Common symptoms are bruising and nosebleeds. Two other disorders of the blood that involve excessive bleeding are _____ and _____. Hemophilia is a hereditary lack of clotting factor VIII (or, in 15% of the cases, a different clotting factor, factor IX). Hemophiliacs can be treated with medications and transfusions. Thrombocytopenia is a bleeding disorder with insufficient platelets to aid in the clotting process. Thrombocytopenia is present in _____, a condition with multiple tiny hemorrhages under the skin.

pancytopenia
[PĂN-sī-tō-PĒ-nē-ă]
erythropenia
[ĕ-rĭth-rō-PĒ-nē-ă]

Small, flat, red spots called *petechiae* may indicate a deficiency in the number of platelets. There are a number of disorders of the blood cells or related substances in the blood. _____ is a condition with a low number of all blood cell components (red blood cells, white blood cells, and thrombocytes). The blood must be supplemented with transfusions. _____ (also called *erythrocytopenia*) is a disorder with an abnormally low number of red blood cells.

polycythemia
[PŎL-ē-sī-THĒ-mē-ă]
hemolysis
[hē-MŎL-ĭ-sĭs]

_____ is a disease that causes an abnormal increase in red blood cells and hemoglobin. Various forms of the disease are associated with conditions such as hypertension and emphysema. _____ is a disorder with breakdowns in the red blood cell membrane.

leukemia
[lū-KĒ-mē-ă]

There are also disorders of white blood cells. The major disease involving white blood cells is _____. This is a general term for a disorder with an excessive increase in white blood cells in the bone marrow and bloodstream. People with leukemia may experience *remissions* (disappearances of the disease) and *relapses* (recurrences of the disease). Some leukemias (acute lymphocytic leukemia and chronic lymphocytic leukemia) occur in the lymph system.

myeloblasts
[MĪ-ĕ-lō-blăsts]

The two most common leukemias of the bone marrow and bloodstream are AML and CML. *Acute myelogenous leukemia (AML)* is a disorder in which immature granulocytes (or _____) invade the bone marrow. *Chronic myelogenous leukemia (CML)* or chronic granulocytic leukemia is a disorder in which mature and immature myeloblasts are present in the bloodstream and marrow. It is usually a slowly developing illness with a reasonably good prognosis. *Acute lymphocytic leukemia (ALL)* is a disorder with an abnormal number of immature lymphocytes. It is usually a disease of childhood and adolescence. The prognosis for recovery is very good. *Chronic lymphocytic leukemia (CLL)* appears mainly in adults and includes an abnormal number of mature lymphocytes.

erythroblastosis fetalis
[ĕ-RĬTH-rō-blăs-TŌ-sĭs
fē-TĂL-ĭs]

_____, or Rh factor incompatibility between the mother and a fetus, can cause death to the fetus or a type of fetal anemia. A blood transfusion or treatment with medication can sometimes save the fetus.

multiple myeloma
[MŬL-tĭ-pl mī-ĕ-LŌ-mă]

_____ is a malignant tumor of the bone marrow. It involves overproduction of certain white blood cells that produce immunoglobulins. The myeloma cells then migrate to different areas of the body where they cause tumors and destroy bony structures.

PRONOUNCE and DEFINE	Pronounce the following terms aloud and write their meaning in the space provided.
myeloblast	[MĪ-ĕ-lō-blăst]
leukemia	[lū-KĒ-mē-ă]
polycythemia	[PŎL-ē-sī-THĒ-mē-ă]
hemolysis	[hē-MŎL-ĭ-sĭs]
purpura	[PŬR-pū-ră]

SPELL and DEFINE	Identify if the following terms are spelled correctly. Correct the words that are spelled incorrectly. Write the definition for each word.	
	Spelling	Definition
hemphilia		
anemia		
pancypenia		
alplastic anemia		
pupura		

UNDERSTAND	Match each term on the left with its definition on the right.

1. _____ dyscrasia   a. low number of red blood cells
2. _____ granulocytosis   b. incompatible disorder between mother and fetus
3. _____ hemolysis   c. disease with abnormal particles in the blood
4. _____ anemia   d. abnormal number of granulocytes in the bloodstream
5. _____ leukemia   e. breakdown of red blood cell membranes
6. _____ erythroblastosis fetalis   f. excessive white blood cells in the bloodstream and bone marrow

APPLY	Describe the cause of each condition.

1. aplastic anemia: _____

_____

2. iron-deficiency anemia: _____

_____

3. pernicious anemia: _____

_____

4. thalassemia: _____

_____

5. sickle cell anemia: _____

_____

LO 10.5 Surgical Terms

Surgery is not generally performed on the blood system. There are two exceptions: bone marrow biopsy and bone marrow transplant.

PRACTICE

Provide the missing term(s) to complete the following sentences.

bone marrow biopsy	A _____ is used in the diagnosis of various blood disorders, such as anemia and leukemia. A needle is introduced into the bone marrow cavity and marrow is extracted for examination.
bone marrow transplant	A _____ is performed for serious ailments, such as leukemia and cancer. In this procedure, a donor's marrow is introduced into the bone marrow of the patient. First, all the diseased cells are killed through extensive radiation and chemotherapy. After the donor's marrow is introduced, successful transplants result in healthy cells taking over the patient's marrow. Unsuccessful transplants may result in rejection of the marrow or a recurrence of the disease.

LO 10.6 Pharmacological Terms

A variety of medications may be used to treat blood disorders and diseases. Medications generally do not cure the disorder; rather, they treat or prevent symptoms.

PRACTICE

Pharmacological

Provide the missing term(s) to complete the following sentences.

anticoagulants [ĂN-tē-kō-ĂG-yū-lĕnts] **thrombolytics** [thrŏm-bō-LĬT-ĭks] **coagulants** [kō-ĂG-yū-lĕnts] **hemostatics** [hē-mō-STĂT-ĭks]	Medications that directly affect the work of the blood system are _____ (to prevent blood clotting); _____ (to dissolve blood clots); _____, or clotting agents (to aid in blood clotting); and _____ (to stop bleeding, such as vitamin K). Anticoagulants are administered before most types of surgeries to prevent emboli. Blood flow is affected by vasoconstrictors and vasodilators, two medications given for cardiovascular problems.
remission [rē-MĬSH-ŭn] **relapse** [RĒ-lăps]	Chemotherapy uses drugs to cause a _____ (disappearance of the disease) in leukemia. Sometimes more treatment is needed when a _____ (recurrence of the disease) occurs.

UNDERSTAND   Complete the following sentences.

1. Hemophiliacs require _____ and _____ to control bleeding.
2. Someone with coronary artery disease might include a(n) _____ to prevent clotting.
3. If medication is not taken regularly, a(n) _____ of a disease might occur and additional treatment will be needed.
4. The disappearance of a disease, called a(n) _____, usually resulting from treatment, can be temporary and unexplained.

Abbreviations

ABBREVIATION REVIEW

Abbreviation	Definition
baso	basophil
BMT	bone marrow transplant
CBC, cbc	complete blood cell count
eos	eosinophil
ESR	erythrocyte sedimentation rate
Hgb, Hb	hemoglobin
mono	monocyte
neut	neutrophil
PT	prothrombin time
PTT	partial thromboplastin time
RBC	red blood cell count
Rh	rhesus
SR	sedimentation rate
WBC	white blood cell count

UNDERSTAND   Match the abbreviation with its definition

1. _____ Rh
2. _____ CBC
3. _____ ESR
4. _____ PTT
5. _____ PT
6. _____ Hgb
7. _____ BMT
8. _____ RBC
9. _____ WBC
10. _____ SR

a. hemoglobin
b. bone marrow transplant
c. sedimentation rate
d. white blood cell count
e. prothrombin time
f. rhesus
g. complete blood count
h. erythrocyte sedimentation rate
i. partial thromboplastin time
j. red blood cell count

APPLY   Read the following scenario and respond accordingly.

The physician has ordered the following diagnostic tests for the patient:

- CBC
- WBC
- ESR
- PT
- PTT

Using terms the patient can understand, explain to the patient what each of these abbreviations means.

_____

_____

_____

Chapter Review

CHAPTER SUMMARY

	Learning Outcome	Summary
10.1	Identify the parts of the blood system and discuss the function of each part.	Blood transports life-sustaining nutrients, oxygen, and hormones to all parts of the body. It prevents toxic buildup, helps maintain the stability of the fluid volume that exists within body tissues, and helps regulate body temperature.
10.2	Recall the major word parts used in building words that relate to the blood system.	Word building requires knowledge of the combining form and meaning.
10.3	Identify the common diagnostic tests, laboratory tests, and clinical procedures used in testing and treating disorders of the blood system.	Diagnostic, procedural, and laboratory findings assist the health care provider in diagnosing medical conditions. Often used in combination, these tests lead to a final diagnosis and assist in treatment planning.
10.4	Define the major pathological conditions of the blood system.	Many diseases and disorders have some effect on the blood, but they are really diseases of other body systems.
10.5	Explain the meaning of surgical terms related to the blood system.	Surgery is not generally performed on the blood system. There are two exceptions: bone marrow biopsy and bone marrow transplant.
10.6	Recognize common pharmacological agents used in treating disorders of the blood system.	A variety of medications may be used to treat blood disorders and diseases. Medications generally do not cure the disorder; rather, they treat or prevent symptoms.
10.7	Identify common abbreviations associated with the blood system.	Abbreviations are used to describe diseases, conditions, procedures, and treatments associated with the blood system.

RECALL

Put the following elements of erythropoiesis formation in order, from beginning to end.

_____ erythrocyte
_____ reticulocyte
_____ progenitor cell
_____ erythroblast
_____ normoblast

Identify if the following terms are spelled correctly. Correct the words that are spelled incorrectly. Write the definition for each word.

	Spelling	Definition
coageulation		
erythrowpoietin		
fibrinogen		
thalassemia		
thrombien		

IMPLEMENT

Match the term in the left column with its correct definition in the right column.

1. _____ coagulation   a. Type of leukocyte
2. _____ heparin   b. A blood protein
3. _____ neutrophil   c. Clumping of incompatible blood cells
4. _____ albumin   d. Process of clotting
5. _____ agglutination   e. Antigen
6. _____ Rh factor   f. Cell that activates clotting
7. _____ erythrocyte   g. An anticoagulant
8. _____ platelet   h. Red blood cell

Fill in the blanks.

1. _____ anemia is a hereditary blood disorder.
2. Anemia occurs when _____ do not transport enough oxygen.
3. Multiple myeloma occurs in the _____.
4. Rh factor incompatibility can cause _____ or _____ of the fetus.
5. Pernicious anemia may result from a deficiency of _____.
6. Leukemia is caused by excessive _____ cells.
7. Hemophilia is due to a lack of _____ factors.

Define the following words using the blood system combining forms listed in this chapter and the prefixes, suffixes, and combining forms from Chapters 1, 2, and 3.

1. agglutinophilic: _____
2. thrombectomy: _____
3. erythroblast: _____
4. hematopathology: _____
5. eosinotaxis: _____
6. lymphoblast: _____
7. phagosome: _____
8. polycythemia: _____
9. cytology: _____
10. leukocyte: _____
11. leukemia: _____
12. thrombocytopenia: _____
13. hematoma: _____
14. erythrocytosis: _____

Dianne Love was admitted to the hospital complaining of respiratory problems and left-sided lower abdominal pain. The physician has reviewed Ms. Love's CBC, WBC, ESR, PTT, and PT. Ms. Love was found to be anemic. The physician has ordered 2 units of O negative blood.

Explain to Ms. Love the reason why each laboratory test was ordered and how she was determined to be anemic.

_____

_____

_____

Reviewing the Terms

Pronounce each of the following terms. Write the definitions on a separate sheet of paper. This review will take you through all the words you learned in this chapter. If you have difficulty with any words, make a flash card for later study. Refer to the English-Spanish and Spanish-English glossaries in the eBook.

agglutin/o [ă-GLŪ-tĭn-ō]

agglutination [ă-glū-tĭ-NĀ-shŭn]

agglutinogen [ă-glū-TĬN-ō-jĕn]

agranulocyte [ā-GRĂN-yū-lō-sīt]

albumin [ăl-BYŪ-mĭn]

anemia [ă-NĒ-mē-ă]

anticoagulant [ĂN-tē-kō-ĂG-yū-lĕnt]

antiglobulin [ĂN-tē-GLŎB-yū-lĭn] **test**

basophils [BĀ-sō-fĭlz]

biochemistry panel

blood [blŭd]

blood chemistry

blood culture

blood indices [ĬN-dĭ-sēz]

blood types or groups

bone marrow biopsy

bone marrow transplant

chemistry profile

coagulant [kō-ĂG-yū-lĕnt]

coagulation [kō-ăg-yū-LĀ-shŭn]

complete blood count (CBC)

dyscrasia [dĭs-KRĀ-zē-ă]

electrophoresis [ē-lĕk-trō-FŌR-ē-sĭs]

eosino [ē-ŏ-SĬN-ō]

eosinophil [ē-ō-SĬN-ō-fĭl]

erythr/o [ĕ-RĬTH-rō]

erythroblastosis fetalis [ĕ-RĬTH-rō-blăs-TŌ-sĭs fē-TĂL-ĭs]

erythrocyte [ĕ-RĬTH-rō-sīt]

erythrocyte sedimentation rate (ESR)

erythropenia [ĕ-rĭth-rō-PĒ-nē-ă]

erythropoietin [ĕ-rĭth-rō-POY-ĕ-tĭn]

fibrin [FĪ-brĭn] **clot**

fibrinogen [fī-BRĬN-ō-jĕn]

gamma globulin [GĂ-mă GLŎB-yū-lĭn]

globin [GLŌ-bĭn]

globulin [GLŎB-yū-lĭn]

granulocyte [GRĂN-yū-lō-sīt]

hematocrit [HĒ-mă-tō-krĭt, HĒM-ă-tō-krĭt]

heme [hēm]

hemo, hemat/o [HĒ-mō, HĒ-mă-tō]

hemoglobin [hē-mō-GLŌ-bĭn]

hemolysis [hē-MŎL-ĭ-sĭs]

hemophilia [hē-mō-FĬL-ē-ă]

hemostatic [hē-mō-STĂT-ĭk]

heparin [HĒP-ă-rĭn]

histamine [HĬS-tă-mēn]

leuk/o [LŪ-kō]

leukemia [lū-KĒ-mē-ă]

leukocyte [LŪ-kō-sīt]

lymphocyte [LĬM-fō-sīt]

megakaryocytes [mĕg-ă-KĀR-ē-ō-sīts]

monocyte [MŎN-ō-sīt]

multiple myeloma [mī-ĕ-LŌ-mă]

myeloblast [MĪ-ĕ-lō-blăst]

neutrophil [NŪ-trō-fĭl]

pancytopenia [PĂN-sī-tō-PĒ-nē-ă]

partial thromboplastin time (PTT)

phag/o [FĂG-ō]

phlebotomy [flĕ-BŎT-ō-mē]

plasma [PLĂZ-mă]

plasmapheresis [PLĂZ-mă-fĕ-RĒ-sĭs]

platelet [PLĀT-lĕt]

platelet count (PLT)

polycythemia [PŎL-ē-sī-THĒ-mē-ă]

prothrombin [prō-THRŎM-bĭn]

prothrombin time (PT)

purpura [PŬR-pū-ră]

red blood cell

red blood cell count

red blood cell morphology

relapse [RĒ-lăps]

remission [rē-MĬSH-ŭn]

reticulocytosis [rĕ-TĬK-yū-lō-sī-TŌ-sĭs]

Rh factor

Rh negative

Rh positive

sedimentation rate (SR)

serum [SĒR-ŭm]

sickle [SĬ-kl] cell anemia

stem cell

thalassemia [thăl-ă-SĒ-mē-ă]

thromb/o [THRŎM-bō]

thrombin [THRŎM-bĭn].

thrombocyte [THRŎM-bō-sīt]

thrombocytopenia [THRŎM-bō-sī-tō-PĒ-nē-ă]

thrombolytic [thrŏm-bō-LĬT-ĭk]

thromboplastin [thrŏm-bō-PLĂS-tĭn]

transfusion [trăns-FYŪ-zhŭn]

venipuncture [VĔN-ĭ-pŭnk-chŭr, VĒ-nĭ-pŭnk-chŭr]

von Willebrand [vŏn WĬL-lĕ-brănd] disease

white blood cell

CHAPTER 11

The Cardiovascular System

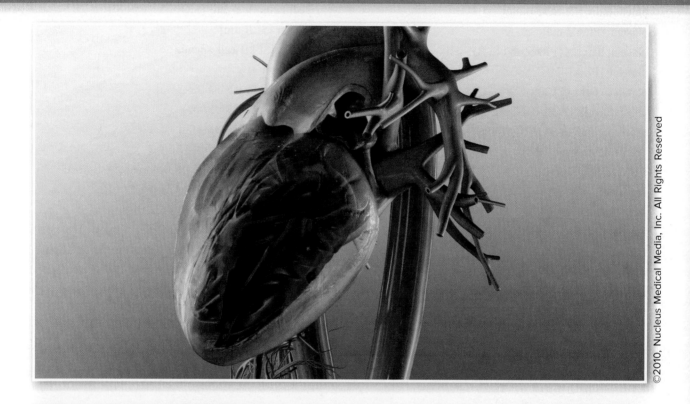

Learning Outcomes

After studying this chapter, you will be able to:

11.1 Identify and discuss the structure and function of the cardiovascular system.

11.2 Define combining forms used in building words that relate to the cardiovascular system.

11.3 Summarize common diagnostic tests, laboratory tests, and clinical procedures used in testing and treating disorders of the cardiovascular system.

11.4 Define the major pathological terms of the cardiovascular system.

11.5 Define surgical terms related to the cardiovascular system.

11.6 Recognize common pharmacological agents used to treat disorders of the cardiovascular system.

11.7 Identify common abbreviations associated with the cardiovascular system.

LO 11.1 Structure and Function of the Cardiovascular System

The function of the cardiovascular system is to deliver blood to tissues within the body. This provides the body with oxygen and nutrients and removes waste materials and carbon dioxide. The heart is the organ that pumps blood throughout the cardiovascular system. It is composed of left and right sides. The left side is responsible for receiving oxygenated blood from the lungs and pumping it out into the body. The right side of the heart receives deoxygenated blood from the body and sends it to the lungs so that the process may reoccur. The following sections provide an overview of cardiovascular terms along with how the cardiovascular system functions. Figure 11-1 shows how the blood circulates through the heart. Figure 11-2 shows the anatomy of the heart.

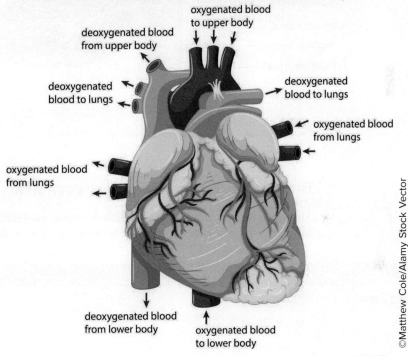

Blood Flow of the Human Heart

oxygenated blood
to upper body

deoxygenated blood
from upper body

deoxygenated
blood to lungs

deoxygenated
blood to lungs

oxygenated blood
from lungs

oxygenated blood
from lungs

deoxygenated blood
from lower body

oxygenated blood
to lower body

©Matthew Cole/Alamy Stock Vector

Figure 11-1 Blood flow in the heart

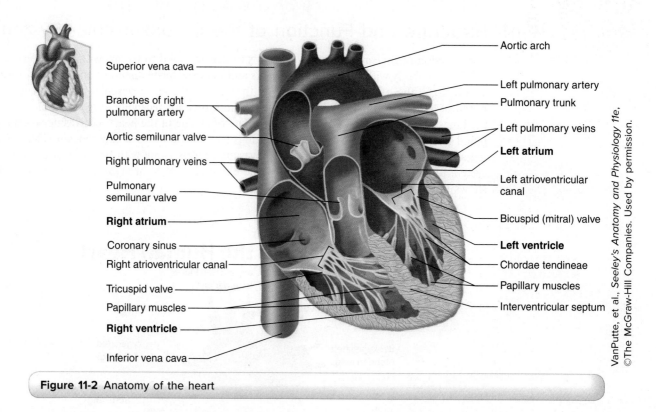

Superior vena cava

Branches of right pulmonary artery

Aortic semilunar valve

Right pulmonary veins

Pulmonary semilunar valve

Right atrium

Coronary sinus

Right atrioventricular canal

Tricuspid valve

Papillary muscles

Right ventricle

Inferior vena cava

Aortic arch

Left pulmonary artery

Pulmonary trunk

Left pulmonary veins

Left atrium

Left atrioventricular canal

Bicuspid (mitral) valve

Left ventricle

Chordae tendineae

Papillary muscles

Interventricular septum

VanPutte, et al., *Seeley's Anatomy and Physiology 11e*, ©The McGraw-Hill Companies. Used by permission.

Figure 11-2 Anatomy of the heart

Building Your Cardiovascular Vocabulary

This section provides an introduction to basic cardiovascular combining terms and their meanings. Review this information prior to moving to the practices.

Combining Form	Meaning
angi/o	blood vessel
aort/o	aorta
arteri/o, arter/o	artery
ather/o	fatty matter
atri/o	atrium
cardi/o	heart
hemangi/o	blood vessel
pericardi/o	pericardium
phleb/o	vein
sphygm/o	pulse
thromb/o	blood clot
vas/o	blood vessel
ven/o	vein

Structure and Function	PRACTICE
	Fill in the correct term(s) to complete the following sentences.
cardiovascular system [KĂR-dē-ō-VĂS-kyū-lăr SĬS-tĕm] **heart** [hărt] **blood** [blŭd] **blood vessels**	The _____ is the body's delivery service. The _____ pumps _____ through the tubular passages through which blood travels, or _____, to all the cells of the body.
	The average adult heart is about 5 inches long and 3.5 inches wide and weighs approximately 300 grams, depending on an individual's size and gender.
	The heart wall consists of a double-layered protective sac and two additional layers (Figure 11-3):
pericardium [pĕr-ĭ-KĂR-dē-ŭm] **epicardium** [ĕp-ĭ-KĂR-dē-ŭm] **myocardium** [mī-ō-KĂR-dē-ŭm] **endocardium** [ĕn-dō-KĂR-dē-ŭm]	1. The protective sac is the _____. It covers the *pericardial cavity,* which is filled with *pericardial fluid,* a lubricant for the membranes of the heart. The pericardium itself consists of the *visceral pericardium* (the inner layer), which is also called the _____ and is attached to the heart wall, and the *parietal pericardium* (the outer portion of the pericardium). 2. The second layer is the _____, a thick layer of muscular tissue. 3. The inner layer, the _____, forms a membranous lining for the chambers and valves of the heart.
	The heart is divided into right and left sides. Each side of the heart pumps blood to a specific area of the body. The right side of the heart pumps deoxygenated blood from the body to the lungs. The left side of the heart pumps oxygenated blood from the lungs to the body, where it delivers nutrients and oxygen.
right atrium [Ā-trē-ŭm] **right ventricle** [VĔN-trĭ-kl] **left atrium** **left ventricle** **septum** [SĔP-tŭm] **septa** [SĔP-tă]	Each side of the heart has two chambers. The _____ and _____ on the right side are separated from the _____ and _____ on the left side by a partition called a _____ (plural, _____). The atria are located in the upper heart chamber; the ventricles are in the lower heart chamber.
atria [Ā-trē-ă] **atrium** [Ā-trē-ŭm] **ventricles** [VĔN-trĭ-klz]	The part of the septum between the two _____ (plural of _____) is called the *interatrial septum;* the part between the two _____ is called the *interventricular septum.*

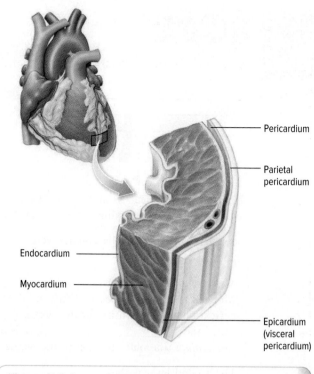

Figure 11-3 Layers of the heart

PRONOUNCE and DEFINE	Pronounce the following terms aloud and write their meaning in the space provided.
cardiovascular	[KĂR-dē-ō-VĂS-kyū-lăr]
pericardium	[pĕr-ĭ-KĂR-dē-ŭm]
epicardium	[ĕp-ĭ-KĂR-dē-ŭm]
endocardium	[ĕn-dō-KĂR-dē-ŭm]
ventricle	[VĔN-trĭ-kl]
septum (pl., septa)	[SĔP-tŭm (SĔP-tă)]

SPELL and DEFINE	Identify if the following terms are spelled correctly. Correct the words that are spelled incorrectly. Write the definition for each word.	
	Spelling	Definition
atreum		
myocardium		
cardiovasculer		
ventricle		
epicardiem		

1. _____ myocardium
2. _____ endocardium
3. _____ blood vessel
4. _____ atria
5. _____ ventricles
6. _____ pericardium

a. Tubular passageways in the cardiovascular system through which blood travels
b. Protective sac of the heart
c. Upper chambers of the heart
d. Muscular layer of heart tissue between the epicardium and the endocardium
e. Lower chambers of the heart
f. Membranous lining of the chambers and valves of the heart; the innermost layer of heart tissue

APPLY   Read the following scenario and answer the questions.

Sarah Schmidt is a student nurse working to help fourth-grade students understand the heart. The diagram they are using identifies the pericardium, epicardium, endocardium, and myocardium. How would you explain each word and break it down for them? How does each of the prefixes add to the meaning?

_____

_____

_____

_____

From the Perspective Of . . .

Who: Josie, Health Care Receptionist

Other Aliases: Medical Secretary, Scheduler, Patient Relations Specialist, Medical Administrative Assistant

Job Duties: Greeting patients; arranging for paperwork to be filled out and processed so the patient can be seen or billed appropriately; answering the phone; operating office equipment (computer, EMR system, fax, copier, postage). A big part of the receptionist's work includes scheduling appointments for patients. This includes translating when and how long the doctor

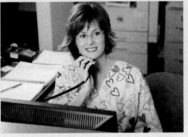
©Lisa F. Young/Shutterstock

has indicated that he/she would like to see the patient and providing directions to testing facilities. When answering the phone, the receptionist often works from a screening flowchart to determine which health care provider needs to take the call or return a call back to the patient. Information, symptoms, and questions need to be spelled and recorded accurately for the physician.

That is why medical terminology is important to me.

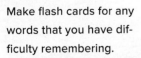

STUDY TIP

Make flash cards for any words that you have difficulty remembering.

Heart Valves

The heart has four chambers. Blood is pumped through the chambers with the assistance of four heart valves. These valves open and close to allow the blood to flow in only one direction. Figures 11-4 and 11-5 show the heart valves.

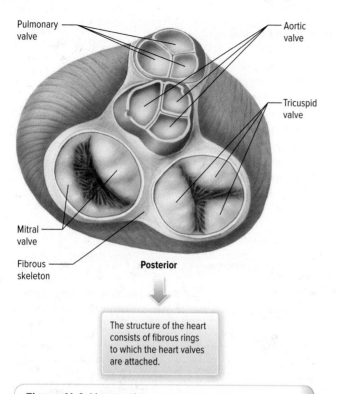

Figure 11-4 Heart valves

Pulmonary valve

Aortic valve

Tricuspid valve

Mitral valve

Fibrous skeleton

Posterior

The structure of the heart consists of fibrous rings to which the heart valves are attached.

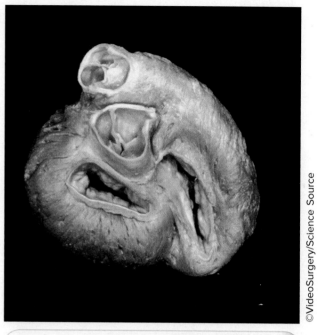

Figure 11-5 Photograph of the heart valves (superior view)

©VideoSurgery/Science Source

Structure and Function	PRACTICE
	Fill in the missing term(s) to complete the following sentences.
valves [vălvz] **arteries** [ĂR-tĕr-ēz], **veins** [vānz]	Blood flows through the chambers of the heart in one direction, with the flow regulated by _____. The blood is pumped throughout the body through the system of _____ and _____.
endothelium [ĕn-dō-THĒ-lē-ŭm] **lumen** [LŪ-mĕn]	Arteries carry oxygenated blood, except in pulmonary circulation, away from the heart. Veins carry deoxygenated blood, except in pulmonary circulation, toward the heart. The arteries have a lining called the _____, which secretes enzymes and other substances into the blood. The space within the arteries through which blood flows is called the _____.
atrioventricular valves [Ā-trē-ō-vĕn-TRĬK-yū-lăr vălvz] **tricuspid valve** [trī-KŬS-pĭd vălv] **bicuspid valve** [bī-KŬS-pĭd vălv] **mitral valve** [MĪ-trăl vălv]	The valves of the heart also control the blood flow through the heart. The two _____—the _____ and the _____ (also called the _____)—control the flow of blood between the atria and ventricles. The tricuspid valve has three cusps (flaps) that open and close to allow blood to flow from the right atrium into the right ventricle. The two cusps of the bicuspid valve are said to resemble a bishop's miter (hat), so this valve is commonly known as the mitral valve. The bicuspid valve controls blood flow on the left side of the heart, from the atrium to the ventricle.
semilunar valves [sĕm-ē-LŪ-năr vălvz] **pulmonary valve** [PŬL-mō-năr-ē vălv] **aortic valve** [ā-ŌR-tĭk vălv]	The two _____—the _____ and the _____—prevent the backflow of blood into the heart.

PRONOUNCE and DEFINE	Pronounce the following terms aloud and write their meaning in the space provided.
atrioventricular valve	[Ā-trē-ō-věn-TRĬK-yū-lăr vălv]
semilunar valve	[sĕm-ē-LŪ-năr vălv]
endothelium	[ĕn-dō-THĒ-lē-ŭm]
bicuspid	[bī-KŬS-pĭd]
veins	[vānz]

SPELL and DEFINE — Identify if the following terms are spelled correctly. Correct the words that are spelled incorrectly. Write the definition for each word.

	Spelling	Definition
endothelum		
tricusped		
atrioventricular		
vien		
aortic valve		

UNDERSTAND — Fill in the blanks.

1. The _____ carry deoxygenated blood.
2. The _____ lines the arteries and secretes substances into the blood.
3. A(n) _____ is a thick-walled vessel that carries oxygenated blood away from the heart.
4. The _____ prevent fluid from flowing backward or forward.
5. _____ is the inside channel of an artery through which blood flows.

APPLY — Read the following scenario and answer the questions.

You are the nurse caring for Mrs. Theresa Taggartis, a 63-year-old white female needing a mitral valve replacement. Mrs. Taggart asks you to explain the different valves and their location and function within the heart.

1. Explain what a mitral valve replacement is and which area of the heart it affects.

_____

_____

2. Lumen is the opening in the vessel. What would remind you of a lumen in the everyday world? (Hint: Think of a tubelike structure with varying openings/sizes.)

_____

_____

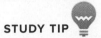

STUDY TIP

To learn the correct spelling of a word, write it ten times.

Vessels of the Cardiovascular System

Blood vessels carry blood within the heart to tissues and organs within the body. There are three types of blood vessels: arteries, veins, and capillaries. Blood vessels will expand to allow more blood to flow through them when needed. The same vessels can constrict to control the flow of blood through the body. Figures 11-6 and 11-7 show the major arteries and veins of the body. Figure 11-8 illustrates blood vessels within the heart.

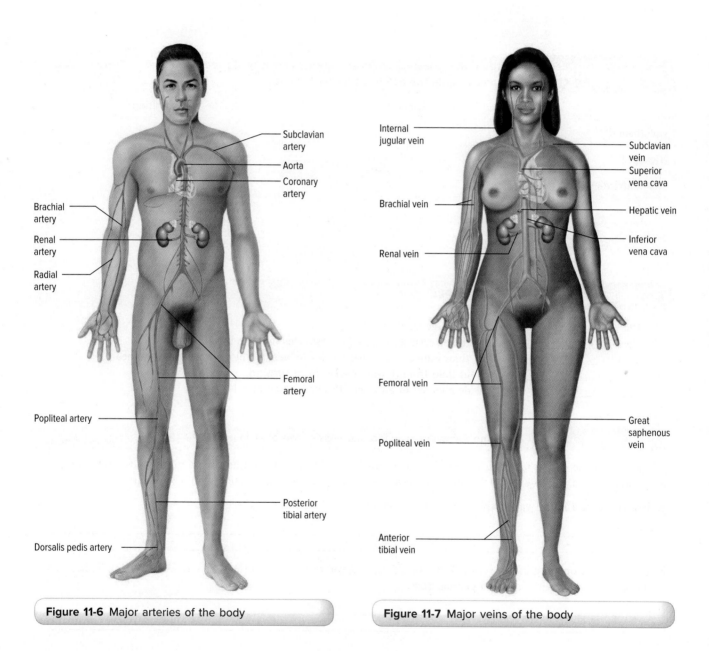

Figure 11-6 Major arteries of the body

Figure 11-7 Major veins of the body

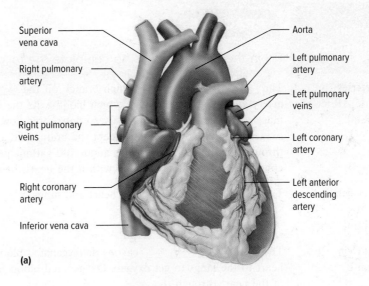

(a)

Superior vena cava

Right pulmonary artery

Right pulmonary veins

Right coronary artery

Inferior vena cava

Aorta

Left pulmonary artery

Left pulmonary veins

Left coronary artery

Left anterior descending artery

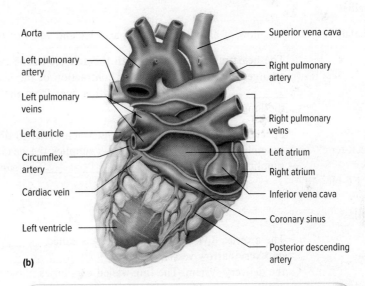

(b)

Aorta

Left pulmonary artery

Left pulmonary veins

Left auricle

Circumflex artery

Cardiac vein

Left ventricle

Superior vena cava

Right pulmonary artery

Right pulmonary veins

Left atrium

Right atrium

Inferior vena cava

Coronary sinus

Posterior descending artery

Figure 11-8 (a) Anterior and (b) posterior blood vessels of the heart

Structure and Function	**PRACTICE**
	Fill in the missing term(s) to complete the following sentences.
	Arteries and veins are the vessels that carry blood throughout the body. This circulation of blood is the essential function of the cardiovascular system, which includes *coronary circulation,* the circulation of blood within the heart; *pulmonary circulation,* the flow of blood between the heart and lungs; and *systemic circulation,* the flow of blood between the heart and the cells of the body.
coronary circulation [KŌR-ō-nār-ē ser-kū-LĀ-shŭn]	The flow of blood within the heart is _____.

continued on next page

Structure and Function	PRACTICE
	Fill in the missing term(s) to complete the following sentences.
coronary arteries [KŌR-ō-nār-ē ĂR-tĕr-ēz] **aorta** [ā-ŌR-tă]	The _____, which branch off the _____ (the body's largest artery and the artery through which blood exits the heart), supply blood to the heart muscle. The aortic semilunar valves control this flow of blood. The heart needs more oxygen than any other organ except the brain. The amount of blood pumped to the heart through the coronary arteries is about 100 gallons per day. The atrioventricular valves control the circulation of blood within the heart, between the atria and the ventricles.
pulmonary circulation [PŬL-mō-nār-ē ser-kū-LĀ-shŭn]	The flow of blood between the heart and lungs is _____.
pulmonary artery [PŬL-mō-nār-ē ĂR-tĕr-ē] **pulmonary veins**	The _____ carries deoxygenated blood from the right ventricle of the heart to the lungs to get oxygen. Oxygenated blood flows from the lungs to the left atrium of the heart through the _____.
systemic circulation	The flow of blood through the arteries and veins of the body is _____.
pulse [pŭls]	The heart pumps blood through the arteries to the cells of the body. The blood moves in a surge caused by the muscular contraction of the heart. This surge is called the _____. The blood that goes from the heart to the cells of the body (except the lungs) is oxygenated.
carotid artery [kă-RŎT-ĭd ĂR-tĕr-ē] **femoral artery** [FĔM-ŏ-răl, FĒ-mŏ-răl] **popliteal artery** [pŏp-LĬT-ē-ăl]	Specialized arteries carry the oxygen-rich blood to different areas of the body. For example, the _____ supplies the head and neck, the _____ supplies the thigh, and the _____ supplies the back of the knee.
arterioles [ăr-TĒ-rē-ōlz] **capillaries** [KĂP-ĭ-lār-ēz] **carbon dioxide, CO₂** **venules** [VĔN-yūlz, VĒ-nūlz]	The arteries divide into smaller vessels called _____, which then divide into very narrow vessels called _____, which act as the transfer station of the delivery system. The thin-walled capillaries allow the essential nutrients to leave the capillaries via osmosis, the movement from a greater concentration to a lesser concentration through a membrane (in this case, the cell wall). The capillaries provide the cells they serve with essential nutrients and, in turn, remove waste products (including _____) from the cells, sending it to the _____, which are small branches of veins.
saphenous veins [să-FĒ-nŭs vānz] **superior vena cava** [VĒ-nă KĂ-vă, KĀ-vă] **inferior vena cava** **venae cavae** [VĒ-nē KĂ-vē, KĀ-vē)] **vena cava**	The veins take deoxygenated blood back to the heart. An example of specialized veins is the _____, which remove oxygen-poor blood from the legs. Veins move the blood by gravity, skeletal muscle contractions, and respiratory activity. The veins contain small valves that prevent the blood from flowing backward. The blood from the upper part of the body is collected and carried to the heart through a large vein called the _____. The blood from the lower part of the body goes to the other large vein, called the _____, and then to the heart. Both of these large veins, the _____ (plural of _____), bring the blood to the right atrium of the heart.

PRONOUNCE and DEFINE	Pronounce the following terms aloud and write their meaning in the space provided.
arterioles	[ăr-TĒ-rē-ōlz]
vena cava (*pl.*, venae cavae)	[VĒ-nă KĂ-vă, KĀ-vă, (VĒ-nē KĂ-vē, KĀ-vē)]
capillaries	[KĂP-ĭ-lār-ēz]
saphenous vein	[să-FĒ-nŭs vān]
aorta	[ā-ŌR-tă]

SPELL and DEFINE	Identify if the following terms are spelled correctly. Correct the words that are spelled incorrectly. Write the definition for each word.	
	Spelling	**Definition**
arterole		
capilarry		
venele		
vena cava		
aerta		

UNDERSTAND	Match each function on the left with its term on the right.

1. _____ Supplies blood to the back of the knee
2. _____ Removes deoxygenated blood from the legs
3. _____ Brings blood into the right atrium of the heart
4. _____ The flow of blood between the heart and lungs
5. _____ Carries deoxygenated blood from the right ventricle of the heart to the lungs

a. Pulmonary circulation
b. Pulmonary artery
c. Popliteal artery
d. Vena cava
e. Saphenous veins

APPLY	Read the following scenario and answer the questions.

Ms. Joanmarie Conaty is the president of the local chapter of the American Heart Association. She has asked you to help provide education to a group that is learning cardiopulmonary resuscitation (CPR) for health care professionals.

1. Beginning with the lungs, trace blood through the heart and back to the lungs.

_____

_____

2. Explain this process to the group utilizing medical terms.

_____

_____

Blood Pressure and Conduction System

Blood pressure measures the pressure of blood within the arteries. Measured with a sphygmomanometer and a stethoscope, it provides information about pressure within the heart before and after the heart contracts. Figure 11-9 illustrates how to take a blood pressure reading.

The conduction system of the heart controls electrical impulses that cause the heart to contract. For most people, the impulse begins in the sinoatrial (SA) node, located in the right atrium, and quickly travels through an electrical pathway into the Purkinje fibers, resulting in coordinated ventricular contraction. Figures 11-10 and 11-11 illustrate the conduction system of the heart.

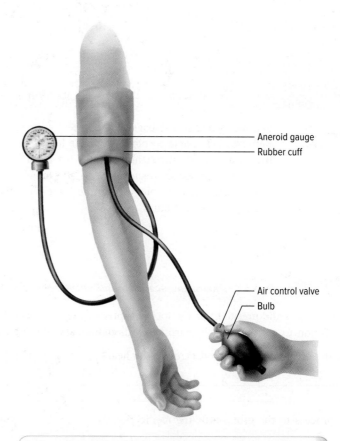

Aneroid gauge
Rubber cuff

Air control valve
Bulb

Figure 11-9 Proper placement of a blood pressure cuff

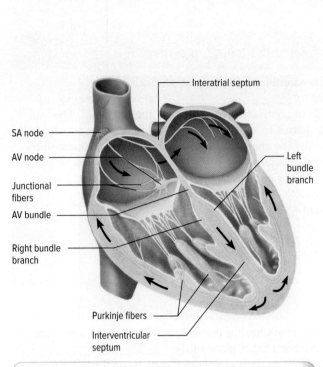

Figure 11-10 Conduction system of the heart

SA node
AV node
Junctional fibers
AV bundle
Right bundle branch
Interatrial septum
Left bundle branch
Purkinje fibers
Interventricular septum

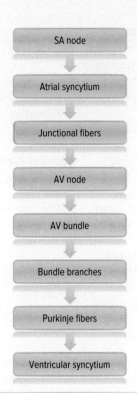

SA node
Atrial syncytium
Junctional fibers
AV node
AV bundle
Bundle branches
Purkinje fibers
Ventricular syncytium

Figure 11-11 Cardiac conduction system

Structure and Function	PRACTICE
	Fill in the missing term(s) to complete the following sentences.
systole [SĬS-tō-lē] **diastole** [dī-ĂS-tō-lē] **blood pressure**	Blood pressure is the force of the blood surging against the walls of the arteries. Each heartbeat consists of two parts. The first is the contraction, called _____, and the second is the relaxation, the _____. _____ is the measurement of the systolic pressure followed by the diastolic pressure. Normal blood pressure for an adult is 120/80. The number 120 represents the pressure within the walls of an artery during systole, or during the contraction; the number 80 represents the pressure within the arterial wall during diastole, or during relaxation. Pulse pressure represents the difference between the diastolic and systolic readings. In blood pressure of 120/80, the pulse pressure is 40, which represents the strength of the left ventricle pumping blood to the body.
conduction system **sinoatrial (SA) node** [sī-nō-Ā-trē-ăl nōd] **pacemaker**	The _____, which controls the impulses that cause the heart to contract, is contained in special heart tissue called conductive tissue in the right atrium. This region is called the _____ and is known as the heart's _____ because its electrical impulse causes the regular contractions that result in a normal heartbeat or pulse.

continued on next page

PRACTICE

Fill in the missing term(s) to complete the following sentences.

polarization
[pō-lăr-ĭ-ZĀ-shŭn]
depolarization
[dē-pō-lă-rĭ-ZĀ-shŭn]
repolarization
[rē-pō-lăr-ĭ-ZĀ-shŭn]
atrioventricular (AV) node
[Ā-trē-ō-vĕn-TRĬK-yū-lăr nōd]
atrioventricular bundle
[Ā-trē-ō-vĕn-TRĬK-yū-lăr bŭn-dl]
bundle of His [hĭz, hĭs]
Purkinje fibers
[per-KĬN-jē FĪ-berz]

The contractions take place in the myocardium, which cycles through _____ (resting state) to _____ (contracting state) to _____ (recharging from contracting to resting) in the heartbeat. The electrical current from the SA node passes to a portion of the interatrial septum called the _____, which sends the charge to a group of specialized muscle fibers called the _____, also called the _____. The bundle of His divides into left and right bundle branches and causes the ventricles to contract, forcing blood away from the heart during systole. At the end of these branches are the _____, specialized fibers that conduct the impulses.

cardiac cycle
[KĂR-dē-ăk SĪ-kl]
sinus rhythm

Heart rate can vary depending on a person's health, physical activity, or emotions at any one time. The repeated beating of the heart takes place in the _____, during which the heart contracts and relaxes as it circulates blood. Normal heart rhythm is called _____.

PRONOUNCE and DEFINE

Pronounce the following terms aloud and write their meaning in the space provided.

polarization	[pō-lăr-ĭ-ZĀ-shŭn]
depolarization	[dē-pō-lă-rĭ-ZĀ-shŭn]
sinoatrial (SA) node	[sī-nō-Ā-trē-ăl nōd]
bundle of His	[BŬN-dl ov hĭz, hĭs]
systole	[SĬS-tō-lē]

SPELL and DEFINE

Identify if the following terms are spelled correctly. Correct the words that are spelled incorrectly. Write the definition for each word.

	Spelling	Definition
diasstole		
repolarization		
sinoatial node		
systole		
kardiac cycle		

Fill in the blanks.

1. _____ is when the heart is in a resting state.
2. _____ is the force of blood against the arterial walls when at rest.
3. _____ is known as the pacemaker of the heart.
4. The _____ sends the electrical charge out to the bundle of His.
5. The heart's normal rhythm is called _____.

APPLY   **Read the following scenario and respond accordingly.**

You are working in an urgent care clinic assisting with a client who has a history of cardiac arrhythmias. The client is a 45-year-old Hispanic male named Mike Ambrosino. The physician just told the client that he was in normal sinus rhythm. The client asks you what this means.

Describe the conduction system to help this client understand the process.

_____

_____

_____

_____

Did you know

High Blood Pressure

High blood pressure is a dangerous condition with virtually no symptoms felt by the client. At almost every doctor visit, blood pressure is measured, usually with a sphygmomanometer. Blood pressure measurements are character-ized as normal, low, or high, but there is dis-agreement as to the ranges of normal. Normal blood pressure for an adult is generally considered 120/80. High blood pressure is sometimes the result of lifestyle factors. Overeating, leading to being overweight; smoking; lack of exercise; and stress are lifestyle factors that affect blood pressure. For high systolic pressures, most doctors recommend lifestyle changes along with medication. *Your doctor should evaluate unusually low readings.*

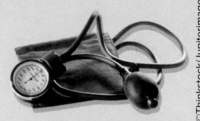

©Thinkstock/Jupiterimages

The American Heart Association (www.americanheart.org) categorizes blood pressure as follows:

Blood Pressure Category	Systolic (mm Hg)		Diastolic (mm Hg)
Normal	less than 120	and	less than 80
Elevated	120–129	and	less than 80
High Blood Pressure Stage 1	130–139	or	80–89
High Blood Pressure Stage 2	140 or higher	or	90 or higher
Hypertensive Crisis	180 or higher	and/or	120 or higher

Fetal Circulation

STUDY TIP 💡

In the fetal heart, the **foramen ovale** allows blood to enter the left atrium from the right atrium. It is one of two shunts, the other being the **ductus arteriosus,** that allows blood entering the right atrium to bypass the pulmonary circulation. In most children, the foramen ovale closes within the first year after birth.

Fetal circulation is the circulatory system of the unborn child. It includes the umbilical cord and the blood vessels within the placenta. Figure 11-12 illustrates structures involved in, and the path of, fetal circulation.

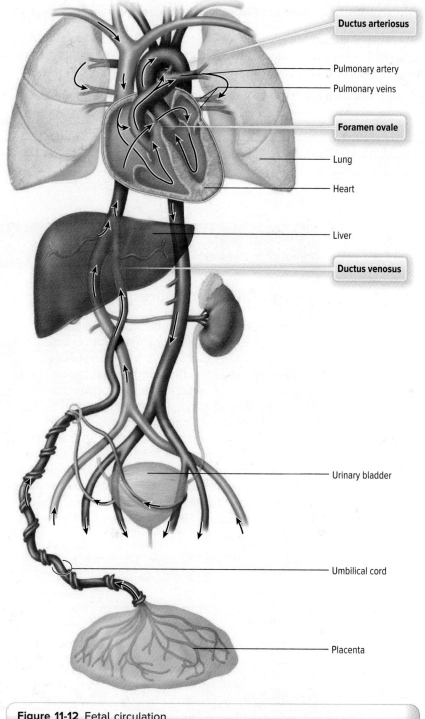

Figure 11-12 Fetal circulation

Structure and Function	**PRACTICE**
	Fill in the missing term(s) to complete the following sentences.
	The circulatory system of the fetus bypasses pulmonary circulation because a fetus's lungs do not function until after birth. The umbilical cord contains arteries and a vein. Fetal blood is transported back and forth to the placenta, where deoxygenated blood is oxygenated and returned to the fetus.
ductus venosus [DŬK-tŭs vĕn-Ō-sŭs] **ductus arteriosus** [DŬK-tŭs ăr-tēr-ē-Ō-sŭs] **foramen ovale** [fō-RĀ-mĕn ō-VĂ-lē]	The _____ is the connection from the umbilical vein to the fetus's inferior vena cava, through which oxygenated blood is delivered to the fetal heart, bypassing the fetal liver. Deoxygenated blood flows from the fetal heart through the _____ and back through the umbilical cord to the placenta, bypassing the fetus's fluid-filled, nonfunctioning lungs. The septum between the atria of the fetal heart has a small opening called the _____, which allows blood to flow from the right atrium into the left atrium. After birth, the opening closes.

PRONOUNCE and DEFINE	Pronounce the following terms aloud and write their meaning in the space provided.
ductus venosus	[DŬK-tŭs vĕn-Ō-sŭs]
ductus arteriosus	[DŬK-tŭs ăr-tēr-ē-Ō-sŭs]
foramen ovale	[fō-RĀ-mĕn ō-VĂ-lē]

SPELL and DEFINE	Identify if the following terms are spelled correctly. Correct the words that are spelled incorrectly. Write the definition for each word.	
	Spelling	**Definition**
foramen ovale		
ductus arteriosus		
ductus venosus		

UNDERSTAND	Match each term on the left to its correct function on the right.

1. _____ foramen ovale

2. _____ ductus arteriosus

3. _____ ductus venosus

a. This structure within fetal circulation allows blood flow to bypass the fetal liver
b. Closes after birth
c. This structure within fetal circulation allows blood flow to bypass the fetal lungs

LO 11.2 Word Building in the Cardiovascular System

Major Terms and Word Building Exercises

Word Building	**PRACTICE**
	Fill in the correct combining form to complete each of the sentences.
angio-gram [AN-jē-ō-gram]	Image of a blood vessel is a(n) _____ gram.
aort-itis [ā-ōr-TĪ-tĭs]	_____ itis is inflammation of the aorta.
arterio-sclerosis [ăr-TĒR-ē-ō-sklĕr-Ō-sĭs]	Hardening of the arteries is _____ sclerosis.
athero-sclerosis [ĂTH-ĕr-ō-sklĕr-ō-sĭs]	_____ sclerosis is hardening of the arteries with irregular plaque deposits.
atrio-ventricular [Ā-trē-ō-vĕn-TRĬK-yū-lăr]	_____ ventricular relates to the atria and ventricles of the heart.
cardio-myopathy [KĂR-dē-ō-mī-ŎP-ă-thē]	Disease of the heart muscle is _____ myopathy.
hemangi-oma [he-MAN-jē-Ō-mă]	An abnormal mass of blood vessels is a(n) _____ oma.
pericard-itis [PĔR-ĭ-kăr-DĪ-tĭs]	_____ itis is inflammation of the pericardium.
phleb-itis [flĕ-BĪ-tĭs]	Inflammation of a vein is _____ itis.
sphygmo-manometer [SFĬG-mō-mă-NŎM-ĕ-tĕr]	A _____ manometer is an instrument used to measure blood pressure.
thrombo-cytosis [THROM-bō-sī-TŌ-sĭs]	_____ cytosis is an abnormal increase in blood platelets in the blood.
vaso-depressor [VĀ-sō-dē-PRES-er]	An agent that lowers blood pressure by relaxing blood vessels is a(n) _____ depressor.
veno-graphy [vē-NŎG-ră-fē]	_____ graphy is radiographic imaging of a vein.

PRONOUNCE and DEFINE	Pronounce the following terms aloud and write their meaning in the space provided.
vasodepressor	[VĀ-sō-dē-PRES-er]
sphygmomanometer	[SFĬG-mō-mă-NŎM-ĕ-tĕr]
arteriosclerosis	[ăr-TĒR-ē-ō-sklĕr-Ō-sĭs]
cardiomyopathy	[KĂR-dē-ō-mī-ŎP-ă-thē]
hemangioma	[hĕ-MAN-jē-Ō-mă]
pericarditis	[PĔR-ĭ-kăr-DĪ-tĭs]

Identify if the following terms are spelled correctly. Correct the words that are spelled incorrectly. Write the definition for each word.

	Spelling	Definition
atriaventricular		
ductus arteriosus		
myocardium		
bundle of His		
sistole		
capillairy		
Purkine fibers		
arteryole		
popliteal		

UNDERSTAND Fill in the blanks.

1. Inflammation of pericardium: _____

2. Hardening of the arteries: _____

3. X-ray of a vein: _____

4. Image of a blood vessel: _____

5. Abnormal mass of blood vessels: _____

6. Abnormal increase of blood platelets: _____

7. Diseased heart muscle: _____

8. Inflammation of a vein: _____

APPLY Read the following scenario and respond accordingly.

Josie, a certified medical assistant (CMA), is working with a client who has a history of cardiomyopathy, atherosclerosis, and arteriosclerosis. The client is being seen today for phlebitis. Venography determines the client has a hemangioma. The client is placed on bedrest to prevent thrombus formation. In layman's terms, explain this to the client.

_____

_____

_____

_____

_____

Diagnostic, Procedural, and Laboratory Terms

Diagnostic, procedural, and laboratory findings assist the physician in diagnosing medical conditions. Often used in combination, these tests lead to a final diagnosis and assist in treatment planning. Figure 11-13 is an example of an electrocardiogram waveform. Figure 11-14 shows an angiogram of coronary arteries.

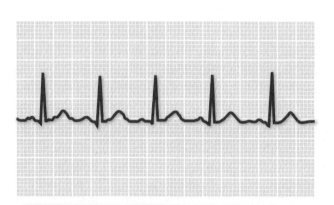

Figure 11-13 Electrocardiogram waveform

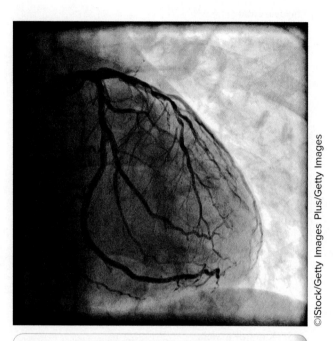

©iStock/Getty Images Plus/Getty Images

Figure 11-14 Angiogram of coronary arteries

Diagnostic	**PRACTICE**
	Fill in the missing term(s) to complete the following sentences.
	Treatment of cardiovascular disease requires a precise understanding of the condition of the heart and of the parts of the body that affect the heart's functioning. Doctors order many types of diagnostic tests based on their observations of a client. They may order clinical procedures whose results will indicate certain specific conditions or they may order laboratory tests to find disease-causing factors or evidence of a specific disease.
cardiologists [KĂR-dē-ŎL-ō-jĭsts] **auscultation** [ăws-kŭl-TĀ-shŭn] **sphygmomanometer** [SFĬG-mō-mă-NŎM-ĕ-tĕr]	Doctors who specialize in the diagnosis and treatment of cardiovascular disease (*cardiology*) are called _____. These specialists usually see clients who already have some type of cardiovascular problem or indication of disease. The cardiologist often starts an examination with _____ (listening to sounds within the body through a stethoscope). Some abnormal sounds a physician may hear are a *murmur,* a *bruit,* or a *gallop.* Each sound is a clue to the client's condition. A _____ is then often used to measure blood pressure.
stress test	One common diagnostic test is a _____. Clients are asked to exercise (for example, on a treadmill) while technicians take certain measurements, such as heart rate and respiration. A stress test may be used to diagnose coronary artery disease or may give a risk factor for heart attack.

electrocardiography [ē-lĕk-trō-kăr-dē-ŎG-ră-fē]	Another common test is _____, which produces an *electrocardiogram* (**ECG, EKG**); this measures the amount of electricity flowing through the heart by means of electrodes placed on the client's skin at specific points surrounding the heart.
Holter monitor [HŌL-tĕr MON-ĭ-ter, -tōr]	A _____ is a portable electrocardiograph, or instrument that performs an electrocardiogram, over a 24-hour period.
angiocardiography [ăn-jē-ō-kăr-dē-ŎG-ră-fē] **angiography** [ăn-jē-ŎG-ră-fē] **arteriography** [ăr-tēr-ē-ŎG-ră-fē] **aortography** [ā-ōr-TŎG-ră-fē] **venography** [vē-NŎG-ră-fē] **phlebography** [flĕ-BŎG-ră-fē]	Various diagnostic procedures can be performed by producing some type of image. Taking x-rays after a dye has been injected is called _____ (x-ray of the heart and its large blood vessels), _____ (x-ray of blood vessels), _____ (x-ray of a specific artery), _____ (x-ray of the aorta), and _____ or _____ (x-ray of a specific vein). These resulting x-ray pictures are called *angiocardiograms, angiograms, arteriograms, aortograms,* and *venograms* or *phlebograms.*
ventriculogram [vĕn-TRĬK-yū-lō-grăm] **ejection fraction**	A _____ is an x-ray showing the ventricles. These tests measure *stroke volume (SV),* the amount of blood leaving a ventricle in one contraction; *cardiac output (CO)* is the amount of blood the ventricle ejects every minute; and the _____, the percentage of volume of the contents of the left ventricle ejected with each contraction.
sonography [sō-NŎG-ră-fē] **Doppler ultrasound** [DŎP-lĕr ŬL-tră-sownd] **echocardiography** [ĔK-ō-kăr-dē-ŎG-ră-fē]	Ultrasound tests, or *ultrasonography* or _____, produce images by measuring the echoes of sound waves against various structures. _____ measures blood flow in certain blood vessels. _____ records sound waves to show the structure and movement of the heart. The test itself is called an *echocardiogram.*
cardiac scan [KĂR-dē-ăk skan] **positron emission tomography (PET) scan** [POZ-ĭ-tron ē-MISH-ŭn tō-MŎG-ră-fē] **multiple-gated acquisition (MUGA) angiography**	Radioactive substances that are injected into the client can provide information in a _____, a test that measures movement of areas of the heart, or in *nuclear medicine imaging.* _____ is one form of nuclear imaging. A PET scan of the heart reveals images of the heart's blood flow and its cellular metabolism. Another form of nuclear imaging is _____. A _____ scan is a non-invasive method of assessing cardiac muscle function.
cardiac MRI	*Magnetic resonance imaging (MRI)* uses magnetic waves to produce images. A _____ provides a detailed image of the heart and shows any lesions in the large blood vessels of the heart.
cardiac catheterization [KĂR-dē-ak kăth-ĕ-tĕr-ĭ-ZĀ-shŭn]	Other procedures require actual insertion of a device, such as a catheter, into a vein or artery, and the device is guided to the heart. _____ allows withdrawal of blood samples from the heart and measures certain pressures and blood flow patterns within the heart. The catheter can be directed to the left side of the heart for measurements and images involving the coronary arteries or to the right side of the heart for measurement of oxygenated blood.

continued on next page

Diagnostic	**PRACTICE**
	Fill in the missing term(s) to complete the following sentences.
	Laboratory tests are crucial for determining what may be happening to a client or for evaluating risk factors for heart disease. Drug therapy, clinical procedures, and lifestyle changes all may be recommended largely on the basis of laboratory test results. All laboratory tests have a range of normal values (see Appendix C). Some of these ranges change as new studies are done and views of what constitutes a healthy value (such as for cholesterol readings) are revised.
cholesterol [kō-LĔS-tĕr-ōl] **triglycerides** [trī-GLĬS-ĕr-īds]	The flow of blood in the arteries is affected by the amount of _____ and _____ (fatty substances or *lipids*) contained in the blood. Lipids are carried through the blood by *lipoproteins. Low-density lipoproteins (LDLs)* and *very low-density lipoproteins (VLDLs)* cause cholesterol to form blockages in the arteries. *High-density lipoproteins (HDLs)* actually remove lipids from the arteries and help protect from the formation of blockages. One factor that increases LDL and VLDL is a diet high in *saturated fats* (animal fats and some vegetable fats that tend to be solid).
lipid profile [LĬP-ĭd PRŌ-fīl]	A _____ (a series of laboratory tests performed on a blood sample) gives the lipid, triglyceride, glucose, and other values that help to evaluate a client's risk factors.
	A laboratory test that can be used to diagnose a myocardial infarction earlier than most other laboratory tests measures the levels of *troponin T* and *troponin I,* proteins found in the heart. As levels of the two rise, it usually indicates the early states of an acute myocardial infarction. If only one level rises, it can indicate a number of conditions not related to the heart, such as kidney failure or muscle trauma.
cardiac enzyme test **serum enzyme test**	Another important laboratory test of blood is the _____ (also called a _____), which measures the levels of enzymes released into the blood by damaged heart muscle during a myocardial infarction. Enzymes that help evaluate the condition of the client are *CPK (creatine phosphokinase)* and *LDH (lactate dehydrogenase)* and the protein **troponin.** The enzymes may indicate the degree of injury to the heart or the seriousness of an attack.

Did you know ❓

Electrocardiograms

The electrocardiograph can have 12 leads, which are placed at specific points on the client's body to monitor electrical activity of the heart. Six of the leads go on the arms and legs and the other six leads go on specific points on the chest. The chest leads are marked with specific codes. For example, V_1 goes in the fourth intercostal space to the right of the sternum. Each lead traces the electrical activity from a different angle.

©Comstock/Alamy

STUDY TIP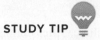

Electrocardiograms identify the cardiac rhythm. The cardiac rhythm provides information on the cardiac conduction system, including depolarization and repolorization.

PRONOUNCE and DEFINE	Pronounce the following terms aloud and write their meaning in the space provided.
electrocardiography	[ē-lĕk-trō-kăr-dē-ŎG-ră-fē]
cholesterol	[kō-LĔS-tĕr-ōl]
auscultation	[ăws-kŭl-TĀ-shŭn]
triglycerides	[trī-GLĬS-ĕr-īdz]
cardiac catheterization	[KĂR-dē-ăk kăth-ĕ-tĕr-ĭ-ZĀ-shŭn]
sphygmomanometer	[SFĬG-mō-mă-NŎM-ĕ-tĕr]

SPELL and DEFINE	Identify if the following terms are spelled correctly. Correct the words that are spelled incorrectly. Write the definition for each word.	
	Spelling	**Definition**
echocardiography		
flebography		
cholesterel		
position emission tomography		
aluscultation		
sphygmometer		

UNDERSTAND	Build a word for each of the following using the combining terms *atrio-*, *phlebo-*, *thrombo-*, and *veno-*.

1. _____ itis, inflammation of a vein
2. _____ ectomy, surgical removal of a thrombus
3. _____ plasty, vein repair
4. _____ megaly, enlargement of the atrium
5. _____ graph, radiograph of veins

Mr. Guy Ashley is a 21-year-old black male who arrives at the cardiology clinic. After examining Mr. Ashley, the physician determines that he may have more than one condition going on. He has ordered the following diagnostic testing for this client.

1. Using correct medical terminology, translate the following:
   a. Blood tests used to determine if the client had a myocardial infarction: _____
   b. Ultrasound test to check blood flow: _____
   c. Test that measures heart rate, blood pressure, and other bodily functions during exercise:
      _____
   d. Device that provides a 24-hour electrocardiogram: _____
   e. Records the electrical currents associated with heart muscle activity for diagnosis:
      _____

2. What conditions would each of these tests screen for?
   _____
   _____

3. What does EKG stand for? What is another abbreviation for this test?
   _____
   _____

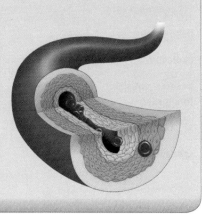

Did you know ?

Cholesterol

Cholesterol is just one of the risk factors for heart disease, but it is one that can be changed by lifestyle and/or medication. That is why many researchers focus on cholesterol levels and ratios. It is generally thought that low LDL levels and high HDL levels are healthier. However, some studies suggest that even HDL levels can get too high.

For more information on cholesterol, go to the Web site of the U.S. Department of Health and Human Services, National Health Information Center: www.healthfinder.gov.

LO 11.4 Pathological Terms

Heart Rhythm

STUDY TIP

Too many PVCs are dangerous, as there is no cardiac perfusion.

Sinus rhythm is the heart's normal rhythm. Due to cardiovascular conditions, the heart can experience abnormal cardiac rhythms. Some of these rhythms are considered an emergency.

Pathological	PRACTICE
	Fill in the missing term(s) to complete the following sentences.
risk factors	Cardiovascular disease (CVD) can have many causes and can take many forms. Some diseases are caused by a congenital anomaly, whereas others may be caused by other pathology or by lifestyle factors (_____), such as poor diet, smoking, and lack of exercise.
arrhythmias [ă-RĬTH-mē-ăz] **bradycardia** [brăd-ē-KĂR-dē-ă] **tachycardia** [TĂK-ĭ-KĂR-dē-ă] **atrial fibrillation** [Ă-trē-ăl fĭ-brĭ-LĀ-shŭn] **fibrillation** [fĭ-brĭ-LĀ-shŭn] **dysrhythmia** [dĭs-RĬTH-mē-ă]	The rhythm of the heart maintains the blood flow through and in and out of the heart. Abnormal rhythms are called _____ . Heart rates may be too slow (_____), too fast (_____), or irregular (also called _____, _____, or _____).
flutter **bruit** [brū-Ē] **murmur**	A _____ is a rapid but regular heartbeat. The heart rate may be regular, but the sound of the heartbeat may be abnormal (_____, heard on auscultation of the carotid artery, or _____ , a soft humming sound, which may indicate valve leakage). A new murmur heard during a heart attack may indicate a rupture of the heart muscle, which is an urgent surgical emergency.
rub **gallop**	Other sounds indicate specific problems; for example, a _____ (a frictional sound) usually indicates a pericardial murmur and a _____ (a triple heart sound) usually indicates serious heart disease.
palpitations [păl-pĭ-TĀ-shŭnz] **atrioventricular block** **heart block** **premature atrial contractions (PACs)** **premature ventricular contractions (PVCs)**	Some pulsations of the heart (_____) can be felt by the client as thumping in the chest. An _____ or _____ is caused by a blocking of impulses from the AV node. The electrical impulses of the heart control contractions. Irregularities in the heart's contractions, such as _____ or _____, can cause palpitations.

PRONOUNCE and DEFINE	Pronounce the following terms aloud and write their meaning in the space provided.
arrhythmias	[ă-RĬTH-mē-ăz]
fibrillation	[fĭ-brĭ-LĀ-shŭn]
bruit	[brū-Ē]
dysrhythmia	[dĭs-RĬTH-mē-ă]
palpitations	[păl-pĭ-TĀ-shŭnz]

SPELL and DEFINE	Identify if the following terms are spelled correctly. Correct the words that are spelled incorrectly. Write the definition for each word.	
	Spelling	Definition
briut		
arterial fibrillation		
palpitashuns		
tachicardia		

UNDERSTAND
Match each term on the left with its correct definition on the right.

1. _____ gallop
2. _____ palpitations
3. _____ fibrillation
4. _____ rub
5. _____ dysrhythmia
6. _____ flutter

a. Abnormally rapid but regular heartbeat
b. Third sound of a heartbeat, usually indicative of serious heart disease
c. Frictional sound heard between heartbeats, usually indicating a pericardial murmur
d. Irregular heart rhythm
e. Uncomfortable pulsations of the heart felt as a thumping in the chest
f. Irregular or abnormal heart rhythm

APPLY
Read the following scenario and answer the questions.

Mrs. Nancy Marr is a 72-year-old black female who has a history of atrial fibrillation and atrial flutter and is now complaining of palpitations. The patient also has uncontrolled diabetes. She is very compliant with the doctor's instructions and sees him regularly.

1. Define the terms *atrial fibrillation* and *atrial flutter*.

_____
_____

2. Explain the connection between atrial fibrillation, atrial flutter, and palpitations.

_____
_____

Blood Pressure

An elevated blood pressure can lead to cardiovascular and other disorders within the body. Unless the client is experiencing symptoms, low blood pressure is usually not treated.

Pathological	PRACTICE
	Fill in the missing term(s) to complete the following sentences.
hypertensive heart disease [HĪ-pĕr-TĔN-sĭv hărt di-ZĔZ] **hypertension (HTN)** [HĪ-pĕr-TĔN-shŭn] **high blood pressure** **hypotension** [HĪ-pō-TĔN-shŭn] **low blood pressure**	Abnormalities in blood pressure (_____) can damage the heart as well as other body systems. If the blood pressure is too high, (_____ or _____) or too low (_____ or _____), the blood vessels do not have the proper pressure of blood flowing through them.

| essential hypertension secondary hypertension | _____ is high blood pressure that is idiopathic, or without any known cause. _____ has a known cause, such as a high-salt diet, renal disease, or adrenal gland disease. |
| | Hypertension is the most common cardiovascular disease. Hypotension often results from another disease process or trauma (as in shock). Hypotension may lead to fainting or becoming unconscious. Extreme hypotension may lead to death. |

PRONOUNCE and DEFINE	Pronounce the following terms aloud and write their meaning in the space.
hypertensive	[HĪ-pĕr-TĔN-sĭv]
hypotension	[HĪ-pō-TĔN-shŭn]

UNDERSTAND — Fill in the blanks.

1. _____ hypertension has no known cause.

2. Hypertension is a blood pressure greater than _____.

3. _____ is heart disease that is worsened by hypertension.

STUDY TIP

Carry flash cards so that you can study when you have a few extra minutes.

Diseases of the Blood Vessels

The blood vessels are responsible for carrying blood throughout the body. If the blood vessel is damaged or diseased, blood flow can be compromised, resulting in decreased oxygen delivered to the tissues and organs. Figure 11-15 shows a normal blood vessel (a) and a blood vessel with plaque buildup (b).

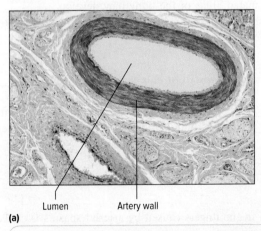

Lumen   Artery wall

(a)

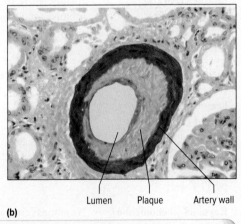

Lumen   Plaque   Artery wall

(b)

©The McGraw-Hill Companies, Inc./Al Telser, photographer

Figure 11-15 (a) Normal blood vessel; (b) blood vessel with plaque buildup

Pathological	PRACTICE
	Fill in the missing term(s) to complete the following sentences.
plaque [plăk] **atheroma** [ăth-ĕr-Ō-mă] **atherosclerosis** [ĂTH-ĕr-ō-sklĕr-Ō-sĭs] **embolus** [ĔM-bō-lŭs] **thrombus** [THRŎM-bŭs]	Blood vessels can become diseased, as when _____, buildup of fatty material, is deposited on the wall of an artery. An _____ is plaque specifically on the wall of an artery, which can build up to cause _____. An _____ is a mass traveling through the bloodstream causing a blockage in the vessel. A _____ is a stationary blood clot, usually formed from elements in the blood.
thrombophlebitis [THRŎM-bō-flĕ-BĪ-tĭs] **thrombosis** [thrŏm-BŌ-sĭs] **deep vein thrombosis** **thrombotic occlusion** [thrŏm-BŎT-ĭk Ŏ-KLŪ-zhŭn]	_____ is an inflammation of a vein with a thrombus. _____ is the presence of a thrombus in a blood vessel. _____ forms in a deep vein or in a vein within a structure rather than one on the surface of a structure. _____ is the occlusion, or closing, of a vessel caused by a thrombus.
constriction [kŏn-STRĬK-shŭn] **occlusion** [ŏ-KLŪ-zhŭn] **aneurysm** [ĂN-yū-rĭzm] **arteriosclerosis** [ăr-TĒR-ē-ō-sklĕr-Ō-sĭs] **claudication** [klăw-dĭ-KĀ-shŭn] **intermittent claudication**	Blood vessels can have a _____, or narrowing, due to contraction. An _____ is the closing off of a blood vessel due to a blockage. A weakness in an artery wall can cause a balloonlike bulge, or _____, which can fatally rupture. Loss of elasticity or hardening of the arteries (_____) can lessen blood flow. Inadequate blood supply, particularly to the blood vessels in the legs, causes _____, limping. _____, irregular attacks of claudication, are helped by resting.
peripheral vascular disease **infarction** [ĭn-FĂRK-shŭn] **necrosis** [nĕ-KRŌ-sĭs] **infarct** [ĬN-fărkt] **perfusion deficit** **ischemia** [ĭs-KĒ-mē-ă] **cyanosis** [sī-ă-NŌ-sĭs]	_____ is a general term for vascular disease in the lower extremities. A sudden drop in the supply of blood to a vessel (an _____) can cause an area of dead tissue, or _____ (an _____). The general term for lack of flow through a blood vessel is _____. An area of blood insufficiency in the body is called _____. Insufficiently oxygenated areas of the body may develop _____, a bluish or purplish discoloration of the skin caused by deficient oxygenation of the blood.
varicose veins [VĂR-ĭ-kōs vānz] **hemorrhoids** [HĔM-ō-roydz] **phlebitis** [flĕ-BĪ-tĭs] **arteritis** [ăr-tĕr-Ī-tĭs] **petechiae** [pĕ-TĒ-kē-ē, pē-TĔK-ē-ē]	Veins sometimes become twisted or enlarged (_____). _____ are varicose veins in the anal region. An inflammation of a vein is called _____. An inflammation of an artery is called _____. Minute hemorrhages in the blood vessels in the skin are called _____.
Raynaud phenomenon [rā-NŌ fĕ-NOM-ĕ-non]	Numbness or pain in the fingers caused by arterial spasms is called _____.

PRONOUNCE and DEFINE	Pronounce the following terms aloud and write their meaning in the space.
varicose	[VĂR-ĭ-kōs]
necrosis	[nĕ-KRŌ-sĭs]
constriction	[kŏn-STRĬK-shŭn]
atheroma	[ăth-ĕr-Ō-mă]
thrombotic occlusion	[thrŏm-BŎT-ĭk Ŏ-KLŪ-zhŭn]
thrombosis	[thrŏm-BŌ-sĭs]

SPELL and DEFINE	Identify if the following terms are spelled correctly. Correct the words that are spelled incorrectly. Write the definition for each word.	
	Spelling	Definition
hemorhoids		
petecheye		
arteritis		
placque		
claudication		

UNDERSTAND Match each term on the left with its definition on the right.

1. _____ cyanosis
2. _____ petechiae
3. _____ ischemia
4. _____ hemorrhoids
5. _____ varicose
6. _____ phlebitis

a. Varicose condition of veins in the anal region
b. Dilated, enlarged, or twisted vein, usually on the leg
c. Inflammation of a vein
d. Bluish or purplish coloration, as of the skin, caused by inadequate oxygenation of the blood
e. Minute hemorrhages in the skin
f. Localized blood insufficiency

APPLY Read the following scenario and answer the questions.

Miss Laurie Ying is a 29-year-old Asian female who was admitted to the hospital yesterday. Ann Thomas, RN, is checking on the client. The client states that when she was up walking today, she experienced pain in her legs that was so severe it made her limp. She shows the nurse an enlarged vein on her left leg. She also states that she has small reddened patches on her chest.

1. What are the medical terms related to the symptoms the patient is describing?

_____

_____

2. How do the symptoms correlate to one another and the patient's condition as a whole?

_____

_____

3. How should Nurse Thomas document this information?

_____

_____

4. Nurse Thomas doesn't know the medical term for reddened patches on the chest. What is it?

_____

_____

Did you know

Raynaud Phenomenon

Raynaud phenomenon may be an indicator of some serious connective tissue or autoimmune diseases. Most often, it is a reaction to cold or to emotional stress. Once a "trigger" starts the phenomenon, three color changes usually take place. First, the finger(s) turn absolutely white when the blood flow is blocked by the spasm; second, the finger becomes cyanotic from the slow return of blood to the site; and third, as blood fills the finger, a darker red color appears. Treatment of Raynaud, when it is not linked to another disease, is usually as simple as wearing gloves when removing items from the freezer and when going out in cold weather.

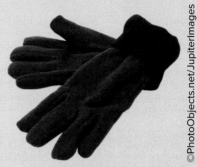

©PhotoObjects.net/JupiterImages

Coronary Artery Disease and General Heart and Lung Disease

The heart and lungs work together to provide oxygenation throughout the body. When the heart is not functioning adequately, it can cause lung disease.

Pathological	PRACTICE
	Fill in the missing term(s) to complete the following sentences.
coronary artery disease (CAD) **aortic stenosis** [ă-OR-tĭk stĕ-NŌ-sĭs] **coarctation of the aorta** [kō-ărk-TĀ-shŭn] **stenosis** [stĕ-NŌ-sĭs] **pulmonary artery stenosis**	_____ refers to any condition that reduces the nourishment the heart receives from the blood flowing through its arteries. Such diseases include _____, or narrowing of the aorta. _____ is also an abnormal narrowing of the aorta. _____ is any narrowing of a blood vessel. _____ slows the flow of blood to the lungs.
angina [ĂN-jĭ-nă, ăn-JĪ-nă] **angina pectoris** [PĔK-tōr-ĭs, pĕk-TŌR-ĭs] **myocardial infarction (MI)**	_____ or _____ (sometimes referred to as cardiac pain) can result from lack of oxygen to the heart muscle. Angina is usually categorized in degrees from class I to class IV. A person with class I angina (able to withstand prolonged exertion) will have no limits to normal activity. Severe angina (class IV) requires strict limitations on any activity except rest.
	When the heart suffers an attack that causes insufficient blood flow to the heart, or ischemia, one is said to have a *coronary* or *heart attack*. These are informal terms for a _____, a disruption in the heart's activity usually caused by blockage (a clot or plaque) of blood flow to a coronary artery. Myocardial infarctions are often classified by the location of the area to which blood flow is restricted; for example, an anterior myocardial infarction is one in which the anterior wall of the heart is affected, and a posterior MI involves the heart's posterior wall.

cardiac arrest **asystole** [ă-SĬS-tō-lē]	_____ or _____ is a sudden stopping of the heart. Such an attack can be fatal or can be a warning to make medical and lifestyle changes to ward off a further attack. Approximately 1.5 million people suffer a heart attack annually. One-third of these people do not survive. Before age 50, men are much more likely to suffer heart attacks than are women, who are thought to be protected by their production of estrogen before menopause. After menopause, the risk for women is approximately the same as for men.
endocarditis [ĔN-dō-kăr-DĪ-tĭs] **myocarditis** [MĪ-ō-kăr-DĪ-tĭs] **pericarditis** [PĔR-ĭ-kăr-DĪ-tĭs] **bacterial endocarditis**	Some diseases of the heart are specific inflammations, such as _____, _____, _____, or _____.
congestive heart failure [kŏn-JĔS-tĭv hărt FĀL-ūr] **pulmonary edema** [PŬL-mō-năr-ē ĕ-DĒ-mă]	Other conditions of the heart have to do with fluid accumulation. _____ occurs when the heart is unable to pump the necessary amount of blood. People suffering from congestive heart failure usually experience shortness of breath, edema, enlarged organs and veins, and irregular breathing patterns. _____, or accumulation of fluid in the lungs, can result from this failure.
intracardiac tumor [ĭn-tră-KĂR-dē-ăk TŪ-mŏr] **cardiomyopathy** [KĂR-dē-ō-mī-ŎP-ă-thē]	An _____ is a tumor in a heart chamber. _____ is disease of the heart muscle.

STUDY TIP

With angina, there is a lack of oxygen. Myocardial cell death occurs with a myocardial infarction.

Did you know ?

Familiar Terms for Heart Disease

Cardiovascular disease is a common ailment of middle and old age. Many familiar terms are used by laypeople to describe common cardiovascular diseases. A myocardial infarction may be called a *coronary* or a *heart attack*. Arteriosclerosis is often referred to as *hardening of the arteries*. Congestive heart failure may be called *heart failure*.

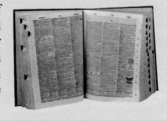

©Burke/Triolo/Brand X Pictures/Jupiterimages

PRONOUNCE and DEFINE	Pronounce the following terms aloud and write their meaning in the space.
cardiomyopathy	[KĂR-dē-ō-mī-ŎP-ă-thē]
myocarditis	[MĪ-ō-kăr-DĪ-tĭs]
asystole	[ă-SĬS-tō-lē]
aortic stenosis	[ă-ŌR-tĭk stĕ-NŌ-sĭs]
coarctation of the aorta	[kō-ărk-TĀ-shŭn]

SPELL and DEFINE	Identify if the following terms are spelled correctly. Correct the words that are spelled incorrectly. Write the definition for each word.	
	Spelling	**Definition**
micarditis		
endocarditis		
peracarditis		
angina		
carchation of aorta		

UNDERSTAND	Fill in the blanks.

1. Abnormal narrowing of the aorta is _____.
2. _____ is due to a lack of oxygen to the heart muscle.
3. Another term for *heart attack* is _____.
4. The heart condition due to excess fluid buildup is _____.
5. _____ occurs when the heart stops.

APPLY	Read the following scenario and answer the questions.

Mr. Matthew Bernard is a 31-year-old white male who presents to the ER with chest pain and the physician has assessed him. The physician tells the client's family that the client had a myocardial infarction and developed congestive heart failure and atrial fibrillation. The client's condition worsened and he experienced asystole, but after resuscitation, the client is now in normal sinus rhythm.

1. What do each of the terms break down to mean?

_____

_____

2. What is the lay term for myocardial infarction?

_____

_____

3. What is the medical term for chest pain?

_____

_____

4. How would you explain what the physician has said to the family in a manner they can understand?

_____

_____

Valve Conditions and Congenital Heart Conditions

The valves are responsible for maintaining blood flow through the heart and into the body. When valves are diseased, cardiovascular symptoms may occur.

Pathological

aortic regurgitation
[ā-OR-tĭk
rē-GŬR-jĭ-TĀ-shŭn]

aortic reflux
[ā-OR-tĭk RĒ-flŭks]

mitral stenosis
[MĪ-trăl stĕ-NŌ-sĭs]

mitral insufficiency
[MĪ-trăl in-sŭ-FISH-en-sē]

mitral reflux
[MĪ-trăl RĒ-flŭks]

mitral valve prolapse
[MĪ-trăl vălv PRŌ-lăps]

tricuspid stenosis

valvulitis
[văl-vyū-LĪ-tĭs]

rheumatic heart disease

vegetation
[vĕj-ĕ-TĀ-shŭn]

congenital heart disease
[kŏn-JĔN-Ĭ-tăl
hărt di-ZĔZ]

patent ductus arteriosus
[PĂ-tĕnt DŬK-tŭs
ăr-tēr-ē-Ō-sŭs]

septal defect
[SĔP-tăl DĔ-fekt]

tetralogy of Fallot
[te-TRAL-ō-jē fă-LŌ]

PRACTICE

Fill in the missing term(s) to complete the following sentences.

The heart valves control the flow of blood into, through, and out of the heart. Valve irregularities affecting the flow of blood can be serious. _____ or _____ is a backward flow of blood through the aortic valve. An abnormal narrowing of the opening of the mitral valve (_____) affects the opening and closing of the valve. _____ or _____ is a backward flow of blood through the mitral valve. Similarly, _____ is a backward flow of blood, but it is due to the abnormal protrusion of one or both of the mitral cusps into the left atrium. _____ is an abnormal narrowing of the opening of the tricuspid valve.

Sometimes, infections or inflammation may cause valve damage. _____ is the general term for a heart valve inflammation. _____ is damage to the heart, usually to the valves, caused by an untreated streptococcal infection. Some infections can cause a clot on a heart valve or opening (_____).

_____ results from a condition present at birth. Some common conditions are _____, a disease in which a small duct remains open at birth; _____, an abnormal opening in the septum between the atria or ventricles; and _____, actually a combination of four congenital heart abnormalities (ventricular septal defect, pulmonary stenosis, incorrect position of the aorta, and right ventricular hypertrophy) that appear together.

PRONOUNCE and DEFINE

Pronounce the following terms aloud and write their meaning in the space.

valvulitis	[văl-vyū-LĪ-tĭs]
vegetation	[vĕj-ĕ-TĀ-shŭn]
patent ductus arteriosus	[PĂ-tĕnt DŬK-tŭs ăr-tēr-ē-Ō-sĭs]

	Spelling	Definition
reumatic heart disease		
tetralogy of Fallot		
patent ductis arterisus		
valvulitis		
aortic regurgition		

Identify if the following terms are spelled correctly. Correct the words that are spelled incorrectly. Write the definition for each word.

UNDERSTAND   Fill in the blanks.

1. Backward flow of blood into the left atrium from the left ventricle is _____.
2. An inflammation of a heart valve is _____.
3. When an infection causes a clot on a heart valve, this is known as _____.
4. When the valve between the right atrium and right ventricle has an abnormal narrowing, this is known as

   _____.
5. Untreated streptoccocal infection can cause _____.

APPLY   Respond to the following:

Using medical terminology, review fetal circulation and its link to congenital heart disease.

_____
_____
_____
_____

LO 11.5 Surgical Terms

Cardiovascular surgery is performed on the heart and/or cardiac vessels. This type of surgery may be done to treat a variety of disorders, including blockages within the cardiac vessels and disorders of the heart valves. Figure 11-16 illustrates angioplasty. Figure 11-17 shows a cardiac stent. Figure 11-18 shows a heart transplant procedure.

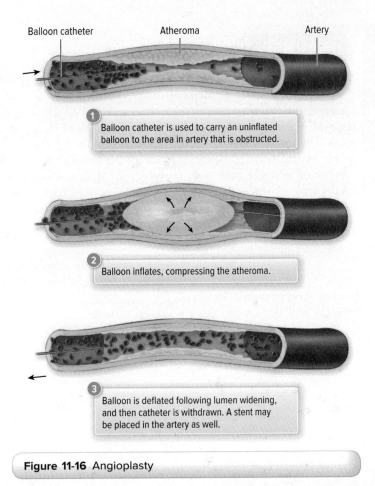

① Balloon catheter is used to carry an uninflated balloon to the area in artery that is obstructed.

Balloon catheter   Atheroma   Artery

② Balloon inflates, compressing the atheroma.

③ Balloon is deflated following lumen widening, and then catheter is withdrawn. A stent may be placed in the artery as well.

Figure 11-16 Angioplasty

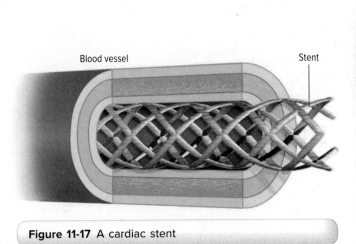

Blood vessel   Stent

Figure 11-17 A cardiac stent

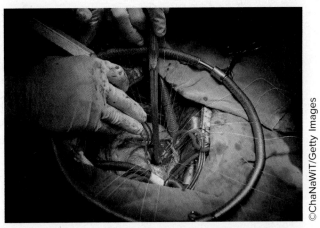

Figure 11-18 Heart transplant

STUDY TIP

Practice saying words aloud with a classmate.

Surgical	**PRACTICE** Fill in the missing term(s) to complete the following sentences.
	Cardiovascular surgery usually involves opening up or repairing blood vessels or valves; removal, repair, or replacement of diseased portions of blood vessels; or bypass of blocked areas. The goal of most cardiovascular surgery is to improve blood flow, thereby allowing proper oxygenation and nourishment of all the cells of the body. Many types of heart surgery are now *minimally invasive procedures*. Most heart operations require opening up the chest to access the heart. However, devices such as lasers, robotic devices, and miniature surgical instruments now allow surgeons to perform certain procedures through a "keyhole," a small opening in the chest.
balloon catheter dilation **percutaneous** **transluminal coronary** **angioplasty** [pĕr-kyū-TĀ-nē-ŭs trăns-LŪ-mĭn-ăl KŌR-ō-năr-ē ĂN-jē-ō-plăs-tē] **(PTCA)** **balloon valvuloplasty** [VĂL-vyū-lō-PLĂS-tē] **angioplasty** [ĂN-jē-ō-plăs-tē] **coronary angioplasty**	A balloon catheter is used in _____ (also called _____ or _____) to open the passageway inside a blood vessel so that blood can flow freely. A _____ involves the use of a balloon catheter to open narrowed cardiac valve openings. Similarly, _____ or _____ is the opening of a blood vessel using a balloon catheter.
	Catheterization is a diagnostic invasive procedure that involves threading a catheter through an artery or vein into the heart to observe blood flow. It is the most common type of procedure performed in the United States.
cardiac angioscopy [KĂR-dē-ăk ăn-jē-ŎS-kō-pē]	_____ uses a fiberoptic catheter to view the interior of a blood vessel.
endovascular surgery [ĕn-dō-VĂS-kyū-lăr SER-jer-ē] **stent** [stĕnt] **intravascular stent** [ĭn-tră-VĂS-kyū-lăr stĕnt]	Surgery that involves the use of cardiac catheterization is called _____. During surgery, a _____ or an _____ may be inserted to hold a blood vessel passageway open. Many stents are now *drug-eluting* stents, meaning that they include slowly released medication that helps to maintain the open passageways. Such procedures also help to break up blockages.
bypass [BĪ-pas] **coronary bypass surgery** **coronary artery bypass** **graft (CABG)** **graft**	Sometimes it becomes necessary to create a detour or a _____ around blockages. _____ or _____ is performed to attach the vessel to be used for the bypass. A _____, particularly of a blood vessel from another part of the body, can be used to bypass an arterial blockage. Saphenous (leg) veins or mammary (chest) arteries are two types of vessels used for this procedure. The number of arteries that are bypassed determines whether a CABG is a triple bypass (when three arteries are bypassed), a quadruple (four-artery) bypass, and so on.
cardiopulmonary bypass [KĂR-dē-ō-PŬL-mŏ-năr-ē BĪ-pas]	Sometimes it is necessary to divert blood flow from the heart during surgery. This procedure, _____ (also called *extracorporeal circulation*), circulates the blood through a heart–lung machine and back into systemic circulation.

heart transplant **valve replacement** **thrombectomy** [thrŏm-BĔK-tō-mē] **embolectomy** [ĕm-bō-LĔK-tō-mē] **atherectomy** [ăth-ĕ-RĔK-tō-mē] **hemorrhoidectomy** [HĔM-ō-roy-DĔK-tō-mē]	Surgical removal and replacement of the entire heart is called a _____. _____ is the removal and replacement of a heart valve. Surgical removal of a thrombus is a _____; of an embolus, an _____; of an atheroma, an _____; and of hemorrhoids, a _____.
endarterectomy [ĕnd-ăr-tēr-ĔK-tō-mē] **arteriotomy** [ăr-tēr-ē-ŏT-ō-mē] **valvotomy** [văl-VŎT-ō-mē]	An _____ removes the diseased lining of an artery; an _____ is an incision into an artery to remove a clot. A _____ is the incision into a cardiac valve to remove an obstruction.
venipuncture [VĔN-ĭ-pŭnk-chŭr, VĒ-nĭ-pŭnk-chŭr] **phlebotomy** [flĕ-BŎT-ō-mē]	_____ is a small puncture of the skin made for the purpose of drawing blood (_____).
valvuloplasty [VĂL-vyū-lō-PLĂS-tē] **anastomosis** [ă-năs-tō-MŌ-sĭs]	Some surgeries are for reconstruction or repair—a _____ is done to reconstruct a cardiac valve. Other surgical procedures, such as _____, are performed to connect blood vessels and to implant devices, such as *pacemakers,* that help regulate body functions. Pacemakers are small computers that provide electrical stimulation to regulate the heart rate. They can be attached temporarily (usually with a small box worn outside the body and a sensor attached to the outside of the chest) or permanently (the lead is surgically inserted into a blood vessel leading to the heart).

PRONOUNCE and DEFINE	Pronounce the following terms aloud and write their meaning in the space.
valvuloplasty	[VĂL-vyū-lō-PLĂS-tē]
anastomosis	[ă-năs-tō-MŌ-sĭs]
endarterectomy	[ĕnd-ăr-tēr-ĔK-tō-mē]
embolectomy	[ĕm-bō-LĔK-tō-mē]
angioplasty	[ĂN-jē-ō-plăs-tē]
cardiopulmonary bypass	[KĂR-dē-ō-PŬL-mŏ-nār-ē BĪ-pas]

SPELL and DEFINE	Identify if the following terms are spelled correctly. Correct the words that are spelled incorrectly. Write the definition for each word.	
	Spelling	**Definition**
thromboctomy		
atherectomy		
arteritomy		
angiascopy		
hemorrhoidectomy		

UNDERSTAND   Define each term in the space provided.

1. anastomosis:

2. valvuloplasty:

3. valvotomy:

4. embolectomy:

5. angioplasty:

APPLY   Read the following scenario and answer the questions.

After the physician used a catheter to visualize the arteries in the heart, he tells the nurse that the client has a fatty deposit on the lining of a coronary artery. The physician wants to insert a balloon catheter into the vessel so that the client can experience increased blood oxygenation.

1. What did the client have done initially?

2. What does the client have in his arteries?

3. What is the procedure the physician wants to perform?

Did you know

Surgical Devices

New surgical devices are being developed all the time. The Da Vinci System is a robotic device that uses a tiny camera with multiple lenses inserted into the client's chest, providing a three-dimensional image of the heart. The surgeon, at a nearby computer workstation, watches through a viewer to see inside the chest as a pair of joysticks control two robotic arms. The arms hold specially designed surgical instruments that mimic the actual movement of the surgeon's hands on the joysticks. This allows for a minimal incision into the client.

LO 11.6 Common Pharmacological Terms and the Cardiovascular System

Medications may be used to treat cardiovascular diseases and symptoms. Many cardiovascular medications may treat more than one cardiovascular disorder. Drug therapy for the cardiovascular system generally treats the following conditions: angina, heart attack, high blood pressure, high cholesterol, congestive heart failure, rhythm disorders, and vascular problems.

Pharmacological	PRACTICE Fill in the missing term(s) to complete the following sentences.
antianginals [ăn-tē-ĂN-jĭ-nălz]	_____ relieve the pain and prevent attacks of angina.
thrombolytics [thrŏm-bō-LĬT-ĭks]	_____ are used to dissolve blood clots in heart attack victims.
antihypertensives [ĂN-tē-hī-per-TEN-sivz] **vasodilators** [VĀ-sō-dī-LĀ-tŏrz] **diuretics** [dī-yū-RĔT-ĭks]	High blood pressure may require treatment with one drug or a combination of drugs. Such drugs are called _____. _____ relax the walls of the blood vessels to regulate blood pressure. Other treatments for high blood pressure include _____, which are used to relieve edema (swelling) and increase kidney function.
cardiotonics [KĂR-dē-ō-TŎN-ĭks] **vasoconstrictors** [VĀ-sō-kŏn-STRĬK-tŏrz]	Congestive heart failure is treated with antihypertensives, diuretics, and _____, which increase myocardial contractions. In certain situations, _____ may be needed to narrow blood vessels.
antiarrhythmics [ăn-tē-ā-RĬTH-mĭks]	Rhythm disorders are treated with a number of medications (some are called _____) that normalize heart rate by affecting the nervous system, which controls the heart rate.
lipid-lowering	Cholesterol is a substance the body needs in certain quantities. Excesses of certain kinds of cholesterol such as LDL can cause fatty deposits or plaque to form on blood vessels. _____ drugs work in various ways (some of which are not understood) to help the body excrete unwanted cholesterol. Blood clotting in vessels can cause dangerous blockages.

continued on next page

PRACTICE

Provide the missing term(s) to complete the following sentences.

anticoagulant
[ĂN-tē-kō-ĂG-yū-lĕnt]

_____, anticlotting, and antiplatelet medications inhibit the ability of the blood to clot. Other medications used for vascular problems may include drugs that decrease the thickness of blood or drugs that increase the amount of blood the heart is able to pump.

PRONOUNCE and DEFINE

Pronounce the following terms aloud and write their meaning in the space.

antiarrhythmics	[ăn-tē-ā-RĬTH-mĭks]
cardiotonics	[KĂR-dē-ō-TŎN-ĭks]
vasoconstrictors	[VĀ-sō-kŏn-STRĬK-tŏrz]
antianginals	[ăn-tē-ĂN-jĭ-nălz]
diuretics	[dī-yū-RĔT-ĭks]

SPELL and DEFINE

Identify if the following terms are spelled correctly. Correct the words that are spelled incorrectly. Write the definition for each word.

	Spelling	Definition
anticoadulant		
thrombolitics		
antiarrhymics		
diuretics		
antianjinals		

UNDERSTAND

Name at least one classification of medication used to treat each of the following conditions.

1. hypertension: _____
2. water retention: _____
3. arrhythmia: _____
4. high cholesterol: _____
5. clotting: _____

APPLY

Read the following scenario and answer the questions.

Mr. Jones has a history of kidney disease. His blood pressure currently is 182/96. Is this blood pressure acceptable? If not, what type of medication might be prescribed for Mr. Jones? What might be the cause of Mr. Jones's high blood pressure?

_____

_____

_____

_____

Abbreviations

REVIEW

Abbreviations	Definition
AV	atrioventricular
BP	blood pressure
CABG	coronary artery bypass graft
CAD	coronary artery disease
CO	cardiac output
CPK	creatine phosphokinase
ECG, EKG	electrocardiogram
HDL	high-density lipoprotein
LDH	lactate dehydrogenase
LDL	low-density lipoprotein
MI	myocardial infarction
MRI	magnetic resonance imaging
PAC	premature atrial contractions
PTCA	percutaneous transluminal coronary angioplasty
PVC	premature ventricular contractions
SA	sinoatrial
SV	stroke volume
VHDL	very high-density lipoprotein
VLDL	very low-density lipoprotein

UNDERSTAND — Match the abbreviation with its definition

1. _____ CAD
2. _____ SA
3. _____ HTN
4. _____ VLDL
5. _____ HDL
6. _____ PAC
7. _____ CPK
8. _____ EKG
9. _____ PTCA
10. _____ CABG

a. coronary artery bypass graft
b. sinoatrial
c. electrocardiogram
d. coronary artery disease
e. hypertension
f. creatine phosphokinase
g. premature atrial contraction
h. high-density lipoprotein
i. percutaneous transluminal coronary angioplasty
j. very low-density lipoprotein

The patient experienced left-sided chest pain. Electrocardiogram identified patient was having a heart attack. Creatine phosphokinase, lactate dehydrogenase, and troponin were indicative of a heart attack. Patient has a history of hypertension and coronary heart disease, with a percutaneous transluminal coronary angioplasty in the past.

_____

_____

_____

CHAPTER SUMMARY

	Learning Outcome	Summary
11.1	Identify and discuss the structure and function of the cardiovascular system.	The function of the cardiovascular system is to deliver blood to tissues within the body. This serves to provide the body with oxygen and nutrients and removes waste materials and carbon dioxide. The heart is the organ that pumps blood throughout the cardiovascular system.
11.2	Define combining forms used in building words that relate to the cardiovascular system.	Word building requires knowledge of the combining form and meaning.
11.3	Summarize common diagnostic tests, laboratory tests, and clinical procedures used in testing and treating disorders of the cardiovascular system.	Diagnostic, procedural, and laboratory findings assist the health care provider in diagnosing medical conditions. Often used in combination, these tests lead to a final diagnosis and assist in treatment planning.
11.4	Define the major pathological terms of the cardiovascular system.	Pathological conditions of the cardiovascular system may affect cardiac rhythm, blood pressure, blood vessels, and coronary arteries and may cause heart and lung disease.
11.5	Define surgical terms related to the cardiovascular system.	Cardiovascular surgery may be performed to treat a variety of disorders, including blockages within the cardiac vessels and disorders of the heart valves.
11.6	Recognize common pharmacological agents used to treat disorders of the cardiovascular system.	Medications may be used to treat cardiovascular diseases and symptoms. Many cardiovascular medications may treat more than one cardiovascular disorder. Drug therapy for the cardiovascular system generally treats the following conditions: angina, heart attack, high blood pressure, high cholesterol, congestive heart failure, rhythm disorders, and vascular problems.
11.7	Identify common abbreviations associated with the cardiovascular system.	Abbreviations are used to describe diseases, conditions, procedures, and treatments associated with the cardiovascular system.

1. Label the parts of the heart using the image provided.

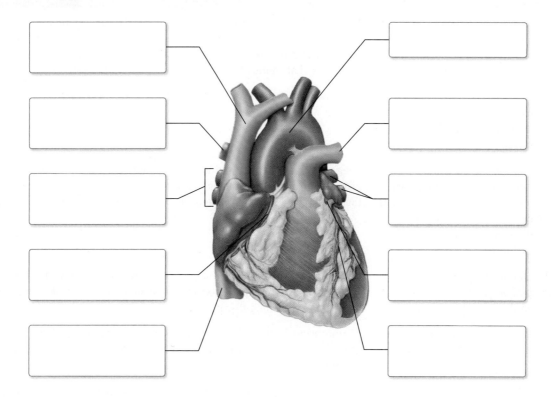

2. Beginning with the lungs and including all valves, identify blood flows into the heart, out to the body, and returned to the heart. Use Figure 11-1 as your guide.

_____

_____

_____

3. Describe how an impulse is conducted through the heart.

_____

_____

_____

Pronounce the following cardiovascular terms aloud and write their meaning in the space.

angiocardiography

cardiomyopathy

patent ductus arteriosus

venule

endocardium

ductus arteriosus

cardiologist

thrombus

sonography

necrosis

Identify if the following terms are spelled correctly. Correct the words that are spelled incorrectly. Write the definition for each word.

	Spelling	Definition
angeografy		
angioscopy		
cardiopulmonary		
ductus venosis		
disrhythmia		
ekhocardiography		
ventrikle		
systole		
indothelum		
tachycardia		

Identify the term that fits each definition. Each term must contain at least one of the combining forms from the previous section. You also may refer to Chapters 1, 2, and 3.

1. Enlargement of the heart: _____
2. Relating to the heart and lungs: _____
3. Establishing an opening into the pericardium: _____
4. Inflammation of the endocardium: _____
5. Repair of a vein: _____
6. Paralysis of a blood vessel: _____
7. Connecting blood vessels: _____

Fill in the Blanks: Complete the sentences by filling in the blanks.

1. A vessel that carries oxygenated blood is a(n) _____.
2. Deoxygenated blood flows through the _____.
3. The innermost layer of heart tissue is called the _____.
4. The two atrioventricular valves control the flow of blood between the _____ and the _____.
5. Carbon dioxide is carried back to the heart via the _____.
6. Three lifestyle factors that may result in high blood pressure are _____, _____, and _____.
7. The fetal circulatory system does not include _____ circulation.
8. The lining of the arteries that secretes substances into the blood is called the _____.
9. Pulmonary circulation is the flow of blood between the _____ and _____.
10. The head and neck receive oxygen-rich blood via the _____.

DECONSTRUCT

The client comes to the physician's office complaining of shortness of breath. He states he has a history of fluid in his lungs and he takes a "water pill" every day. Both legs are swollen. His blood pressure is 168/98 and his pulse is 144 beats per minute. Upon listening to his heart with a stethoscope, a third heart sound is noted. Discuss all of this information with the physician using correct medical terminology.

_____

_____

_____

_____

Reviewing the Terms

Pronounce each of the following terms. Write the definitions on a separate sheet of paper. This review will take you through all the words you learned in this chapter. If you have difficulty with any words, make a flash card for later study. Refer to the English-Spanish and Spanish-English glossaries in the eBook.

anastomosis [ă-năs-tō-MŌ-sĭs]

aneurysm [ĂN-yū-rĭzm]

angi/o [ĂN-jē-ō]

angina [ĂN-jĭ-nă, ăn-JĪ-nă]

angina pectoris [PĔK-tōr-ĭs, pĕk-TŌR-ĭs]

angiocardiography [ăn-jē-ō-kăr-dē-ŎG-ră-fē]

angiography [ăn-jē-ŎG-ră-fē]

angioplasty [ĂN-jē-ō-plăs-tē]

angioscopy [ăn-jē-ŎS-kō-pē]

angiotensin [ăn-jē-ō-TĔN-sĭn] **converting enzyme (ACE) inhibitor**

antianginal [ăn-tē-ĂN-jĭ-năl]

antiarrhythmic [ăn-tē-ă-RĬTH-mĭk]

anticlotting

anticoagulant [ĂN-tē-kō-ĂG-yū-lĕnt]

antihypertensive [ĂN-tē-hī-per-TEN-siv]

aort/o [ā-ŌR-tō]

aorta [ā-ŌR-t ă]

aortic [ā-ŌR-tĭk] **valve**

aortic regurgitation [rē-GŬR-jĭ-TĀ-shŭn] **or reflux** [RĒ-flŭks]

aortic stenosis [stĕ-NŌ-sĭs]

aortography [ā-ŏr-TŎG-ră-fē]

arrhythmia [ā-RĬTH-mē-ă]

arter/o [ăr-tĕr-Ō]

arteri/o [ăr-TĒR-ē-ō]

arteriography [ăr-tĕr-ē-ŎG-ră-fē]

arteriole [ăr-TĒ-rē-ōl]

arteriosclerosis [ăr-TĒR-ē-ō-sklĕr-Ō-sĭs]

arteriotomy [ăr-tĕr-ē-ŎT-ō-mē]

arteritis [ăr-tĕr-Ī-tĭs]

artery [ĂR-tĕr-ē]

asystole [ă-SĬS-tō-lē]

ather/o [ĂTH-ĕr-ō]

atherectomy [ăth-ĕ-RĔK-tō-mē]

atheroma [ăth-ĕr-Ō-mă]

atherosclerosis [ĂTH-ĕr-ō-sklĕr-Ō-sĭs]

atri/o [Ā-trē-ō]

atrial fibrillation [Ā-trē-ăl fĭ-brĭ-LĀ-shŭn]

atrioventricular [Ā-trē-ō-vĕn-TRĬK-yū-lăr] (AV) node

atrioventricular block [Ā-trē-ō-vĕn-TRĬK-yū-lăr blok]

atrioventricular [Ā-trē-ō-vĕn-TRĬK-yū-lăr] bundle

atrioventricular [Ā-trē-ō-vĕn-TRĬK-yū-lăr] valve

atrium (pl., atria) [Ā-trē-ŭm (Ā-trē-ă)]

auscultation [ăws-kŭl-TĀ-shŭn]

bacterial endocarditis [EN-dō-car-DĪ-tĭs]

balloon catheter dilation

balloon valvuloplasty [VĂL-vyū-lō-PLĂS-tē]

beta [BĀ-tă] blocker

bicuspid [bĭ-KŬS-pĭd] valve

blood [blŭd]

blood pressure

blood vessel

bradycardia [brăd-ē-KĂR-dē-ă]

bruit [brū-Ē]

bundle of His [hĭz, hĭs]

bypass [BĪ-pas]

calcium channel blocker

capillary [KĂP-ĭ-lār-ē]

carbon dioxide, CO$_2$

cardi/o [KĂR-dē-ō]

cardiac arrest

cardiac catheterization [kăth-ĕ-tĕr-ĭ-ZĀ-shŭn]

cardiac cycle

cardiac enzyme tests/studies

cardiac MRI

cardiac scan

cardiac tamponade [tăm-pō-NĀD]

cardiologist [KĂR-dē-ŎL-ō-jĭst]

cardiomyopathy [KĂR-dē-ō-mī-ŎP-ă-thē]

cardiopulmonary [KĂR-dē-ō-PŬL-mŏ-nār-ē] bypass

cardiotonic [KĂR-dē-ō-TŎN-ĭk]

cardiovascular [KĂR-dē-ō-VĂS-kyū-lĕr]

carotid [kă-RŎT-ĭd] artery

cholesterol [kō-LĔS-tĕr-ōl]

claudication [klăw-dĭ-KĀ-shŭn]

coarctation [kō-ărk-TĀ-shŭn] of the aorta

conduction system

congenital [kŏn-JĔN-Ĭ-tăl] heart disease

congestive [kŏn-JĔS-tĭv] heart failure

constriction [kŏn-STRĬK-shŭn]

coronary [KŌR-ō-nār-ē] artery

coronary angioplasty [ĂN-jē-ō-plăs-tē]

coronary artery bypass graft (CABG)

coronary artery disease (CAD)

coronary bypass surgery

cyanosis [sī-ă-NŌ-sĭs]

deep vein thrombosis [thrŏm-BŌ-sĭs]

depolarization [dē-pō-lă-rĭ-ZĀ-shŭn]

diastole [dī-ĂS-tō-lē]

digital subtraction angiography (DSA)

diuretic [dī-yū-RĔT-ĭk]

Doppler ultrasound [DŎP-lĕr ŬL-tră-sownd]

ductus arteriosus [DŬK-tŭs ăr-tēr-ē-Ō-sŭs]

ductus venosus [vĕn-Ō-sŭs]

dysrhythmia [dĭs-RĬTH-mē-ă]

echocardiogram [ĕk-ō-KĂR-dē-ō-grăm]

echocardiography [ĔK-ō-kăr-dē-ŎG-ră-fē]

ejection fraction

electrocardiography [ē-lĕk-trō-kăr-dē-ŎG-ră-fē]

embolectomy [ĕm-bō-LĔK-tō-mē]

embolus [ĔM-bō-lŭs]

endarterectomy [ĕnd-ăr-tēr-ĔK-tō-mē]

endocarditis [ĔN-dō-kăr-DĪ-tĭs]

endocardium [ĕn-dō-KĂR-dē-ŭm]

endothelium [ĕn-dō-THĒ-lē-ŭm]

endovascular [ĕn-dō-VĂS-kyū-lăr] surgery

epicardium [ĕp-ĭ-KĂR-dē-ŭm]

essential hypertension

femoral [FĔM-Ŏ-răl, FĒ-mŏ-r ăl] artery

fibrillation [fĭ-brĭ-LĀ-shŭn]

flutter

foramen ovale [fō-RĀ-mĕn ō-VĂ-lē]

gallop

graft

heart [hărt]

heart block

heart transplant

hemangi/o [hĕ-MĂN-jē-ō]

hemorrhoidectomy [HĔM-ō-roy-DĔK-tō-mē]

hemorrhoids [HĔM-ō-roydz]

heparin [HĔP-ă-rĭn]

high blood pressure

Holter [HŌL-tĕr] monitor

hypertension [HĪ-pĕr-TĔN-shŭn]

hypertensive heart disease

hypotension [HĪ-pō-TĔN-sŭn]

infarct [ĬN-fărkt]

infarction [ĭn-FĂRK-shŭn]

inferior vena cava [VĒ-nă KĂ-vă, KĀ-vă]

intermittent claudication

intracardiac [ĭn-tră-KĂR-dē-ăk] tumor

intravascular stent [ĭn-tră-VĂS-kyū-lăr stĕnt]

ischemia [ĭs-KĒ-mē-ă]

left atrium [Ā-trē-ŭm]

left ventricle [VĔN-trĭ-kl]

lipid [LĬP-ĭd] profile

lipid-lowering

low blood pressure

lumen [LŪ-mĕn]

mitral [MĪ-trăl] insufficiency or reflux

mitral stenosis [MĪ-trăl stĕ-NŌ-sĭs]

mitral [MĪ-trăl] valve

mitral valve prolapse [PRŌ-lăps]

multiple-gated acquisition (MUGA) angiography

murmur

myocardial infarction (MI)

myocarditis [MĪ-ō-kăr-DĪ-tĭs]

myocardium [mī-ō-KĂR-dē-ŭm]

necrosis [nĕ-KRŌ-sĭs]

nitrate [NĪ-trāt]

occlusion [Ŏ-KLŪ-zhŭn]

pacemaker

palpitations [păl-pĭ-TĀ-shŭnz]

patent ductus arteriosus [PĀ-tĕnt DŬK-tŭs ăr-tēr-ē-Ō-sŭs]

percutaneous transluminal [pĕr-kyū-TĀ-nē-ŭs trăns-LŪ-mĭn-ăl] coronary angioplasty (PTCA)

perfusion deficit

pericardi/o [PĔR-ĭ-KĂR-dē-ō]

pericarditis [PĔR-ĭ-kăr-DĪ-tĭs]

pericardium [pĕr-ĭ-KĂR-dē-ŭm]

peripheral vascular disease

petechiae (sing., petechia) [pĕ-TĒ-kē-ē, pē-TĔK-ē-ē, (pĕ-TĒ-kē-ă, pē-TĔK-ē-ă)]

phleb/o [FLĔB-ō]

phlebitis [flĕ-BĪ-tĭs]

phlebography [flĕ-BŎG-ră-fē]

phlebotomy [flĕ-BŎT-ō-mē]

plaque [plăk]

polarization [pō-lăr-ĭ-ZĀ-shŭn]

popliteal [pŏp-LĬT-ē-ăl] artery

positron emission tomography [tō-MŎG-ră-f ē] (PET) scan

premature atrial contractions (PACs)

premature ventricular contractions (PVCs)

pulmonary [PŬL-mō-nār-ē] artery

pulmonary artery stenosis

pulmonary edema [ĕ-DĒ-mă]

pulmonary valve

pulmonary vein

pulse [pŭls]

Purkinje fibers [per-KĬN-jē FĪ-berz]

Raynaud [rā-NŌ] phenomenon

repolarization [rē-pō-lăr-ĭ-ZĀ-shŭn]

rheumatic heart disease

right atrium [Ā-trē-ŭm]

right ventricle [VĔN-trĭ-kl]

risk factor

rub

saphenous [să-FĒ-nŭs] veins

secondary hypertension

semilunar [sĕm-ē-LŪ-năr] valve

septal [SĔP-tăl] defect

septum (pl., septa) [SĔP-tŭm (SĔP-tă)]

serum enzyme tests

sinoatrial [sī-nō-Ā-trē-ăl] (SA) node

sinus rhythm

sonography [sō-NŎG-ră-fē]

sphygm/o [SFĬG-mō]

sphygmomanometer [SFĬG-mō-mă-NŎM-ĕ-tĕr]

statins [STĂ-tĭnz]

stenosis [stĕ-NŌ-sĭs]

stent [stĕnt]

stress test

superior vena cava [VĒ-nă KĂ-vă, KĀ-vă]

systole [SĬS-tō-lē]

tachycardia [TĂK-ĭ-KĂR-dē-ă]

tetralogy [te-TRAL-ō-jē] of Fallot [fă-LŌ]

thromb/o [THRŎM-bō]

thrombectomy [thrŏm-BĔK-tō-mē]

thrombolytic [thrŏm-bō-LĬT-ĭk]

thrombophlebitis [THRŎM-bō-flĕ-BĪ-tĭs]

thrombosis [thrŏm-BŌ-sĭs]

thrombotic [thrŏm-BŎT-ĭk] occlusion

thrombus [THRŎM-bŭs]

tricuspid stenosis [trī-KŬS-pĭd stĕ-NŌ-sĭs]

tricuspid [trī-KŬS-pĭd] valve

triglyceride [trī-GLĬS-ĕr-īd]

valve [vălv]

valve replacement

valvotomy [văl-VŎT-ō-mē]

valvulitis [văl-vyū-LĪ-tĭs]

valvuloplasty [VĂL-vyū-lō-PLĂS-tē]

varicose [VĂR-ĭ-kōs] vein

vas/o [VĀ-sō]

vasoconstrictor [VĀ-sō-kŏn-STRĬK-tŏr]

vasodilator [VĀ-sō-dī-LĀ-tŏr]

vegetation [vĕj-ĕ-TĀ-shŭn]

vein [vān]

ven/o [VĒ-nō]

vena cava (*pl.*, venae cavae) [VĒ-nă KĂ-vă, KĀ-vă (VĒ-nē KĂ-vē, KĀ-vē)]

venipuncture [VĔN-ĭ-pŭnk-chŭr, VĒ-nĭ-pŭnk-chŭr]

venography [vē-NŎG-ră-fē]

ventricle [VĔN-trĭ-kl]

ventriculogram [vĕn-TRĬK-yū-lō-grăm]

venule [VĔN-yūl, VĒ-nūl]

The Respiratory System

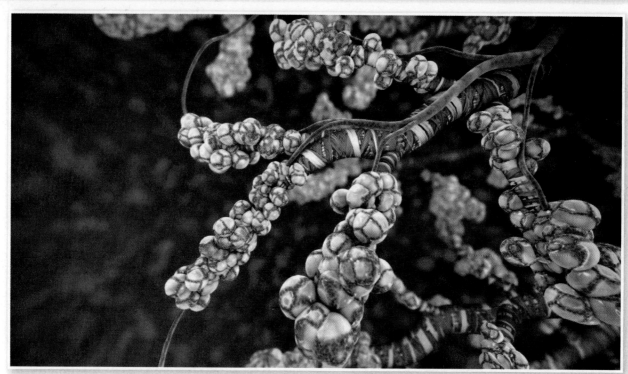

Learning Outcomes

After studying this chapter, you will be able to:

12.1 Identify the parts of the respiratory system and discuss the function of each part.

12.2 Recognize the major word parts used in building words that relate to the respiratory system.

12.3 Identify common diagnostic tests, laboratory tests, and clinical procedures used in testing and treating disorders of the respiratory system.

12.4 Define the major pathological conditions of the respiratory system.

12.5 Explain the meaning of surgical terms related to the respiratory system.

12.6 Recognize common pharmacological agents used in treating disorders of the respiratory system.

12.7 Identify common abbreviations associated with the respiratory system.

LO 12.1 Structure and Function of the Respiratory System

The **respiratory system** is the body's system for breathing. The respiratory system consists of the upper and lower tracts. Its primary function involves the exchange of oxygen and carbon dioxide between the atmosphere, the body, and its cells. Figure 12-1 shows the upper and lower respiratory tracts. Figure 12-2 shows the structure of the lungs.

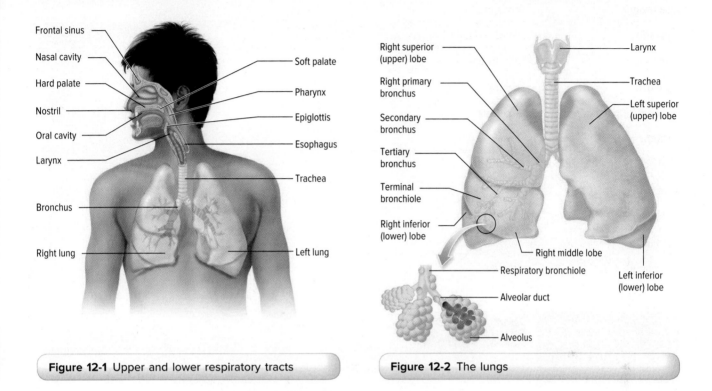

Figure 12-1 Upper and lower respiratory tracts

Figure 12-2 The lungs

Building Your Respiratory Vocabulary

The following sections provide an introduction to basic respiratory combining terms and their meanings. Review this information prior to moving to the practices.

Combining Form	Meaning
adenoid/o	adenoid
alveol/o	alveolus
bronch/o, bronchi/o	bronchus
bronchiol/o	bronchiole
capn/o	carbon dioxide
epiglott/o	epiglottis
laryng/o	larynx
lob/o	lobe of the lung
mediastin/o	mediastinum
nas/o	nose

continued on next page

Combining Form	Meaning
or/o	mouth
ox/o, oxi-, oxy-	oxygen
pharyng/o	pharynx
phon/o	voice, sound
phren/o	diaphragm
pleur/o	pleura
pneum/o, pneumon/o	air, lung
rhin/o	nose
spir/o	breathing
steth/o	chest
thorac/o	thorax, chest
tonsill/o	tonsils
trache/o	trachea

Structure and Function

PRACTICE

Provide the missing term(s) to complete the following sentences.

respiratory system [RĔS-pĭ-ră-tōr-ē, rĕ-SPĪR-ă-tōr-ē]	The _____ is the body's breathing system.
external respiration	_____, breathing or exchanging air between the body and the outside environment, is accomplished within the structures of the respiratory system. In this type of respiration, air from the atmosphere is inhaled and, later, carbon dioxide is exhaled.
internal respiration	Another type of respiration, _____, the bringing of oxygen to the cells and removing carbon dioxide from them, happens in the circulation of blood throughout the body. The carbon dioxide is removed from the body during exhalation.
lungs [lŭngz] respiratory tract	The respiratory system includes the _____ (organs where oxygenation of blood takes place), the _____ (passageways through which air moves in and out of the lungs), and the muscles that move air into and out of the lungs.

PRONOUNCE and DEFINE

Pronounce the following terms aloud and write their meaning in the space provided.

respiratory	[RĔS-pĭ-ră-tōr-ē, rĕ-SPĪR-ă-tōr-ē]
lungs	[lŭngz]

Match each term on the left to its description on the right.

1. _____ lungs
2. _____ internal respiration
3. _____ external respiration
4. _____ respiratory tract

a. Air between the body and environment are exchanged
b. The passageway for air
c. Oxygenation occurs
d. Oxygen is exchanged for carbon dioxide

APPLY **Read the following scenario and respond accordingly.**

You have been asked to teach a group of elementary children how oxygenation occurs. Explain it in a way that they can understand.

_____

_____

_____

From the Perspective Of . . .

Who: Clinical Certified Medical Assistant [CMA (AAMA)]

Other Aliases: Medical Office Assistant, Clinical Assistant, Back Office Assistant, Patient Care Assistant

Job Duties: Greeting patients; escorting patients to the exam area; obtaining vital signs, height, weight; documenting chief complaint; assisting with the examination; relaying instructions; scheduling tests; relaying results (per provider orders).

That is why medical terminology is important to me.

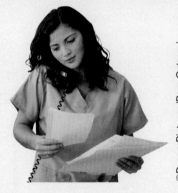

©DreamPictures/Pam Ostrow/Blend Images LLC

STUDY TIP

Remember, breathing is an involuntary process.

The Respiratory Tract

The respiratory system is divided into the upper and lower tracts. The upper respiratory tract includes the nose, nasal cavity, sinuses, and pharynx. The lower respiratory tract includes the larynx, trachea, bronchial tree, and lungs. Both the upper and lower respiratory tracts assist in the exchange of gases. Figure 12-3 illustrates open and closed vocal cords. Figures 12-4 and 12-5 provide details of the bronchioles and alveoli.

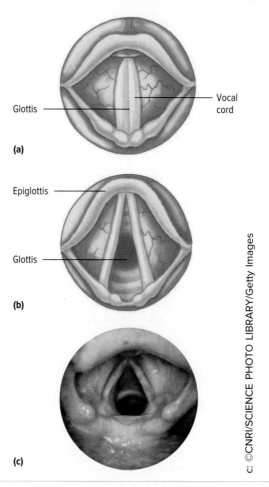

Glottis — Vocal cord

(a)

Epiglottis —

Glottis —

(b)

(c)

c: ©CNRI/SCIENCE PHOTO LIBRARY/Getty Images

Figure 12-3 Open and closed vocal cords. The vocal chords as viewed from above with the glottis (a) closed and (b) open. (c) Photograph of the glottis and vocal chords.

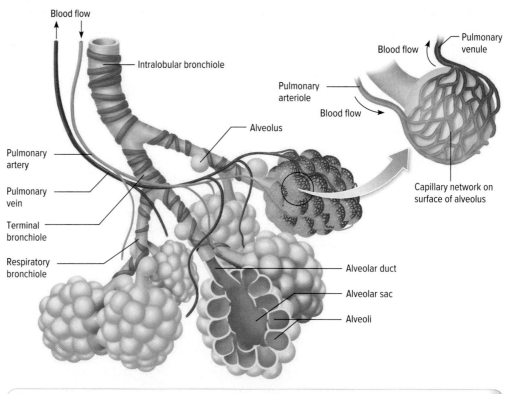

Blood flow

Intralobular bronchiole

Pulmonary artery

Pulmonary vein

Terminal bronchiole

Respiratory bronchiole

Alveolus

Blood flow — Pulmonary venule

Pulmonary arteriole

Blood flow

Capillary network on surface of alveolus

Alveolar duct

Alveolar sac

Alveoli

Figure 12-4 Bronchioles and alveoli

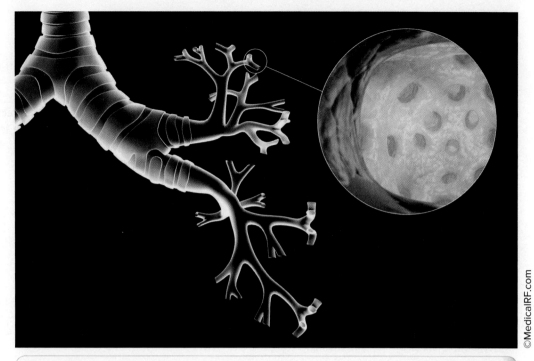

©MedicalRF.com

Figure 12-5 The bronchiole tree

PRACTICE

Provide the missing term(s) to complete the following sentences.

The respiratory tract is also known as the *airway,* the route through which air enters the lungs and the route via which air exits the body.

inspiration
[ĭn-spĭ-RĀ-shŭn]
inhalation
[ĭn-hă-LĀ-shŭn]
nose
[nōz]
nostrils
[NŎS-trĭlz]
external nares
[ĕks-TER-năl NĀR-ēz]
nasal septum
[NĀ-zăl SĔP-tŭm]
nasal cavity
[NĀ-zăl KĂV-ĭ-tē]
cilia
[SĬL-ē-ă]

_____ (breathing in or _____) brings air from the outside environment into the _____ or mouth. The nose has three functions: to warm, filter, and moisten the air. The _____ (also called _____) are the two external openings at the base of the external portion of the nose. The external nose is supported by the nasal bones and is divided into two halves by the _____, a strip of cartilage. After air enters the nose, it passes into the _____, where it is warmed by blood in the mucous membranes that line these areas. _____ (hairs) in the nasal cavity filter out foreign bodies.

continued on next page

pharynx [FĂR-ĭngks] **throat** [thrōt] **nasopharynx** [NĀ-zō-FĂR-ĭngks] **soft palate** [sŏft PĂL-ăt] **pharyngeal tonsils** [fă-RĬN-jē-ăl TŎN-sĭlz] **adenoids** [ĂD-ĕ-noydz]	Next, the air reaches the _____ (_____), which is a passageway for both air and food. The pharynx is divided into three sections. The _____ lies above the _____, which is a flexible muscular sheet that separates the nasopharynx from the rest of the pharynx. The nasopharynx contains the _____, more commonly known as the _____, which aid in the body's immune defense.
oropharynx [ŌR-ō-FĂR-ĭngks] **palatine tonsils** [PĂL-ă-tīn TŎN-sĭlz]	The next division of the pharynx is the _____, the back portion of the mouth. It contains the _____, lymphatic tissue that works as part of the immune system. The oropharynx is part of the mechanism of the mouth that triggers swallowing.
laryngopharynx [lă-RĬNG-gō-făr-ĭngks] **larynx** [LĂR-ĭngks] **voice box** **trachea** [TRĀ-kē-ă] **windpipe**	The bottom and third section of the pharynx is the _____. It is at this point that the respiratory tract divides into the esophagus, the passageway for food, and the _____ or _____, through which air passes to the _____ or _____.
epiglottis [ĕp-ĭ-GLŎT-ĭs] **glottis** [GLŎT-ĭs]	Food is prevented from going into the larynx by the _____, a movable flap of cartilage that covers the opening to the larynx (called the _____) every time one swallows. Food then passes only into the esophagus. Occasionally, a person may swallow and inhale at the same time, allowing some food to be pulled (or *aspirated*) into the larynx. Usually, a strong cough forces out the food, but sometimes the food particle blocks the airway and the food must be dislodged with help from another person in a technique called the abdominal thrust maneuver. This technique is also called the *Heimlich maneuver*. It has saved many people from choking to death.
vocal cords **thyroid cartilage** [THĪ-royd KĂR-tĭ-lĭj] **Adam's apple**	Air goes into the larynx, which serves both as a passageway to the trachea and as the area where the sounds of speech are produced. The larynx contains _____, strips of epithelial tissue that vibrate when muscular tension is applied. The size and thickness of the cords determine the pitch of the sound. The male's thicker and longer vocal cords produce a lower pitch than do the shorter and thinner vocal cords of most women. Children's voices tend to be higher in pitch because of the smaller size of their vocal cords. Sound volume is regulated by the amount of air that passes over the vocal cords. The larynx is supported by various cartilaginous structures, one of which consists of two disks joined at an angle to form the _____ or _____ (larger in males than females).

| trachea
[TRĀ-kē-ă]
bronchi
[BRŎNG-kī]
bronchus
[BRŎNG-kŭs]
mediastinum
[MĒ-dē-ăs-TĬ-nŭm]
septum [SĔP-tŭm]
expiration
[ĕks-pĭ-RĀ-shŭn]
exhalation
[ĕks-hă-LĀ-shŭn] | The _____ is a cartilaginous and membranous tube that connects the larynx to the right and left _____ (plural of _____), the tubular branches into which the larynx divides. The trachea contains about 20 horseshoe-shaped structures that provide support so that it will not collapse, similar to the way a vacuum cleaner hose acts during use. The point at which the trachea divides is called the _____, a general term for a median area, especially one with a _____, or cartilaginous division. The median portion of the thoracic cavity, which contains the heart, esophagus, trachea, and thymus gland, is called the mediastinum. Both bronchi contain cartilage and mucous glands and are the passageways through which air enters the right and left lungs. Air that is pushed out of the lungs travels up through the respiratory tract during _____ (breathing out or _____), where it is expelled into the environment. |
| bronchioles
[BRŎNG-ē-ōlz]
alveolus
[ăl-VĒ-ō-lŭs]
alveoli
[ăl-VĒ-ō-lī] | The bronchi further divide into many smaller branches called _____. Inside the lungs, the structures resemble tree branches, with smaller parts branching off. At the end of each bronchiole is a cluster of air sacs. Each air sac is called an _____ (plural, _____). There are about 300 million alveoli in the lungs. The one-celled, thin-walled alveoli are surrounded by capillaries, with which they exchange gases. |

Did you know

Aspiration

Occasionally, food or saliva can be aspirated by inhaling, laughing, or talking with food, gum, or fluid in the mouth. An unconscious person who is lying on his or her back may aspirate some saliva or possibly blood, as in a trauma. The body's automatic response to aspiration is violent coughing or choking in an attempt to expel the material. If total obstruction occurs, then the abdominal thrust maneuver (also known as the Heimlich maneuver) must be used. It is important to remove the object so oxygen can get into the lungs to keep the alveoli from collapsing.

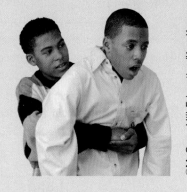

©McGraw-Hill Education/Ken Karp, photographer

PRONOUNCE and DEFINE	Pronounce the following terms aloud and write their meaning in the space provided.
cilia	[SĬL-ē-ă]
trachea	[TRĀ-kē-ă]
epiglottis	[ĔP-ĭ-GLŎT-ĭs]
alveolus	[ăl-VĒ-ō-lŭs]
pharynx	[FĂR-ĭngks]

Identify if the following terms are spelled correctly. Correct the words that are spelled incorrectly. Write the definition for each word.

	Spelling	Definition
bronchioldes		
larygopharynx		
nasopharynx		
orapharynx		
exhaleation		

UNDERSTAND   Match each term on the left to its description on the right.

1. _____ soft palate
2. _____ trachea
3. _____ pharynx
4. _____ cilia
5. _____ exhalation

a. Passageway at back of mouth
b. Sweeps foreign particles away
c. Airway from larynx into bronchi
d. Separates nasopharynx from rest of pharynx
e. Breathing out

APPLY   Read the following scenario and answer the questions.

Kate Bartell is a first-grade teacher at a local elementary school. She has asked you to come to the classroom and explain how the respiratory system works. One of the children believes that food and air go "down the same tube."

1. How would you explain the process of breathing to this group?
   _____
   _____

2. How would you explain the process of breathing to an adult group?
   _____
   _____

3. How would you explain the process of breathing to a group of medical professionals?
   _____
   _____

Lungs

The lungs are the essential respiratory organ. Their primary function is to carry oxygen from the atmosphere into the bloodstream and to release carbon dioxide from the bloodstream into the atmosphere. Figure 12-6 identifies the lobes of the lungs.

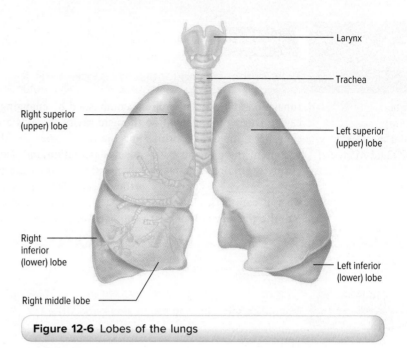

Larynx

Trachea

Right superior (upper) lobe

Left superior (upper) lobe

Right inferior (lower) lobe

Left inferior (lower) lobe

Right middle lobe

Figure 12-6 Lobes of the lungs

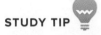

STUDY TIP

Are your flash cards up to date?

Structure and Function	PRACTICE
	Provide the missing term(s) to complete the following sentences.
thorax [THŌ-răks] **pleura** [PLŪR-ă] **pleurae** [PLŪR-ē] **parietal pleura** [pă-RĪ-ĕ-tăl PLŪR-ă] **visceral pleura** [VĬS-ĕr-ăl PLŪR-ă] **pleural cavity** [PLŪR-ăl KĂV-ĭ-tē]	The lungs take up most of the thoracic cavity (or _____), reaching from the collarbone to the diaphragm. The outside of the lungs has a moist, double layer of membrane called the _____ (plural, _____). The outer layer, the _____, lines the thoracic cavity, the inside of the ribs. The inner layer, the _____, covers the surface of the lungs. The space between the two pleura is called the _____. This space is filled with fluid. This pleural fluid prevents contact between the lungs and the ribs to avoid the inflammation that would be caused by friction.
apex [Ā-pĕks] **hilum** [HĪ-lŭm] **hilus** [HĪ-lŭs] **base** [bās] **superior lobe** **middle lobe** **inferior lobe**	Each lung has an _____, or topmost section; a middle area called the _____ or _____; and a lower section called the _____. The hilum is the area where the bronchi, blood vessels, and nerves enter the lungs. The right, larger lung is divided into three lobes: a _____, a _____, and an _____. The left lung is divided into two lobes: a superior and an inferior. Humans can function with one or more lobes removed or even an entire lung removed, as is necessary in some cases of lung cancer.

Breathing is the inhalation of oxygen into the lungs. Oxygen is then exchanged from the alveoli into the capillaries of the bloodstream and carbon dioxide is returned from the capillaries into the alveoli. Oxygen is then delivered to the body's other cells. This process is called internal respiration. This type of respiration is affected by how well the cardiovascular system supplies oxygenated blood. Carbon dioxide is expelled back up through the respiratory tract during expiration. |

continued on next page

PRACTICE

Provide the missing term(s) to complete the following sentences.

diaphragm
[DĪ-ă-frăm]
intercostal muscles
[ĭn-tĕr-KŎS-tăl MŬS-ĕlz]

Inhalation and exhalation are accomplished by changing the capacity of the thoracic cavity. During inhalation, the thoracic cavity expands and the lungs fill with air. During exhalation, the cavity shrinks and the lungs expel air. Muscular contractions enlarge the volume of the thoracic cavity during inspiration and decrease the volume when they relax during expiration. The major muscles that contract are the _____ and the _____ (the muscles between the ribs). The diaphragm lowers itself when it contracts, allowing more space in the thoracic cavity, and the intercostal muscles pull the ribs upward and outward when they contract, also enlarging the thoracic cavity.

PRONOUNCE and DEFINE

Pronounce the following terms aloud and write the meaning in the space provided.

thorax	[THŌ-răks]
pleura	[PLŪR-ă]
intercostal muscles	[ĭn-tĕr-KŎS-tăl MŬS-ĕlz]
visceral pleura	[VĬS-ĕr-ăl PLŪR-ă]

SPELL and DEFINE

Identify if the following terms are spelled correctly. Correct the words that are spelled incorrectly. Write the definition for each word.

	Spelling	Definition
diafragm		
helum		
pleurae		

UNDERSTAND

Fill the blanks.

1. The bottom of the lung is the _____.
2. The visceral pleura make up the _____ layer.
3. _____ muscles are located between the ribs.
4. The chest cavity is also known as the _____.
5. The superior lobe is located on the _____ of each lung.

Mr. Rick Fritzringer is a 55-year-old black male who has a tumor in his lung. He has a 40-year history of smoking a pack of cigarettes per day. The surgeon tells you that he wants to perform a lobectomy and asks you to explain the procedure to the patient. Mr. Fritzringer is concerned that he will have only one lung remaining and he will not be able to get enough oxygen to breathe.

1. As the medical professional, how will you respond to Mr. Fritzringer's concerns?

   _____

   _____

   _____

2. How would you explain the procedure in lay terms to him?

   _____

   _____

   _____

Did you know ?

Lung Capacity

Normal inspiration brings about 500 mL of air into the lungs. Normal expiration expels about the same amount from the lungs. Forced inspiration brings extra air (up to six times the normal amount) into the lungs. Forced expiration can expel up to three times the normal amount of air from the lungs. Some quantity of air always remains in the lungs so that newly inhaled air mixes with the remaining air. This helps to maintain the proper concentration of oxygen and carbon dioxide in the lungs.

Posterior internal intercostal muscles pull ribs down and inward

Diaphragm

Abdominal organs force diaphragm higher

Abdominal wall muscles contract and compress abdominal organs

LO 12.2 Word Building in the Respiratory System

Word Building	PRACTICE
	Provide the correct combining form to complete the following sentences.
epiglott-itis [ĕp-ĭ-glŏt-Ī-tĭs]	Inflammation of the epiglottis is _____ itis.
phono-meter [fō-NŎM-ĕ-tĕr]	A _____ meter is an instrument for measuring sounds.
rhin-itis [rī-NĪ-tĭs]	_____ itis is inflammation of the nose.

continued on next page

Word Building	PRACTICE
	Provide the correct combining form to complete the following sentences.
adenoid-ectomy [ĂD-ĕ-noy-DĔK-tō-mē]	An operation for removal of adenoid growths is an _____ ectomy.
pleur-itis [plū-RĪ-tĭs]	_____ itis is inflammation of the pleura.
capno-gram [KAP-nō-gram]	A _____ gram is a continuous recording of the carbon dioxide in expired air.
naso-gastric [nā-zō-GAS-trik]	Relating to the nasal passages and the stomach is _____ gastric.
tonsill-ectomy [TŎN-sĭ-LĔK-tō-mē]	_____ ectomy is removal of one entire tonsil or of both tonsils.
bronch-itis [brŏng-KĪ-tĭs]	Inflammation of the lining of the bronchial tubes is _____ itis.
pneumo-lith [NŪ-mō-lĭth]	_____ lith is calculus in the lungs.
oro-pharynx [ŌR-ō-FĂR-ĭngks]	The part of the pharynx that lies behind the mouth is the _____ pharynx
tracheo-scopy [trā-kē-OS-kŏ-pē]	_____ scopy is inspection of the interior of the trachea.
mediastin-itis [MĒ-dē-as-ti-NĪ-tis]	Inflammation of the tissue of the mediastinum is _____ itis.
alveol-itis [AL-vē-ō-LĪ-tis]	_____ itis is inflammation of the alveoli.
stetho-scope [STETH-ō-skōp]	An instrument used to listen to sounds in the chest is a _____ scope.
lob-ectomy [lō-BĔK-tō-mē]	Removal of a lung lobe is a _____ ectomy.
pneumon-itis [nū-mō-NĪ-tĭs]	Inflammation of the lungs is _____ itis.
phren-itis [fre-NĪ-tĭs]	_____ itis is inflammation of the diaphragm.
laryngo-scope [lă-RING-gō-skōp]	A device used to examine the larynx through the mouth is a _____ scope.
spiro-meter [spī-RŎM-ĕ-tĕr]	A _____ meter is an instrument used to measure respiratory gases.
bronchiol-itis [brŏng-kē-ō-LĪ-tĭs]	Inflammation of the bronchioles is _____ itis.
oxi-meter [ok-SIM-ĕ-tĕr]	An instrument for measuring oxygen saturation of blood is an _____ meter.
thoraco-tomy [thōr-ă-KŎT-ō-mē]	_____ tomy is an incision into the chest wall.
pharyng-itis [făr-ĭn-JĪ-tĭs]	_____ itis is inflammation in the pharynx.

	Spelling	Definition
nasopharyngx		
trachae		
resperation		
alveoli		
diagphram		
epiglottus		
pharinx		
mediastinum		
tonsills		
bronchis		

UNDERSTAND   Match the description on the left to its term on the right.

1. _____ Inflammation of the lungs
2. _____ Instrument used to listen to the heart
3. _____ Instrument used to examine the larynx
4. _____ Inflammation of the nose
5. _____ Used to measure oxygen saturation
6. _____ Incision into the chest wall
7. _____ Inflammation of the pharynx
8. _____ Instrument used to measure sounds
9. _____ Inflammation of the bronchial tubes
10. _____ Continuous graphing of carbon dioxide in expired air

a. bronchitis
b. capnogram
c. laryngoscope
d. pneumonitis
e. oximeter
f. pharyngitis
g. phonometer
h. thoracotomy
i. rhinitis
j. stethoscope

APPLY   Read the following scenario and answer the questions.

Mrs. Melony Henshaw is an 83-year-old white female. She comes into the clinic complaining of continuous shortness of breath (says she "can't seem to catch her breath"), weakness, and increasing fatigue. She has a history of a thoracotomy and a lobectomy. The physician refers her to a pulmonologist.

1. What testing might the physician order?

_____

_____

2. What are a thoracotomy and a lobectomy? How might this impact breathing?

_____

_____

3. What is a pulmonologist, and why would the doctor refer Mrs. Henshaw to one?

_____

_____

LO 12.3 Diagnostic, Procedural, and Laboratory Terms

Diagnostic, procedural, and laboratory findings assist in diagnosing medical conditions. Often used in combination, these tests lead to a diagnosis and assist in treatment planning. Figure 12-7 shows an x-ray of the sinuses. Figure 12-8 depicts spirometer testing. Figure 12-9 illustrates a throat culture test. Figure 12-10 compares a radiograph of healthy lungs to those with tuberculosis.

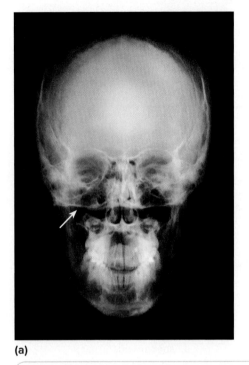

(a)

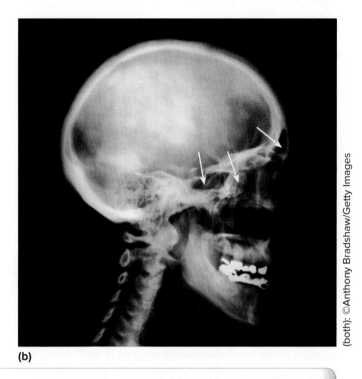

(b)

(both): ©Anthony Bradshaw/Getty Images

Figure 12-7 X-ray of the sinuses: (a) anterior, (b) lateral

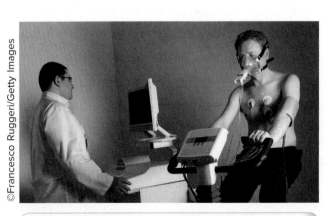

©Francesco Ruggeri/Getty Images

Figure 12-8 Spirometry testing in an office setting

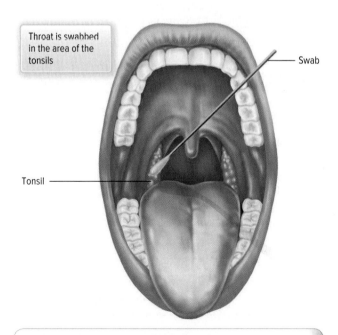

Throat is swabbed in the area of the tonsils

Swab

Tonsil

Figure 12-9 Throat culture test

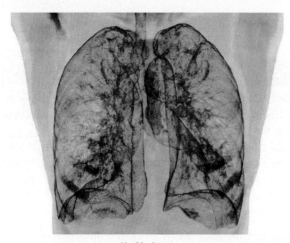

Healthy lungs

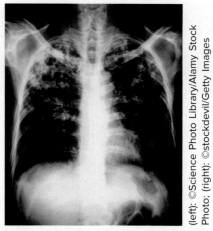

Tuberculosis

Figure 12-10 Healthy lungs appear dark and clear on a radiograph. Lungs with tuberculosis have cloudy areas where fibrous tissue grows, walling off infected areas.

STUDY TIP

When assessing patients, remember to inspect, auscultate, and then percuss.

Diagnostic	PRACTICE
	Provide the missing term(s) to complete the following sentences.
auscultation [ăws-kŭl-TĀ-shŭn] **percussion** [pĕr-KŬSH-ŭn]	Disorders of the respiratory system can be diagnosed in several ways. First, a physician usually listens to the lungs with a stethoscope, a process called _____. Next, the respiratory rate is determined by counting the number of respirations per minute. One inhalation and one exhalation equal a single respiration. Adult respirations normally range from 15 to 20 per minute. The physician may use _____, tapping over the lung area, to see if the lungs are clear (a hollow sound) or filled with fluid (a dull sound). Sputum can be observed for its color. Pus in sputum usually causes a greenish or yellowish color and indicates infection. Blood in the sputum may indicate tuberculosis.
pulmonary function tests **peak flow meter** **spirometer** [spī-RŎM-ĕ-tĕr]	_____ measure the mechanics of breathing. Breathing may be tested by a _____. Asthmatics often use this type of measuring device to check breathing capacity; they can then take medicine if an attack seems imminent. A _____ is a machine that tests pulmonary function by measuring the lungs' volume and capacity (*spirometry*). This machine measures the *forced vital capacity (FVC)*, or highest breathing capacity, of the lungs when the patient takes the deepest breath possible. Other breathing measurements such as *forced expiratory volume (FEV)* show capacity at different parts of the respiratory cycle.
	Tuberculosis is a disease of the respiratory system. Tests for tuberculosis were discussed in Chapter 5, The Integumentary System, because reactions on the surface of the skin indicate a positive result for a tuberculosis test.

continued on next page

Diagnostic	PRACTICE
	Provide the missing term(s) to complete the following sentences.
bronchography [brŏng-KŎG-ră-fē]	Visual images of the chest and parts of the respiratory system play an important role in diagnosing respiratory ailments. Chest x-rays, MRIs, and lung scans can detect abnormalities such as masses and restricted blood flow within the lungs. A _____ provides a radiological picture of the trachea and bronchi. A thoracic CT scan shows a cross-sectional view of the chest that can reveal tissue masses. A pulmonary angiography is an x-ray of the blood vessels of the lungs taken after dye is injected into a blood vessel. A lung scan or *ventilation/perfusion (V/Q) scan* is a recording of radioactive material, injected or inhaled, to show air flow and blood supply in the lungs.
endoscope [ĔN-dō-skōp] **bronchoscope** [BRŎNG-kō-skōp] **nasopharyngoscopy** [NĀ-zō-fă-rĭng-GŎS-kō-pē] **laryngoscopy** [LĂR-ĭng-GŎS-kō-pē] **mediastinoscopy** [MĒ-dē-ăs-tĭ-NŎS-kō-pē]	Parts of the respiratory system also can be observed by *endoscopy,* insertion of an _____ (a viewing tube) into a body cavity. A _____ is used for *bronchoscopy.* In _____, a flexible endoscope is used to examine nasal passages and the pharynx. _____ is the procedure for examining the mouth and larynx, and _____, for examining the mediastinum area and all the organs within it. Such diagnostic testing can reveal structural abnormalities, tumors, and irritations.
	**Laboratory Tests**
throat cultures **sputum sample** [SPŪ-tŭm SAM-pel] **sputum culture** **arterial blood gases (ABGs)** [ăr-TĒR-ē-ăl blŭd GAS-ĕz] **sweat test**	_____ are commonly used to diagnose streptococcal infections. A swab is passed over a portion of the throat and the swab is then put in contact with a culture. If a strep infection is present, the culture will show certain bacteria. A _____ or _____ may be taken and cultured to identify any disease-causing organisms. _____ measure the levels of pressure of oxygen (O_2) and carbon dioxide (CO_2) dissolved in the plasma of arterial blood. These measurements help diagnose heart and lung functions. A _____ measures the amount of salt in sweat and is used to confirm cystic fibrosis.

PRONOUNCE and DEFINE	Pronounce the following terms aloud and write their meaning in the space provided.
bronchoscope	[BRŎNG-kō-skōp]
percussion	[pĕr-KŬSH-ŭn]
spirometer	[spī-RŎM-ĕ-tĕr]
sputum sample	[SPŪ-tŭm SAM-pel]
bronchography	[brŏng-KŎG-ră-fē]

SPELL and DEFINE	Identify if the following terms are spelled correctly. Correct the words that are spelled incorrectly. Write the definition for each word.	
	Spelling	**Definition**
endoscope		
nasapharyngoscopy		
spirameter		
mediastinoscopie		
laryngoscopy		

UNDERSTAND — Fill in the blanks.

1. If the physician wants to measure the lung's volume and capacity, a _____ would be ordered.
2. A sweat test is used to diagnose what condition? _____
3. An asthmatic would use a _____ to measure breathing capacity.
4. Which type of endoscope would the physician use to view the nasal passages and pharynx? _____
5. Which diagnostic test measures the blood's pH, oxygen, and carbon dioxide levels? _____

APPLY — Read the following scenario and answer the questions.

Mr. Steven Phillips is a 35-year-old white male who was admitted to Midvale Hospital from the emergency room. His medical record reads as follows:

A chest x-ray showed a pneumonic infiltrate in the left lower lobe with some parapneumonic effusion. Follow-up chest x-rays showed progression of infiltrate and then slight clearing. Serial ECGs (ECGs given one after another in succession) were compatible with ischemia or a pericardial process. Labs were normal. Arterial blood gases were ordered. Sputum culture could not be obtained.

1. Explain in lay terms what this record means?

_____

_____

2. Why do you think blood gas tests were ordered for Mr. Phillips?

_____

_____

Did you know

Streptococcal Infections

Throat cultures are commonly ordered for children with sore throats. The presence of a streptococcal infection is usually treated with antibiotics because the infection can cause health problems (such as heart and kidney damage) if left unchecked.

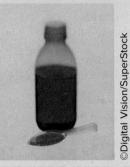

©Digital Vision/SuperStock

LO 12.4 Pathological Terms

Inflammations

Respiratory inflammatory conditions are the body's attempt to protect itself from infection and other harmful substances. Inflammation can occur in both the upper and lower respiratory tracts.

Pathological	PRACTICE
	Provide the missing term(s) to complete the following sentences.
	The respiratory system is the site for many inflammations, disorders, and infections. This system must contend with foreign material coming into the body from outside, as well as internal problems that may affect any of its parts. Each of its parts may become inflamed.
pharynx [FĂR-ĭngks] **pharyngitis** [făr-ĭn-JĪ-tĭs]	A sore throat is an inflammation of the _____, called _____.
rhinitis [rī-NĪ-tĭs]	_____ is nasal inflammation.
laryngotracheobronchitis [lă-RĬNG-gō-TRĀ-kē-ō-brŏng-KĪ-tĭs]	Inflammation of the larynx, trachea, and bronchi is _____.
adenoiditis [ĂD-ĕ-noy-DĪ-tĭs]	_____ is inflammation of the adenoids.
pneumonitis [nū-mō-NĪ-tĭs]	Inflammation of the lung is _____.
bronchitis [brŏng-KĪ-tĭs] **chronic bronchitis**	_____ is inflammation of the bronchi; recurring or long-lasting bouts are called _____.
tonsillitis [TŎN-sĭ-LĪ-tĭs]	Inflammation of the tonsils is _____.
pleurisy [PLŪR-ĭ-sē] **pleuritis** [plŭ-RĪ-tĭs]	Inflammation of the pleura is _____ or _____.
epiglottitis [ĕp-ĭ-glŏt-Ī-tĭs]	_____ is inflammation of the epiglottis.
tracheitis [trā-kē-Ī-tĭs]	Inflammation of the trachea is _____.
laryngitis [lăr-ĭn-JĪ-tĭs]	Inflammation of the larynx is _____.
nasopharyngitis [NĀ-zō-fă-rĭn-JĪ-tĭs]	_____ is inflammation of the nose and pharynx.
sinusitis [sī-nū-SĪ-tĭs]	_____ is inflammation of sinuses.

STUDY TIP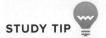

Inflammation of the pleura is called pleurisy (or, sometimes, pleuritis). Pleurisy is often very painful and is intensified by coughing or breathing. Often, analgesics or nonsteroidal anti-inflammatory medications are prescribed.

PRONOUNCE and DEFINE	Pronounce the following terms aloud and write their meaning in the space provided.
laryngotracheobronchitis	[lă-RĬNG-gō-TRĀ-kē-ō-brŏng-KĪ-tĭs]
adenoiditis	[ĂD-ĕ-noy-DĪ-tĭs]
rhinitis	[rī-NĪ-tĭs]
epiglottitis	[ĕp-ĭ-glŏt-Ī-tĭs]
nasopharyngitis	[NĀ-zō-fă-rĭn-JĪ-tĭs]

SPELL and DEFINE	Identify if the following terms are spelled correctly. Correct the words that are spelled incorrectly. Write the definition for each word.	
	Spelling	Definition
pleuritis		
tonsillites		
pneumonitis		
fharyngitis		
sinusites		

UNDERSTAND	Fill in the blanks

1. Inflammation of the throat is called _____.
2. A physician would diagnose inflamed sinuses as _____.
3. Rhinitis is a _____.
4. Inflammation of the larynx, trachea, and bronchi is _____.
5. When the client has recurrent bronchitis, it is known as _____.

Jack Lamborn is a 7-year-old black male who presents to the ER with his mother. The mother explains that the patient has a history of "sore throats," difficulty and painful swallowing, and excessive snoring at night. The physician tells the client (and his mother) that he has sinusitis, tonsillitis, and pneumonitis.

1. What are the medical terms for the symptoms that the mom has relayed to the physician?

   _____

   _____

2. Explain to the client what he has.
   a. What is sinusitis? _____
   b. What is tonsillitis? _____
   c. What is pneumonitis? _____

3. What word part does each share? How are the terms similar and what does each word break down to mean?

   _____

   _____

Breathing Problems and Conditions Related to Irregular Breathing Patterns

Clients can experience a variety of breathing disorders that may be related to a disease or condition. Breathing disorders can affect the ability of the body to provide adequate oxygenation.

Pathological	PRACTICE Provide the missing term(s) to complete the following sentences.
eupnea [yūp NĒ-ă]	Normal breathing (_____) may become affected by diseases or conditions and change to one of the following breathing difficulties:
apnea [ĂP-nē-ă]	Absence of breathing is _____.
tachypnea [tăk-ĭp-NĒ-ă]	Fast breathing is _____.
hyperpnea [hī-pĕrp-NĒ-ă]	Abnormally deep breathing is _____.
orthopnea [ōr-thŏp-NĒ-ă, ōr-THŎP-nē-ă]	Difficulty in breathing, especially while lying down, is _____. Physicians determine the degree of orthopnea by the number of pillows required to allow the patient to breathe easily (e.g., two-pillow orthopnea, three-pillow orthopnea).
bradypnea [brăd-ĭp-NĒ-ă]	Slow breathing is _____.
dyspnea [dĭsp-NĒ-ă, DĬSP-nē-ă]	Difficult breathing is _____.
hypopnea [hī-PŎP-nē-ă]	Shallow breathing is _____.

Cheyne-Stokes respiration [chān stōks rĕs-pĭ-RĀ-shŭn]	_____, for example, is an irregular breathing pattern with a period of apnea followed by deep, labored breathing that becomes shallow, then apneic.
crackles [KRĂK-lz] **rales** [răhlz] **wheezes** [HWĒZ-ĕz] **rhonchi** [RŎNG-kī] **stridor** [STRĪ-dōr] **dysphonia** [dĭs-FŌ-nē-ă]	Irregular sounds usually indicate specific disorders: _____ or _____ are popping sounds heard in lung collapse and other conditions, such as congestive heart failure and pneumonia. _____ or _____ occur during attacks of asthma or emphysema; _____ is a high-pitched crowing sound; and _____ is hoarseness, often associated with laryngitis.
hyperventilation [HĪ-pĕr-vĕn-tĭ-LĀ-shŭn] **hypoventilation** [HĪ-pō-ven-tĭ-LĀ-shŭn] **hypercapnia** [hī-pĕr-KĂP-nē-ă] **hypoxemia** [hī-pŏk-SĒ-mē-ă] **hypoxia** [hī-PŎK-sē-ă]	_____, excessive breathing in and out, may be caused by anxiety or overexertion. _____, abnormally low movement of air in and out of the lungs, may cause excessive buildup of carbon dioxide in the lungs, or _____. _____ is a deficient amount of oxygen in the blood and _____ is a deficient amount of oxygen in tissue.

STUDY TIP

Clients experiencing hypoxemia or hypoxia may experience confusion or a change in the level of consciousness due to decreased oxygenation.

PRONOUNCE and DEFINE	Pronounce the following terms aloud and write their meaning in the space provided.
Cheyne-Stokes respiration	[chān stōks rĕs-pĭ-RĀ-shŭn]
eupnea	[yūp-NĒ-ă]
hypopnea	[hī-PŎP-nē-ă]
hyperpnea	[hī-pĕrp-NĒ-ă]
hypoxia	[hī-PŎK-sē-ă]

Identify if the following terms are spelled correctly. Correct the words that are spelled incorrectly. Write the definition for each word.

	Spelling	Definition
rails		
dysfonia		
dispnea		
bradypnea		
Strider		

UNDERSTAND   Match each term on the left to its description on the right.

1. _____ apnea
2. _____ orthopnea
3. _____ hypopnea
4. _____ dyspnea
5. _____ hyperpnea

a. Shallow breathing
b. Abnormally deep breathing
c. Difficulty breathing while lying down
d. Cessation of breathing
e. Difficult breathing

APPLY   Read the following scenario and answer the questions.

Ms. Michelle Lopane is a 35-year-old Hispanic female who presents to the urgent care center. She states that she is having difficulty breathing but cannot get many words out to explain further. The nurse is performing a respiratory assessment on Ms. Lopane. The following information is gathered:

- Whistling sound on inspiration
- Popping sound throughout lungs
- Fast, shallow respiratory rate and rhythm
- Discomfort in chest due to hiccups for 3 days

1. Is this a priority? Why?

_____

_____

2. How would you document the nurse's findings using medical terminology?

_____

_____

3. How can incorrect pronunciation and spelling impact the patient's outcome adversely?

_____

_____

4. What reference material would you use to "look up" a word you don't know or remember?

_____

_____

The respiratory system can experience a wide variety of diseases and disorders. Figure 12.11 shows what happens in cystic fibrosis. Figure 12.12 illustrates blockage of the airway during an asthma attack.

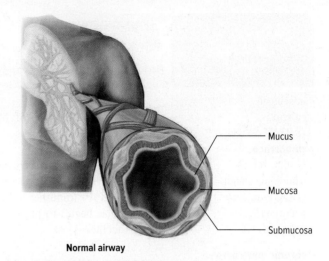

Normal airway

- Mucus
- Mucosa
- Submucosa

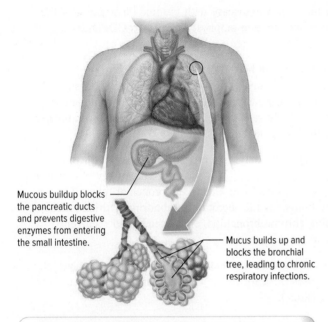

Mucous buildup blocks the pancreatic ducts and prevents digestive enzymes from entering the small intestine.

Mucus builds up and blocks the bronchial tree, leading to chronic respiratory infections.

Figure 12-11 Cystic fibrosis

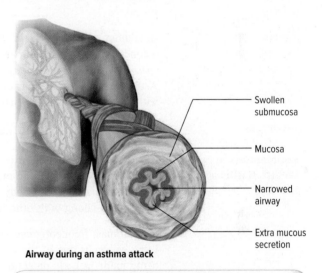

Airway during an asthma attack

- Swollen submucosa
- Mucosa
- Narrowed airway
- Extra mucous secretion

Figure 12-12 Blockage of airway during an asthma attack

Pathological	PRACTICE
upper respiratory infection **croup** [krūp] **diphtheria** [dĭf-THĒR-ē-ă]	Provide the missing term(s) to complete the following sentences. _____ is a term that covers an infection of some or all of the upper respiratory tract. Other disorders of the tract include _____, acute respiratory syndrome in children and infants, and _____, acute infection of the throat and upper respiratory tract.

continued on next page

Pathological	PRACTICE

Provide the missing term(s) to complete the following sentences.

Term	Sentence
nosebleed epistaxis [ĔP-ĭ-STĂK-sĭs] rhinorrhea [rīn-nō-RĒ-ă] whooping cough [HŎOP-ĭng kăwf] pertussis [pĕr-TŬS-ĭs]	_____ or _____ results from a trauma to, or a spontaneous rupture of, blood vessels in the nose; _____ is nasal discharge usually caused by an inflammation or infection; and _____ or _____ is a severe infection of the pharynx, larynx, and trachea caused by *Bordetella pertussis* bacteria. Diphtheria and pertussis have virtually disappeared in the United States since the regular administration of DPT (DTaP) (diphtheria, pertussis, tetanus) vaccines to most infants. However, pertussis has begun to make a comeback as some children are not receiving that part of the vaccine.
chronic obstructive pulmonary disease (COPD)	_____ is a term for any disease with chronic obstruction of the bronchial tubes and lungs. Chronic bronchitis and emphysema are two COPD disease processes.
asthma [ĂZ-mă]	In addition to bronchitis, the bronchial tubes can be the site of _____, a condition of bronchial airway obstruction, causing an irritable airway prone to spasm; this spasm is called a *bronchospasm.* The underlying cause is allergic inflammation of lung tissue. Asthma can be very serious and is even fatal in rare cases. However, it is usually controllable with the use of inhalers, called *bronchodilators,* and steroids.
hemoptysis [hē-MŎP-tĭ-sĭs] cystic fibrosis [SĬS-tĭk fī-BRŌ-sĭs]	_____ is a lung or bronchial hemorrhage that results in the coughing up of blood. _____ involves chronic airway obstruction caused by disease of the exocrine glands, which also affects the bronchial tubes. The predominant characteristic of cystic fibrosis is the secretion of abnormally thick mucus in various places in the body, causing chronic bronchitis, emphysema, and recurrent pneumonia, along with other ailments.
	Carcinomas, frequently caused by smoking, also can be found in the respiratory system. Lung cancer is one of the leading causes of death in the United States, but advances are being made in early detection and treatment.
	Some disorders in newborns, such as *hyaline membrane disease* or *respiratory distress syndrome (RDS),* occur most frequently in premature babies and are often the result of underdeveloped lungs. *Adult respiratory distress syndrome (ARDS)* may have a number of causes, especially injury to the lungs.
atelectasis [ăt-ĕ-LĔK-tă-sĭs] emphysema [ĕm-fă-SĒ-mă, ĕm-fă-ZĒ-mă] pneumonia [nū-MŌ-nē-ă]	Lung disorders may occur in the alveoli: for example, _____, an incomplete expansion of the lung or part of a lung; _____, hyperinflation of the air sacs often caused by smoking; and _____, acute infection of the alveoli. Pneumonia is a term used for a number of infections. Such infections typically affect bedridden and frail people whose internal respiration is compromised.
tuberculosis [tū-bĕr-kyū-LŌ-sĭs] bacilli [bă-SĬL-ī] pulmonary abscess [PŬL-mō-nār-ē ĂB-sĕs] pulmonary edema [PŬL-mō-nār-ē ĕ-DĒ-mă]	_____ is a highly infectious disease caused by rod-shaped bacteria (_____) that invade the lungs and cause small swellings and inflammation. Many forms of tuberculosis have become drug resistant. A _____ is a large collection of pus in the lungs and _____ is a buildup of fluid in the air sacs and bronchioles, usually caused by failure of the heart to pump enough blood to and from the lungs.

pneumoconiosis [NŪ-mō-kō-nē-Ō-sĭs] **black lung** **anthracosis** [ăn-thră-KŌ-sĭs] **asbestosis** [ăs-bĕs-TŌ-sĭs]	Several environmental agents cause _____, a lung condition caused by dust in the lungs. _____, or _____, is caused by coal dust and is, therefore, a threat to coal miners; _____ is caused by inhalation of asbestos particles released during construction of ships and buildings.
pneumothorax [nū-mō-THŌR-ăks] **empyema** [ĕm-pī-Ē-mă] **hemothorax** [hē-mō-THŌR-ăks] **pleural effusion** [PLŬR-ăl ĕ-FYŪ-zhŭn] **mesothelioma** [MĔZ-ō-thē-lē-Ō-mă]	Disorders of the pleura, other than pleurisy, include _____, an accumulation of air or gas in the pleural cavity; _____, pus in the pleural cavity; _____, blood in the pleural cavity; _____, an escape of fluid into the pleural cavity; and, rarely, _____, a cancer associated with asbestosis.
bronchospasms [BRŎNG-kō-spăzmz] **laryngospasms** [lă-RĬNG-gō-spăzmz]	The respiratory system may be disturbed by spasms that cause coughing or constriction. When severe, these spasms can be life threatening. _____ occur in the bronchi (as seen in asthma) and _____ occur in the larynx.

PRONOUNCE and DEFINE	**Pronounce the following terms aloud and write their meaning in the space provided.**
mesothelioma	[MĔZ-ō-thē-lē-Ō-mă]
pneumothorax	[nū-mō-THŌR-ăks]
atelectasis	[ăt-ĕ-LĔK-tă-sĭs]
hemoptysis	[hē-MŎP-tĭ-sĭs]
croup	[krūp]

SPELL and DEFINE	**Identify if the following terms are spelled correctly. Correct the words that are spelled incorrectly. Write the definition for each word.**	
	Spelling	**Definition**
empiema		
abestosis		
emphysema		
laryngospasm		
bacilli		

Match each term on the left to its description on the right.

1. _____ pleurisy, pleuritis   a. Whooping cough
2. _____ epistaxis   b. Deficient oxygen in blood
3. _____ dysphonia   c. Black lung
4. _____ hypoxemia   d. Pleural inflammation
5. _____ hypercapnia   e. Hoarseness
6. _____ anthracosis   f. Chronic bronchitis and emphysema
7. _____ pleural effusion   g. Nosebleed
8. _____ pertussis   h. Fast breathing
9. _____ tachypnea   i. Too much carbon dioxide
10. _____ COPD   j. Fluid in the pleural cavity

APPLY   **Read the following scenario and answer the questions.**

Mr. Adam Boyle is a 41-year-old, white, married male who has worked in the coal mining industry for 20 years. He has five children. He also did construction on old buildings as an extra job. He states that he drinks two alcoholic beverages per day after work. Today he presents to the physician's office with a persistent cough and is complaining of coughing up blood. He denies a runny nose or bleeding from his nose.

1 Using medical terminology, how would you describe the client's history to the physician?

_____

_____

2. What information is important to relay to the doctor and what is not essential to the patient's care? Why?

_____

_____

3. What tests may the physician order based on the symptoms?

_____

_____

4. How would you schedule those tests? What would you say?

_____

_____

Did you know ?

Severe Acute Respiratory Syndrome (SARS)

SARS first appeared in Asia in 2003 and was fairly quickly contained by a worldwide cooperative response. Either travel to and from countries where SARS first appeared was restricted or people were checked before and after travel. In general, people with the disease were quarantined. SARS begins with a high fever (temperature greater than 100.4°F [>38.0°C]). Other symptoms may include headache and body aches. After 2 to 7 days, SARS patients may develop a dry cough. Most patients develop pneumonia. It is hoped that a vaccine can be developed before the next outbreak.

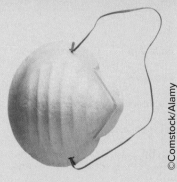

©Comstock/Alamy

LO 12.5   Surgical Terms

Surgery may be performed on the respiratory system depending upon the disease or condition. Figure 12-13 shows a healthy lung and a cancerous lung. Figure 12-14 illustrates a tracheostomy.

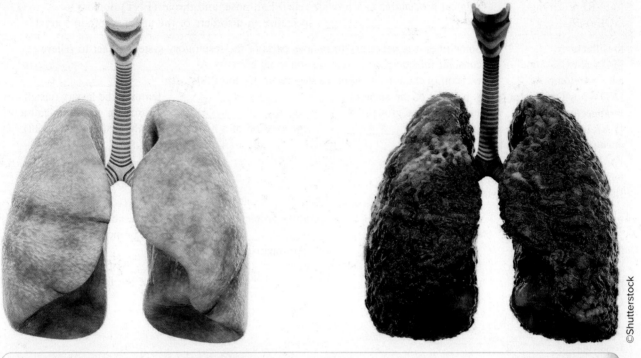

©Shutterstock

Figure 12-13 (left) Healthy lung; (right) cancerous lung

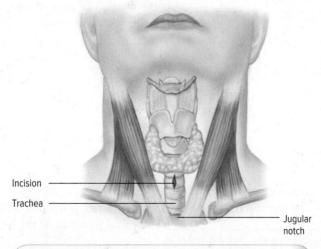

Incision

Trachea

Jugular notch

Figure 12-14 A tracheostomy is an incision into the trachea, usually to provide an airway.

Term	Practice
otorhinolaryngologists [ō-tō-RĪ-nō-lăr-ĭng-GŎL-ō-jĭsts]	When breathing is disrupted or chronic infections of the respiratory tract occur, surgical procedures can provide relief. Ear, nose, and throat (ENT) doctors, or _____, specialize in disorders of the upper respiratory tract.
tonsillectomy [TŎN-sĭ-LĔK-tō-mē] **adenoidectomy** [ĂD-ĕ-noy-DĔK-tō-mē] **laryngectomy** [LĂR-ĭn-JĔK-tō-mē] **pneumonectomy** [NŪ-mō-NĔK-tō-mē] **lobectomy** [lō-BĔK-tō-mē]	Sometimes it is necessary to remove parts of the respiratory system, either to relieve constant infections or to remove abnormal growths. A _____ is excision of the tonsils (often to stop recurrent tonsillitis). An _____ is removal of the adenoids; a _____ removes the larynx (usually to stop cancerous growth); a _____ is the excision of a lung; and a _____ is the excision of a lung lobe (as when cancer is present).
bronchoplasty [BRŎNG-kō-plăs-tē] **laryngoplasty** [lă-RĬNG-gō-plăs-tē] **rhinoplasty** [RĪ-nō-plăs-tē] **septoplasty** [SĔP-tō-plăs-tē] **tracheoplasty** [TRĀ-kē-ō-plăs-tē]	Surgical repair can relieve respiratory problems caused by trauma, abnormalities, growths, or infections. A _____ is the repair of a bronchus; _____ is the repair of the larynx; _____ is the repair of the bones of the nose; _____ is the repair of the nasal septum; and _____ is the repair of the trachea.
thoracic sugeons [thō-RĂS-ĭk SER-jŭnz] **laryngotracheotomy** [lă-RĬNG-gō-trā-kē-ŎT-ō-mē] **septostomy** [sĕp-TŎS-tō-mē] **sinusotomy** [sĭn-ŭ-SŎT-ō-mē] **thoracotomy** [thŏr-ă-KŎT-ō-mē] **thoracostomy** [thŏr-ă-KŎS-tō-mē] **tracheotomy** [trā-kē-ŎT-ō-mē]	Incisions into parts of the respiratory system are sometimes necessary. _____ are the specialists who usually perform such procedures. A _____ is an incision of the larynx and trachea. _____ is the creation of an opening in the nasal septum; _____ is an incision of a sinus; _____ is an incision into the chest cavity; _____ is the establishment of an opening in the chest cavity to drain fluid; and _____ is an incision into the trachea, usually to provide an airway.
laryngocentesis [lă-RĬNG-gō-sĕn-TĒ-sĭs] **pleurocentesis** [PLŪR-ō-sĕn-TĒ-sĭs] **thoracentesis** [THŎR-ă-sĕn-TĒ-sĭs]	Surgical punctures provide a means to aspirate or remove fluid. _____ is a surgical puncture of the larynx; while the surgical puncture of the pleural space is _____; and the surgical puncture of the chest cavity is _____.

tracheostomy [TRĀ-kē-ŎS-tō-mē] **laryngostomy** [LĂR-ĭng-GŎS-tō-mē] **endotracheal intubation (ET)** [ĔN-dō-TRĀ-kē-ăl ĭn-tū-BĀ-shŭn]	Artificial openings into the respiratory tract may allow for alternative airways, as in a _____ (artificial tracheal opening) or a _____ (artificial laryngeal opening). An _____ is the insertion of a tube through the nose or mouth, pharynx, and larynx and into the trachea to establish an airway.

PRONOUNCE and DEFINE

Pronounce the following terms aloud and write their meaning in the space provided.

rhinoplasty	[RĪ-nō-plăs-tē]
septoplasty	[SĔP-tō-plăs-tē]
tracheoplasty	[TRĀ-kē-ō-plăs-tē]
adenoidectomy	[ĂD-ĕ-noy-DĔK-tō-mē]
laryngectomy	[LĂR-ĭn-JĔK-tō-mē]

SPELL and DEFINE

Identify if the following terms are spelled correctly. Correct the words that are spelled incorrectly. Write the definition for each word.

	Spelling	Definition
plurocentesis		
thoracentesis		
laringostome		
bronkhoplasty		
tracheostomy		

UNDERSTAND

Match each term on the left to its description on the right.

1. _____ rhinoplasty
2. _____ pleurocentesis
3. _____ adenoidectomy
4. _____ tracheostomy
5. _____ tracheotomy
6. _____ laryngectomy
7. _____ lobectomy
8. _____ laryngostomy

a. Artificial laryngeal opening
b. Removal of a lobe of the lung
c. Puncture of the pleura
d. Incision into the trachea
e. Artificial tracheal opening
f. Removal of the adenoids
g. Repair of the nose
h. Removal of the larynx

Ten-year-old Susan Jones is admitted to the emergency department with an acute asthma attack. She has had tonsillitis three times in the last 5 months that has caused inflammation of her upper respiratory tract. She has been to the emergency department twice in the last month for an asthma attack. Her physician, an ENT, is also a surgeon.

1. Why is it important that her physician is a surgeon?

_____

_____

2. How might surgery help avoid future upper respiratory infections?

_____

_____

LO 12.6 Pharmacological Terms

Pharmacological	PRACTICE
	Provide the missing term(s) to complete the following sentences.
bronchodilators [brŏng-kō-dī-LĀ-tŏrz] **expectorants** [ĕk-SPĔK-tō-rănts] **antitussives** [ăn-tē-TŬS-sĭvz] **decongestants** [dē-kŏn-JĔST-ănts]	Antibiotics, antihistamines, and anticoagulants are used for respiratory system disorders just as with other system disorders. Specific to respiratory problems are _____, drugs that dilate the walls of the bronchi (as during an asthmatic attack), and _____, drugs that promote coughing and the expulsion of mucus. _____ relieve coughing and _____ help congestion of the upper respiratory tract.
ventilators [VĔN-tĭ-lā-tŏrz] **nebulizers** [NĔB-yū-līz-ĕrz]	Two mechanical devices aid in breathing. Mechanical _____ actually serve as a breathing substitute for patients who cannot breathe on their own. _____ deliver medication through the nose or mouth to ease breathing problems. Some nebulizers and MDIs (metered dose inhalers) deliver a specific amount of spray with each puff of the inhaler.

1. Coughing can be controlled with _____.
2. Insufficiently dilated bronchi can be treated with _____.
3. Productive coughing is helped with _____.
4. Medication is delivered in a fine spray by means of a _____.
5. A person who cannot breathe on his or her own may be assisted with breathing by a _____.

Mr. Johnson has COPD. He does not want to take any medications to treat his disease. Explain to Mr. Johnson why it is important to take his medications as ordered.

_____

_____

_____

_____

Abbreviations

ABBREVIATION REVIEW

Abbreviation	Definition
ABG	arterial blood gas
AFB	acid-fast bacillus
ARDS	acute respiratory distress syndrome or adult respiratory distress syndrome
COPD	chronic obstruction pulmonary disease
CPAP	continuous positive airway pressure
LRT	lower respiratory tract
MDI	metered dose inhaler
PFT	pulmonary function test
SIDS	sudden infant death syndrome
SOB	shortness of breath
TB	tuberculosis
URT	upper respiratory tract

UNDERSTAND   **Using abbreviations, rewrite the note.**

The patient was admitted with chronic obstructive pulmonary disease. He was exhibiting severe shortness of breath. Arterial blood gases were abnormal upon admission. Family stated that the patient had been using his nebulizer, metered dose inhaler, and continuous airway pressure machine at home with no result. Past pulmonary function tests were abnormal. No history of tuberculosis. Will continue to monitor for shortness of breath.

_____

_____

_____

_____

CHAPTER SUMMARY

	Learning Outcome	Summary
12.1	Identify the parts of the respiratory system and discuss the function of each part.	The respiratory system is the body's system for breathing.
12.2	Recognize the major word parts used in building words that relate to the respiratory system.	Word building requires knowledge of the combining form and meaning.
12.3	Identify common diagnostic tests, laboratory tests, and clinical procedures used in testing and treating disorders of the respiratory system.	Diagnostic, procedural, and laboratory findings assist the health care provider in diagnosing medical conditions. Often used in combination, these tests lead to a final diagnosis and assist in treatment planning.
12.4	Define the major pathological conditions of the respiratory system.	Respiratory inflammatory conditions are the body's attempt to protect the body from infection and other harmful substances. Inflammation can occur in both the upper and lower respiratory tracts. Breathing disorders can affect the ability of the body to provide adequate oxygenation to the body.
12.5	Explain the meaning of surgical terms related to the respiratory system.	Surgery may be performed on the respiratory system depending upon the disease or condition.
12.6	Recognize common pharmacological agents used in treating disorders of the respiratory system.	Medications may be used to treat symptoms related to infection, cough, and other breathing disorders.
12.7	Identify common abbreviations associated with the respiratory system.	Abbreviations are used to describe diseases, conditions, procedures, and treatments associated with the respiratory system.

Use the following figure to identify the parts of the upper and lower respiratory system.

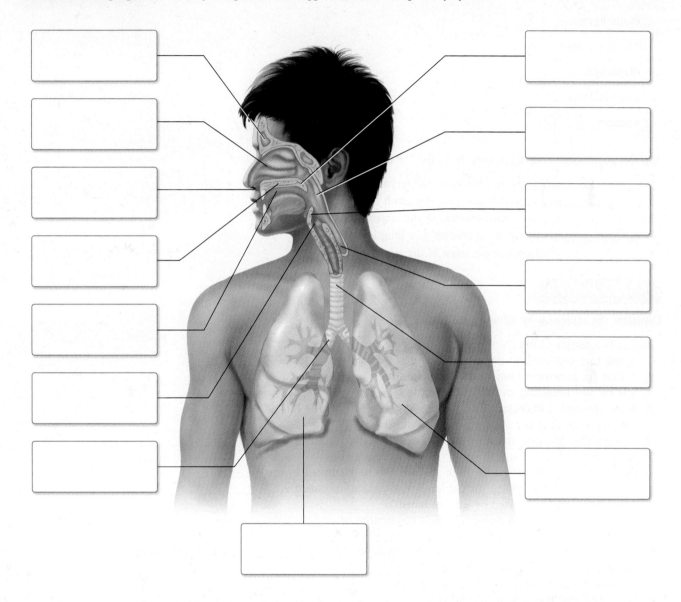

Pronounce the following terms aloud and write their meaning in the space provided.

cystic fibrosis

decongestants

diaphragm

mesothelioma

wheezes

Add the appropriate combining form from the list in this chapter.

1. _____ scopy means viewing of the larynx.
2. _____ gram means a measure of carbon dioxide in expired air.
3. _____ ectomy means removal of the larynx.
4. _____ itis means inflammation of a lung lobe.
5. _____ plegia means paralysis of the larynx.

Complete the sentences by filling in the blanks.

1. The mechanics of breathing are measured by _____ tests.
2. A test that can confirm the presence of cystic fibrosis is called a(n) _____.
3. A tube for viewing a body cavity is called a(n) _____.
4. The highest breathing capacity is called the _____ capacity.
5. A stethoscope is necessary for _____, listening to the lungs.
6. Streptococcal infections can be detected in a(n) _____.
7. Tapping the skin over the lung area to check whether the lungs are clear is called _____.
8. Asthmatics often use a(n) _____ to check breathing capacity.
9. Disease-causing organisms found in sputum can be identified in a(n) _____.
10. A device that measures the lung volume and capacity is called a(n) _____.
11. Any lung condition caused by dust is called _____.
12. Chronic bronchial airway obstruction is a symptom of _____.
13. The sounds heard in atelectasis are _____ or _____.
14. Many respiratory conditions are caused or made worse by _____, an addictive habit.
15. An incision into the chest cavity is a(n) _____.
16. An airway can be provided by an emergency _____.
17. Cancer of the lung may require a(n) _____.
18. Surgically attaching the pleura in place is called _____.

Complete the following sentences.

1. Foreign material comes into the body during _____.
2. Dysphonia is associated with _____.
3. Diphtheria, pertussis, and tuberculosis are all caused by _____.
4. A pleural effusion is _____.
5. Respiratory spasms may cause _____.
6. Bronchospasms occur during _____.
7. _____ can be passed from one person to another.
8. Atelectasis is another name for _____.
9. Inflammation of the voice box is called _____.
10. Hypopnea is abnormally _____ breathing.

DECONSTRUCT

The physician tells the family that the client is on a breathing machine due to chronic obstruction of his bronchial tubes and lungs. The physician states the client is having spasms within his airways and, upon listening to breath sounds, there is absence of airflow from parts of the lung due to a failure of the lung to expand. The physician states that the biggest concern is that the client's heart will fail to pump adequately and that fluid will accumulate in the air sacs and bronchioles.

Using medical terminology, write what the physician has told the family regarding the client.

_____
_____
_____
_____

Reviewing the Terms

Pronounce each of the following terms. Write the definitions on a separate sheet of paper. This review will take you through all the words you learned in this chapter. If you have difficulty with any words, make a flash card for later study. Refer to the English-Spanish and Spanish-English glossaries in the eBook.

Adam's apple
adenoid/o [ĂD-ĕ-noy-dō]
adenoidectomy [ĂD-ĕ-noy-DĔK-tō-mē]
adenoiditis [ĂD-ĕ-noy-DĪ-tĭs]
adenoids [ĂD-ĕ-noydz]
alveol/o [ăl-VĒ-ō-lō]
alveolus (pl., alveoli) [ăl-VĒ-ō-lŭs (ăl-VĒ-ō-lī)]
anthracosis [ăn-thră-KŌ-sĭs]
antitussives [ăn-tē-TŬS-sĭvs]
apex [Ā-pĕks]
apnea [ĂP-nē-ă]
arterial [ăr-TĒR-ē-ăl] blood gases (ABGs)
asbestosis [ăs-bĕs-TŌ-sĭs]
asthma [ĂZ-mă]
atelectasis [ăt-ĕ-LĔK-tă-sĭs]

auscultation [ăws-kŭl-TĀ-shŭn]
bacilli (sing., bacillus) [bă-SĬL-ī (bă-SĬL-ŭs)]
base [bās]
black lung
bradypnea [brăd-ĭp-NĒ-ă]
bronch/o, bronchi/o [BRŎNG-kō, BRŎNG-kē-ō]
bronchial alveolar lavage [BRŎNG-kē-ăl ăl-VĒ-ō-lăr lă-VĂZH]
bronchial brushing
bronchiol/o [brŏng-KĒ-ō-lō]
bronchiole [BRŎNG-kē-ōl]
bronchitis [brŏng-KĪ-tĭs]
bronchodilators [brŏng-kō-dī-LĀ-tŏrz]
bronchography [brŏng-KŎG-ră-fē]
bronchoplasty [BRŎNG-kō-plăs-tē]

bronchoscope [BRŎNG-kō-skōp]

bronchospasm [BRŎNG-kō-spăzm]

bronchus (pl., bronchi) [BRŎNG-kŭs (BRŎNG-kī)]

capn/o [KĂP-nō]

Cheyne-Stokes respiration [chān stōks rĕs-pĭ-RĀ-shŭn]

chronic bronchitis

chronic obstructive pulmonary disease (COPD)

cilia [SĬL-ē-ă]

crackles [KRĂK-lz]

croup [krūp]

cystic fibrosis [SĬS-tĭk fī-BRŌ-sĭs]

decongestants [dē-kŏn-JĔST-ănts]

diaphragm [DĬ-ă-frăm]

diphtheria [dĭf-THĔR-ē-ă]

dysphonia [dĭs-FŌ-nē-ă]

dyspnea [dĭsp-NĒ-ă, DĬSP-nē-ă]

emphysema [ĕm-fă-SĒ-mă, ĕm-fă-ZĒ-mă]

empyema [ĕm-pī-Ē-mă]

endoscope [ĔN-dō-skōp]

endotracheal intubation (ET) [ĔN-dō-TRĀ-kē-ăl ĭn-tū-BĀ-shŭn]

epiglott/o [ĕp-ĭ-GLŎT-ō]

epiglottis [ĕp-ĭ-GLŎT-ĭs]

epiglottitis [ĕp-ĭ-glŏt-Ī-tĭs]

epistaxis [ĔP-ĭ-STĂK-sĭs]

eupnea [yūp-NĒ-ă]

exhalation [ĕks-hă-LĀ-shŭn]

expectorants [ĕk-SPĔK-tō-rănts]

expiration [ĕks-pĭ-RĀ-shŭn]

external nares [NĀR-ēz]

external respiration

glottis [GLŎT-ĭs]

hemoptysis [hē-MŎP-tĭ-sĭs]

hemothorax [hē-mō-THŌR-ăks]

hilum [HĪ-lŭm]

hilus [HĪ-lŭs]

hypercapnia [hī-pĕr-KĂP-nē-ă]

hyperpnea [hī-pĕrp-NĒ-ă]

hyperventilation [HĪ-pĕr-vĕn-tĭ-LĀ-shŭn]

hypopnea [hī-PŎP-nē-ă]

hypoventilation [HĪ-pō-ven-tĭ-LĀ-shŭn]

hypoxemia [hī-pŏk-SĒ-mē-ă]

hypoxia [hī-PŎK-sē-ă]

inferior lobe [ĭn-FĒ-rē-ōr lōb]

inhalation [ĭn-hă-LĀ-shŭn]

inspiration [ĭn-spĭ-RĀ-shŭn]

intercostal muscles [ĭn-tĕr-KŎS-tăl MŬS-ĕlz]

internal respiration

laryng/o [lă-RĬNG-gō]

laryngectomy [LĂR-ĭn-JĔK-tō-mē]

laryngitis [lăr-ĭn-JĪ-tĭs]

laryngocentesis [lă-RĬNG-gō-sĕn-TĒ-sĭs]

laryngopharynx [lă-RĬNG-gō-făr-ĭngks]

laryngoplasty [lă-RĬNG-gō-plăs-tē]

laryngoscopy [LĂR-ĭng-GŎS-kō-pē]

laryngospasm [lă-RĬNG-gō-spăzm]

laryngostomy [LĂR-ĭng-GŎS-tō-mē]

laryngotracheobronchitis [lă-RĬNG-gō-TRĀ-kē-ō-brŏng-KĪ-tĭs]

laryngotracheotomy [lă-RĬNG-gō-trā-kē-ŎT-ō-mē]

larynx [LĂR-ĭngks]

lob/o [LŌ-bō]

lobectomy [lō-BĔK-tō-mē]

lung [lŭng]

mediastin/o [MĒ-dē-ăs-TĪ-nō]

mediastinoscopy [MĒ-dē-ăs-tĭ-NŎS-kō-pē]

mediastinum [MĒ-dē-ăs-TĪ-nŭm]

mesothelioma [MĔZ-ō-thē-lē-Ō-mă]

middle lobe

nas/o [NĀ-zō]

nasal cavity [NĀ-zăl KĂV-ĭ-tē]

nasal septum [SĔP-tŭm]

nasopharyngitis [NĀ-zō-făr-ĭn-JĪ-tĭs]

nasopharyngoscopy [NĀ-zō-fă-rĭng-GŎS-kō-pē]

nasopharynx [NĀ-zō-FĂR-ĭngks]

nebulizers [NĔB-yū-līz-ĕrz]

nose [nōz]

nosebleed

nostrils [NŎS-trĭlz]

or/o [ŌR-ō]

oropharynx [ŌR-ō-FĂR-ĭngks]

orthopnea [ōr-thŏp-NĒ-ă, ōr-THŎP-nē-ă]

otorhinolaryngologist [Ō-tō-RĪ-nō-lăr-ĭng-GŎL-ō-jĭst]

ox/o, oxi-, oxy- [ŎK-sō, ŎK-sĭ, ŎK-sē]

palatine tonsils [PĂL-ă-tīn TŎN-sĭlz]

pansinusitis [păn-sī-nŭ-SĪ-tĭs]

parietal pleura [pă-RĪ-ĕ-tăl PLŪR-ă]

paroxysmal [păr-ŏk-SĬZ-măl]

peak flow meter

percussion [pĕr-KŬSH-ŭn]

pertussis [pĕr-TŬS-ĭs]

pharyng/o [fă-RĬNG-gō]

pharyngeal tonsils [fă-RĬN-jē-ăl TŎN-sĭlz]

pharyngitis [făr-ĭn-JĪ-tĭs]

pharynx [FĂR-ĭngks]

phon/o [FŌ-nō]

phren/o [FRĔN-ō]

pleur/o [PLŪR-ō]

pleura (pl., pleurae) [PLŪR-ă (PLŪR-ē)]

pleural cavity [PLŪR-ăl KĂV-ĭ-tē]

pleural effusion [PLŪR-ăl ĕ-FYŪ-zhŭn]

pleuritis, pleurisy [plū-RĪ-tĭs, PLŪR-ĭ-sē]

pleurocentesis [PLŪR-ō-sĕn-TĒ-sĭs]

pneum/o [NŪ-mō]

pneumon/o [nū-MŌ-nō]

pneumobronchotomy [NŪ-mō-brŏng-KŎT-ō-mē]

pneumoconiosis [NŪ-mō-kō-nē-Ō-sĭs]

pneumonectomy [NŪ-mō-NĔK-tō-mē]

pneumonia [nū-MŌ-nē-ă]

pneumonitis [nū-mō-NĪ-tĭs]

pneumothorax [nū-mō-THŌR-ăks]

pulmonary abscess [PŬL-mō-nār-ē ĂB-sĕs]

pulmonary edema [PŬL-mō-nār-ē ĕ-DĒ-mă]

pulmonary function tests

rales [răhlz]

respiratory [RĔS-pĭ-ră-tōr-ē, rĕ-SPĪR-ă-tōr-ē] system

respiratory tract

rhin/o [RĪ-nō]

rhinitis [rī-NĪ-tĭs]

rhinoplasty [RĪ-nō-plăs-tē]

rhinorrhea [rīn-nō-RĒ-ă]

rhonchi [RŎNG-kī]

septoplasty [SĔP-tō-plăs-tē]

septostomy [sĕp-TŎS-tō-mē]

septum [SĔP-tŭm]

severe acute respiratory syndrome (SARS)

silicosis [sĭl-ĭ-KŌ-sĭs]

sinusitis [sī-nŭ-SĪ-tĭs]

sinusotomy [sīn-ŭ-SŎT-ō-mē]

soft palate [sŏft PĂL-ăt]

spir/o [SPĪ-rō]

spirometer [spī-RŎM-ĕ-tĕr]

sputum [SPŪ-tŭm] sample or culture

steth/o [STĔTH-ō]

stridor [STRĪ-dōr]

superior lobe

sweat test

tachypnea [tăk-ĭp-NĒ-ă]

thorac/o [THŌR-ă-kō]

thoracic [thō-RĂS-ĭk] surgeon

thoracentesis [THŌR-ă-sĕn-TĒ-sĭs]

thoracostomy [thōr-ă-KŎS-tō-mē]

thoracotomy [thōr-ă-KŎT-ō-mē]

thorax [THŌ-răks]

throat [thrōt]

throat culture

thyroid cartilage [THĪ-royd KĂR-tĭ-lĭj]

tonsill/o [TŎN-sĭ-lō]

tonsillectomy [TŎN-sĭ-LĔK-tō-mē]

tonsillitis [TŎN-sĭ-LĪ-tĭs]

trache/o [TRĀ-kē-ō]

trachea [TRĀ-kē-ă]

tracheitis [trā-kē-Ī-tĭs]

tracheoplasty [TRĀ-kē-ō-plăs-tē]

tracheostomy [TRĀ-kē-ŎS-tō-mē]

tracheotomy [trā-kē-ŎT-ō-mē]

tuberculosis [tū-bĕr-kyū-LŌ-sĭs]

upper respiratory infection

ventilators [VĔN-tĭ-lā-tŏrz]

visceral pleura [VĬS-ĕr-ăl PLŪR-ă]

vocal cords

voice box

wheezes [HWĒZ-ĕz]

whooping cough [HŎOP-ĭng kăwf]

windpipe

CHAPTER 13

The Lymphatic System and Body Defense

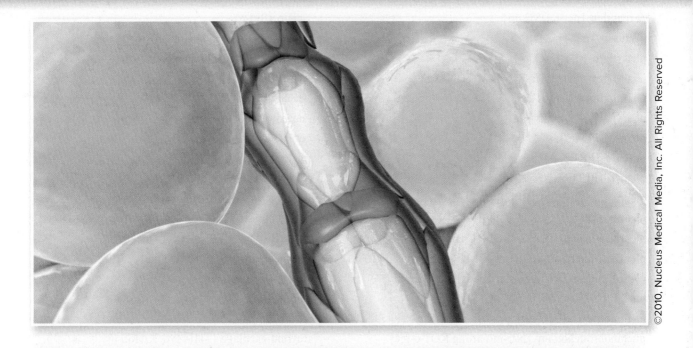

Learning Outcomes

After studying this chapter, you will be able to:

13.1 Identify the parts of the lymphatic and immune systems and discuss the function of each part.

13.2 Recognize the major word parts used in building words that relate to the lymphatic and immune systems.

13.3 Identify the common diagnostic tests, laboratory tests, and clinical procedures used in testing and treating disorders of the lymphatic and immune systems.

13.4 Define the major pathological conditions of the lymphatic and immune systems.

13.5 Explain the meaning of surgical terms related to the lymphatic and immune systems.

13.6 Recognize common pharmacological agents used in treating disorders of the lymphatic and immune systems.

13.7 Identify common abbreviations associated with the lymphatic and immune systems.

LO 13.1 Structure and Function of the Lymphatic and Immune Systems

The lymphatic and immune systems share some of the same structures and functions. The immune system uses other systems to maintain its functions. Both the lymphatic and immune systems contain the lymph nodes, spleen, thymus gland, and some of the disease-fighting immune cells. The lymphatic system provides the location to gather and concentrate foreign substances present in the body so that lymphocytes circulating through the lymphatic organs and vessels are able to destroy and remove them.

The lymphatic system has the following functions:

- It reduces tissue edema by removing fluid from capillary beds.
- It returns the proteins from the fluids to the blood.
- It traps and filters cellular debris, such as cancer cells and microbes, with the help of cells called macrophages.
- It recycles body fluid to various parts of the body.
- It circulates lymphocytes to assist with the immune response.
- It moves fats from the gastrointestinal (GI) tract to the blood.

The immune system is the body's defense system and has the following functions:

1. It protects the body against foreign body invasion.
2. In normal function, it coordinates activities in the blood, body tissues, and the lymphatic system to protect the body from foreign body invasion.
3. It fights off infections and protects against future infections by producing a variety of immune responses.
4. It produces antibodies (immunoglobulins).

Figure 13-1 shows the major location of lymph nodes. Figure 13-2 shows how lymph circulates throughout the body. Figure 13-3 illustrates the lymphatic vessels and capillaries. Figure 13-4 shows a lymph node. Figure 13-5 shows the location of the spleen and thymus.

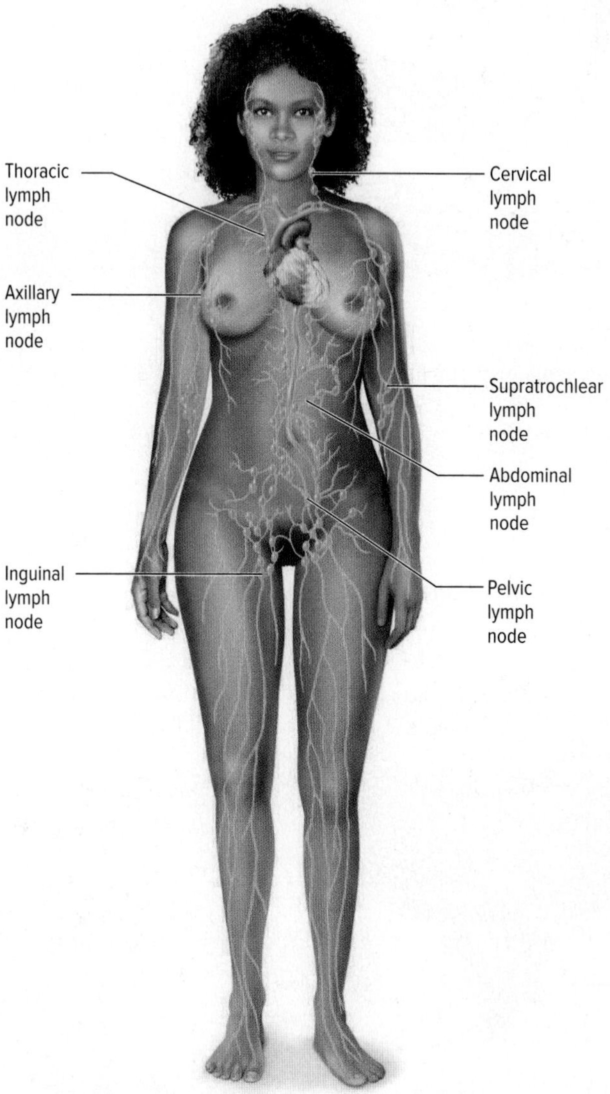

Thoracic lymph node

Axillary lymph node

Inguinal lymph node

Cervical lymph node

Supratrochlear lymph node

Abdominal lymph node

Pelvic lymph node

Figure 13-1 Location of lymph nodes

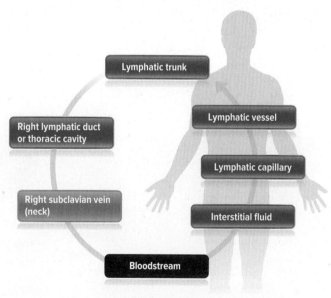

Lymphatic trunk

Right lymphatic duct or thoracic cavity

Lymphatic vessel

Lymphatic capillary

Right subclavian vein (neck)

Interstitial fluid

Bloodstream

Figure 13-2 Lymph circulation throughout the body

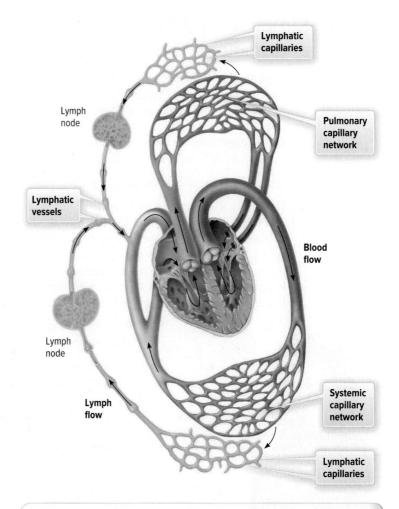

Lymphatic capillaries

Lymph node

Pulmonary capillary network

Lymphatic vessels

Blood flow

Lymph node

Systemic capillary network

Lymph flow

Lymphatic capillaries

Figure 13-3 Lymphatic vessels and capillaries

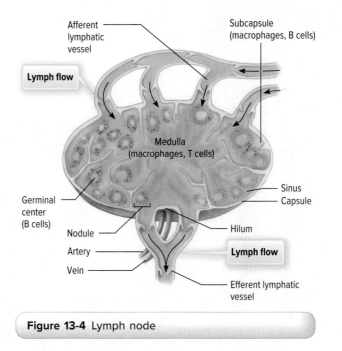

Afferent lymphatic vessel

Subcapsule (macrophages, B cells)

Lymph flow

Medulla (macrophages, T cells)

Germinal center (B cells)

Sinus

Capsule

Nodule

Hilum

Artery

Lymph flow

Vein

Efferent lymphatic vessel

Figure 13-4 Lymph node

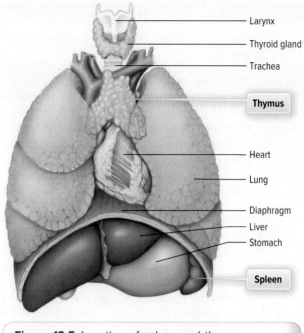

Larynx

Thyroid gland

Trachea

Thymus

Heart

Lung

Diaphragm

Liver

Stomach

Spleen

Figure 13-5 Location of spleen and thymus

Lymphatic Organs and Structures

The lymphatic system is similar to both the cardiovascular and blood systems in that it involves a network of vessels that transports fluid around the body. The liquid part of the blood, plasma, has the ability to leave the blood capillaries and enter the cellular areas of the body. Once plasma leaves the vascular system, it is known as interstitial fluid. This interstitial fluid provides nutrients and performs other functions in the exchange of fluids to and from the cells. The lymphatic system serves as a drainage system to remove fluid from the cellular areas. It concentrates foreign substances to assist the immune system. Figure 13-6 shows how lymph enters and leaves a lymph node through lymphatic vessels. The lymphatic system consists of the following:

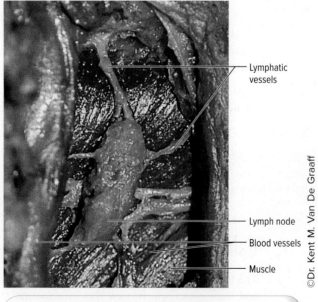

Lymphatic vessels

Lymph node

Blood vessels

Muscle

©Dr. Kent M. Van De Graaff

Figure 13-6 Lymph enters and leaves a lymph node through lymphatic vessels

lymph [lĭmf]	Fluid that contains white blood cells and other substances and flows in the lymphatic vessels.
lymphatic **pathways** [lĭm-FĂD-ĭk PARH-wā] **lymphatic vessels**	The vessels that transport lymph (the fluid of the lymphatic system) around the body. The smallest parts of these pathways are the *microscopic capillaries* located in the capillary beds of the body. The capillary beds are thin-walled vessels that receive fluid and debris from the bloodstream. Once inside the beds, the fluid is known as lymph. The lymph travels throughout the lymphatic vessels in one direction only—back toward the heart. Lymphatic vessels contain valves that prevent backflow of lymph. As the vessels approach the heart, they carry more fluid and are larger in size. Figure 13-2 illustrates the flow of lymph through the body.
lymph node	Specialized organ that filters harmful substances from the tissues and assists in the immune response. The lymph passes through many lymph nodes for filtering so that it is ready for transferring back to the vascular system. By the time the fluid reaches the thoracic cavity, it has been filtered many times. The lymph nodes contain special cells (macrophages) that devour foreign substances. Lymph nodes become swollen with *lymphocytes* (lymph cells) and macrophages. Lymph nodes are located throughout the body except in the central nervous system. They are quite numerous near the joints of the body. The major groups of lymph nodes are located in the throat (the tonsils and adenoids are actually lymph tissue), neck, axilla (armpit), mediastinum, and groin.
spleen [splēn]	Organ of lymph system that filters and stores blood, removes old red blood cells, and activates lymphocytes. The largest lymphatic organ, it is located in the upper left portion of the abdominal cavity, where, unfortunately, it easily can be injured and ruptured. In such cases, it must be repaired or removed (its functions are taken over by the lymph nodes, liver, and bone marrow). The function of the spleen is to filter foreign material from the blood, store blood, remove damaged or old red blood cells, and activate lymphocytes that destroy some of the foreign substances filtered from the blood (see Figure 13-5). The spleen is important not only to the lymphatic system, but also to the circulatory system; its association with the circulatory system is similar to the association of the lymph node to the lymphatic system. The spleen is also a major site for immunoglobulin (antibody) production by *B lymphocytes* that have differentiated into antibody-producing plasma cells.
thymus gland [THĪ-mŭs glănd]	Soft gland with two lobes that is involved in immune responses; located in mediastinum. It is large during infancy and early childhood when immunity is most crucial, but gradually shrinks until it becomes connective tissue in adulthood (when the body has acquired other types of immunities).
T cells (T lymphocytes)	Specialized white blood cells that receive markers in the thymus, are responsible for cellular immunity, and assist with humoral immunity.
B lymphocytes (B cells) [LĬM-fō-sīts]	A kind of lymphocyte that manufactures antibodies.
thymosin [THĪ-mō-sĭn]	Hormone secreted by the thymus gland that aids in distribution of thymocytes (T lymphocytes) and lymphocytes.

Building Your Lymphatic and Immune Vocabulary

The following sections provide an introduction to basic lymph and immune combining terms and their meanings. Review this information prior to moving to the practices.

Combining Form	Meaning
aden/o	gland
immun/o	immunity
lymph/o	lymph
lymphaden/o	lymph nodes
lymphangi/o	lymphatic vessels
splen/o	spleen
thym/o	thymus
tox/o, toxi-, toxico-	poison

Structure and Function

PRACTICE

Provide the missing term(s) to complete the following sentences.

lymph [lĭmf]	The *lymphatic pathways* are the vessels that transport _____ (the fluid of the lymphatic system) around the body.
lymph nodes	Located along the lymphatic vessels are the _____, small lumps of lymphatic tissue that serve as collecting points to filter the lymph.
spleen [splēn]	The largest lymphatic organ, the _____, is located in the upper left portion of the abdominal cavity, where, unfortunately, it easily can be injured and ruptured.
thymus gland [THĪ-mŭs glănd] **T lymphocytes** [LĬM-fō-sīts] **T cells** **B lymphocytes** [LĬM-fō-sīts] **B cells** **thymosin** [THĪ-mō-sĭn]	The _____ is a two-lobed, soft gland located in the thoracic cavity. The thymus gland contains a high number of _____, or _____, and a decreased number of _____, or _____. After being produced in the bone marrow, some of the lymphocytes (immature T cells) migrate through the thymus gland, where they acquire the marker that identifies them as T lymphocytes. Other lymphocytes become B cells. T cells provide immunity after they leave the thymus. Their movement is aided by _____, a hormone secreted by the thymus.

PRONOUNCE and DEFINE

Pronounce the following terms aloud and write their meaning in the space provided.

spleen	[splēn]
lymph	[lĭmf]

1. _____ T cells
2. _____ lymph node
3. _____ B lymphocytes
4. _____ thymosin

a. Manufacture antibodies
b. Aids in distribution of thymocytes and lymphocytes
c. Filters toxins
d. Aid in cellular and humoral immunity

APPLY   **Read the following scenario and respond accordingly.**

You are doing a presentation on the structure and function of the lymphatic system. Explain it in a method that everyone can understand.

_____

_____

_____

The Immune System

The immune system relies on several other systems to accomplish its duties. The *reticuloendothelial system (RES)*, hematopoietic system, *mononuclear phagocytic system* (or *phagocytic system*), and *lymphoid system* play significant roles in the functions of the immune system. The hematopoietic system is responsible for the production of the blood cells in the bone marrow. The blood cells include the erythrocytes (red blood cells), leukocytes (white blood cells), and thrombocytes (platelets). The immune system shares several parts with the lymphatic system (lymph nodes, spleen, and thymus gland). These parts serve as defense mechanisms protecting the body. Parts of other systems, such as the skin and tonsils, also play an important role in protecting the body from disease. The immune system of the body consists of all the processes that perform a series of defenses to protect from and respond to disease. Figure 13-7 depicts a cross section of the spleen.

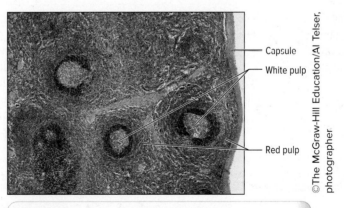

Capsule
White pulp
Red pulp

©The McGraw-Hill Education/Al Telser, photographer

Figure 13-7 The spleen resembles a large lymph node

STUDY TIP

After answering all of the questions, review the ones that you missed and write the correct spelling of the terms.

Structure and Function	PRACTICE
	Provide the missing term(s) to complete the following sentences.

lymphocytes
[LĬM-fō-sīts]

macrophages
[MĂK-rō-fāj-ĕz]

microphages
[MĬK-rō-fāj-ĕz]

phagocytosis
[FĂG-ō-sī-TŌ-sĭs]

The leukocytes include _____, monocytes, and granulocytes (*polymorphonucleated cells* or *PMN*). The RES and phagocytic systems provide the phagocytes of the tissues and the phagocytes of the blood that are called _____ and _____. Phagocytes remove foreign particles from the body by the process of _____, the internalization or "eating" of the particles and the digestion of the particles for presentation to the appropriate cells of the immune system. The immune response is divided into two kinds: the *cellular response* and the *humoral* or *immunoglobulin (antibody) response*.

antibodies
[ĂN-tē-bŏd-ēz]

The B cells are responsible for the production of _____ (also called immunoglobulins), that is, the humoral response.

pathogens
[PĂTH-ō-jĕnz]

The human body includes a number of mechanical, chemical, and other defenses against disease. When disease-causing agents, _____, try to enter the body, they often are stopped by the skin, the cilia in the nostrils, and various mucous membranes—all of which are mechanical barriers to intrusion.

antigens
[ĂN-tĭ-jĕnz]

In the bloodstream, certain substances called _____ may provoke an immune response to certain diseases.

PRONOUNCE and DEFINE	Pronounce the following words aloud and write their meaning in the space provided.
antibodies	[ĂN-tē-bŏd-ēz]
pathogens	[PĂTH-ō-jĕnz]
lymphocytes	[LĬM-fō-sīts]

SPELL and DEFINE	Identify if the following terms are spelled correctly. Correct the words that are spelled incorrectly. Write the definition for each word.

	Spelling	Definition
fagocytosis		
macrofages		
lymphocytes		

UNDERSTAND	Fill in the blanks.

1. The special cells that ingest foreign substances are called _____.
2. A pathogen is _____.
3. The tonsils and skin serve to _____ from disease.
4. The T cells signal the B cells to _____.

The body has just been invaded by a foreign substance. Describe what happens.

_____

_____

_____

_____

The Immune Process

Structure and Function	PRACTICE — Provide the missing term(s) to complete the following sentences.
immunity [ĭ-MYŪ-nĭ-tē]	Mechanical or chemical defenses work together to avert or attack disease. In addition, the body has specific defenses of the immune system called _____ that provide resistance to particular pathogens. There are three major types of immunity: natural immunity, acquired active immunity, and acquired passive immunity.
	Natural Immunity
natural immunity	_____ is the human body's natural resistance to certain diseases.
	Acquired Active Immunity
acquired active immunity **immunization** [ĬM-yū-nĭ-ZĀ-shŭn] **vaccination** [VĂK-sĭ-NĀ-shŭn] **antigen** [ĂN-tĭ-jĕn] **vaccine** [văk-SĒN, VĂK-sēn]	The body develops _____ either by having a disease and producing natural antibodies to it or by being vaccinated against the disease. _____ or _____ is the injection of an _____, a substance that provokes an immune response from an organism that causes active immunity via the production of antibodies. This substance is called a _____.
humoral immunity [HYŪ-mōr-ăl ĭ-MYŪ-nĭ-tē] **plasma cells** [PLĂZ-mă sĕlz] **immunoglobulins** [ĬM-yū-nō-GLŎB-yū-lĭnz]	Acquired active immunity is further divided into two types. The first, _____, is immunity provided by _____, which produce antibodies called _____. There are five major types of immunoglobulins: • _Immunoglobulin G (IgG)_ is effective against bacteria, viruses, and toxins. • _Immunoglobulin A (IgA)_ is common in exocrine gland secretions, such as breast milk, tears, nasal fluid, and gastric juice. IgA transfers immunity from mother to infant through breast milk. • _Immunoglobulin M (IgM)_ develops in the blood plasma in response to certain antigens within the body or from foreign sources. It is the first antibody to be produced after infection. • _Immunoglobulin D (IgD)_ is important in B-cell activation, which helps immunity by transforming itself into a plasma cell in the presence of a specific type of antigen. • _Immunoglobulin E (IgE)_ appears in glandular secretions and is associated with allergic reactions.

cell-mediated immunity interferons [ĭn-tĕr-FĒR-ŏnz] interleukins [ĭn-tĕr-LŪ-kĭnz]	The second type of acquired active immunity, or _____, is provided by the action of T cells. The T cells respond to antigens by multiplying rapidly and producing proteins called lymphokines (e.g., _____ and _____) that have antiviral properties or properties that affect the actions of other cells in the body. T cells also produce substances to stimulate B cells to differentiate into plasma cells and to produce antibodies.
helper cells cytotoxic cells [sī-tō-TŎK-sĭk sĕlz] suppressor cells [sŭ-PRĔS-ōr sĕlz]	Three types of other specialized T cells are • _____ or CD4 cells that stimulate the immune response. • _____ or CD8 cells that help in the destruction of infected cells. • _____ or T cells (mainly CD8 and some CD4) that suppress B cells and other immune cells.
Acquired Passive Immunity	
acquired passive immunity antitoxin [ăn-tē-TŎK-sĭn] gamma globulin [GĂ-mă GLŎB-yū-lĭn]	_____ is immunity provided in the form of antibodies or antitoxins that have been developed in another person or another species. Acquired passive immunity is necessary in cases of snakebite and tetanus or any problem where immediate immunity is needed. In such cases, a dose of _____ (antibody directed against specific toxins) is given to provide antibodies. Passive immunity also may be administered to lessen the chance of catching a disease or to lessen the severity of the course of the disease. _____ is a preparation of collected antibodies given to prevent or lessen certain diseases, such as hepatitis A, varicella, and rabies.

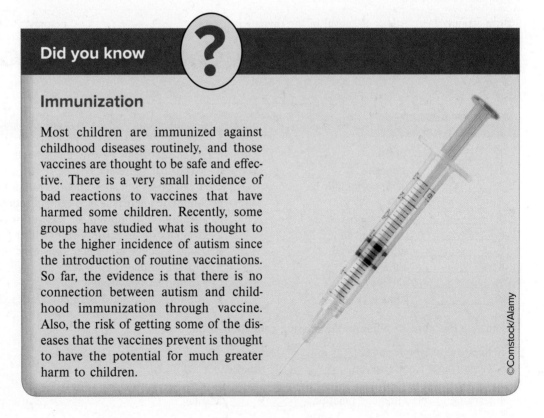

Did you know ?

Immunization

Most children are immunized against childhood diseases routinely, and those vaccines are thought to be safe and effective. There is a very small incidence of bad reactions to vaccines that have harmed some children. Recently, some groups have studied what is thought to be the higher incidence of autism since the introduction of routine vaccinations. So far, the evidence is that there is no connection between autism and childhood immunization through vaccine. Also, the risk of getting some of the diseases that the vaccines prevent is thought to have the potential for much greater harm to children.

©Comstock/Alamy

Word Building in the Lymphatic
and Immune Systems

Word Building	**PRACTICE**
	Provide the correct combining form to complete the following sentences.
splen-ectomy [splē-NEK-tō-mē]	_____ ectomy is removal of the spleen.
immuno-suppressor [ĬM-yū-nō-sŭ-PRĔS-ōr]	An agent that suppresses the immune response is an _____ suppressor.
lymphang-itis [lĭm-fan-JĪ-tĭs]	Inflammation of the lymphatic vessels is _____ itis.
adeno-carcinoma [ĂD-ĕ-nō-kar-sĭ-NŌ-mă]	Glandular cancer is _____ carcinoma.
lympho-cyte [LĬM-fō-sīt]	A _____ cyte is a white blood cell associated with the immune response.
toxi-cosis [tŏk-sĭ-KŌ-sĭs]	Systemic poisoning is _____ cosis.
lymphadeno-pathy [lĭm-făd-ĕ-NOP-ă-thē]	_____ pathy is a disease affecting the lymph nodes.
thym-ectomy [thī-MĔK-tō-mē]	Removal of the thymus is a _____ ectomy.

UNDERSTAND	Match each term in the left column with its correct definition in the right column.

1. _____ T cell
2. _____ pathogen
3. _____ immunoglobulin E
4. _____ IgD
5. _____ helper cell
6. _____ cytotoxic cell
7. _____ suppressor cell
8. _____ antitoxin
9. _____ antibody
10. _____ gamma globulin

a. T cell that helps destroy foreign cells or substances
b. T cell that supresses B cells
c. T cell that stimulates immune response
d. Antibody important in B-cell activation
e. Agent given to prevent or lessen disease
f. Lymphocyte associated with cellular immunity
g. Helps produce immediate resistance to a disease or a poison
h. Protein produced by B cells that fight foreign cells
i. Disease-causing agent
j. Antibody associated with allergic reaction

Complete the word by filling in the missing combining form.

1. Removal of lymph nodes: _____ ectomy
2. Hemorrhage from a spleen: _____ rrhagia
3. Tumor of the thymus: _____ oma
4. Lacking in some immune function: _____ deficient
5. Cell of a gland: _____ cyte
6. Skin disease caused by a poison: _____ derma
7. Dilation of the lymphatic vessels: _____ ectasis
8. Resembling lymph: _____ oid

Some hospitals are part of large university complexes. These hospitals often do many kinds of research and offer tertiary care, medical care at a center that has a unit specializing in certain diseases. They may provide data on drug trials. They may work on improving diagnostic testing. Some research is focused on diseases that are infectious and for which there is not yet a cure. The goal of many studies is to produce a vaccine.

1. Why would researchers want to produce a vaccine?

_____

_____

2. What form of immunity might a vaccination provide?

_____

_____

LO 13.3 Diagnostic, Procedural, and Laboratory Terms

Diagnostic, procedural, and laboratory findings assist in the diagnosing of medical conditions. Often used in combination, these tests can lead to a final diagnosis and assist in treatment planning. Figure 13-8 shows a lymphangiogram of the lymphatic vessels and lymph nodes of the pelvic region. Figure 13-9 shows a scanning electron micrograph of a circulating lymphocyte.

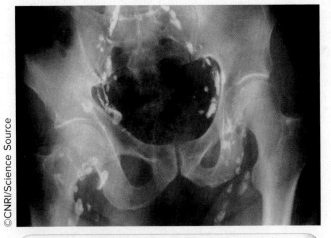

Figure 13-8 A lymphangiogram of the lymphatic vessels and lymph nodes of the pelvic region

©CNRI/Science Source

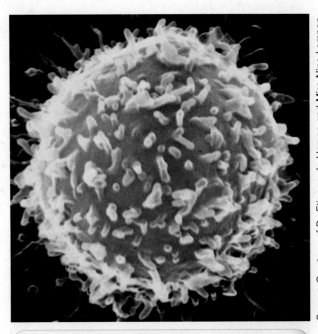

Figure 13-9 Falsely colored scanning electron micrograph of a circulating lymphocyte.

Source: Courtesy of Dr. Etienne de Harven and Miss Nina Lampen, from the Sloan-Kettering Institute for Cancer Research

PRACTICE

Provide the missing term(s) to complete the following sentences.

enzyme-linked immunosorbent assay (ELISA) or enzyme immunoassay (EIA) [ĬM-yū-nō-SŌR-bent, ĕ-LĪ-ză, ĕ-LĪ-să] [ĬM-yū-nō-ĂS-ā, ĭm-YŪ-nō-ĂS-ā] **Western blot**	Abnormalities of lymph organs can be checked in a CAT scan. Several blood tests that indicate the number and condition of white blood cells are used in diagnosing lymph and immune systems diseases. Human immunodeficiency virus (HIV) infection is diagnosed mainly with two blood serum tests: _____ and _____. ELISA tests blood for the antibody to the HIV virus (as well as antibodies to other specific viruses, such as hepatitis B) and the Western blot is a confirming test for the presence of HIV antibodies. A diagnosis of acquired immune deficiency syndrome (AIDS) is made based on the presence of opportunistic infections and T-cell counts in specified ranges.
	Allergy tests are performed by an allergist. Tests usually consist of some form of exposure to a small amount of the suspected allergen to see if a reaction occurs. Now there are even home allergy tests available that can detect allergies by testing a small amount of blood.

UNDERSTAND

Complete the following sentences.

1. The ELISA tests for _____.
2. A Western blot determines if _____ is present.
3. An analysis of _____ blood cells can help diagnose lymph and immune system diseases.

LO 13.4 Pathological Terms

Diseases of the lymph and immune systems include diseases that attack lymph tissue itself, diseases that are spread through the lymphatic pathways, and diseases that flourish because of a suppression of the immune response. Disorders of the lymph and immune systems can be caused by an overly vigorous response to an immune system invader. This is the case with some diseases of other body systems, such as multiple sclerosis, in which the immune system attacks some of the nervous system's protective covering, myelin. Figure 13-10 shows the human immunodeficiency virus (HIV). Figure 13-11 shows T- and B-cell activation. Figure 13-12 is a photograph of Kaposi sarcoma.

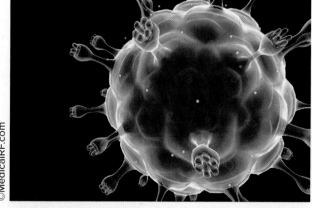

©MedicalRF.com

Figure 13-10 The human immunodeficiency virus (HIV)

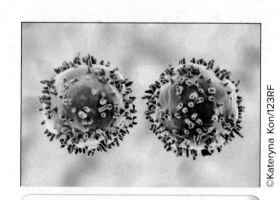

©Kateryna Kon/123RF

Figure 13-11 T- and B-cell activation

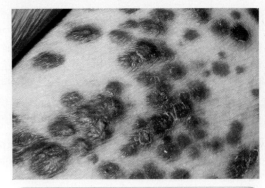

Figure 13-12 Kaposi sarcoma

Pathological	**PRACTICE** Provide the missing term(s) to complete the following sentences.
allergy [ĂL-ĕr-jē]	A(n) _____ is an immune overresponse to a stimulus.
human immunodeficiency virus (HIV) [ĬM-yū-nō-dē-FĬSH-ĕn-sē VĪ-rŭs]	The most widespread virus that attacks the immune system is the _____, a virus spread by sexual contact, exchange of bodily fluids, or intravenous exposure. A person may be *HIV positive,* meaning that the person carries HIV, but has not yet come down with HIV infections (diseases that tend to occur in HIV-positive people) or has not been given a diagnosis of AIDS. Many people are HIV positive without knowing it; only a test can make that diagnosis when there are no symptoms.
AIDS [ādz] **acquired immunodeficiency syndrome** [ĬM-yū-nō-dē-FĬSH-ĕn-sē] **immunosuppressive disease** [ĬM-yū-nō-sŭ-PRĔS-ĭv di-ZĒZ] **retrovirus** [rĕ-trō-VĪ-rŭs]	_____ or _____ is the most widespread _____, a disease that suppresses the ability of the immune system to defend against infection. AIDS is a complex of symptoms caused by HIV, which is a type of _____, a ribonucleic acid (RNA) that causes reversal of normal cell copying. The word part *retro-* ("reverse") refers to its being the opposite of the ordinary method of DNA copying itself onto RNA.
opportunistic infections [ŏp-pōr-tū-NĬS-tĭk in-FEK-shŭnz]	AIDS patients are subject to a number of _____, infections that a healthy immune system can easily fight off but that take hold because of the lowered immune response. Many of these infections are present in other body systems. Table 13-1 lists some opportunistic infections commonly present in AIDS patients and the parts of the body affected. AIDS affects the entire body, with diseases such as herpes, candidiasis, and Kaposi's sarcoma appearing on the skin and *Pneumocystis carinii* (proposed new name *Pneumocystis jiroveci*) pneumonia (PCP) appearing in the lungs. Opportunistic infections also attack the immune systems of people with immunosuppressive disorders other than AIDS. Any recipient of an organ transplant must take immunosuppressive drugs to avoid organ rejection. These drugs leave the patient open to opportunistic infections. There are a number of other immunosuppressive disorders. Some are congenital and may be inherited. Others are a result of disease; for example, a severe case of diabetes can weaken the immune system.

1. Allergies involve a(n) _____ response.
2. Multiple sclerosis is a disease in which the _____ attack some of the body's cells.
3. AIDS is a disease of the _____ system.

APPLY   **Read the following scenario and respond accordingly.**

Mrs. Jones was diagnosed with AIDS approximately 6 months ago. She now presents with PCP and herpes. She states she does not understand how she got these infections as she has been working hard to stay healthy. Explain to Mrs. Jones why these infections occur.

_____

_____

TABLE 13-1	Opportunistic Malignancies and Infections That Often Accompany AIDS	
Opportunistic Infection	**Type of Malignancy or Infection**	**Areas Affected**
candidiasis	caused by the fungus *Candida albicans*	digestive tract, respiratory tract, skin, and some reproductive organs (particularly the vagina)
cytomegalovirus	Herpesviridae	can infect various cells or organs (e.g., the eyes); causes swelling
Kaposi sarcoma	malignancy arising from capillary linings	skin and lymph nodes
Mycobacterium avium-intracellulare (MAI)	caused by a bacterium found in soil and water	systemic infection with fever, diarrhea, lung and blood disease, and wasting
Pneumocystis jiroveci	caused by fungus, formerly known as *Pneumocystis carinii*	lungs—a particularly dangerous type of pneumonia

Did you know

Contracting AIDS

When the AIDS epidemic began in the United States, many people feared that HIV could be spread by casual contact. In fact, time has shown that there are very few specific ways it can be transmitted. These are the ways that AIDS is transmitted and how it is not transmitted.

How HIV Is Transmitted

- Sexual contact, particularly vaginal, anal, and oral intercourse
- Contaminated needles (intravenous drug use, accidental needle stick in medical setting)
- During birth from an infected mother
- Receiving infected blood or other tissue (rare; precautions usually prevent this)

How HIV Is Not Transmitted

- Casual contact (social kissing, hugging, handshakes)
- Objects: toilet seats, deodorant sticks, doorknobs
- Mosquitoes
- Sneezing and coughing
- Sharing food
- Swimming in the same water as an infected person

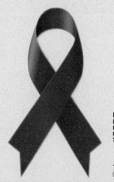

©dvarg/123RF

Other Immune System Disorders

Pathological

Provide the missing term(s) to complete the following sentences.

lymphoma
[lĭm-FŌ-mă]
Hodgkin lymphoma
Hodgkin disease
non-Hodgkin lymphoma
metastasis
[mĕ-TĂS-tă-sĭs]

_____, cancer of the lymph nodes, is a relatively common cancer with high cure rates. Some AIDS patients are especially susceptible to lymphomas because of their lowered immune systems. There are many different types of lymphomas. Two of the most common are _____ (_____), a type of lymph cancer of uncertain origin that generally appears in early adulthood, and _____, a cancer of the lymph nodes with some cells resembling healthy cells and spreading in a diffuse pattern. It usually appears in midlife. Depending on how far the disease has spread (_____), both types can be arrested with chemotherapy and radiation. Surgery (bone marrow transplantation) is also useful in Hodgkin lymphoma.

thymoma
[thī-MŌ-mă]
splenomegaly
[splēn-ō-MĔG-ă-lē]
hypersplenism
[hī-pĕr-SPLĒN-ĭzm]
lymphocytic lymphoma
[lĭm-fō-SĬT-ĭk
lĭm-FŌ-mă]
histiocytic lymphoma
[HĬS-tē-ō-SĬT-ĭk
lĭm-FŌ-mă]

Malignant tumors appear in many places in the lymph system. A _____ is a tumor of the thymus gland. Hodgkin lymphoma is a malignancy of the lymph nodes and spleen. Enlarged lymph nodes, enlarged spleen (_____), and overactive spleen (_____) characterize this disease. Non-Hodgkin lymphoma is a disease with malignant cells that resemble large lymphocytes (_____) or large macrophages called histiocytes (hence the name _____).

sarcoidosis
[săr-koy-DŌ-sĭs]
lymphadenopathy
[lĭm-făd-ĕ-NŎP-ă-thē]
infectious mononucleosis
[MŎN-ō-nū-klē-Ō-sĭs]

Nonmalignant lesions on the lymph nodes, lungs, spleen, skin, and liver can indicate the presence of _____, an inflammatory condition that can affect lung function. Swollen lymph nodes (_____) also can indicate the presence of _____, an acute infectious disease caused by the Epstein-Barr virus. Infectious mononucleosis is often called the "kissing disease" because it is usually transmitted through mouth-to-mouth contact during kissing, sharing drinks, and sharing eating utensils. Rest is generally the only cure.

PRONOUNCE and DEFINE

Pronounce the following terms aloud and write their meaning in the space provided.

thymoma	[thī-MŌ-mă]
splenomegaly	[splēn-ō-MĔG-ă-lē]
sarcoidosis	[săr-koy-DŌ-sĭs]
lymphadenopathy	[lĭm-făd-ĕ-NŎP-ă-thē]
hypersplenism	[hī-pĕr-SPLĒN-ĭzm]

	Spelling	Definition
lymphoma		
mononuclosis		
metastases		
histiocetic lymphoma		
lymphocytic lymphoma		

SPELL and DEFINE — Identify if the following terms are spelled correctly. Correct the words that are spelled incorrectly. Write the definition for each word.

UNDERSTAND — Fill in the blanks.

1. Sarcoidosis is an inflammatory condition of the _____ system.
2. Splenomegaly is a(n) _____ .
3. This disease is caused by the Epstein-Barr virus: _____ .
4. _____ is the spread of the disease.

APPLY — Read the following scenario and respond accordingly.

The client has been diagnosed with non-Hodgkin lymphoma. Explain to the client and family the difference between Hodgkin lymphoma and non-Hodgkin lymphoma.

_____

_____

_____

The Allergic Response and Autoimmune Disorders

Allergies are a disorder of the immune system that affect millions of people every year. Figure 13-13 shows some common allergens. Figure 13-14 illustrates an immediate-reaction allergy.

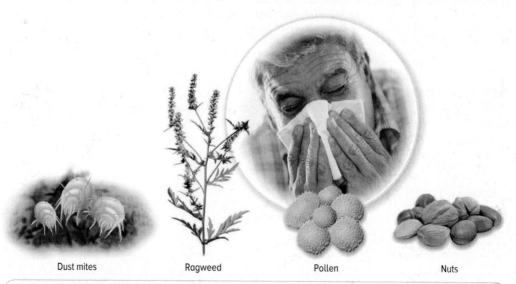

Dust mites   Ragweed   Pollen   Nuts

Figure 13-13 Common allergens

(Man sneezing): ©Tim Pannell/Corbis

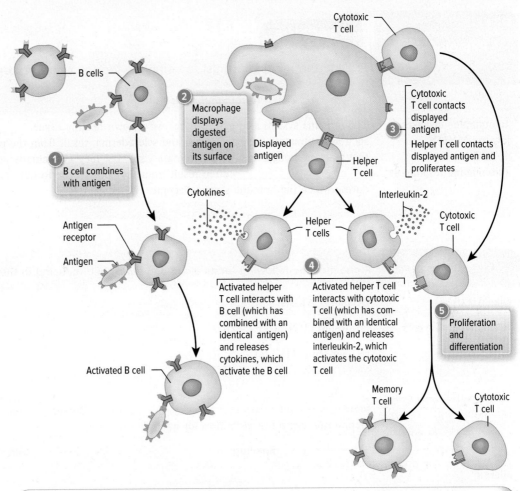

Figure 13-14 T- and B-cell activation: During an infection, macrophages bind to helper T cells, activating them to trigger other immune defenses.

Pathological	PRACTICE
	Provide the missing term(s) to complete the following sentences.

	The Allergic Response
allergen [ĂL-ĕr-jĕn]	Allergies are a problem of the immune system that affect millions of people. They are due to the production of IgE antibodies against an _____, an allergy-causing substance. Antibodies and some antigens cause a histamine to be released into the tissues. This histamine release is the cause of allergy symptoms.
hypersensitivity [HĪ-pĕr-sĕn-sĭ-TĬV-ĭ-tē] **anaphylaxis** [ĂN-ă-fĭ-LĂK-sĭs]	Allergies vary for different people depending on time of year, amount of exposure to different allergens, and other immunological problems. _____ increases as exposure increases, sometimes resulting in _____ (or anaphylactic reaction or shock), a reaction so severe that it can be life-threatening by decreasing blood pressure, affecting breathing, and causing loss of consciousness. Some people are extremely allergic to peanuts. A person with a severe peanut allergy who ingests even a tiny amount of peanuts (as in a cookie) will immediately go into an anaphylactic reaction. Some people are allergic in the same way to other foods and to bee stings. Most severely allergic people carry a dose of epinephrine to slow the reaction.

continued on next page

PRACTICE

Provide the missing term(s) to complete the following sentences.

Autoimmune Disorders	
autoimmune diseases [ăw-tō-ĭ-MYŪN di-ZĒZ-ĕz] **autoimmune responses**	The immune system also can turn against its own healthy tissue. _____, such as rheumatoid arthritis, lupus, and scleroderma, result from the proliferation of T cells that react as though they were fighting a virus, but they are actually destroying healthy cells. _____ often result from the body's need to fight an actual infection, during which the immune system becomes overactive.

PRONOUNCE and DEFINE

Pronounce the following terms aloud and write their meaning in the space provided.

anaphylaxis	[ĂN-ă-fĭ-LĂK-sĭs]
autoimmune diseases	[ăw-tō-ĭ-MYŪN di-ZĒZ-ĕz]
hypersensitivity	[HĬ-pĕr-sĕn-sĭ-TĬV-ĭ-tē]

SPELL and DEFINE

Identify if the following terms are spelled correctly. Correct the words that are spelled incorrectly. Write the definition for each word.

	Spelling	Definition
allergin		
audoimune		
anneflaxis		

UNDERSTAND

Fill in the blanks.

1. Allergies involve a(n) _____ response.
2. _____ occur when the immune system attacks healthy tissue.
3. If someone is highly allergic to bee stings, _____ can occur.

APPLY

Read the following scenario and answer the question.

You are explaining to the parents of a child with a peanut allergy the importance of watching his diet very closely and the need to recognize an allergic reaction. What symptoms will you tell the child's parents to look for?

_____

_____

_____

_____

LO 13.5 Surgical Terms

Surgery of the lymphatic system is usually related to a diagnosis of cancer. It is done to determine the stage of the cancer so that the appropriate level of treatment may be initiated.

PRACTICE

Provide the missing term(s) to complete the following sentences.

lymph node dissection
lymphadenectomy
[lǐm-făd-ĕ-NĔK-tō-mē]
lymphadenotomy
[lǐm-făd-ĕ-NŎ-tō-mē]
splenectomy
[splĕ-NĔK-tō-mē]
thymectomy
[thī-MĔK-tō-mē]

Cancers of the lymph system may require a _____, removal of cancerous lymph nodes for microscopic examination. A _____ is the removal of a lymph node and a _____ is an incision into a lymph node. A _____ is removal of the spleen, which is usually required if it is ruptured. Other organs of the body, such as the liver, will take over the functions of the spleen if it is removed. A _____ is removal of the thymus gland, which is very important to the maturation process but not as serious once a patient reaches adulthood.

UNDERSTAND

Write and define the lymph and immune system combining forms that can be found in the following words.

1. splenectomy: _____
2. lymphadenotomy: _____
3. thymectomy: _____
4. lymphangioma: _____

Did you know (?)

Lymph Node Surgery

A person with a malignant neoplasm in the breast must have further tests to determine if the cancer has metastasized. In the past, biopsies included removal of many lymph nodes until one without cancer was found. Now, a procedure called sentinel node biopsy is commonly used. A contrast medium is injected into the area around the tumor. The first node it reaches is the sentinel node. It is checked for malignancy. If that node is clean, then no further biopsy is done on the other lymph nodes and the patient is spared painful surgical side effects.

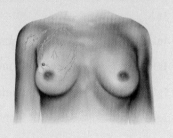

LO 13.6 Pharmacological Terms

Diseases of the lymphatic and immune systems are often treated with relatively high doses of chemotherapy and/or radiation. Autoimmune diseases are often managed for symptoms, although some newer drugs have been able to slow the advance of such diseases. Advances in AIDS research have made it possible to manage this disease (i.e., to prolong a patient's life) once thought fatal. A "cocktail" of anti-HIV drugs (such as HAART—highly active, antiretroviral therapy), a potential AIDS vaccine, and other newer drug compounds are bringing hope for long-term vitality to people with AIDS. Other drug compounds have been developed to fight opportunistic infections. A wide variety of antiviral drugs have been developed that are used to block virus growth and a particular antimicroorganism agent—*pentamidine*–is used to prevent PCP.

Allergic reactions are treated with antihistamines, many of which are available over the counter. Certain antihistamines are abused so that even over-the-counter sales may be limited.

UNDERSTAND **Fill in the blanks.**

1. AIDS patients often have to take many medications, including some to avoid _____ infections.
2. Lymphomas are generally treatable with _____ and _____.

LO 13.7 Abbreviations

Abbreviation	ABBREVIATION REVIEW Definition
AB	antibiotic
AIDS	acquired immunodeficiency syndrome
EIA	enzyme immunoassay
ELISA	enzyme-linked immunosorbent assay
HIV	human immunodeficiency virus
Ig	immunoglobulin
IgA	immunoglobulin A
IgD	immunoglobulin D
IgE	immunoglobulin E
IgG	immunoglobulin G
IgM	immunoglobulin M
PCP	*Pneumocystis carinii* pneumonia
PMN	polymorphonucleated cells
RES	reticuloendothelial system

APPLY **Read the following scenario and respond accordingly.**

You are teaching a community group about immunoglobulins. Using a method everyone can understand, describe the purpose of IgG, IgA, IgM, IgD, and IgE.

_____

_____

_____

Chapter Review

CHAPTER SUMMARY

	Learning Outcome	Summary
13.1	Identify the parts of the lymphatic and immune systems and discuss the function of each part.	The lymphatic and immune systems share some of the same structures and functions. Both the lymphatic and immune systems contain the lymph nodes, spleen, thymus gland, and some of the disease-fighting immune cells. The lymphatic system provides the location to gather and concentrate foreign substances present in the body so that lymphocytes circulating through the lymphatic organs and vessels are able to destroy and remove them from the body. The immune system is the body's defense system.
13.2	Recognize the major word parts used in building words that relate to the lymphatic and immune systems.	Word building requires knowledge of the combining form and meaning.
13.3	Identify the common diagnostic tests, laboratory tests, and clinical procedures used in testing and treating disorders of the lymphatic and immune systems.	Diagnostic, procedural, and laboratory findings assist the health care provider in diagnosing medical conditions. Often used in combination, these tests lead to a final diagnosis and assist in treatment planning.
13.4	Define the major pathological conditions of the lymphatic and immune systems.	Diseases of the lymphatic and immune systems include diseases that attack lymph tissue itself, diseases that are spread through the lymphatic pathways, and diseases that flourish because of a suppression of the immune response. Disorders of the lymphatic and immune systems can be caused by an overly vigorous response to an immune system invader.
13.5	Explain the meaning of surgical terms related to the lymphatic and immune systems.	Surgery of the lymphatic system is usually related to a diagnosis of cancer. It is performed to determine the stage of the cancer so that the appropriate level of treatment may be initiated.
13.6	Recognize common pharmacological agents used in treating disorders of the lymphatic and immune systems.	Diseases of the lymphatic and immune systems are often treated with relatively high doses of chemotherapy and/or radiation. Autoimmune diseases are often managed for symptoms, although some newer drugs have been able to slow the advance of such diseases.
13.7	Identify common abbreviations associated with the lymphatic and immune systems.	Abbreviations are used to describe diseases, conditions, procedures, and treatments associated with the lymphatic and immune systems.

Identify the location of the major lymph nodes throughout the body on the following figure.

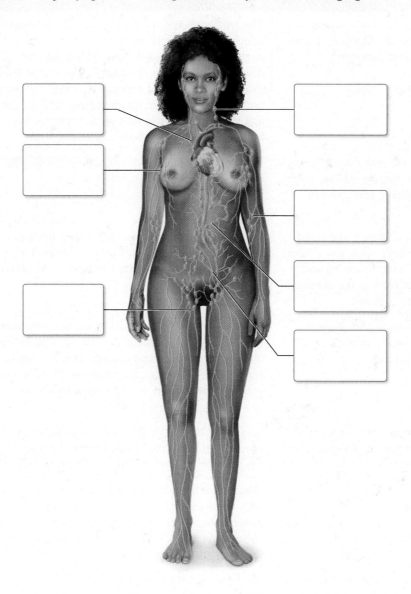

Identify if the following terms are spelled correctly. Correct the words that are spelled incorrectly. Write the definition for each word.

	Spelling	Definition
1. retorvirus		
2. immunosuppressive		
3. imunodeficiency		
4. sarcodosis		
5. lumphoma		
6. mononucleosis		
7. anphylaxis		
8. histocytic		
9. metastasis		
10. thimoma		

IMPLEMENT

Fill in the blanks.

1. People are born with some _____ immunity.
2. Vaccinations give _____ immunity.
3. Antitoxins give _____ immunity.
4. The special cells that ingest foreign substances are called _____.
5. Lymph contains _____ blood cells.
6. The thymus gland provides markers for cells that become _____.
7. Agents of T cells that destroy disease-causing cells are _____ and _____.
8. The fluid that contains white blood cells and other substances and flows in the lymphatic vessels is called

_____.

Find a Match: Match each term on the left with its correct definition on the right.

1. _____ toxicologist	a.	anemia resulting from a poison
2. _____ splenomegaly	b.	malignancy in the lymphatic vessels
3. _____ lymphangiosarcoma	c.	cystic mass containing lymph
4. _____ splenomyelomalacia	d.	inflammation of a lymph node
5. _____ lymphocele	e.	spleen enlargement
6. _____ lymphadenitis	f.	expert in the science of poisons
7. _____ toxanemia	g.	softening of the spleen and bone marrow

John Latella, a patient with AIDS, came to the hospital's clinic for his monthly T-cell test and to review the medications he is taking. He seems to be feeling more energetic, so John believes his T-cell test will show improvement. During the examination, however, the doctor notices an enlargement in John's lymph nodes. He sends John to the outpatient surgical unit for a biopsy. Mr. Latella's biopsy reveals that the node is not malignant. The swelling is thought to be an infection. Further blood tests show that it is. John already takes a number of prophylactic medications aimed at preventing infection. For this infection, he is put on a course of antibiotics.

1. If the node was malignant, what kind of surgery would most likely be performed?

_____

_____

2. A malignancy may have to be treated with radiation and/or chemotherapy, both of which destroy some healthy cells at the same time that they destroy malignant cells. Why would such treatment be especially risky for an AIDS patient?

_____

_____

3. Why does John find it difficult to fight infections?

_____

_____

4. What results are the antibiotics supposed to provide?

_____

_____

Reviewing the Terms

Pronounce each of the following terms. Write the definitions on a separate sheet of paper. This review will take you through all the words you learned in this chapter. If you have difficulty with any words, make a flash card for later study. Refer to the English-Spanish and Spanish-English glossaries in the eBook.

acquired active immunity

acquired immunodeficiency [ĬM-yū-nō-dē-FĬSH-ĕn-sē] **syndrome (AIDS)** [ādz]

acquired passive immunity

aden/o [ĂD-ĕ-nō]

allergen [ĂL-ĕr-jĕn]

allergy [ĂL-ĕr-jē]

anaphylaxis [ĂN-ă-fĭ-LĂK-sĭs]

antibody [ĂN-tē-bŏd-ē]

antigen [ĂN-tĭ-jĕn]

antitoxin [ăn-tē-TŎK-sĭn]

autoimmune [ăw-tō-ĭ-MYŪN] **diseases**

autoimmune responses

B lymphocytes [LĬM-fō-sīts], **B cells**

cell-mediated immunity

cytotoxic [sī-tō-TŎK-sĭk] **cell**

enzyme-linked immunosorbent assay (ELISA) [ĕ-LĪ-ză, ĕ-LĪ-să], or **enzyme immunoassay (EIA)**

gamma globulin [GĂ-mă GLŎB-yū-lĭn]

helper cell

histiocytic [HĬS-tē-ō-SĬT-ĭk] **lymphoma**

Hodgkin lymphoma, Hodgkin disease

human immunodeficiency [ĬM-yū-nō-dē-FĬSH-ĕn-sē] **virus (HIV)**

humoral [HYŪ-mōr-ăl] **immunity**

hypersensitivity [HĪ-pĕr-sĕn-sĭ-TĬV-ĭ-tē]

hypersplenism [hī-pĕr-SPLĒN-ĭzm]

immun/o [ĬM-yū-nō]

immunity [ĭ-MYŪ-nĭ-tē]

immunization [ĬM-yū-nī-ZĀ-shŭn]

immunoglobulin [ĬM-yū-nō-GLŎB-yū-lĭn]

immunosuppressive [ĬM-yū-nō-sŭ-PRĚS-ĭv] disease

infectious mononucleosis [MŎN-ō-nū-klē-Ō-sĭs]

interferon [ĭn-tĕr-FĚR-ŏn]

interleukin [ĭn-tĕr-LŪ-kĭn]

lymph [lĭmf]

lymph node

lymph node dissection

lymph/o [LĬM-fō]

lymphaden/o [lĭm-FĂD-ĕ-nō]

lymphadenectomy [lĭm-făd-ĕ-NĚK-tō-mē]

lymphadenopathy [lĭm-făd-ĕ-NŎP-ă-thē]

lymphadenotomy [lĭm-făd-ĕ-NŎ-tō-mē]

lymphangi/o [lĭm-FĂN-jē-ō]

lymphatic [lĭm-FĂD-ĭk] pathways

lymphatic vessels

lymphocyte [LĬM-fō-sīt]

lymphocytic [lĭm-fō-SĬT-ĭk] lymphoma

lymphoma [lĭm-FŌ-mă]

macrophage [MĂK-rō-fāj]

metastasis [mĕ-TĂS-tă-sĭs]

microphage [MĪK-rō-fāj]

natural immunity

non-Hodgkin lymphoma

opportunistic [ŏp-pōr-tū-NĬS-tĭk] infection

pathogen [PĂTH-ō-jĕn]

phagocytosis [FĂG-ō-sī-TŌ-sĭs]

plasma [PLĂZ-mă] cell

retrovirus [rĕ-trō-VĪ-rŭs]

sarcoidosis [săr-koy-DŌ-sĭs]

spleen [splēn]

splen/o [SPLĒ-nō]

splenectomy [splē-NĚK-tō-mē]

splenomegaly [splēn-ō-MĚG-ă-lē]

suppressor [sŭ-PRĚS-ōr] cell

T cells

T lymphocytes

thym/o [THĪ-mō]

thymectomy [thī-MĚK-tō-mē]

thymoma [thī-MŌ-mă]

thymosin [THĪ-mō-sĭn]

thymus [THĪ-mŭs] gland

tox/o, toxi-, toxico- [TŎK-sō, TŎK-sĭ, TŎK-sĭ-kō]

vaccination [VĂK-sĭ-NĀ-shŭn]

vaccine [văk-SĒN, VĂK-sēn]

Western blot

CHAPTER 14

The Digestive System and Body Metabolism

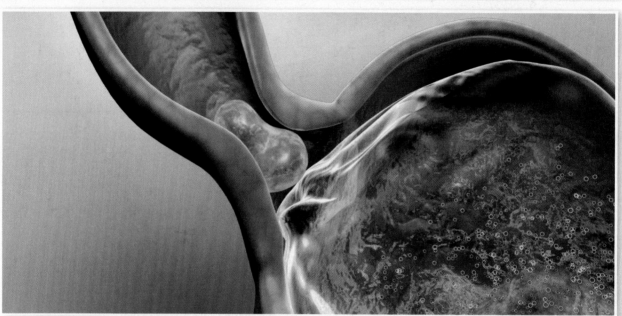

©2010, Nucleus Medical Media, Inc. All Rights Reserved

Learning Outcomes

After studying this chapter, you will be able to:

14.1 Describe the basic function and structure of the digestive system and body metabolism.

14.2 Recognize the major word parts used in building words that relate to the digestive system.

14.3 Recall the common diagnostic tests, laboratory tests, and clinical procedures used in treating disorders of the digestive system.

14.4 Define the major pathological conditions of the digestive system.

14.5 Define surgical terms related to the digestive system.

14.6 Recognize common pharmacological agents used in treating disorders of the digestive system.

14.7 Identify common abbreviations associated with the digestive system.

LO 14.1 Structure and Function of the Digestive System

The study of the digestive system is called **gastroenterology,** which is a breakdown of the combining forms *gastro-* ("stomach"), *entero-* ("intestines"), and *-ology* ("the study of"). The digestive system (also known as the alimentary system) is comprised of several organs and processes that break down, metabolize, and supply nutrients to the body. Gastroenterology consists of the nature in which food proceeds through the body via peristalsis, or the wavelike muscle contractions that move food to different processing stations in the digestive tract.

Figure 14-1 shows the major parts of the digestive (gastrointestinal [GI]) system and accessory organs. The major organs of the alimentary system are common and recognizable to most people. Most students learn about them in elementary school, but when we look at the accessory organs, we might not associate them with digestion. The accessory organs are a vital part of the system and metabolism would not be possible without them.

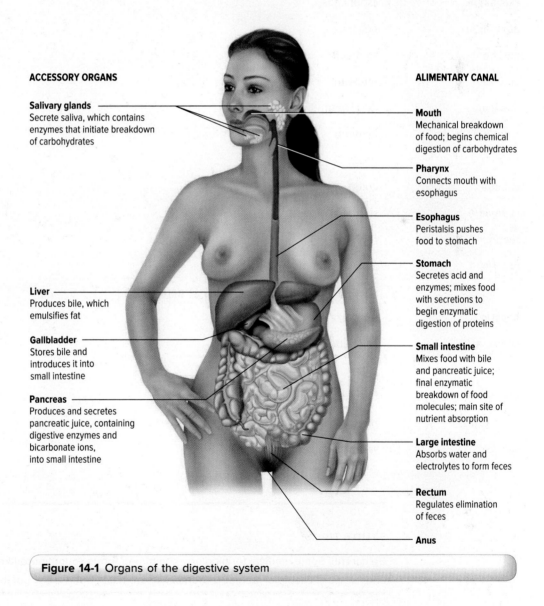

ACCESSORY ORGANS

Salivary glands
Secrete saliva, which contains enzymes that initiate breakdown of carbohydrates

Liver
Produces bile, which emulsifies fat

Gallbladder
Stores bile and introduces it into small intestine

Pancreas
Produces and secretes pancreatic juice, containing digestive enzymes and bicarbonate ions, into small intestine

ALIMENTARY CANAL

Mouth
Mechanical breakdown of food; begins chemical digestion of carbohydrates

Pharynx
Connects mouth with esophagus

Esophagus
Peristalsis pushes food to stomach

Stomach
Secretes acid and enzymes; mixes food with secretions to begin enzymatic digestion of proteins

Small intestine
Mixes food with bile and pancreatic juice; final enzymatic breakdown of food molecules; main site of nutrient absorption

Large intestine
Absorbs water and electrolytes to form feces

Rectum
Regulates elimination of feces

Anus

Figure 14-1 Organs of the digestive system

Building Your Digestive Vocabulary

Combining Form	Meaning
stomat/o	mouth
dent/o, odont/o	teeth
gloss/o, lingu/o	tongue
cheil/o	lips
gingiv/o	gums
esophag/o	esophagus
pharyng/o	pharynx
gastr/o	stomach
enter/o	intestine
duoden/o	duodenum
jejun/o	jejunum
ile/o	ileum
colon/o	colon
sigmoid/o	sigmoid colon
rect/o	rectum
proct/o	anus and rectum
Accessory Organs	
hepat/o	liver
cholecyst/o	gallbladder
chole	gall
cyst/o	bladder
pancreat/o	pancreas
saliv/o	salivary glands

STUDY TIP

Be careful! Some medical terminology combining forms sound more like a lay term for another part. Example: stomat/o sounds like stomach, but it is the combining form for mouth!

Structure and Function	**PRACTICE**

The three basic functions of the digestive system are as follows:

digestion [dī-JĔS-chŭn]	1. _____ is the process of breaking down foods into nutrients that can be absorbed by cells.
absorption [ăb-SŌRP-shŭn]	2. _____ is the passing of digested nutrients into the bloodstream. This primarily occurs in the small intestines.
elimination [ē-lĭm-ĭ-NĀ-shŭn]	3. _____ is the conversion of any residual material from a liquid to a solid and removal of that material from the alimentary canal via defecation.
alimentary canal [ăl-ĭ-MĔN-tĕr-ē kă-NĂL] **mouth** **pharynx** [FĂR-ĭngks] **esophagus** [ĕ-SŎF-ă-gŭs] **stomach** [STŎM-ăk] **small intestine** **large intestine** **bowels** [bŏw-lz] **anal canal** [Ā-năl kă-NĂL]	The digestive system consists of the _____ (digestive tract or gastrointestinal tract) and several accessory organs. Food enters the alimentary canal through the _____, passes through the _____ and _____ into the _____, then into the _____ and _____ or _____, and then into the _____ (Figure 14-2).
anus [Ā-nŭs] **peristalsis** [pĕr-ĭ-STĂL-sĭs]	The alimentary canal is a tube that extends from the mouth to the _____. The wall of the alimentary canal has four layers that aid in the _____ of food that passes through it.
enzymes [ĔN-zīmz] **amino acids** [ă-MĒ-nō ĂS-ĭdz] **glucose** [GLŪ-kōs] **fatty acids**	Digestive _____ convert complex proteins into _____, compounds that can be absorbed by the body. Complex sugars are reduced to _____ and other simpler sugars, and fat molecules are reduced to _____ and other substances through the action of the digestive enzymes.

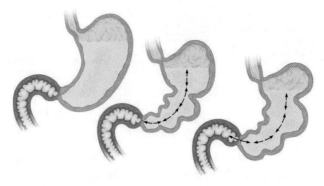

(a)

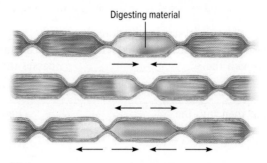

Digesting material

(b)

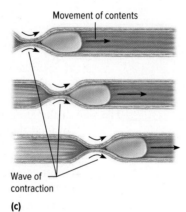

Movement of contents

Wave of
contraction

(c)

Figure 14-2 Movement of food through the alimentary canal

Did you know **?**

Food Digestion

It takes an average of just 20 to 48 hours for food to travel from the mouth through the digestive system and pass from the body. During that time, the stomach processes food particles for only 3 to 5 hours. The remainder of the time it is processing through the intestinal tracts.

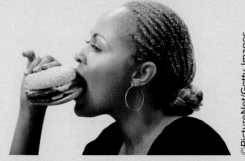

PRONOUNCE and DEFINE	Pronounce the following terms aloud and write the definition.
peristalsis	[pĕr-ĭ-STĂL-sĭs]
elimination	[ē-lĭm-ĭ-NĀ-shŭn]
enzymes	[ĔN-zīmz]
alimentary canal	[ăl-ĭ-MĔN-tĕr-ē kă-NĂL]

SPELL	Write the correct spelling of the related term.
digestive tract (two words)	
movement of digestion	
convert proteins	
end of the alimentary canal	

UNDERSTAND   Match each term on the left to its description on the right.

1. _____ cheilitis
2. _____ small intestine
3. _____ large intestine
4. _____ glucose
5. _____ pharyngeal
6. _____ peristalsis

a. Complex sugars are made into this for the body to use
b. Nutrients are broken down for absorption here
c. Inflammation of the lips
d. Final processing of food occurs here
e. How food moves through the body
f. Pertaining to the pharynx

APPLY   Read the following scenario and answer the questions.

Mr. Tom DiPietropolo, a 19-year-old Italian immigrant male, presents to the Community Care Clinic complaining of the following symptoms: upset stomach, difficulty swallowing, and diarrhea.

1. Which digestive parts are affected?

_____
_____
_____

2. Are any ancillary organs involved?

_____
_____
_____

3. What would the terms be for the symptoms he is having?

_____
_____
_____

4. Draw a diagram that shows peristalsis from mouth to anus.

_____
_____
_____

From the Perspective Of . . .

Who: Licensed Practical Nurse

Other Aliases: LPN, LVN, Office Nurse, Clinical Care Assistant, Patient Care Nurse, Clinical Support Nurse

Job Duties: Greeting and escorting patients to designated areas; obtaining vital signs; assessment of patient status; gathering health history, allergies, and medications. The licensed practical nurse assists the physician with procedures and provides care for the patient after, instructs the patient on side effects and disease/conditions, and administers medication. The licensed practical nurse also provides routine patient care in long-term health care facilities.

Licensed practical nurses work in several care settings including doctors' offices, nursing homes, home health care, and residential facilities.

Based on the above, why would it be important for a licensed practical nurse to understand medical terminology, speak clearly, and communicate effectively?

That is why medical terminology is important to me.

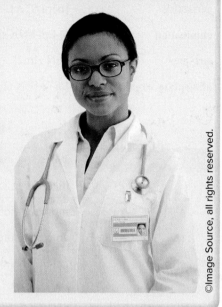

STUDY TIP

Digestion actually begins in the mouth. After you take a bite of food, your body starts the process in motion by stimulating and releasing saliva, which chemically reacts with the food particles.

The Mouth, Pharynx, and Esophagus

Digestion begins in the mouth, pharynx, and esophagus (Figure 14-3). The medical term for mouth is **stomat/o,** which can easily be confused with stomach. The medical term for pharynx is **pharyng/o** and esophagus is **esophag/o.** After the choice of which food to eat is made, the mouth (with help from the tongue, teeth, and lips) breaks down the food into smaller particles while mixing it with saliva, which is secreted from the salivary glands. This process is called **mastication.**

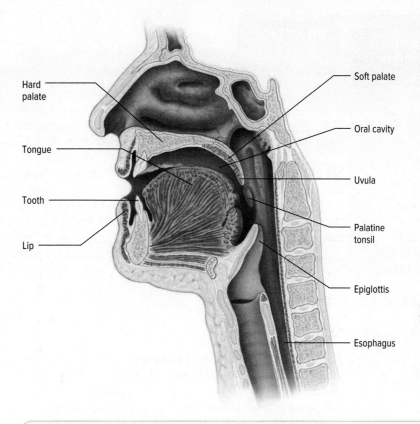

Hard palate

Tongue

Tooth

Lip

Soft palate

Oral cavity

Uvula

Palatine tonsil

Epiglottis

Esophagus

Figure 14-3 Sagittal section of the mouth, nasal cavity, and pharynx

Did you know

Teeth

Teeth are a very important part of digestion. If teeth are not cared for now, many systemic problems may develop, some of which can be life threatening, including infection, heart disease, and malnutrition. Dental researchers are looking into ways that stem cells taken from one's teeth could be used to "grow" replacement teeth for people.

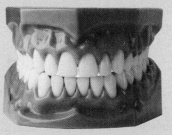

©Comstock/Alamy

PRACTICE

Provide the missing term(s) to complete the following sentences.

Mouth

lips

cheeks

tongue
[tŭng]

mastication
[măs-tĭ-KĀ-shŭn]

deglutition
[dē-glū-TĬSH-ŭn]

papilla (*pl.,* **papillae**)
[pă-PĬL-ă (pă-PĬL-ē)]

frenulum
[FRĔN-yū-lŭm]

lingual tonsils
[LĬNG-gwăl TŎN-sĭlz]

The _____ sense the food that is about to enter the mouth. Once food is taken into the oral cavity (mouth), it is chewed with the help of the muscles of the _____ (the walls of the oral cavity) and the _____ (which moves food during _____ (chewing)). The last mechanical process that takes place in the mouth is _____ (swallowing). The tongue has _____, small raised areas that contain the taste buds (cells that provide the sensation of taste). The tongue is connected to the floor of the mouth by a mucous membrane called a _____. At the back of the tongue, _____ form two rounded mounds of lymphatic tissue that play an important role in the immune system (see Chapter 13) (Figure 14-4).

hard palate
[hard PĂL-ăt]

rugae
[RŪ-gē]

soft palate
[soft PĂL-ăt]

uvula
[YŪ-vyū-lă]

palatine tonsils
[PĂL-ă-tīn TŎN-sĭlz]

gums
[gŭmz]

The roof of the mouth is formed by the _____, the hard anterior part of the palate with irregular ridges of mucous membranes called _____, and the _____, the soft posterior part of the palate. At the back of the soft palate is a downward cone-shaped projection called the _____. On either side of the back of the mouth are rounded masses of lymphatic tissue called the _____. The mouth also contains the _____, the fleshy sockets that hold the teeth.

salivary glands
[SĂL-ĭ-văr-ē glăndz]

saliva
[să-LĪ-vă]

amylase
[ĂM-ĭl-ās]

Digestion of food begins in the mouth with mastication. In addition, the three sets of _____ surrounding the oral cavity secrete _____, a fluid containing enzymes (such as _____, an enzyme that begins the digestion of carbohydrates) that aid in breaking down food.

Pharynx

pharynx
[FĂR-ĭngks]

epiglottis
[ĕ-pĭ-GLŎT-ĭs]

From the mouth, food travels through the throat (_____). Both food and air share this passageway. When we eat and swallow food, a flap of tissue (the _____) covers the trachea until the food is moved into the esophagus.

Esophagus

reflux
[RĒ-flŭks]

emesis
[ĕ-MĒ-sĭs]

regurgitation
[rē-GŬR-jĭ-TĀ-shŭn]

As the swallowed food is advanced toward the stomach by the peristaltic wave, the cardiac sphincter will open briefly. Once the food is in the stomach, it will close. This prevents _____ (backflow) and _____ or _____ (vomiting). Every time more food comes through the esophagus to the stomach, the muscles relax and allow the food to pass.

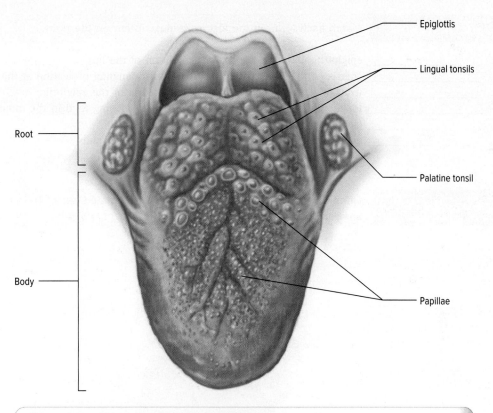

Root

Body

Epiglottis

Lingual tonsils

Palatine tonsil

Papillae

Figure 14-4 Superior view: tongue, epiglottis, and tonsils

PRONOUNCE and DEFINE	Pronounce the following terms aloud and write the definition.
mastication	[măs-tĭ-KĀ-shŭn]
papilla (*pl.*, **papillae**)	[pă-PĬL-ă (pă-PĬL-ē)]
uvula	[YŪ-vyū-lă]
regurgitation	[rē-GŬR-jĭ-TĀ-shŭn]

SPELL	Write the correct spelling of the related term.
	throat
	backflow
	vomiting
	chewing
	swallowing

Match each term on the left to its description on the right.

1. _____ epiglottitis
2. _____ emesis
3. _____ uvula
4. _____ tongue
5. _____ cheilosis
6. _____ gingival

a. Condition of the lips
b. Downward dangling projection at the back of the soft palate
c. Inflammation of the epiglottis
d. Assists with moving food in the mouth
e. Vomiting
f. Pertaining to the gums

APPLY

Label the diagram of the mouth with its associated parts. Then read the scenario and answer the question.

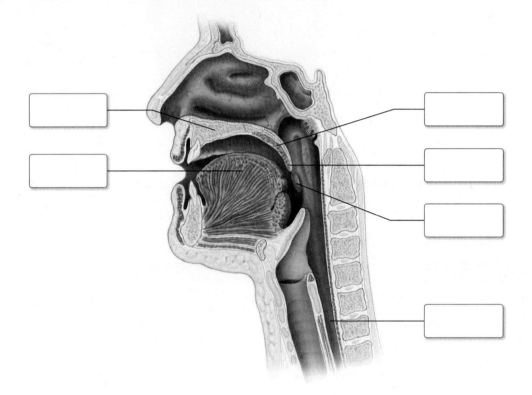

Ms. Lara Kempton is a 30-year-old African-American female who presents to the Dearborn Family Medical Center with sores in her mouth and a history of reflux. You have weighed her and she has lost 17 pounds since her last visit a month ago.

Which digestive parts are affected?

_____

_____

STUDY TIP

An adult's stomach can hold about 1.5 liters of contents and the stomach acts like a washing machine, churning and mixing food contents. Very little actual absorption of nutrients occurs in the stomach.

The Stomach

Once food leaves the mouth and passes through the esophagus, it reaches the stomach (Figure 14-5). The medical term for stomach is **gastr/o.** The stomach's main function is to further break down food particles; initiate protein digestion; and mix it, much like a washing machine, with needed enzymes before moving on to the small intestine. The stomach is a pouchlike organ that typically holds more than 1 liter of food contents. **Gastropathy** is the medical term for any disease of the stomach.

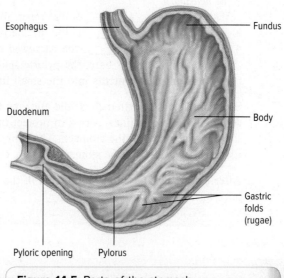

Figure 14-5 Parts of the stomach

Did you know

Mucous Lining

The human stomach produces an entirely new mucous lining approximately every 2 weeks so it is protected from digesting itself due to the hydrochloric acid that it uses to break down food.

Structure and Function	PRACTICE
	Provide the missing term(s) to complete the following sentences.
pepsin [PĔP-sĭn]	The enzyme _____ in the gastric juice begins protein digestion. Gastric juice is produced by the gastric glands, which are stimulated to produce this substance continuously but in varying amounts depending on the amount of food being absorbed.

continued on next page

Provide the missing term(s) to complete the following sentences.

fundus [FŬN-dŭs] **body** **pylorus** [pī-LŌR-ŭs]	The stomach has four regions. 1. The *cardiac region,* the region closest to the heart, is where the cardiac sphincter allows food to enter the stomach and prevents regurgitation. If the cardiac sphincter does not close completely, or if it fails to remain closed, stomach juices can splash into the esophagus where there is no protective lining. This causes extreme burning known as *heartburn.* 2. The _____ is the upper, rounded portion of the stomach. 3. The _____ is the middle portion. 4. The _____, the narrowed bottom part of the stomach, has a powerful, circular muscle at its base, the pyloric sphincter. This sphincter controls the emptying of the stomach's contents into the small intestine.
	Stomach juices are extremely acidic allowing them to digest food. The lining of the stomach (and of the intestines) serves to protect the cells of the lining from being affected by the digestive juices in the stomach. The lining is relatively thick with many folds of mucous tissue called *rugae.* As the stomach fills up, the wall distends and the folds disappear.
chyme [kīm]	After eating, the muscular movements of the stomach and the mixing of food with gastric juice form a semifluid mass called _____.

Pronounce the following terms aloud and write the definition.

chyme	[kīm]
pylorus	[pī-LŌR-ŭs]
pepsin	[PĔP-sĭn]
fundus	[FŬN-dŭs]

Write the correct spelling of the related term.

	Semifluid food mass
	Enzyme in gastric juice
	Narrowed bottom part of stomach
	Top part of stomach

Match each term on the left to its description on the right.

1. _____ pepsin
2. _____ pylorus
3. _____ chyme
4. _____ fundus
5. _____ gastropathy
6. _____ gastritis

a. Inflammation of the stomach
b. Narrowed bottom portion of the stomach
c. Upper portion of the stomach
d. The semifluid mass after food is mixed with gastric juices
e. Enzyme in gastric juice
f. Condition of the stomach

APPLY

Label the three parts of the stomach on the figure. Then read the scenario and answer the questions.

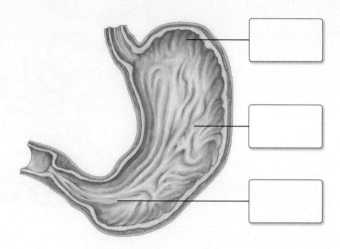

Mr. Scott Woodall is a 67-year-old Caucasian male who has come into the ER holding his stomach after eating a large meal. The doctor has examined him and determined that he has a history of stomach discomfort. The doctor diagnoses him with dyspepsia and gastralgia that has resulted in a peptic ulcer.

1. Which digestive parts are affected?

   _____

   _____

2. What are the lay terms for his symptoms?

   _____

   _____

3. How did you break down the word parts?

   _____

   _____

STUDY TIP

The entire alimentary canal is a muscular tube that is an average 8 meters, or 27 feet, long.

Small and Large Intestines

The small intestine is a tubelike organ that extends from the pylorus to the beginning of the large intestine or colon (Figure 14-6). It is the longest tube in the body and takes up the majority of the abdominal cavity. This is where the majority of nutrient absorption in the body occurs. There are three sections to the small intestine: the duodenum, jejunum, and ileum. The medical term for intestine is **enter/o** and the terms for the three sections are **duoden/o, jejun/o,** and **ile/o.**

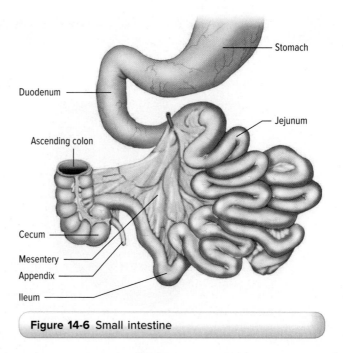

Figure 14-6 Small intestine

The large intestine, or colon, is larger in diameter than the small intestine and extends to the rectum (Figure 14-7). The main purpose of the colon is to reabsorb the water, salts, water-soluble nutrients, and electrolytes from digested and undigested food particles. The remaining solid waste, or feces, is then excreted from the body. There are three main sections to the colon: the ascending, transverse, and descending colon. The medical term for large intestine is **colon/o.** The beginning of the colon is the cecum, and the medical term is **cec/o.** The end section of the colon is the sigmoid colon, and the medical term is **sigmoid/o.**

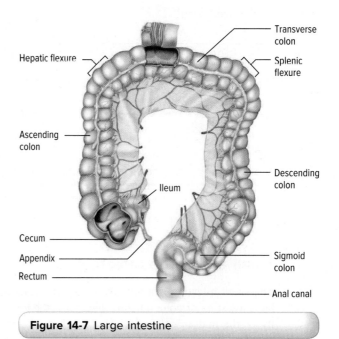

Figure 14-7 Large intestine

Structure and Function	**PRACTICE**

Provide the missing term(s) to complete the following sentences.

Small Intestine

duodenum [dū-ō-DĒ-nŭm] **glycogen** [GLĪ-kō-jĕn] **villi** [VĬL-ī] **villus** [VĬL-ŭs]	The small intestine has the following three parts: 1. The _____ is only about 10 inches long. In it, chyme mixes with bile to aid in fat digestion; with pancreatic juice to aid in digestion of starch, proteins, and fat; and with intestinal juice to aid in digesting sugars (glucose). Glands in the walls of the small intestine excrete intestinal juice. The juices also help change starch (_____) into glucose. The entire small intestine is lubricated by secretions from mucous glands. The small intestine is lined with _____ (singular, _____), tiny, one-cell-thick fingerlike projections with capillaries through which digested nutrients are absorbed into the bloodstream and lymphatic system.
jejunum [jĕ-JŪ-nŭm]	2. The _____ is an 8-foot-long section of the small intestine in which the digestive process continues.
ileum [ĬL-ē-ŭm]	3. The _____ connects the small intestine to the large intestine. Located at the bottom of the ileum is the ileocecal sphincter muscle that relaxes to allow undigested and unabsorbed food material into the large intestine in fairly regular waves. Other muscular contractions segment the ileum and prevent waste material in the large intestine from backing up into the small intestine.
mesentery [MĔS-ĕn-tĕr-ē, MĔZ-ĕn-tĕr-ē]	Together, the three sections of the small intestine are about 20 feet long from the stomach to the large intestine. The small intestine lies within the abdominopelvic cavity, where it is held in place by the _____, a membranous tissue that attaches both the small and large intestines to the muscle wall at the dorsal part of the abdomen. Absorption (passage of material through the walls to the bloodstream) begins in the small intestines. Chyme takes from 1 to 6 hours to travel through the small intestine before it enters the large intestine. The length of time for digestion varies depending on the food being digested and the health of the digestive system.

Large Intestine

	The large intestine, which is about 5 feet long, has the following four parts:
cecum [SĒ-kŭm] **appendix** [ă-PĔN-dĭks] **appendage** [ă-PĔN-dĭj]	1. The _____ is a pouch attached to the bottom of the ileum of the small intestine. It has three openings: one from the ileum into the cecum, one from the cecum into the colon, and another from the cecum into a wormlike pouch on the side, the _____ (also called the *vermiform appendix*). The appendix is filled with lymphatic tissue but is considered an _____, an accessory part of the body that has no central function, because it no longer has a role in the digestive process. The appendix can, however, become inflamed and may require surgical removal. Within the cecum, the process of turning waste material into semisolid waste (*feces*) begins, as water and certain necessary substances are absorbed back into the bloodstream. As the water is removed, a semisolid mass is formed and moved into the colon.

continued on next page

PRACTICE

Provide the missing term(s) to complete the following sentences.

colon
[KŌ-lŏn]

2. The next section is the _____. It is further divided into three parts: the *ascending colon,* the *transverse colon,* and the *descending colon.* The ascending colon extends upward from the cecum to a place under the liver, where it makes a right-angle bend known as the *hepatic flexure.* After the bend, the transverse colon continues across the abdomen from right to left, where it makes a right-angle bend (the *splenic flexure*) toward the spleen. After the bend, the descending colon extends down to the rim of the pelvis, where it connects to the sigmoid colon.

sigmoid colon
[SĬG-moyd KŌ-lŏn]

3. The _____ is an S-shaped body that goes across the pelvis to the middle of the sacrum, where it connects to the rectum.

rectum
[RĔK-tŭm]

feces
[FĒ-sēz]

stool
[stūl]

defecation
[dĕ-fĕ-KĀ-shŭn]

4. The _____ attaches to the *anal canal.* _____ (_____) then pass from the anal canal into the anus. The anus and anal canal open during the release of feces from the body (_____).

The entire large intestine forms a rectangle around the tightly packed small intestine. Undigestible waste products from digestion usually remain in the large intestine from 12 to 24 hours.

PRONOUNCE and DEFINE

Pronounce the following terms aloud and write the definition.

sigmoid colon	[SĬG-mŏyd KŌ-lŏn]
duodenum	[dū-ō-DĒ-nŭm]
jejunum	[jĕ-JŪ-nŭm]
defecation	[dĕ-fĕ-KĀ-shŭn]

SPELL

Write the correct spelling of the related term.

First section of the small intestine	
Second section of the small intestine	
Third section of the small intestine	
First section of the large intestine (attaches to small)	
Attaches to anal canal	

1. _____ ascending colon
2. _____ jejunum
3. _____ cecum
4. _____ feces
5. _____ sigmoid
6. _____ ileum

a. Attached to bottom of ileum
b. Waste product
c. End section of the large intestine that connects to rectum
d. Extends upward from cecum to just under the liver
e. Connects small intestine to large intestine
f. Middle section of the small intestine that is about 8 feet long

APPLY | **Read the following scenario and respond accordingly.**

You have been asked to teach a group of high school students about the parts of the large and small intestines and their functions. Explain it in a way the students can understand.

_____

_____

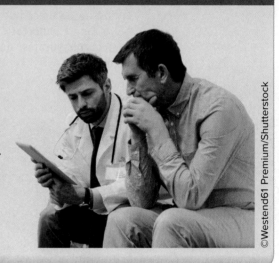

Did you know **?**

Colon Cancer

Most cases of colon cancer could have been prevented with a colonoscopy. If colon cancer runs in your family, it is very important to eat a high-fiber diet and have regular colon screenings after the age of 40, according to the American College of Gastroenterology.

©Westend61 Premium/Shutterstock

STUDY TIP

The liver is a vital organ that has many jobs, some of which include producing bile to aid in digestion, detoxification, and blood filtering. It is the largest single organ in the body, and survival is not possible without it.

Digestive Accessory Organs

In addition to the major parts of the digestive system, the accessory organs play a big role in digestion. Absorption of nutrients would not be accomplished without their help.

The liver is the largest abdominal organ in the body (Figure 14-8). It has many functions, but the most important digestive function is bile secretion. The liver lies in the upper right abdominal cavity just below the diaphragm. The medical term for liver is **hepat/o.**

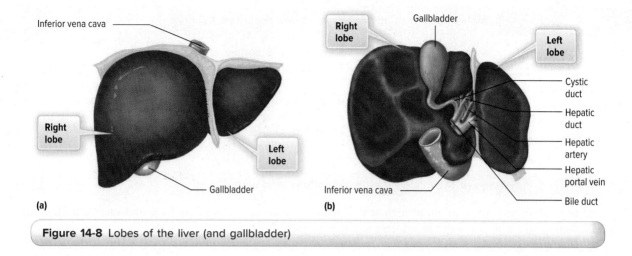

Figure 14-8 Lobes of the liver (and gallbladder)

The gallbladder is a small pear-shaped sac that lies protected against the inside surface of the liver. It acts as a storage area for bile until it is needed for digestion. The medical term for gallbladder is taken from two word parts: **chole** (= gall) and **cyst/o** (= bladder).

The pancreas also has many roles in the human body. It is mainly discussed in the endocrine system, but it is closely attached to the small intestine and responsible for secretion of pancreatic juice. Pancreatic juice is comprised of enzymes that metabolize fats, carbohydrates, and proteins. The medical term for pancreas is **pancreat/o.** See Figure 14-9.

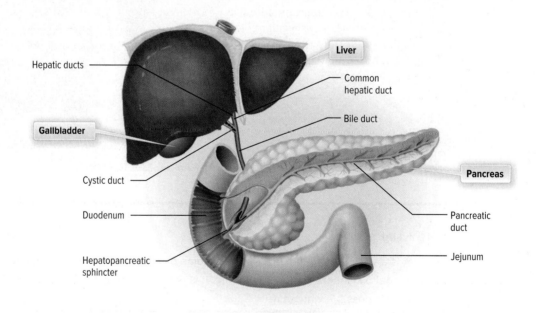

Figure 14-9 The liver, pancreas, and gallbladder

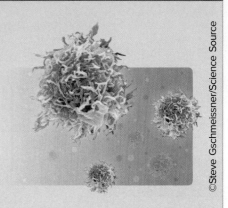
Structure and Function

PRACTICE

Provide the missing term(s) to complete the following sentences.

	Liver
liver [LĬV-ĕr]	The _____ is an important digestive organ located in the right upper quadrant of the abdominal cavity.
bile [bīl] **bilirubin** [bĭl-ĭ-RŪ-bĭn]	Aside from changing food nutrients into usable substances, the liver also secretes _____ (a yellowish-brown to greenish fluid), which is stored in the gallbladder for use in breaking down fats and other digestive functions. It stores glucose and certain vitamins for release when the body needs them. The liver also secretes _____, a bile pigment that is combined with bile and excreted into the duodenum.
	Gallbladder
gallbladder [GĂWL-blăd-ĕr]	The bile released from the liver to the *hepatic duct* is then released into the *cystic duct,* which brings the substance into the _____. This organ is involved in the production, storage and transportation of bile.
emulsification [ĕ-MŬL-sĭ-fĭ-KĀ-shŭn]	At the entrance to the duodenum, bile mixes with pancreatic juices and enters the duodenum from the common bile duct. There the bile aids in _____, the breaking down of fats.
	Pancreas
pancreas [PĂN-krē-ăs] **lipase** [LĬP-ās]	The chyme that empties into the small intestine mixes with secretions from the pancreas and liver. The _____ is 5 to 6 inches long and lies across the posterior side of the stomach. The pancreas is a digestive organ in that it secretes digestive fluids into the small intestine through its system of ducts. The digestive fluid is called *pancreatic juice,* which includes various enzymes such as *amylase* and _____.

The Pancreas

The actual size of the human pancreas is approximately 7 in. (17.5 cm) long and 1.5 in. (3.8 cm) wide and it is yellowish in color. With the help of modern medicine, it is possible to sustain life without a pancreas and pancreatic transplants are becoming more successful.

PRONOUNCE and DEFINE	Pronounce the following terms aloud and write the definition.
lipase	[LĬP-ās]
emulsification	[ĕ-MŬL-sĭ-fĭ-KĀ-shŭn]
bile	[bīl]
bilirubin	[bĭl-ĭ-RŪ-bĭn]

SPELL	Write the correct spelling of the medical term related to the definition. (Remember to use prefixes/suffixes as necessary.)
	Inflammation of the liver
	Enlarged pancreas
	Gallbladder condition/disease
	Bile pigment secreted by liver
	Pancreatic juice

UNDERSTAND	Match each term on the left to its description on the right.

1. _____ lipase
2. _____ liver
3. _____ gallbladder
4. _____ emulsification
5. _____ pancreas
6. _____ bilirubin

a. Process of breaking down fats
b. Part of the endocrine system; produces "juice"
c. Pancreatic fluid
d. Small sac that stores bile
e. Bile pigment
f. Largest abdominal organ

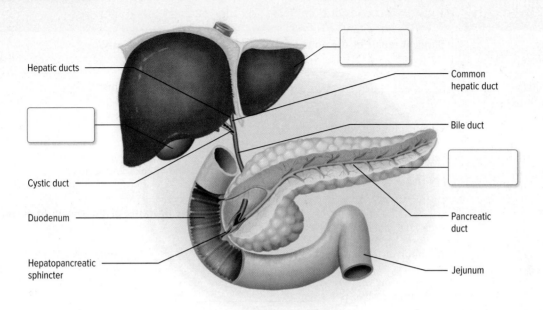

Hepatic ducts

Common hepatic duct

Bile duct

Cystic duct

Duodenum

Pancreatic duct

Hepatopancreatic sphincter

Jejunum

Mrs. Jennifer Pierce is an 18-year-old French female who doesn't speak English. She has come into the ER holding her right side and wincing in pain. The emergent care nurse practitioner has determined that she may have acute cholecystitis.

1. What is cholecystitis?

_____

_____

_____

2. Where is the gallbladder located?

_____

_____

3. Why would it be important to have further testing done? What other organs are in that region?

_____

_____

_____

LO 14.2 Word Building in the Digestive System

Now that the digestive and accessory anatomy has been covered, it is time to practice word building. Following are some medical terms and combinations common to the digestive system.

As you work through this practice, try to mix and match or associate various word roots with different prefixes/suffixes to extend your knowledge and vocabulary.

ano-plasty [Ā-nō-plăs-tē]	Surgical repair of the anus is _____ plasty.
appendic-itis [ă-pĕn-dĭ-SĪ-tĭs]	_____ itis is inflammation of the appendix.
bili-verdin [bĭl-ĭ-VER-dĭn]	Green bile pigment is _____ verdin.
bucco-gingival [bŭk-ō-JIN-ji-văl]	_____ gingival pertains to the cheeks and gums.
ceco-pexy [SĒ-kō-pek-sē]	_____ pexy is surgical repair or fixing of the cecum to correct excessive mobility.
celi-oma [sē-lē-Ō-mă]	A tumor in the abdomen is a(n) _____ oma.
chole-ic [kō-LĒ-ik]	Pertaining to bile is _____ ic.
cholangio-gram [kō-LAN-jē-ō-gram]	A _____ gram is an x-ray image of the bile vessels.
cholecyst-ectomy [KŌ-lē-sĭs-TĔK-tō-mē]	Removal of the gallbladder is _____ ectomy.
choledocho-tomy [kō-led-ō-KOT-ō-mē]	_____ tomy is an incision into the common bile duct.
col-ectomy [kō-LĔK-tō-mē]	_____ ectomy is removal of all or part of the colon.
duoden-itis [dū-od-ĕ-NĪ-tĭs]	Inflammation of the duodenum is _____ itis.
entero-pathy [en-tĕr-OP-ă-thē]	_____ pathy is any intestinal disease.
esophago-scopy [ĕ-sŏf-ă-GŎS-kō-pē]	Examination of the interior of the esophagus is _____ scopy.
gastr-algia [gas-TRAL-jē-ă]	_____ algia is a stomach ache.
glosso-pharyngeal [GLOS-ō-fă-RIN-jē-ăl]	_____ pharyngeal relates to the tongue and pharynx.
gluco-genesis [gloo-kō-JEN-ĕ-sĭs]	The formation of glucose is _____ genesis.
glycos-uria [glī-kō-SŪ-rē-ă]	_____ uria is abnormal excretion of carbohydrates in urine.
glycogeno-lysis [GLĪ-kō-jĕ-NOL-ĭ-sĭs]	The breakdown of glycogen to glucose is _____ lysis.

hepat-itis [hĕp-ă-TĪ-tĭs]	_____ itis is liver disease or inflammation of the liver.
ile-itis [ĬL-ē-Ī-tĭs]	Inflammation of the ileum is _____ itis.
jejun-ostomy [je-jū-NOS-tō-mē]	_____ ostomy is a surgical opening to the outside of the body for the jejunum.
labio-plasty [LĀ-bē-ō-plas-tē]	Surgical repair of the lips is _____ plasty.
linguo-dental [LĬNG-gwō-DĔN-tal]	Pertaining to the tongue and teeth is _____ dental.
oro-facial [ōr-ō-FĀ-shăl]	_____ facial pertains to the mouth and face.
pancreat-itis [PĂN-krē-ă-TĪ-tĭs]	_____ itis is inflammation of the pancreas.
periton-itis [PĔR-ĭ-tō-NĪ-tĭs]	Inflammation of the peritoneum is _____ itis.
pharyngo-tonsillitis [fă-RING-gō-ton-si-LĪ-tĭs]	Inflammation of the tonsils and pharynx is _____ tonsillitis.
procto-logist [prok-TOL-ō-jist]	A specialist in the study and treatment of diseases of the anus and rectum is a _____ logist.
pyloro-spasm [pī-LŌ-rō-spazm]	_____ spasm is involuntary contraction of the pylorus.
recto-abdominal [REK-tō-ab-DOM-i-năl]	_____ abdominal relates to the rectum and abdomen.
sial-ism [SĪ-ă-lizm]	Excessive secretion of saliva is _____ ism.
sialaden-itis [SĪ-ă-lō-ăd-ē-NĪ-tĭs]	_____ itis is inflammation of the salivary glands.
sigmoido-scopy [SĬG-moy-DŎS-kō-pē]	Visual examination of the sigmoid colon is _____ scopy.
steato-rrhea [STĒ-ă-tō-RĒ-ă]	Greater than normal amounts of fat in the feces is _____ rrhea.
stomat-itis [stō-mă-TĪ-tĭs]	Inflammation of the lining of the mouth is _____ itis.

PRONOUNCE and DEFINE	Pronounce the following terms aloud and write the definition.
peritonitis	[PĔR-ĭ-tō-NĪ-tĭs]
choledochotomy	[kō-led-ō-KOT-ō-mē]
linguodental	[LĬNG-gwō-DĔN-tal]
anoplasty	[Ā-nō-plăs-tē]

SPELL and DEFINE	Identify if the following terms are spelled correctly. Correct the words that are spelled incorrectly. Write the definition for each word.	
	Spelling	Definition
pantcreatus		
esophagectomy		
hepotology		
pharingoplegia		
choledochotomy		

UNDERSTAND Match each term on the left to its description on the right.

1. _____ linguodental
2. _____ pancreatitis
3. _____ anoplasty
4. _____ colectomy
5. _____ ileitis
6. _____ jejunitis

a. Inflammation of ileum
b. Surgical repair of the anus
c. Inflammation of the pancreas
d. Pertaining to teeth and tongue
e. Removal of colon (part or all)
f. Inflammation of the jejunum

APPLY Read the following scenario and answer the questions.

Miss Red Feather is a 15-year-old Native American female patient who is reviewing her past history with you in her medical record. Her past illnesses and procedures include proctitis, colitis, rectorrhagia, partial colectomy, and anoplasty.

1. Using nonmedical terminology, what are her past conditions?

_____

_____

2. Using nonmedical terminology, what are her past procedures?

_____

_____

3. Separate the word parts to define them.

_____

_____

LO 14.3 Diagnostic, Procedural, and Laboratory Terms

Although there are several test mechanisms available to the provider caring for patients with gastroenterological conditions, the most common procedure is entering and viewing the alimentary canal with a scope. Because the GI system is essentially a long tube, scopes are the least risky and most cost-effective way to evaluate the system. There are various scopes used in GI examination, including enteroscopy, proctoscopy or sigmoidoscopy, and colonoscopy. **Proct/o** = rectum and anus + **-scopy** = viewing using a scope. Figure 14-10 illustrates an endoscopy.

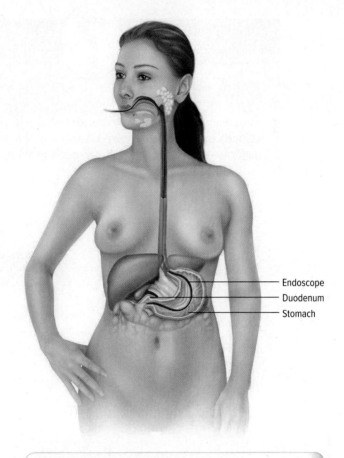

Figure 14-10 Endoscopy

PRACTICE

Provide the missing term(s) to complete the following sentences.

Diagnostic	
esophagoscopy [ĕ-sŏf-ă-GŎS-kō-pē] **gastroscopy** [găs-TRŎS-kō-pē] **colonoscopy** [kō-lŏn-ŎS-kō-pē] **proctoscopy** [prŏk-TŎS-kō-pē] **sigmoidoscopy** [SĬG-moy-DŎS-kō-pē] **peritoneoscopy** [PĔR-ĭ-tō-nē-ŎS-kō-pē]	An _____ is the use of an *esophagoscope* to illuminate the esophagus as it is passed through the mouth and into the esophagus. When ulcers are seen in the digestive system through the endoscope, a diagnosis of *H. pylori (Helicobacter pylori)*, bacteria that cause ulcers, is given. This is usually treated with an antibiotic and dietary modification. A *gastroscope* is used to examine the stomach in _____. A _____ is the use of an endoscope to examine the colon. A *proctoscope* is used to examine the rectum and anus in a _____. A *sigmoidoscope* is used to examine the sigmoid colon in _____. *Endoscopic retrograde cholangiopancreatography (ERCP)* is a procedure used to examine the biliary ducts with x-ray, a contrast medium, and the use of an endoscope. _____ or *laparoscopy* is the examination of the abdominal cavity with an instrument called a *peritoneoscope* or a *laparoscope*.
cholangiography [kō-lăn-jē-ŎG-ră-fē] **cholecystography** [kō-lē-sĭs-TŎG-ră-fē]	A *cholangiogram* is an image of the bile vessels taken in _____, an x-ray of the bile ducts. A *cholecystogram* is an image of the gallbladder taken in _____, an x-ray of the gallbladder taken after the patient swallows iodine. A liver scan, done after injection of radioactive material, can reveal abnormalities. Ultrasound is used to provide images of the entire abdominal area, as in *abdominal ultrasonography*.

Did you know

Colon Polyps

Thousands of colon polyps are identified and removed each year during a screening colonoscopy. Not every polyp is cancerous, but many gastroenterologists agree that the majority of colon polyps will become cancerous over time if left in the colon.

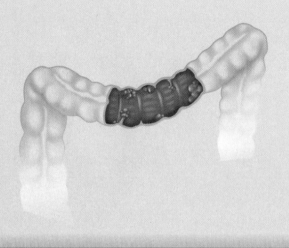

PRONOUNCE and DEFINE	Pronounce the following terms aloud and write the definitions.
cholangiography	[kō-lăn-jē-ŎG-ră-fē]
esophagoscopy	[ĕ-sŏf-ă-GŎS-kō-pē]
cholecystography	[kō-lē-sĭs-TŎG-ră-fē]
peritoneoscopy	[PĔR-ĭ-tō-nē-ŎS-kō-pē]

SPELL	Write the correct spelling of the related term.
	Scope of the esophagus, stomach, and duodenum
	Scope of the rectum and anus
	Scope to examine the last section of the colon only
	Scope to examine the stomach only

1. _____ colonoscopy

2. _____ esophagoscopy

3. _____ choleangiography

4. _____ cholecystography

5. _____ gastroscopy

6. _____ protocoscopy

a. Scope of the esophagus

b. X-ray test of the gallbladder

c. Scope of the stomach

d. Scope of the rectum and anus

e. X-ray test of the bile ducts

f. Scope of the large intestine

APPLY APPLY   Read the following scenario and answer the questions.

You are reviewing the medical record of Mr. John Jones, a 57-year-old African-American male. His recent hospitalization lists several procedures. His main complaint is abdominal pain. The tests are as follows: esophagoscopy with gastroscopy, cholangiography, cholecystography, laparoscopy, and colonoscopy. He eventually had a cholecystectomy.

1. What does each of the tests discover?

_____

_____

2. Write a "story" in lay terms of what happened to the patient during his recent hospitalization.

_____

_____

LO 14.4   Pathological Terms

Eating disorders are the most common pathological conditions associated with the digestive system. Females are diagnosed with eating disorders twice as often as males, but that number is on the rise in recent years. Although eating disorders are related to the digestive system, there are many different specialty physicians who are involved in the diagnosis and treatment of patients with these conditions.

The medical term *anorexia* by itself means, simply, to not eat. Many patients could therefore be anorexic. However, it becomes an eating disorder when the term *nervosa* is added to the end. Figure 14-11 describes several different types of eating disorders.

Binge eating and then purging the contents before the calories can be absorbed is also a popular and dangerous fad of young girls today. Many of them realize how dangerous this is to their health and get help before it is too late. Schools and teen outreach programs are showcasing the risks of these eating disorders and giving people the knowledge and tools to get help and treatment.

STUDY TIP

Body mass index (BMI) is a measurement that compares weight and height calculations in a chart that defines obesity. Patients are preobese if their BMI is between 25 and 29 kg/m^2 and morbidly obese when it is greater than 30 kg/m^2. For a free BMI calculator, go to http://www.aarp.org/health/fitness/info-05-2010/bmi_calculator.html.

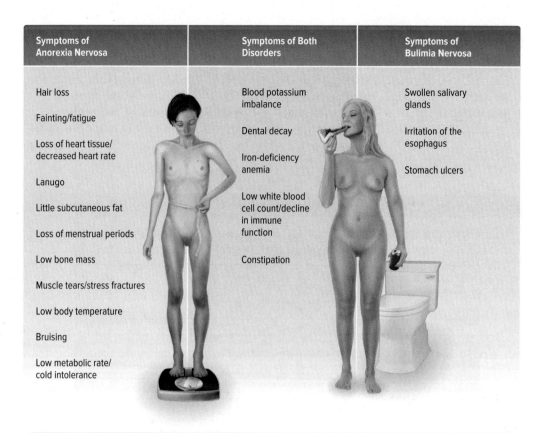

Symptoms of Anorexia Nervosa	Symptoms of Both Disorders	Symptoms of Bulimia Nervosa
Hair loss	Blood potassium imbalance	Swollen salivary glands
Fainting/fatigue	Dental decay	Irritation of the esophagus
Loss of heart tissue/ decreased heart rate	Iron-deficiency anemia	Stomach ulcers
Lanugo	Low white blood cell count/decline in immune function	
Little subcutaneous fat		
Loss of menstrual periods	Constipation	
Low bone mass		
Muscle tears/stress fractures		
Low body temperature		
Bruising		
Low metabolic rate/ cold intolerance		

Figure 14-11 Eating disorders

Eating Disorders

This table introduces terms for various eating disorders.

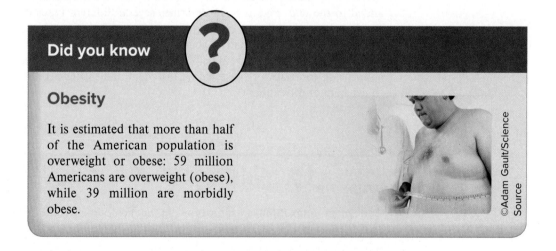

Did you know ?

Obesity

It is estimated that more than half of the American population is overweight or obese: 59 million Americans are overweight (obese), while 39 million are morbidly obese.

©Adam Gault/Science Source

Pathological	PRACTICE
	Provide the missing term(s) to complete the following sentences.
	The digestive system is both the site and the source of many diseases and disorders. What we take into our mouths determines the type of nutrition our body receives. Eating disorders can be the catalyst for disease processes to start.
anorexia nervosa [ăn-ō-RĔK-sē-ă něr-VŌ-să] **bulimia** [bū-LĒM-ē-ă]	Anorexia is a loss of appetite. In its most severe form, _____, it is a morbid refusal to eat because the person wishes to be dangerously thin. _____ is a disease wherein bingeing on food and then purposely purging or vomiting is also a quest for abnormal weight loss. Both anorexia nervosa and bulimia can produce many health problems and symptoms, such as hair loss, amenorrhea, and heart damage.
obesity [ō-BĒS-ĭ-tē]	_____ is often the result of overeating, although recent gene studies indicate a possible hereditary defect in many obese people. Obesity can be one of the factors in many health problems, such as heart disease and diabetes. Many eating disorders can be treated with psychological counseling; some, such as anorexia nervosa, may result in death if the patient is not treated at an eating disorder unit or clinic.

PRONOUNCE and DEFINE	Pronounce the following terms aloud and write the definition.
anorexia nervosa	[ăn-ō-RĔK-sē-ă něr-VŌ-să]
bulimia	[bū-LĒM-ē-ă]

SPELL	Write the correct spelling of the related term.
	Eating disorder of not eating or eating very little
	Eating disorder of bingeing and purging
	Eating disorder that has caused additional health problems
	Over the target weight for height and weight

UNDERSTAND	Match each term on the left to its description on the right.

1. _____ anorexia nervosa
2. _____ anorexia
3. _____ bulimia
4. _____ obesity
5. _____ morbid obesity

a. Eating disorder that causes a pathological condition
b. Eating disorder by bingeing and purging
c. Eating disorder by limiting food
d. Simple term for not eating/not hungry
e. Abnormal accumulation of fat

Miss Katherine Marx is a 16-year-old Caucasian female who has just expired suddenly in the ER. When filing her paperwork with the morgue, you are to review to ensure that all of her health history is included for the coroner to perform an autopsy. Upon admission, her weight was 94 pounds and her height was 5'7". Depression, acute anxiety, and body image disorder are listed as her diagnoses. She stated several times that she wasn't hungry, but her family reported they did occasionally see her eating, and although she was thin, they "didn't worry."

1. What eating disorder(s) could she have had?

_____

_____

_____

2. Based on the information, could an eating disorder be the cause of death?

_____

_____

_____

Disorders of the Mouth, Pharynx, and Esophagus

Typical disorders of the mouth, pharynx, and esophagus are usually secondary, or caused by some other mechanism that has caused symptoms in these areas. The most common culprits for mouth sores are allergic reactions, viruses, or bacterial infections caused by poor dental care. **Pharyng/o, cheil/o, stomat/o,** and **esophag/o** are all word roots used for disorders of the mouth, pharynx, and esophagus. Figure 14-12 shows canker sores of the mouth.

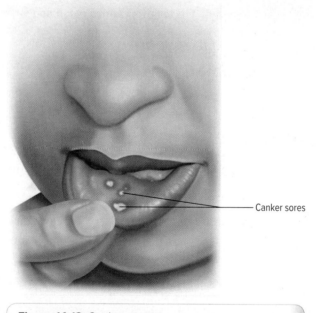

Canker sores

Figure 14-12 Canker sores

STUDY TIP

Ankyloglossia is a birth defect where the tissue that attaches the tongue to the bottom of the mouth (lingual frenulum) is abnormally short. The affected person may have extreme difficulty with eating and speech due to the inability to move the tongue normally.

PRACTICE

Provide the missing term(s) to complete the following sentences.

Mouth

cheilitis
[kī-LĪ-tĭs]

glossitis
[glŏ-SĪ-tĭs]

sialoadenitis
[SĪ-ă-lō-ăd-ĕ-NĪ-tĭs]

parotitis
[păr-ō-TĪ-tĭs]

parotiditis
[pă-rŏt-ĭ-DĪ-tĭs]

halitosis
[hăl-ĭ-TŌ-sĭs]

ankyloglossia
[ĂNG-kĭ-lō-GLŎS-ē-ă]

aphagia
[ă-FĀ-jē-ă]

dysphagia
[dĭs-FĀ-jē-ă]

Areas in the mouth can become inflamed from an infection, allergy, injury, or internal disorder. _____ occurs on the lips; _____ occurs on the tongue; _____ occurs in the salivary glands; and _____ or _____ occurs in the parotid glands. Various other dental disorders may similarly cause inflammation. _____ is unusually foul mouth odor, which may be caused by poor dental hygiene, gum disease, certain foods, or an internal disorder such as a sinus infection. _____ is a condition in which the tongue is partially or completely attached to the floor of the mouth, thereby preventing normal movement. Normal swallowing is an important part of maintaining good nutrition. People with swallowing disorders usually require diet supplementation via a tube. _____ is an inability to swallow; _____ is difficulty in swallowing.

Pharynx

Diseases of the pharynx are discussed in Chapter 12 as part of the respiratory system. Food travels into the mouth, through the pharynx, and into the esophagus.

Esophagus

esophagitis
[ĕ-sŏf-ă-JĪ-tĭs]

Esophageal varices are twisted veins in the esophagus that are prone to hemorrhage and ulcers. _____ is any inflammation of the esophagus. Gastroesophageal reflux disease (GERD) or esophageal reflux involves malfunctioning of the sphincter muscle at the bottom of the esophagus. It opens at the wrong time to allow backflow of stomach contents into the esophagus, causing irritation of the esophageal lining.

achalasia
[ăk-ă-LĀ-zē-ă]

_____ is the failure of the same esophageal sphincter to relax during swallowing and allow food to pass easily from the esophagus into the stomach to continue the digestive process. This disorder interferes with the intake of normal amounts of nutrients.

Did you know

Esophagus Diameter

The diameter of the esophagus is 24 mm, or the size of a quarter. It is common for young children to put objects in their mouths and many children swallow coins without any adverse outcome. Even so, it is always better to play it safe and keep small objects out of their reach!

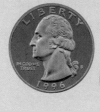
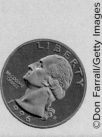

©Don Farrall/Getty Images

PRONOUNCE and DEFINE	Pronounce the following terms aloud and write the definition.
achalasia	[ăk-ă-LĀ-zē-ă]
dysphagia	[dĭs-FĀ-jē-ă]
aphagia	[ă-FĀ-jē-ă]
ankyloglossia	[ĂNG-kĭ-lō-GLŎS-ē-ă]

SPELL and DEFINE	Identify if the following terms are spelled correctly. Correct the words that are spelled incorrectly. Write the definition for each word.	
	Spelling	**Definition**
parotaditis		
ankyloglossia		
sialoadenitis		
acholasia		
cheiloitis		

UNDERSTAND	Match each term on the left to its description on the right.

1. _____ esophageal varices
2. _____ cheilitis
3. _____ dysphagia
4. _____ aphagia
5. _____ halitosis

a. Unable to swallow
b. Difficulty swallowing
c. Bad breath
d. Inflammation of lips
e. Large veins in the esophagus

APPLY	Read the following scenario and answer the questions.

You are coding physician notes for billing of services for Ms. Marion Mayweather, a 78-year-old Caucasian female. The physician has dictated the following: halitosis, dysphagia, cheilitis, and esophageal varices.

1. What is the definition of each of the terms listed?

_____

_____

2. How do they relate to one another?

_____

_____

3. What testing would the physician do to look at these areas? (Remember to reference the procedures.)

_____

_____

Stomach Disorders

The stomach ache, or **gastralgia/gastrodynia,** is probably the most common problem that everyone experiences sometime in life. Because eating is something that everyone does, every day, stomach issues are more noticeable and many people try to self-treat with over-the-counter products. A common stomach disorder is **dyspepsia,** or indigestion. Dyspepsia can be caused be several different issues. Stress, overeating, and peptic ulcers all can play a role in causing dyspepsia.

STUDY TIP

Commonly viral enteritis, or stomach flu, is contracted through contact with an infected person or consuming contaminated water or food. Most people recover quickly and without complication. For those with compromised immune systems, however, viral enteritis can be deadly.

Pathological	PRACTICE
	Provide the missing term(s) to complete the following sentences.
	The stomach is the site of many disorders. Some people are sensitive to various foods (such as very spicy dishes) or have allergies (such as to milk products or shellfish).
achlorhydria [ā-klōr-HĪ-drē-ă] **dyspepsia** [dĭs-PĔP-sē-ă] **gastritis** [găs-TRĪ-tĭs] **gastroenteritis** [GĂS-trō-ĕn-tĕr-Ī-tĭs]	_____ is the lack of hydrochloric acid in the stomach, a chemical necessary for digestion. _____ is difficulty in digesting food, particularly in the stomach. _____ is any stomach inflammation. _____ is an inflammation of both the stomach and small intestine.
flatulence [FLĂT-yū-lĕns] **eructation** [ē-rŭk-TĀ-shŭn] **nausea** [NĂW-zē-ă]	_____ is an accumulation of gas in the stomach or intestines. _____ may release some of this gas through the mouth. _____ is a sick feeling in the stomach caused by illness or the ingestion of spoiled food. It also may be felt in certain situations such as early pregnancy or when repetitive motion causes discomfort, as in car sickness or sea sickness.
hematemesis [hē-mă-TĔM-ĕ-sĭs] **peptic ulcer** **hiatal hernia** [hī-Ā-tăl HĔR-nē-ă]	_____ is the vomiting of blood from the stomach, usually a sign of a severe disorder. *Stomach ulcers* or gastric ulcers are a type of _____, a sore on the mucous membrane of any part of the gastrointestinal system (see Figure 14-13). A _____ is a protrusion of the stomach through an opening in the diaphragm called the hiatal opening.

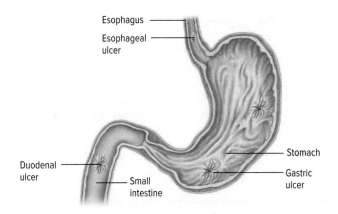

Esophagus

Esophageal ulcer

Stomach

Duodenal ulcer

Small intestine

Gastric ulcer

Figure 14-13 Peptic ulcers

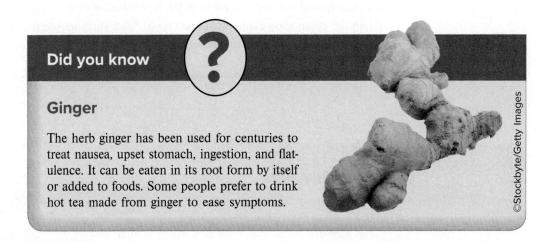

Did you know ?

Ginger

The herb ginger has been used for centuries to treat nausea, upset stomach, ingestion, and flatulence. It can be eaten in its root form by itself or added to foods. Some people prefer to drink hot tea made from ginger to ease symptoms.

©Stockbyte/Getty Images

PRONOUNCE and DEFINE	Pronounce the following terms aloud and write the definition.
gastroenteritis	[GĂS-trō-ĕn-tĕr-Ī-tĭs]
hematemesis	[hē-mă-TĔM-ĕ-sĭs]
achlorhydria	[ā-klōr-HĪ-drē-ă]
eructation	[ē-rŭk-TĀ-shŭn]

SPELL	Write the correct spelling of the related term.
	Sore on the stomach membrane
	Result of gas in the intestines
	Protrusion of the stomach into the esophagus
	Lack of hydrochloric acid in the stomach

UNDERSTAND	Match each term on the left to its description on the right.

1. _____ hiatal hernia
2. _____ dyspepsia
3. _____ nausea
4. _____ hematemesis
5. _____ eructation

a. Feeling of upset stomach
b. Protrusion of stomach into esophagus
c. "Burping"
d. Vomiting blood
e. Difficult digestion

Your neighbor, Mrs. Mary Teegarden, is a 58-year-old widow who likes to talk about her health problems. She tells you that she has had "awful, upset stomach, burping, and feels like her food sits in her stomach like a rock." She is worried because she has "spit up a little bit of pink" and she wonders if it could be blood. Of course, you tell her to see her doctor right away.

1. What are the medical terms for all of her symptoms?

_____

_____

2. How do they relate to one another?

_____

_____

3. How would you write this entire case study in medical terms?

_____

_____

Disorders of the Liver, Pancreas, and Gallbladder

Gallstones, or **cholelithiasis,** are a common disorder of the gallbladder (see Figure 14-14). They are caused from an abnormal production of calcium deposits in the gallbladder. The stones can be asymptomatic in many people but can cause pain when trying to pass, or they can block the normal flow of bile and result in a life-threatening condition called **choledocholithiasis.**

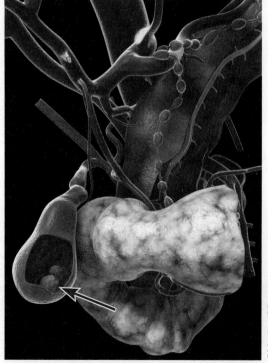

©MedicalRF.com

Figure 14-14 Gallstones

PRACTICE

Provide the missing term(s) to complete the following sentences.

jaundice [JĂWN-dĭs] **icterus** [ĬK-tĕr-ŭs] **hyperbilirubinemia** [HĪ-pĕr-BĬL-ĭ-rū-bĭ-NĒ-mē-ă]	Secretions of the liver, pancreas, and gallbladder mix with the stomach contents that move into the duodenum. The liver can be the site of _____ or _____, when excessive bilirubin in the blood (_____) causes a yellow discoloration of the skin. Newborn jaundice may be a result of liver disease or many other factors. It is sometimes treated with exposure to artificial lights or sunlight.
hepatomegaly [HĔP-ă-tō-MĔG-ă-lē] **hepatopathy** [hĕp-ă-TŎP-ă-thē] **hepatitis** [hĕp-ă-TĪ-tĭs]	_____ is an enlarged liver. _____ is a general term for liver disease, and _____ is a term for several types of contagious diseases, some of which are sexually transmitted.
cirrhosis [sĭr-RŌ-sĭs] **pancreatitis** [PĂN-krē-ă-TĪ-tĭs]	_____ is a chronic liver disease usually caused by poor nutrition and excessive alcohol consumption. _____ is an inflammation of the pancreas. (Other pancreatic diseases are discussed in Chapter 9.)
gallstones **cholelithiasis** [KŌ-lē-lĭ-THĪ-ă-sĭs] **cholangitis** [kō-lăn-JĪ-tĭs] **cholecystitis** [KŌ-lē-sĭs-TĪ-tĭs]	The gallbladder can be the site of calculi (_____ or _____) that block the bile from leaving the gallbladder. The presence of gallstones in the common bile duct is called *choledocholithiasis*. _____ is any inflammation of the bile ducts. _____ is any inflammation of the gallbladder, either acute or chronic.
duodenal ulcers [DŪ-ō-DĒ-năl ŬL-sĕrz] **appendicitis** [ă-pĕn-dĭ-SĪ-tĭs]	The duodenum can be the site of _____. These are a type of peptic ulcer and are thought to be bacterial (*H. pylori*) in origin. This discovery has led to the widespread use of antibiotics to treat many types of ulcers. On the side of the duodenum lies the appendix, which can become inflamed if gastric substances leak into it from the duodenum. This condition is called _____, which usually requires surgery to prevent the appendix from bursting.

Hepatitis

Hepatitis is the simple medical term for inflammation of the liver: **hepat/o** = liver + **-itis** = inflammation. Although hepatitis by itself sounds pretty general and could be caused from a number of conditions, there are viral types of hepatitis that are classified by the letters A, B, C, D, and E. They are much more threatening and specific diseases. Some are **acute,** or emergent/short term, and others are **chronic,** or long term.

Table 14-1 lists each of the specific types of viral hepatitis, its mode of transmission, and whether a vaccine is available to prevent it. *Note:* Hepatitis A, D, and E are not common to the United States, but hepatitis C infection is on the rise, even in groups with no history of risk behaviors.

TABLE 14-1	Types of Hepatitis			
Type	**Description**	**Incubation**	**Mode of Transmission**	**Vaccination**
Hepatitis A (HAV)	A viral infection of the liver that can cause jaundice, fatigue, nausea, vomiting, and fever for at least 1 month.	14–50 days	Fecal/oral: Virus is shed through the feces and is spread by improper hand washing. Also spread through contaminated food (e.g., undercooked fruits, vegetables, and shellfish [particularly raw and undercooked shellfish]) and ice and water.	Yes ©McGraw-Hill Education
Hepatitis B (HBV)	A viral infection of the liver. It can be acute or chronic. Transmission routes include sexual or close household contact, mother to baby, IV drug use, or nosocomial exposure.	60–90 days	Parenteral/sexual/perinatal: Body substances capable of transmitting the virus include blood and blood products; saliva; cerebrospinal fluid; peritoneal, pleural, pericardial, and synovial fluid; amniotic fluid; semen and vaginal secretions; and any other body fluid containing blood.	Yes ©Ingram Publishing/SuperStock
Hepatitis C (HCV)	A virus that causes inflammation of the liver.	2 weeks–6 months; commonly 6-9 weeks. Chronic infection can persist up to 20 years before the onset of cirrhosis or hepatoma	Blood: Spread by direct blood contact, usually through IV drug use. Prior to 1990, many cases of hepatitis C were spread through the use of blood or blood products. It is rare but possible for it to spread through unprotected sex, mother to baby, or accidental needlestick.	No ©Chris Holthof/Shutterstock
Hepatitis D (HDV)	A viral infection of the liver. It is always associated with a current infection of hepatitis B.	2-8 weeks	Parenteral/sexual/perinatal	No
Hepatitis E (HEV)	A viral infection of the liver. Outbreaks of hepatitis E and sporadic cases occur over a wide geographical area, primarily in countries with inadequate environmental sanitation.	26–42 days	Fecal/oral: Fecally contaminated drinking water is the most commonly documented vehicle of transmission. The fatality rate is similar to that of hepatitis A, except in pregnant women, where it may reach 20% among those infected during the third trimester of pregnancy.	No ©Filipe B. Varela/Shutterstock

Did you know

Jaundice

Jaundice, or yellowing of the skin color, is a relatively common occurrence in newborns. It is caused by an excessive amount of bilirubin in the baby's skin. The bilirubin is the result of overproduction of red blood cells that the baby's immature liver cannot break down and usually resolves with light exposure within a few days after birth.

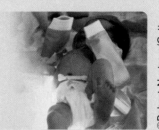

©Robert Nystrom/Getty Images

PRONOUNCE and DEFINE	Pronounce the following terms aloud and write the definition.
hepatitis	[hĕp-ă-TĪ-tĭs]
cholelithiasis	[KŌ-lē-lĭ-THĪ-ă-sĭs]
cirrhosis	[sĭr-RŌ-sĭs]
hepatomegaly	[HĔP-ă-tō-MĔG-ă-lē]

SPELL	Write the correct spelling of the related term.
	Yellowing of the skin
	Inflammation of the pancreas
	Gallstones
	Inflammation of the appendix
	Enlarged liver

UNDERSTAND	Match each term on the left to its description on the right.

1. _____ cholelithiasis a. Condition of the liver
2. _____ hepatopathy   b. Inflammation of the gallbladder
3. _____ appendicitis   c. Inflammation of the appendix
4. _____ hyperbilirubinemia d. Gallstones
5. _____ cholecystitis   e. High level of bilirubin

Mr. Kyle Martin is a 55-year-old hemophiliac patient who has come into the clinic for a blood transfusion. He also has hepatitis C and is complaining of nausea, indigestion, emesis, and right-sided pain.

1. Why is he having right-sided pain?

_____

_____

2. What are the risk factors for contracting hepatitis C?

_____

_____

Intestinal Disorders

Colitis is the general term for inflammation of the colon; however, there are several forms of colitis. The most common two are chronic diseases that can severely impact a patient's health and quality of life. These are ulcerative colitis and Crohn disease (Figure 14-15). A gastroenterologist cannot always distinguish which disease by visualizing alone and must perform a biopsy of the affected tissue. The biopsy is gathered frequently during a diagnostic **colonoscopy.**

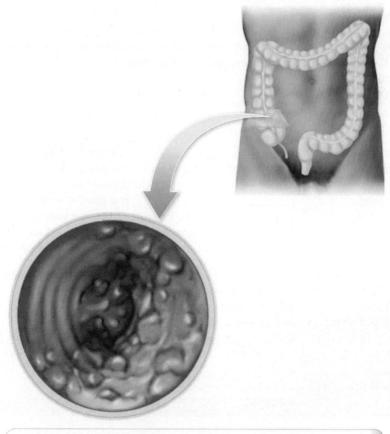

STUDY TIP

Colic is a pattern of excessive crying, not an illness or disease. Babies affected by colic are generally healthy with no physical or mental development issues. There is no evidence that colic has any long-term effect on babies.

Figure 14-15 Crohn disease

Pathological	
	Provide the missing term(s) to complete the following sentences.
ileus [ĬL-ē-ŭs] **enteritis** [ĕn-tĕr-Ī-tĭs] **colitis** [kō-LĪ-tĭs]	The small and large intestines can have ulcers, obstructions, irritations, inflammations, abnormalities, and cancer. An _____ is an intestinal blockage, which may be caused by lack of sufficient moisture to move waste material through the system or by an internal disorder. _____ and _____ are general terms for inflammations in the small intestine.
ulcerative colitis [ŬL-sĕr-ă-tiv kō-LĪ-tĭs]	_____ is a chronic type of inflammatory bowel disease with recurring ulcers and inflammations. Other symptoms may include cramping, abdominal pain, and diarrhea.
Crohn disease [krōn di-ZĒZ] **fistulas** [FŬS-tyū-lăz]	_____ is another type of inflammatory bowel disease with symptoms similar to ulcerative colitis but lacking ulcers and sometimes having _____, abnormal passages or openings in tissue walls.
colic [KŎL-ĭk]	_____ is a condition (usually in infants) of gastrointestinal distress due to allergies, an underdeveloped digestive tract, or other conditions that prevent easy digestion of food. In infants, colic usually resolves itself within a few months as the infant matures.
diverticulosis [DĪ-vĕr-tĭk-yū-LŌ-sĭs] **diverticula** [dī-vĕr-TĬK-yū-lă] **diverticulitis** [DĪ-vĕr-tĭk-yū-LĪ-tĭs] **ileitis** [ĬL-ē-Ī-tĭs]	_____ is a condition in which _____, small pouches in the intestinal wall, trap food or bacteria. _____ is an inflammation of the diverticula (see Figure 14-16). _____ is an inflammation of the ileum.
dysentery [DĬS-ĕn-tĕr-ē] **polyposis** [PŎL-ĭ-PŌ-sĭs]	_____ is a general term for irritation of the intestinal tract with loose stools and other symptoms, such as abdominal pain and weakness. It often is caused by bacteria such as those found in many underdeveloped countries. _____ is a general term for a condition in which polyps develop in the intestinal tract. Polyps can become cancerous so they are often checked or removed to detect any abnormalities at an early stage. Colonic polyposis is polyps in the colon, which have a high likelihood of changing to colorectal cancer.
volvulus [VŎL-vyū-lŭs] **intussusception** [ĬN-tŭs-sŭ-SĔP-shŭn] **ascites** [ă-SĪ-tēz] **peritonitis** [PĔR-ĭ-tō-NĪ-tĭs]	A _____, an intestinal blockage caused by twisting of the intestine on itself, requires emergency surgery. An _____ is the telescoping of the intestine. One section prolapses (collapses) into a neighboring part. The abdominal and peritoneal regions surrounding the intestinal tract can become filled with fluid (_____) or inflamed (_____).

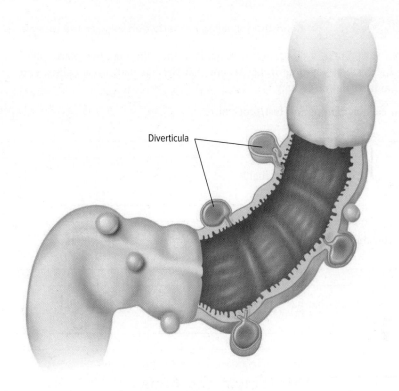

Diverticula

Figure 14-16 Diverticulitis, abnormal pouches in the colon that have become infected

PRONOUNCE and DEFINE	Pronounce the following terms aloud and write the definition.
polyposis	[PŎL-ĭ-PŌ-sĭs]
colitis	[kō-LĪ-tĭs]
volvulus	[VŎL-vyū-lŭs]
diverticulosis	[DĪ-vĕr-tĭk-yū-LŌ-sĭs]

SPELL	Write the correct spelling of the related term.
	General term for irritation of intestinal tract with diarrhea
	Twisting intestinal blockage
	Condition of small growths in the intestine
	Intestinal blockage caused by lack of moisture
	Abnormal pouches in the colon

UNDERSTAND	Match each term on the left to its description on the right.

1. _____ ascites
2. _____ polyposis
3. _____ diverticula
4. _____ enteritis
5. _____ peritonitis

a. Excessive fluid in the abdominal cavity
b. Pouches in the colon wall
c. Polyps on the colon wall
d. Inflammation of the intestine
e. Inflammation of the abdominal regions

Miss Karen Carpointer, a 60-year-old female, is at the clinic for her yearly physical recheck appointment. When reviewing her history, you note in her record that she has had diverticulitis, enteritis, abdominal pain, laparoscopy, polyposis, and partial colectomy.

1. Explain each symptom and test/procedure.

_____

_____

2. How do they relate to one another?

_____

_____

3. What procedures did she have?

_____

_____

4. Write a "story" of what has happened to her using lay terms to explain.

_____

_____

STUDY TIP

In general, anal fistulas result from a previous abscess. Inside the anus there are small glands, and when clogged, the gland becomes infected and can result in an abscess. Fistulas connect infected anal glands to the skin on the outside of the anus.

The Rectum and Anus

There are several common disorders of the rectum and anus. It is a region of the body that is very active and controls bowel evacuation. A common disorder that affects both men and women is **hemorrhoids.** Hemorrhoids are essentially varicose veins of the rectum (see Figure 14-17). They can be caused from heredity, repeated strain, and/or sitting for long periods of inactivity, which puts pressure on the rectal area. Sometimes they are **asymptomatic,** but the majority of patients state they have discomfort and swelling as a result.

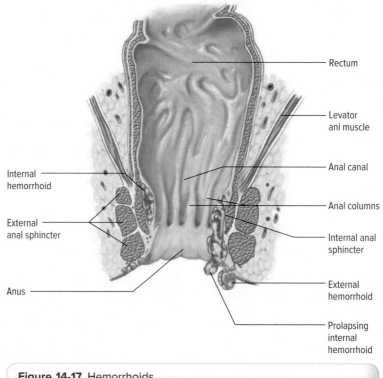

Figure 14-17 Hemorrhoids

PRACTICE

Provide the missing term(s) to complete the following sentences.

proctitis
[prŏk-TĪ-tĭs]

constipation
[kŏn-stĭ-PĀ-shŭn]

diarrhea
[dī-ă-RĒ-ă]

flatus
[FLĀ-tŭs]

The rectum, anus, and stool may play a role in some disorders. _____ is an inflammation of the rectum and anus. _____ is a condition with infrequent or difficult release of bowel movements, sometimes the result of insufficient moisture to soften and move stools. _____ is loose, watery stools that may be the result of insufficient roughage or of an internal disorder. _____ is the release of gas through the anus.

melena
[mĕ-LĒ-nă]

hematochezia
[HĒ-mă-tō-KĒ-zē-ă]

steatorrhea
[STĒ-ă-tō-RĒ-ă]

The analysis of stool for blood, bacteria, and other elements can provide a clue to various ailments. _____ is a condition in which blood that is not fresh appears in the stool as a black, tarry mass. _____ is bright red blood in the stool. _____ is fat in the stool.

anal fistula
[Ā-năl FĬS-tyū-lă]

hemorrhoids
[HĔM-ō-roydz]

A small opening in the anal canal is called an _____. Waste material can enter the abdominal cavity through a fistula. The anus may be the site of _____, swollen, twisted veins that can cause great discomfort.

PRONOUNCE and DEFINE

Pronounce the following terms aloud and write the definition.

hematochezia	[HĒ-mă-tō-KĒ-zē-ă]
melena	[mĕ-LĒ-nă]
steatorrhea	[STĒ-ă-tō-RĒ-ă]

SPELL and DEFINE

Identify if the following terms are spelled correctly. Correct the words that are spelled incorrectly. Write the definition for each word.

	Spelling	Definition
hemorroids		
diarrhea		
hematachezia		
steatorhhea		

UNDERSTAND

Match each term on the left to its description on the right.

1. _____ hemorrhoids
2. _____ hematochezia
3. _____ anal fistula
4. _____ proctitis
5. _____ steatorrhea
6. _____ melena

a. Bright red blood in the stool
b. Black, tarry, "old" blood in the stool
c. Inflammation of rectum/anus
d. Fat in the stool
e. Swollen, twisted veins in the rectum
f. Small opening in the anal canal

You are working in the lab of a large hospital. You note that several stool samples have come in for analysis labeled below. Note: Some may be normal.

- B.R. = bright red stripes in stool
- G.T. = dark coffee-ground-looking stool; black
- H.L. = greenish-brown stool
- C.C. = fatty, oily concentrations in the stool

1. What is the medical term for the type of stool that B.R. has?

   _____

   _____

2. What is the medical term for the type of stool that G.T. has?

   _____

   _____

3. What is the medical term for the type of stool that C.C. has?

   _____

   _____

Hernias

A hernia is any loop or twist of an intestine or other organ not positioned correctly in the abdomen. There are many types of hernias. Some common ones are as follows:

- A *hiatal hernia* is the protrusion of the stomach into the esophagus.
- An *inguinal hernia* is a protrusion of the intestine through a weakness in the abdominal wall.
- A *strangulated hernia* is one in which blood flow is restricted or absent. *It may be life threatening!*
- A *femoral hernia* is a protrusion of a loop of intestine into the femoral canal.
- An *umbilical hernia* is a protrusion of part of the intestine into the umbilicus.

Did you know ?

Inguinal Hernias

Inguinal hernias are most often associated with a person who has strained and caused stress to an area as a result of heavy lifting, but children and babies also can develop inguinal hernias. If the muscle wall is underdeveloped or weak, part of the small intestine can slip through and therefore cause a hernia, which usually requires surgical repair.

LO 14.5 Surgical Terms

Gastroenterologists and surgeons work closely together because the GI system disorders frequently require surgical intervention to reach a cure or remissive state. In some rural areas, the same physician is trained in both specialties. In other cases, there are surgeons who specialize only in particular GI cases, such as **gastric** bypass or **colorectal** surgery.

STUDY TIP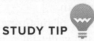

Abdominocentesis is a procedure where the abdomen is surgically punctured to create a hole to draw fluid for pathology (looking for disease or cancer) or as a comfort measure to relieve pressure of fluid accumulation caused most often as a result of cancer or disease.

Surgical	**PRACTICE**
	Provide the missing term(s) to complete the following sentences.
	Treating the digestive tract often includes biopsies, surgeries, and observation using endoscopes. The following is a list of some of the surgical procedures performed on the digestive system.
abdominocentesis [ăb-DŎM-ĭ-nō-sĕn-TĒ-sĭs] **paracentesis** [PĂR-ă-sĕn-TĒ-sĭs]	_____ or _____ is a surgical puncture to remove fluid or relieve pressure in the abdominal cavity, as in ascites.
cholelithotomy [KŌ-lē-lĭ-THŎT-ō-mē] **choledocholithotomy** [kō-LĔD-ō-kō-lĭ-THŎT-ō-mē] **cholelithotripsy** [kō-lē-LĬTH-ō-trĭp-sē]	_____ is an incision for the removal of stones. _____ is an incision for the removal of stones in the common bile duct. _____ is the crushing of gallstones using sound waves or other techniques.
glossorrhaphy [glŏ-SŌR-ă-fē] **esophagoplasty** [ĕ-SŎF-ă-gō-plăs-tē] **proctoplasty** [PRŎK-tō-plăs-tē]	Surgical repair of the digestive tract includes _____ (tongue suturing); _____ (esophagus repair); and _____ (repair of the rectum and anus).

continued on next page

glossectomy [glŏ-SĔK-tō-mē] **polypectomy** [pŏl-ĭ-PĔK-tō-mē] **appendectomy** [ăp-pĕn-DĔK-tō-mē] **cholecystectomy** [KŌ-lē-sĭs-TĔK-tō-mē] **diverticulectomy** [dī-vĕr-tĭk-ū-LĔK-tō-mē] **gastrectomy** [găs-TRĔK-tō-mē] **gastric resection** **gastric bypass** **colectomy** [kō-LĔK-tō-mē] **pancreatectomy** [PĂN-krē-ă-TĔK-tō-mē] **hemorrhoidectomy** [HĔM-ō-roy-DĔK-tō-mē] **hepatic lobectomy** [hĕ-PĂT-ĭk lō-BĔK-tō-mē] **liver biopsy** **anal fistulectomy** [Ā-năl fĭs-tyū-LĔK-tō-mē] **Billroth I** [BĬLL-rŏth] **Billroth II**	Some parts of the digestive tract may require partial or complete removal because of malignancies or chronic inflammation. A _____ is removal of the tongue. A _____ is the removal of polyps, particularly in areas such as the colon, which are susceptible to cancer. An _____ is the removal of a diseased appendix that is in danger of rupturing. A _____ is the removal of the gallbladder, particularly one that is constantly inflamed and susceptible to painful bouts of gallstones. A _____ is removal of diverticula. A _____ is removal of some or all of the stomach. It may be followed by a gastric resection, to repair the remaining part of the stomach. A _____ or _____ removes a portion of the stomach to limit overeating as a treatment for obesity. A _____ is the removal of some or all of the colon. This may be a temporary operation that is followed by a surgical reconnection of parts of the colon or it may require the use of a colostomy bag. A _____ is removal of the pancreas, usually only in cases with malignancy. A _____ is the removal of hemorrhoids, which are sometimes treated by laser cauterization. A _____ is removal of one or more lobes of the liver. It is usually preceded by a _____ to determine the type and extent of disease. People can live with only part of a liver. However, if a person with a completely diseased liver does not receive an organ transplant, he or she will usually die. An anal fistula is removed in an _____. _____ and _____ are two types of operations. The first is the excision of the pylorus, and the second is the resectioning of the pylorus with the stomach.
anastomosis (*pl.,* **anastomses**) [ă-năs-tō-MŌ-sĭs (ă-năs-tō-MŌ-sēz)]	An _____, a surgical union of two hollow tubes, is sometimes used to bypass parts of the intestines, as in the case of removal of a section of the intestines. There are many types of anastomoses used in various body systems. There are a number of ways that anastomoses can correct digestive disorders. An *ileorectal anastomosis* is the connection of the ileum and the rectum after a total colectomy. An *end-to-side anastomosis* is a connection of the end of one vessel to the side of a larger one.
ileostomy [ĬL-ē-ŌS-tō-mē] **colostomy** [kō-LŎS-tō-mē]	Openings may have to be made in the gastrointestinal tract. Sometimes they are temporary to allow evacuation of waste material. In some cases, they are permanent, as when intestinal parts cannot be reconnected. An _____ is the creation of an opening in the abdomen that is attached to the ileum to allow fecal matter to discharge into a bag outside the body. A _____ is an opening in the colon to the abdominal wall to create a place for waste to exit the body other than through the anus. A colostomy is sometimes required in the case of diseases such as cancer and ulcerative colitis.

Abdominal Surgery

The first known doctor to perform abdominal surgery using a general anesthetic was a Chinese physician named Hua T'o. This surgery occurred sometime between 170 and 180 AD. He used a mixture of hemp and strong wine to render his patients unconscious and achieve general anesthesia. There is no mention of success or failure with this surgery in curing the patient.

PRONOUNCE and DEFINE	Pronounce the following surgical terms aloud and write the definition.
ileostomy	[ĬL-ē-ŎS-tō-mē]
cholelithotomy	[KŌ-lē-lĭ-THŎT-ō-mē]
hepatic lobectomy	[hĕ-PĂT-ĭk lō-BĔK-tō-mē]

SPELL	Write the correct spelling of the related term.
	Surgical union of two tubes
	Removal of the appendix
	Removal of the gallbladder
	Surgical opening from the colon into the abdomen
	Lip repair

UNDERSTAND	Match each term on the left to its description on the right.

1. _____ anastomosis   a. Tongue suturing
2. _____ cholecystectomy   b. Creating an opening in the colon
3. _____ colectomy   c. Removal of part or all of colon
4. _____ colostomy   d. Removal of the gallbladder
5. _____ glossorrhaphy   e. Surgical union of two tubes

A group of surgical technology students is studying for a test on the various procedures that a GI surgeon would perform. They need to know them to assist appropriately and provide the correct instruments: colostomy, colectomy, hepatic lobectomy, esophagectomy, ileostomy, small intestinal anastomosis, and hemorrhoidectomy.

1. What is the difference between a colostomy and a colectomy?

_____

_____

2. What organ is a hepatic lobectomy performed on and what is it?

_____

_____

3. How would an ileostomy and small intestinal anastomosis relate to each other?

_____

_____

4. Where is a hemorrhoidectomy performed and what is it?

_____

_____

LO 14.6 Pharmacological Terms

The majority of pharmacological agents associated with the digestive system are used to remedy symptoms, and many are sold over the counter. Laxatives and medications to ease indigestion are common; however, there are other systemic medications that are sometimes used to treat more complex diseases. Steroids are used in the treatment of autoimmune disorders such as Crohn disease to suppress inflammation.

Some digestive medications serve more than one purpose and can be used for different ailments. The patient needs to be cautious because if the medication is effective for both antacid and laxative use, and the patient wants relief from acid indigestion (dyspepsia), diarrhea also may develop.

Pharmacological	PRACTICE
	Provide the missing term(s) to complete the following sentences.
antacids [ănt-ĂS-ĭds] **antiemetics** [ĂN-tē-ĕ-MĔT-ĭks] **antispasmodics** [ĂN-tē-spăz-MŎD-ĭks] **laxative** [LĂK-să-tĭv] **cathartic** [kă-THĂR-tĭk] **antidiarrheal** [ĂN-tē-dī-ă-RĒ-ăl]	Aside from treatments for cancer, medications for the digestive tract counteract situations that occur in various parts of the tract. _____ neutralize stomach acid. Many antacids are taken before meals to prevent the buildup of excess stomach acids. Others are taken after symptoms appear. _____ prevent vomiting. _____ relieve spasms in the gastrointestinal tract. A _____ stimulates movement of bowels. A _____ induces vomiting. An _____ helps to control loose, watery stools.

PRONOUNCE and DEFINE	Pronounce the following terms aloud and write the definition.
antiemetic	[ĂN-tē-ĕ-MĚT-ĭk]
cathartic	[kă-THĂR-tĭk]
antispasmodic	[ĂN-tē-spăz-MŎD-ĭk]

SPELL	Write the correct spelling of the related term.
	Stimulates bowel movements
	Neutralizes stomach acid
	Induces vomiting
	Prevents vomiting
	Acts like natural cortisone

UNDERSTAND	Match each term on the left to its description on the right.

1. _____ antacid
2. _____ cathartic
3. _____ antispasmodic
4. _____ antiemetic
5. _____ antidiarrheal

a. Neutralizes acid
b. Prevents vomiting
c. Induces vomiting
d. Controls loose stools
e. Relieves cramps in the intestinal tract

APPLY	Read the following scenario and respond accordingly.

Mr. Cole Smith is a pharmacy technician who works part time at a local pharmacy. The pharmacist has asked him to restock the shelves based on the medication type. All medications are available over the counter (OTC) and include Pepto-Bismol®, Tums®, ex-lax®, Imodium®, and ipecac. Arrange the preceding medications in order by type using the classification below (you may have to research the OTC drugs if you are not familiar with them).

1. antacid
2. cathartic
3. antispasmodic
4. antiemetic
5. antidiarrheal

Abbreviations

ABBREVIATION REVIEW

Abbreviation	Definition
ALT	alanine aminotransferase
AST	aspartate aminotransferase
BM	bowel movment
BMI	body mass index
EGD	esophagogastroduodenoscopy
GB	gallbladder
GI	gastrointestinal
HAV	hepatitis A
HBV	hepatitis B
HCV	hepatitis C
HDV	hepatitis D
HEV	hepatitis E
IBD	inflammatory bowel disease
IBS	irritable bowel syndrome
LFT	liver function test
NG	nasogastric
PUD	peptic ulcer disease
SGOT	serum glutamic oxaloacetic transaminase
SGPT	serum glutamic pyruvic transaminase
TPN	total parental nutrition
UGI	upper gastrointestinal

APPLY   Rewrite the note using abbreviations.

This patient is experiencing gastrointestinal upset and is jaundiced, with nausea, vomiting, and fatigue. Last bowel movement was 3 days ago. The physician has ordered liver function tests, serum glutamic oxaloacetic transaminase, serum glutamic pyruvic transaminase, alanine aminotransferase, aspartate aminotransferase, and upper gastrointestinal testing. Suspects hepatitis A.

_____

_____

_____

CHAPTER SUMMARY

	Learning Outcome	Summary
14.1	Describe the basic function and structure of the digestive system and body metabolism.	The digestive system is comprised of major organs and accessory organs that function to work together to process and metabolize food products and provide nutrients to the body.
14.2	Recognize the major word parts used in building words that relate to the digestive system.	Word building requires knowledge of word parts and their corresponding meanings to form medical terms within the digestive system.
14.3	Recall the common diagnostic tests, laboratory tests, and clinical procedures used in treating disorders of the digestive system.	Diagnostic, procedural, and laboratory findings assist the health care provider in diagnosing medical conditions. Often used in combination, these tests lead to a final diagnosis and assist in treatment planning.
14.4	Define the major pathological conditions of the digestive system.	Knowledge and understanding of diseases and conditions of the digestive system, including acute and chronic diseases, structure, repair and treatment to promote function, and cancer increase critical thinking related to pathological medical terms.
14.5	Define surgical terms related to the digestive system.	Surgical procedures within the digestive system revolve closely around repair of damaged or nonfunctioning structures and treatment of cancer within the system.
14.6	Recognize common pharmacological agents used in treating disorders of the digestive system.	Primary and common pharmacological agents used in the digestive system are symptomatic relief agents, peristalsis-promoting or -inhibiting agents, and corticosteroids.
14.7	Identify common abbreviations associated with the digestive system.	Abbreviations are used to describe diseases, conditions, procedures, and treatments associated with the digestive system.

RECALL

1. Identify the parts of the main digestive system.

_____

_____

_____

_____

2. Identify the parts of the accessory digestive system.

_____

_____

_____

_____

Identify if the following terms are spelled correctly. Correct the words that are spelled incorrectly. Write the definition for each word.

	Spelling	Definition
hemmorrhoid		
diarhea		
cathartic		
anal fistulectomy		
alimentary canal		
mastecation		
emulsfication		
colecystectomy		

Pronounce the above terms aloud.

Complete the words using the appropriate combining forms learned in this chapter.

1. _____ scopy means viewing the stomach.
2. _____ gram means a measure of the gallbladder.
3. _____ ectomy means removal of the ileum.
4. _____ itis means inflammation of the liver.
5. _____ plegia means paralysis of the colon.

Complete the sentences by filling in the blanks.

1. _____ is the creation of an opening in the abdomen, which is attached to the ileum to allow fecal matter to discharge into a bag outside the body.
2. _____ is a repair of the rectum and anus.
3. _____ is the removal of a diseased appendix that is in danger of rupturing.
4. _____ is a condition in which blood that is not fresh appears in the stool as a black, tarry mass.
5. A small opening in the anal canal is called a(n) _____.
6. _____ is a general term for a condition in which polyps develop in the intestinal tract.
7. _____ is the vomiting of blood from the stomach.
8. _____ is an incision for the removal of gallstones.
9. _____ is a chronic liver disease usually caused by poor nutrition and excessive alcohol consumption.
10. A *cholangiogram* is an image of the bile vessels taken in _____, an x-ray of the bile ducts.
11. Inflammation of the esophagus is _____.
12 _____ is an inability to swallow; _____ is difficulty in swallowing.
13. A(n) _____ is the use of an endoscope to examine the colon.
14. _____ is an enlarged liver.
15. A(n) _____ is an intestinal blockage, which may be caused by lack of sufficient moisture to move waste material through the system or by an internal disorder.
16. Suture of the stomach is called _____.
17. _____ is a specialist in the study of diseases and treatment of the rectum and anus.
18. Inflammation of the lips is _____.
19. Pertaining to the tongue and teeth is _____.
20. Removal of the gallbladder is _____.

The physician tells the family that the client has had some upper GI bleeding that has caused her to vomit blood and he will need to perform a procedure to explore the area from the throat to the stomach to find out where the bleeding is coming from. If it is coming from the esophagus, he may need to repair the area. If the bleeding is coming from the stomach, he may need to take a small amount of tissue to check for cancer and other conditions.

Using medical terminology, write what the physician has told the family regarding the client.

_____

_____

_____

_____

Reviewing the Terms

Pronounce each of the following terms. Write the definitions on a separate sheet of paper. This review will take you through all the words you learned in this chapter. If you have difficulty with any words, make a flash card for later study. Refer to the English-Spanish and Spanish-English glossaries in the eBook.

abdominocentesis [ăb-DŎM-ĭ-nō-sĕn-TĒ-sĭs]

absorption [ăb-SŎRP-shŭn]

achalasia [ăk-ă-LĀ-zē-ă]

achlorhydria [ā-klōr-HĪ-drē-ă]

alimentary [ăl-ĭ-MĔN-tĕr-ē] **canal**

amino [ă-MĒ-nō] **acid**

amylase [ĂM-ĭl-ās]

an/o [Ā-nō]

anal [Ā-năl] **canal**

anal fistula [Ā-năl FĬS-tyū-lă]

anal fistulectomy [Ā-năl fĭs-tyū-LĔK-tō-mē]

anastomosis [ă-năs-tō-MŌ-sĭs]

ankyloglossia [ĂNG-kĭ-lō-GLŎS-ē-ă]

anorexia nervosa [ăn-ō-RĔK-sē-ă nĕr-VŌ-să]

antacid [ănt-ĂS-ĭd]

antidiarrheal [ĂN-tē-dī-ă-RĒ-ăl]

antiemetic [ĂN-tē-ĕ-MĔT-ĭk]

antispasmodic [ĂN-tē-spăz-MŎD-ĭk]

anus [Ā-nŭs]

aphagia [ă-FĀ-jē-ă]

append/o, appendic/o [ă-PĔN-dō, ă-PĔN-dĭ-kō]

appendage [ă-PĔN-dĭj]

appendectomy [ăp-pĕn-DĔK-tō-mē]

appendicitis [ă-pĕn-dĭ-SĪ-tĭs]

appendix [ă-PĔN-dĭks]

ascites [ă-SĪ-tēz]

bil/o, bili [bĭl-ō, bĭl-ĭ]

bile [bīl]

bilirubin [bĭl-ĭ-RŪ-bĭn]

Billroth I [BĬLL-rŏth]

Billroth II

body

bowel [bŏw-l]

bucc/o [bŭk-ō]

bulimia [bū-LĒM-ē-ă]

cathartic [kă-THĂR-tĭk]

cec/o [SĒ-kō]

cecum [SĒ-kŭm]

celi/o [SĒ-lē-ō]

cheeks

cheilitis [kī-LĪ-tĭs]

cheiloplasty [KĪ-lō-plăs-tē]

chol/e, cholo [KŌ-lē, KŎL-ō]

cholangi/o [kō-LĂN-jē-ō]

cholangiography [kō-lăn-jē-ŎG-ră-fē]

cholangitis [kō-lăn-JĪ-tĭs]

cholecyst/o [kō-lē-SĬS-tō]

cholecystectomy [KŌ-lē-sĭs-TĔK-tō-mē]

cholecystitis [KŌ-lē-sĭs-TĪ-tĭs]

cholecystography [kō-lē-sĭs-TŎG-ră-fē]

choledoch/o [kō-LĔD-ō-kō]

choledocholithotomy [kō-LĔD-ō-kō-lǐ-THŎT-ō-mē]

cholelithiasis [KŌ-lē-lǐ-THĪ-ǎ-sǐs]

cholelithotomy [KŌ-lē-lǐ-THŎT-ō-mē]

cholelithotripsy [kō-lē-LĬTH-ō-trǐp-sē]

chyme [kīm]

cirrhosis [sǐr-RŌ-sǐs]

col/o, colon/o [KŌ-lō, kō-LŎN-ō]

colectomy [kō-LĔK-tō-mē]

colic [KŎL-ǐk]

colitis [kō-LĪ-tǐs]

colon [KŌ-lŏn]

colonoscopy [kō-lŏn-ŎS-kō-pē]

colostomy [kō-LŎS-tō-mē]

constipation [kŏn-stǐ-PĀ-shŭn]

Crohn [krōn] **disease**

defecation [dĕ-fĕ-KĀ-shŭn]

deglutition [dē-glū-TĬSH-ŭn]

diarrhea [dī-ǎ-RĒ-ǎ]

digestion [dī-JĔS-chŭn]

diverticula [dī-vĕr-TĬK-yū-lǎ]

diverticulectomy [dī-vĕr-tĭk-ū-LĔK-tō-mē]

diverticulitis [DĪ-vĕr-tĭk-yū-LĪ-tǐs]

diverticulosis [DĪ-vĕr-tĭk-yū-LŌ-sǐs]

duoden/o [dū-ō-DĒ-nō]

duodenal [DŪ-ō-DĒ-nǎl] **ulcers**

duodenum [dū-ō-DĒ-nŭm]

dysentery [DĬS-ĕn-tĕr-ē]

dyspepsia [dǐs-PĔP-sē-ǎ]

dysphagia [dǐs-FĀ-jē-ǎ]

elimination [ē-lǐm-ǐ-NĀ-shŭn]

emesis [ĕ-MĒ-sǐs]

emulsification [ĕ-MŬL-sǐ-fǐ-KĀ-shŭn]

enter/o [ĔN-tĕr-ō]

enteritis [ĕn-tĕr-Ī-tǐs]

enzyme [ĔN-zīm]

epiglottis [ĕ-pǐ-GLŎT-ǐs]

eructation [ē-rŭk-TĀ-shŭn]

esophag/o [ĕ-SŎF-ǎ-gō]

esophagitis [ĕ-sŏf-ǎ-JĪ-tǐs]

esophagoplasty [ĕ-SŎF-ǎ-gō-plǎs-tē]

esophagoscopy [ĕ-sŏf-ǎ-GŎS-kō-pē]

esophagus [ĕ-SŎF-ǎ-gŭs]

fatty acid

feces [FĒ-sēz]

fistula [FĬS-tyū-lǎ]

flatulence [FLĂT-yū-lĕns]

flatus [FLĀ-tŭs]

frenulum [FRĔN-yū-lŭm]

fundus [FŬN-dŭs]

gallbladder [GĂWL-blǎd-ĕr]

gallstones

gastr/o [GĂS-trō]

gastrectomy [gǎs-TRĔK-tō-mē]

gastric resection or **gastric bypass**

gastritis [gǎs-TRĪ-tǐs]

gastroenteritis [GĂS-trō-ĕn-tĕr-Ī-tǐs]

gastroscopy [gǎs-TRŎS-kō-pē]

gloss/o [GLŎS-ō]

glossectomy [glŏ-SĔK-tō-mē]

glossitis [glŏ-SĪ-tǐs]

glossorrhaphy [glŏ-SŌR-ǎ-fē]

gluc/o [GLŪ-kō]

glucose [GLŪ-kōs]

glyc/o [GLĪ-kō]

glycogen [GLĪ-kō-jĕn]

glycogen/o [GLĪ-kō-jĕn-ō]

gums [gŭmz]

halitosis [hǎl-ǐ-TŌ-sǐs]

hard palate [PĂL-ǎt]

hematemesis [hē-mǎ-TĔM-ĕ-sǐs]

hematochezia [HĒ-mǎ-tō-KĒ-zē-ǎ]

hemorrhoidectomy [HĔM-ō-roy-DĔK-tō-mē]

hemorrhoids [HĔM-ō-roydz]

hepat/o [hĕ-PĂT-ō]

hepatic lobectomy [hĕ-PĂT-ǐk lō-BĔK-tō-mē]

hepatitis [hĕp-ǎ-TĪ-tǐs]

hepatomegaly [HĔP-ǎ-tō-MĔG-ǎ-lē]

hepatopathy [hĕp-ă-TŎP-ă-thē]

hiatal hernia [hī-Ā-tăl HĔR-nē-ă]

hyperbilirubinemia [HĪ-pĕr-BĬL-ĭ-rū-bĭ-NĒ-mē-ă]

icterus [ĬK-tĕr-ŭs]

ile/o [ĬL-ē-ō]

ileitis [ĬL-ē-Ī-tĭs]

ileostomy [ĬL-ē-ŎS-tō-mē]

ileum [ĬL-ē-ŭm]

ileus [ĬL-ē-ŭs]

intussusception [ĬN-tŭs-sŭ-SĔP-shŭn]

jaundice [JĂWN-dĭs]

jejun/o [jĕ-JŪ-nō]

jejunum [jĕ-JŪ-nŭm]

labi/o [LĀ-bē-ō]

large intestine

laxative [LĂK-să-tĭv]

lingu/o [LĬNG-gwō]

lingual tonsils [LĬNG-gwăl TŎN-sĭlz]

lipase [LĬP-ās]

lips

liver [LĬV-ĕr]

liver biopsy

mastication [măs-tĭ-KĀ-shŭn]

melena [mĕ-LĒ-nă]

mesentery [MĔS-ĕn-tĕr-ē, MĔZ-ĕn-tĕr-ē]

mouth

nausea [NĂW-zē-ă]

obesity [ō-BĒS-ĭ-tē]

or/o [ŌR-ō]

palatine [PĂL-ă-tīn] tonsils

pancreas [PĂN-krē-ăs]

pancreat/o [PĂN-krē-ăt-ō]

pancreatectomy [PĂN-krē-ă-TĔK-tō-mē]

pancreatitis [PĂN-krē-ă-TĪ-tĭs]

papilla (pl., papillae) [pă-PĬL-ă (pă-PĬL-ē)]

paracentesis [PĂR-ă-sĕn-TĒ-sĭs]

parotitis, parotiditis [păr-ō-TĪ-tĭs, pă-rŏt-ĭ-DĪ-tĭs]

pepsin [PĔP-sĭn]

peptic ulcer

peristalsis [pĕr-ĭ-STĂL-sĭs]

periton/eo [PĔR-ĭ-tō-NĒ-ō]

peritoneoscopy [PĔR-ĭ-tō-nē-ŎS-kō-pē]

peritonitis [PĔR-ĭ-tō-NĪ-tĭs]

pharyng/o [FĂR-ĭng-kō]

pharynx [FĂR-ĭngks]

polypectomy [pŏl-ĭ-PĔK-tō-mē]

polyposis [PŎL-ĭ-P-sĭs]

proct/o [PRŎK-tō]

proctitis [prŏk-TĪ-tĭs]

proctoplasty [PRŎK-tō-plăs-tē]

proctoscopy [prŏk-TŎS-kō-pē]

pylor/o [pī-LŌR-ō]

pylorus [pī-LŌR-ŭs]

rect/o [RĔK-tō]

rectum [RĔK-tŭm]

reflux [RĒ-flŭks]

regurgitation [rē-GŬR-jĭ-TĀ-shŭn]

rugae [RŪ-gē]

saliva [să-LĪ-vă]

salivary [SĂL-ĭ-vār-ē] glands

sial/o [SĪ-ă-lō]

sialaden/o [SĪ-ă-lăd-ĕ-nō]

sialoadenitis [SĪ-ă-lō-ăd-ĕ-NĪ-tĭs]

sigmoid [SĬG-moyd] colon

sigmoid/o [SĬG-moyd-ō]

sigmoidoscopy [SĬG-moy-DŎS-kō-pē]

small intestine

soft palate [PĂL-ăt]

steat/o [STĒ-ă-tō]

steatorrhea [STĒ-ă-tō-RĒ-ă]

stomach [STŎM-ăk]

stomat/o [STŌ-mă-tō]

stool [stūl]

throat [thrōt]

tongue [tŭng]

ulcerative colitis [kō-LĪ-tĭs]

uvula [YŪ-vyū-lă]

villi (sing., villus) [VĬL-ī (VĬL-ŭs)]

volvulus [VŎL-vyū-lŭs]

The Urinary System

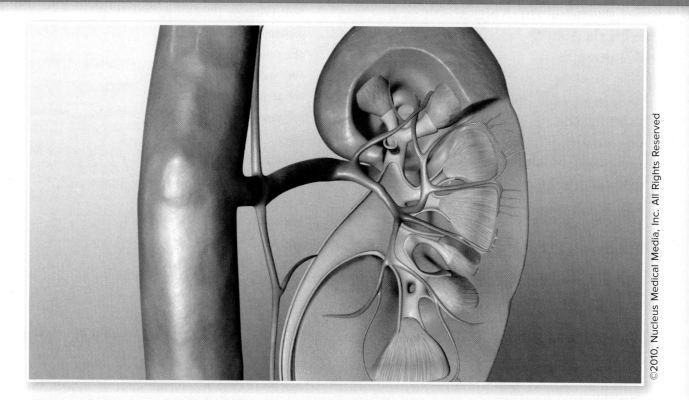

Learning Outcomes

After studying this chapter, you will be able to:

15.1 Describe the parts of the urinary system and discuss the function of each part.

15.2 Recognize the major word parts used in building words that relate to the urinary system.

15.3 Identify and understand the common diagnostic tests, laboratory tests, and clinical procedures used in testing and treating disorders of the urinary system.

15.4 Define the major pathological conditions of the urinary system.

15.5 Define the surgical terms related to the urinary system.

15.6 Recognize common pharmacological agents used in treating disorders of the urinary system.

15.7 Identify common abbreviations associated with the urinary system.

LO 15.1 Structure and Function of the Urinary System

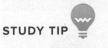
The urinary system (also called the *renal system* or *excretory system*) maintains the proper amount of water in the body and removes waste products from the blood by excreting them in the urine (Figure 15-1). The medical term for the study of the urinary system is **urology.**

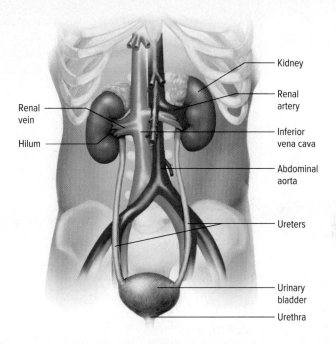

Renal vein —
Hilum —
Kidney
Renal artery
Inferior vena cava
Abdominal aorta
Ureters
Urinary bladder
Urethra

Figure 15-1 The urinary system

The urinary system is composed of kidneys, ureters, urinary bladder, and urethra. The two kidneys [**nephr/o**] are located in the posterior midtrunk. The kidneys' main purpose is to filter toxins and substances from the blood to make urine. The kidneys also assist in regulation of blood pressure through the production of renin, produce erythropoietin for erythrocyte production, produce prostaglandins, and help metabolize vitamin D. Next are the two ureters, which carry the urine from each kidney to the urinary bladder. The bladder's only function is to store the urine until it is released from the body through the urethra.

Structure and Function	PRACTICE
	Provide the missing term(s) to complete the following sentences.
urinary system [YŪR-ĭ-nār-ē SĬS-těm]	The _____ consists of:
kidneys [KĬD-nēz]	1. Two _____, organs that remove dissolved waste and other substances from the blood and urine.
ureters [yū-RĒ-těrz]	2. Two _____, tubes that transport urine from the kidneys to the bladder.
bladder [BLĂD-ěr]	3. The _____, the organ that stores urine.
urethra [yū-RĒ-thră] **meatus** [mē-Ā-tŭs]	4. The _____, a tubular structure that transports urine through the _____, the external opening of a canal, to the outside of the body.

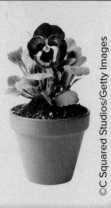
PRONOUNCE and DEFINE	Pronounce the following urinary terms aloud and write the definition.
ureter	[yū-RĒ-tĕr]
urethra	[yū-RĒ-thră]
meatus	[mē-Ā-tŭs]
urology	[yū-RŎL-ō-jē]

SPELL	Write the correct spelling of the related term.
	One of two tubes that lead to the bladder
	Specialty that studies the bladder
	Organ that stores urine
	External opening of a canal

UNDERSTAND Match each term on the left to its description on the right.

1. _____ urology
2. _____ urethra
3. _____ ureter
4. _____ meatus
5. _____ bladder

a. Tube that carries urine to the outside
b. Tube that carries urine to the bladder
c. Opening to the outside
d. Saclike structure that stores urine
e. Study of the urinary system

APPLY Read the following scenario and answer the questions.

Mrs. Betty Garble is a 46-year-old mother of five whom your physician has referred to see a urologist. She is having trouble controlling her urine output.

1. What is a urologist?

_____

_____

2. What is the structure that controls the output of urine?

_____

_____

Major Word Parts of the Urinary System

Combining Form/Suffix	Meaning
cali/o, calic/o	calyx
cyst/o	bladder, especially the urinary bladder
glomerul/o	glomerulus
meat/o	meatus
nephr/o	kidney
pyel/o	renal pelvis
ren/o	kidney
trigon/o	trigone
ur/o, urin/o	urine
ureter/o	ureter
urethr/o	urethra
-uria	of urine
vesic/o	bladder, generally used when describing something in relation to a bladder

STUDY TIP

Each human kidney is approximately 4 to 5 in. (12–14 cm) long and 3 in. (7–8 cm) wide and weighs between 5 and 7 ounces. In comparison, it is similar to the average computer mouse.

Kidneys

The kidneys are bean-shaped organs that are housed on either side of the mid- to lumbar area of the back (Figure 15-2). They perform several functions for the body. The main function is the life-sustaining process of filtering the blood and regulating fluids.

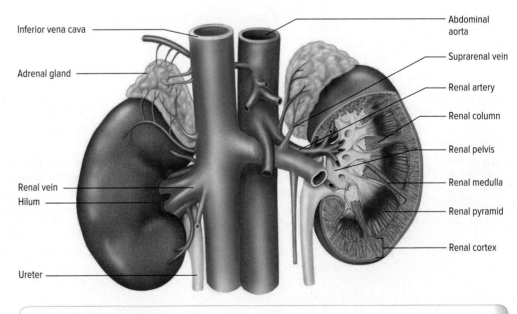

Figure 15-2 The kidneys

The kidneys have mechanisms to maintain homeostasis (equilibrium) in the filtration rate of the glomeruli. The constant flow of water and its substances back into the bloodstream and the flow of water and waste substances into the renal tubule maintain the body's balance of water, salts (the most common salt in the body is sodium chloride), sugars (the most common sugar in the body is glucose), and other substances (Figure 15-3). To do this, the kidneys have two lines of defense. The first is the automatic dilating and constricting of the arterioles as needed to increase or decrease the flow of blood into the glomeruli. The second is to release renin to increase the blood pressure and thus the filtration rate of blood to maintain a constant supply. Maintaining homeostasis affects blood pressure either by lowering it when blood is flowing too quickly or by increasing it when blood is flowing too slowly. Some forms of high blood pressure are caused by the effort of poorly functioning kidneys to maintain homeostasis.

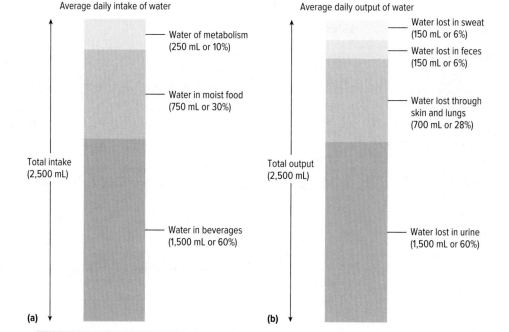

Figure 15-3 Water balance in the body

STUDY TIP

Urine is mostly comprised of water, salts, and nitrogenous waste. It also can contain medication components that were not metabolized by the body if filtration occurred in the kidneys.

Structure and Function	PRACTICE
	Provide the missing term(s) to complete the following sentences.
retroperitoneal [RĔ-trō-PĔR-ĭ-tō-NĒ-ăl]	Each kidney is a bean-shaped organ about the size of a human fist. The kidneys are located in the _____ (posterior to the peritoneum) space behind the abdominal cavity on either side of the vertebral column. The kidneys sit against the deep muscles of the back surrounded by fatty and connective tissue. The left kidney is usually slightly higher than the right one.
reabsorption [rē-ăb-SŌRP-shŭn]	The kidneys serve two functions—to form urine for excretion and to retain essential substances the body needs in the process called _____.

filtration [fĭl-TRĀ-shŭn] **urea** [yū-RĒ-ă] **creatine** [KRĒ-ă-tēn] **creatinine** [krē-ĂT-ĭ-nēn] **uric acid** [YŪR-ĭk ĂS-ĭd]	Urine is produced by _____ of water, salts, sugar, _____, and other nitrogenous waste materials such as _____ (and its component _____) and _____. The excretion rate of creatinine is measured in urinary tests because it is an indicator of how the kidneys are functioning. In the average adult, kidneys will filter about 1,700 liters of blood per day. Urine output is the only means for the body to remove toxic nitrogenous wastes from the body.
cortex [KŌR-tĕks] **medulla** [mĕ-DŪL-ă] **hilum** [HĪ-lŭm]	The kidneys have an outer protective portion, the _____, and an inner soft portion, the _____ (a term used for the inner, soft portion of any organ). In the middle of the concave side of the kidney is a depression, the _____, through which the blood vessels, the nerves, and the ureters enter and exit the kidney.
nephron [NĔF-rŏn] **urine** [YŪR-ĭn]	The functional unit of the kidney is the _____. The nephron removes waste products from the blood and produces _____. Each kidney contains about 1 million nephrons, more nephrons than one person needs. That is why people can live a normal life with only one kidney.
glomerulus [glō-MĂR-yū-lŏs] **glomeruli** [glō-MĂR-yū-lī] **renin** [RĔ-nĭn] **Bowman's capsule** [BŌ-mănz KAP-sūl]	Blood enters each kidney through the *renal artery* and leaves through the *renal vein*. Once inside the kidney, the renal artery branches into smaller arteries called *arterioles*. Each arteriole leads into a nephron. Each nephron contains a *renal corpuscle* made up of a group of capillaries called a _____ (*pl.,* _____). The glomerulus filters fluid from the blood and is the first place where urine is formed in the kidney. Each nephron also contains a *renal tubule*, which carries urine to ducts in the kidney's cortex. Blood flows through the kidneys at a constant rate. If the blood flow is decreased, the kidney automatically produces _____, a substance that causes an increase in the blood pressure to maintain the filtration rate of blood. The wall of each glomerulus is thin enough to allow water, salts, sugars, urea, and certain wastes to pass through. Each glomerulus is surrounded by a capsule, _____, where this fluid collects. The filtered substances that are removed from the blood then pass into the renal tubules.
renal pelvis **calices** [KĂL-ĭ-sēz] **calyces** [KĂL-ĭ-sēz] **calyx** [KĀ-lĭks]	Substances held in the renal tubule that can be used by the body are reabsorbed back to the bloodstream. During this reabsorption, most of the water, nutrients including glucose, and selected electrolytes move back to the blood. Any substance not reabsorbed will become urine. Urine travels to the _____, a collecting area in the center of the kidney. Pelvis is a general term for the collecting area of an organ or system. The renal pelvis contains small cuplike structures called _____ (also spelled _____; singular _____) that collect urine.

Did you know ?

Survival Without Kidneys

A human is able to function normally with only 50% of one kidney. It is possible to survive without kidney(s) with the help of medical treatments and dialysis to remove and filter toxins.

PRONOUNCE and DEFINE	Pronounce the following terms aloud and write the definition.
glomerulus	[glō-MĀR-yū-lŏs]
nephron	[NĔF-rŏn]
hilum	[HĪ-lŭm]
retroperitoneal	[RĔ-trō-PĔR-ĭ-tō-NĒ-ăl]

SPELL	Write the correct spelling of the related term.
	Capsule that surrounds each glomerulus
	Excretion rate of this is measured to assess kidney function
	When blood flow is decreased, a kidney produces this
	Collecting center in the kidney
	Outer protective portion of the kidney

UNDERSTAND   Match each term on the left to its description on the right.

1. _____ calyces
2. _____ cortex
3. _____ renin
4. _____ nephron
5. _____ urea

a. Cuplike structures
b. Causes increase in blood pressure
c. Removes waste products from the blood
d. A component of urine
e. Outer protective portion of the kidney

APPLY   Read the following scenario and answer the questions.

Mr. Mark Grey, a third-grade teacher, has asked you to explain the structure and function of the kidneys to his class.

1. What are the main components of the kidneys?

_____

_____

2. What is in urine?

_____

_____

3. How does urine progress?

_____

_____

4. Draw an illustration of the kidney (without looking at the pictures) that the students would understand.

_____

_____

Ureters, Bladder, and Urethra

The ureter is a tube that is approximately 22 cm in length and extends from the kidney (renal pelvis) to the urinary bladder. Because there are two kidneys, there are two ureters.

The urinary bladder (we must use "urinary" at the front because there are other types of bladders) is a saclike structure that sits in the pelvis. It is muscular in nature, as it needs to force urine into the urethra.

The urethra (there is only one) extends from the urinary bladder to the meatus, which then allows the body to control when urine is released.

The urinary system is the same in males and females with the exception of the prostate gland. Males alone have this additional gland, which is housed connecting the urethra and the ejaculatory duct. Figure 15-4 illustrates the ureter, bladder, and urethra.

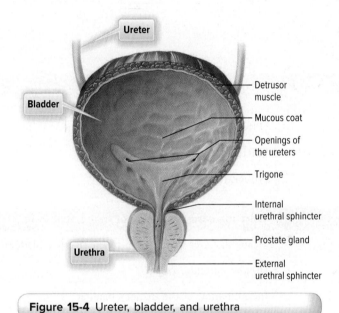

Figure 15-4 Ureter, bladder, and urethra

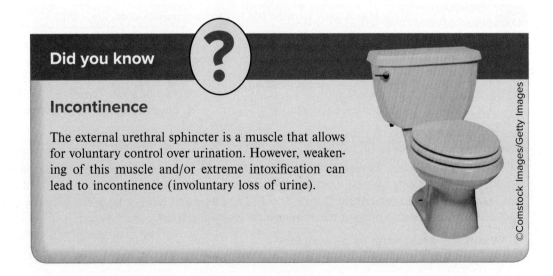

Did you know ?

Incontinence

The external urethral sphincter is a muscle that allows for voluntary control over urination. However, weakening of this muscle and/or extreme intoxification can lead to incontinence (involuntary loss of urine).

©Comstock Images/Getty Images

Structure and Function	**PRACTICE** Provide the missing term(s) to complete the following sentences.
ureters [yū-RĒ-tĕrz] **urinary bladder** [YŬR-ĭ-nār-ē BLĂD-ĕr]	The _____ transport urine to the _____ .
urinary bladder [YŬR-ĭ-nār-ē BLĂD-ĕr] **trigone** [TRĪ-gōn]	The _____ is a hollow, muscular organ that stores urine until it is ready to be excreted from the body. The base of the bladder contains a triangular area, the _____ , where the ureters enter the bladder and the urethra exits it.
urethra [yū-RĒ-thră] **prostate gland** [PRŎS-tāt glănd]	The _____ and ejaculatory duct meet at the _____ .

PRONOUNCE and DEFINE	**Pronounce the following terms aloud and write the definition.**
prostate	[PRŎS-tāt] (Be careful; there is no second "R" in this term. It is often mispronounced!)
trigone	[TRĪ-gōn]
urethra	[yū-RĒ-thră]

SPELL	**Write the correct spelling of the related term.**
	Triangular area at the base of the urinary bladder
	Hollow muscular organ
	Inflammation of the urinary bladder
	External tube carrying urine to the outside of the body

UNDERSTAND   **Match each term on the left to its description on the right.**

1. _____ prostate gland   a. Area at the base of the bladder where ureters enter
2. _____ urethra   b. This meets at the urethra on males
3. _____ ureter   c. Muscular organ that stores urine
4. _____ trigone   d. Two of them; carry urine to bladder
5. _____ urinary bladder   e. Single tube that carries urine to the meatus

APPLY   **Read the following scenario and answer the questions.**

Mr. Matthew Webber is a 43-year-old Caucasian male who has come into the office requesting a yearly recheck of his physical status. His only complaint is the urgency to urinate often and moderately high blood pressure. The doctor has examined him and determined that he would like to have you recheck his blood pressure and schedule a PSA (prostate screening antigen) blood test to screen for prostate cancer.

1. What is the medical term for his symptom?

_____

_____

2. Based on structure and function, what do you think could be causing him to have urinary urgency?

_____

_____

LO 15.2 Word Building in the Urinary System

Now that the urinary anatomy has been covered, it is time to practice word building. The following practice lists some medical terms and combinations common to the urinary system. As you work through the practice, try to mix and match or associate various word roots with different prefixes/suffixes to extend your knowledge and vocabulary (also see Table 15-1).

TABLE 15-1	Cystitis vs. Pyelonephritis	
Cystitis: Superficial Infection	**Pyelonephritis**	
Intracellular, biofilm-like pods	Invasion of kidney, +/− bloodstream	
Dysuria, urgency, frequency	Fever, chill, flank pain, tenderness, increased WBC	

Source: Gregory G. Anderson, Joseph J. Palermo, Joel D. Schilling, Robyn Roth, John Heuser, Scott J. Hultgren, "Intracellular Bacterial Biofilm-Like Pods in Urinary Tract Infections," *Science*, 04 Jul 2003: Vol. 301, Issue 5629, pp. 105–107.

Word Building	PRACTICE
	Provide the correct combining form to complete the sentences.
trigon-itis [TRĪ-gō-NĪ-tĭs]	Inflammation of the trigone of the bladder is _____ itis.
meato-tomy [mē-ă-TŎT-ō-mē]	Surgical enlargement of the meatus is _____ tomy.
cyst-itis [sĭs-TĪ-tĭs]	Inflammation of the bladder is _____ itis.
urethro-rrhea [yū-rē-thrō-RĒ-ă]	Abnormal discharge from the urethra is _____ rrhea.
nephr-itis [nĕ-FRĪ-tĭs]	Inflammation of the kidney is _____ itis.
calio-plasty [KĀ-lē-ō-plăs-tē]	_____ plasty is surgical reconstruction of a calix.
an-uria [ăn-YŪ-rē-ă]	Lack of urine formation is an _____.
ur-emia [yū-RĒ-mē-ă]	Excess urea and other nitrogenous wastes in the blood is _____ emia.
pyelo-plasty [PĪ-ĕ-lō-plăs-tē]	_____ plasty is surgical repair of the renal pelvis.
glomerul-itis [glō-MĂR-yū-LĪ-tĭs]	_____ itis is inflammation of the glomeruli.

continued on next page

Word Building	**PRACTICE**
	Provide the correct combining form to complete the sentences.
vesico-abdominal [VĔS-ĭ-kō-ăb-DŎM-ĭ-năl]	_____ abdominal relates to the urinary bladder and the abdominal wall.
reno-megaly [RĒ-nō-MĔG-ă-lē]	_____ megaly is enlargement of the kidney.
uretero-stenosis [yū-RĒ-tĕr-ō-stĕ-NŌ-sĭs]	Narrowing of a ureter is _____ stenosis.

Did you know

UTIs

Bacterial infections in the urinary tract are often the cause of urinary tract infections (UTIs). Though less common, cystitis also can occur due to a reaction to medication, radiation therapy, irritants, or illness.

PRONOUNCE and DEFINE	Pronounce the following terms aloud and write the meaning.
urethrorrhea	[yū-rē-thrō-RĒ-ă]
renomegaly	[RĒ-nō-MĔG-ă-lē]
pyeloplasty	[PĬ-ĕ-lō-plăs-tē]
meatotomy	[mē-ă-TŎT-ō-mē]

SPELL	Identify if the following terms are spelled correctly. Correct the words that are spelled incorrectly. Write the definition for each word.	
	Spelling	**Definition**
urethrorrhea		
nephroitis		
glomerulitis		
meatomy		
cystectomy		
anouria		

Match each term on the left to its description on the right.

1. _____ meatotomy
2. _____ nephromegaly
3. _____ urethrostenosis
4. _____ uremia
5. _____ cystitis

a. Inflammation of the bladder
b. Excess of wastes in the blood
c. Narrowing of the urethra
d. Incision into the opening to the outside
e. Enlargement of the kidney

APPLY   **Read the following scenario and answer the questions.**

Mrs. Jocelyn Workus is a 25-year-old woman with a history of diabetes. The diabetes has damaged her kidneys and Mrs. Workus is on a waiting list for a kidney transplant. Her diagnoses are listed as the following in her medical record: nephromegaly, nephritis, uremia, anuria, and trigonitis. She is scheduled for a nephrectomy.

1. What is nephromegaly? Nephritis?

_____

_____

2. What is uremia? Anuria?

_____

_____

3. What is a nephrectomy?

_____

_____

LO 15.3 Diagnostic, Procedural, and Laboratory Terms

STUDY TIP

Understanding common lab tests can help with studying terms and being able to relate them in practice. For instance, routine urinalysis can detect many potential problems not only in the urinary system but also dehydration, potential diabetes, and more.

There are several mechanisms that are used when a physician is diagnosing urinary symptoms, conditions, and diseases. The majority of them are generalized as the urine not only can signal urinary disorders but also can provide information on other systems. The most common diagnostic test is a **urinalysis** (Figure 15-5), which is the term used for inspecting a urine sample for abnormalities using either a microscope or a machine.

Dr. Joel Chorzik
1420 Glen Road
Meadowvale, OK 44444
111-222-3333

Run Date: 09/22/XX

Run Time: 1507

Patient: James Delgado	Acct #1: A994584732	Loc: ED	U#:
Reg Dr: S. Anders, M.D,	Age/Sex: 55/M	Room:	Reg: 09/22/XX
	Status: Reg ER	Bed:	Des:

Spec #: 0922 : U0009A	Coll: 09/22//XX	Status Comp:	Req #: 77744444
	Reed: 09/22//XX	Suben Dr:	

Entered: 09/22/XX-0841   Other Dr:

Ordered: UA with micro

Comments: Urine Description: Clean catch urine

Test	Result	Flag	Reference
Urinalysis			
UA with micro			
COLOR	YELLOW		
APPEARANCE	HAZY	..	
SP GRAVITY	1.018		1.001–1.030
GLUCOSE	NORMAL		NORMAL mg/dl
BILIRUBIN	NEGATIVE		NEG
KETONE	NEGATIVE		NEG mg/dl
BLOOD	2+	..	NEG
FH	5.0		4.5–8.0
PROTEIN	TRACE	..	NEG mg/dl
UROBILINOGEN	NORMAL		NORMAL –1.0 mg/dl
NITRITES	NEGATIVE		NEG
LEUKOCYTES	2+	..	NEG
WBC	20–50	..	0–5/HPF
RBC	2–5		0–5/HPF
EPI CELLS	20–50		/HPF
BACTERIA	2+	..	
MUCUS			

Specimen Report	Patient 1	Page 1

Figure 15-5 Urinalysis report

Urine is typically **sterile** before leaving the body, so for critical or important results, it is customary to obtain a sterile specimen via catheter to prevent any outside contaminants from interfering with results.

However, urinalysis also is done via "clean catch" when the provider decides it is not necessary to obtain a sterile sample, often for less critical diagnostic conditions.

Diagnostic	PRACTICE
urinalysis [yū-ri-NĂL-i-sis]	_____ is the examination of urine for its physical, chemical, and microscopic properties. Urine is gathered from a client who voids, or urinates, into a specimen bottle or whose urine is obtained by *urinary catheterization,* the insertion of a flexible tube through the meatus and into the urinary bladder.
Foley catheter [FŌ-lē KĂTH-ĕ-tĕr] **indwelling** [ĬN-dwĕ-lĭng] **condom catheter** [KŎN-dŏm KĂTH-ĕ-tĕr]	Some patients do not have bladder control or may have certain conditions that require catheters to aid in urination. A _____ is _____ (left in the bladder) and is held in place by a balloon inflated in the bladder. Foley catheters (Figure 15-6) are also known as *retention catheters.* Foley catheters are used when intake and output (I&O) are required to be monitored closely. A _____ (also called a *Texas catheter, external urinary drainage [EUD] catheter,* or *latex catheter*) consists of a rubber sheath placed over the penis with tubing connected to a drainage or leg bag where the urine collects (Figure 15-7).
	There are three phases of a complete urinalysis (for references on ranges, see Appendix C):
specific gravity	1. The first phase is the *macroscopic* or *physical phase.* During this phase, the color, turbidity (cloudiness caused by suspended sediment), and _____ (ratio of density of a substance) of urine give certain diagnostic clues.
pH	2. The second phase is the *chemical phase,* which determines the types of chemicals present in the urine. It also determines the _____ range of urine (see Appendix C for chemical analyses and ranges commonly used in urinalysis).
casts	3. The third phase is the *microscopic phase,* during which urine sediment is examined for solids (including cellular material) or _____, which are formed when protein accumulates in the urine.
acetone [ĂS-ĕ-tōn] **ketones** [KĒ-tōnz] **albumin** [ăl-BYŪ-mĭn] **glucose** [GLŪ-kōs] **bilirubin** [bĭl-ĭ-RŪ-bĭn]	In addition, tests of urine are designed to detect various substances indicative of specific conditions. The presence of high quantities of _____ usually occurs in diabetes. _____ in the urine may indicate starvation or diabetes. Ketones in the urine can lead to dangerously high levels of acid in the blood, which is a potential cause of coma and/or death. The presence of serum protein _____ in urine may indicate a leakage of blood proteins through the renal tubules, an indicator of nephron disease. _____ in the urine usually indicates diabetes. Pus in the urine makes the urine cloudy and indicates an infection or inflammation in the urinary system. Bacteria in the urine elevates the nitrite result on the urinalysis. This indicates a urinary tract infection. Blood in the urine usually indicates bleeding in the urinary tract. Calcium in the urine is abnormal and indicates one of several conditions, such as rickets. _____ in the urine indicates liver disease, such as obstructive disease of the biliary tract or liver cancer.
	Blood Tests: Two important blood tests for kidney function are the *blood urea nitrogen (BUN)* and the *creatinine clearance test.* The presence of high amounts of urea or creatinine in the kidney shows that the kidney is not filtering and removing these toxic substances from the blood. If this is not treated and kidney failure persists, death may result.
phenylketones [FĔN-ĭl-KĒ-tōnz]	_____ in the blood show a lack of an important enzyme that can lead to mental retardation in infants unless a strict diet is followed into adulthood. Infants are routinely tested for this deficiency at birth by taking a blood sample (using a heel stick), which is analyzed for presence of the enzyme.

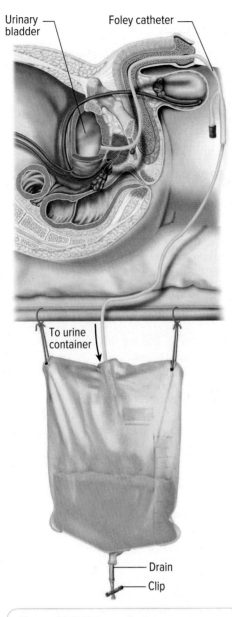

Urinary bladder

Foley catheter

To urine container

Drain

Clip

Figure 15-6 Foley catheter

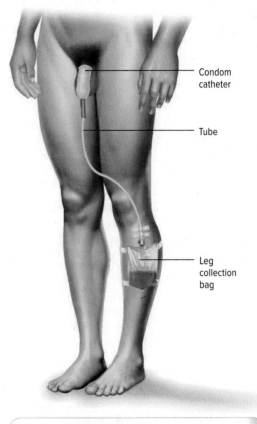

Condom catheter

Tube

Leg collection bag

Figure 15-7 Condom catheter

Did you know ?

Asparagus

Many people notice that directly after eating asparagus, their urine smells exactly like the vegetable did before it was eaten. The body excretes the same element that produces the smell in the urine.

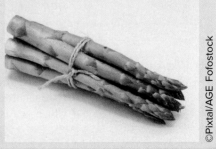

©Pixtal/AGE Fofostock

PRONOUNCE and DEFINE	Pronounce the following terms aloud and write the definition.
albumin	[ăl-BYŪ-mĭn]
urinalysis	[yū-rĭ-NĂL-ĭ-sĭs]
phenylketones	[FĔN-ĭl-KĒ-tōnz]
acetone	[ĂS-ĕ-tōn]

SPELL	Write the correct spelling of the related term.
	Sugar in the urine
	Usually occurs in diabetes
	Indicates liver disease
	May indicate starvation
	Range of urine
	Produced from a presence of serum protein

UNDERSTAND — Match each term on the left to its description on the right.

1. _____ urinalysis
2. _____ phenylketones
3. _____ specific gravity
4. _____ acetone
5. _____ glucose

a. Examination of urine
b. Ratio of density of a substance
c. This is checked for in infants
d. If found in urine, may indicate diabetes
e. May indicate starvation or diabetes

APPLY — Read the following scenario and answer the questions.

Brad Leighton is an 11-year-old with juvenile diabetes as his main diagnosis. The doctor has ordered a urinalysis to be done. He wants it tested for acetones, ketones, glucose, specific gravity, and pH.

1. What is a urinalysis?

_____

_____

2. What are ketones?

_____

_____

3. What is specific gravity?

_____

_____

4. Is glucose normally present in urine?

_____

_____

Imaging Tests and Urinary Tract Procedures

Every specialty relies on imaging tests and procedures to evaluate a patient's condition and/or provide treatment to an existing condition. **Urology** is no different. The physician listens to the patient, reads the previous history, and determines which tests/procedures to order based on that information to provide the best picture of what is really going on inside the patient's body.

A common imaging test in the urinary system is a **KUB** x-ray. (KUB stands for kidney/ureter/bladder.) The patient is positioned midabdominal view so the provider is able to see any structural abnormalities within those organs. It is also possible to detect obstruction and determine bladder fullness.

An **ultrasound** is another imaging test that is used often in the urinary system. One popular question people ask is why the technician always tells the patient to drink a lot of water prior to the procedure. Sound travels better through fluid, and it is easier to see key areas when the bladder is full and distended out of the way.

Diagnostic	**PRACTICE** Provide the missing term(s) to complete the following sentences.
	Imaging Tests: Various tests are used to visually diagnose stones, growths, obstructions, and abnormalities in the urinary system.
cystoscopy [sĭs-TŎS-kō-pē] **cystoscope** [SĬS-tō-skōp] **kidney, ureter, bladder (KUB)**	_____ is the insertion of a tubular instrument (a _____) to examine the bladder with a light. An *intravenous pyelogram (IVP)* and an *intravenous urogram* are x-rays of the urinary tract after a contrast medium is injected into the bloodstream. A _____ is an x-ray of three parts of the urinary tract. A *renal angiogram* is an x-ray of the renal artery after a contrast medium has been injected into the artery.
retrograde pyelogram (RP) [RĔT-rō-grād PĪ-ĕl-ō-grăm] **voiding cystogram (VCG), voiding (urinating) cystourethrogram (VCUG)** [VOYD-ĭng sĭs-tō-yū-RĒ-thrō-grăm]	A _____ is an x-ray of the kidney, bladder, and ureters taken after a cystoscope is used to introduce a contrast medium. A _____ is an x-ray taken during urination to examine the flow of urine through the system. An *abdominal sonogram* is the production of an image of the urinary tract using sound waves.
renogram [RĒ-nō-grăm]	Radioactive imaging is also used to diagnose kidney disorders via a renal scan. A _____ is used to study kidney function.
	Urinary Tract Procedures
dialysis [dī-ĂL-ĭ-sĭs] **hemodialysis** [HĒ-mō-dī-ĂL-ĭ-sĭs] **peritoneal dialysis** [PĔR-ĭ-tō-NĒ-ăl dī-ĂL-ĭ-sĭs]	Certain procedures, particularly _____, can mechanically maintain kidney or renal function when kidney failure occurs. _____ is the process of filtering blood outside the body in an artificial kidney machine and returning it to the body after filtering. _____ is the insertion and removal of a dialysis solution into the peritoneal cavity. (See Figure 15-8.)
extracorporeal shock wave lithotripsy (ESWL) [ĔKS-tră-kōr-PŌR-ē-ăl shŏk wāv LĪTH-ō-trĭp-sē]	_____ is the breaking up of urinary stones by using shock waves from outside the body. (See Figure 15-9.)

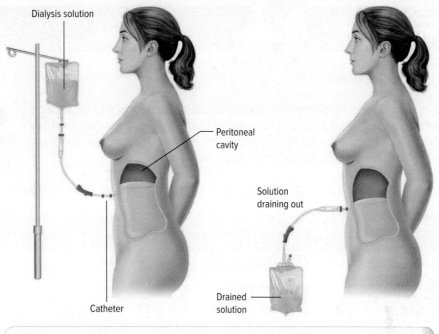

Figure 15-8 Peritoneal dialysis

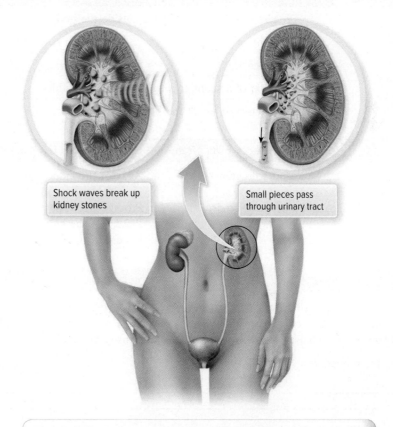

Figure 15-9 Extracorporeal shock wave lithotripsy

Kidney Stones

Kidney stones can be different colors or variegated throughout with interesting shapes and sizes. Some cultures have made necklaces and jewelry out of them due to the attractiveness of the coloring and/or shape. It is also a testimony to surviving the painful state of passing them.

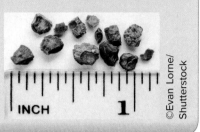

©Evan Lorne/ Shutterstock

PRONOUNCE and DEFINE	Pronounce the following terms aloud and write the definition.
peritoneal dialysis	[PĔR-ĭ-tō-NĒ-ăl dī-ĂL-ĭ-sĭs]
renogram	[RĒ-nō-grăm]
cystoscopy	[sĭs-TŎS-kō-pē]
cystourethrogram	[sĭs-tō-yū-RĒ-thrō-grăm]

SPELL	Write the correct spelling of the related term.
	Process of filtering the blood outside the body
	Breaking of stones
	Urinating
	Insertion of a scope to view the urinary bladder
	Radioactive image of the kidney

UNDERSTAND   Match each term on the left to its description on the right.

1. _____ cystourethrogram
2. _____ hemodialysis
3. _____ peritoneal dialysis
4. _____ renogram
5. _____ KUB

a. X-ray of the kidney, ureter, bladder
b. Insertion and removal of dialysis solution into the peritoneum
c. Process of filtering the blood outside the body
d. Picture of the kidney
e. Picture of the bladder and urethra

APPLY   Read the following scenario and answer the questions.

You are entering information from a paper chart into an electronic medical record for Mr. Harvey Mews, a 90-year-old black male who has a complex medical history. There are several notations in his chart, which include renogram, cystitis, diabetes, hemodialysis, KUB, cystoscopy, cystourethrogram, and cystotomy.

1. Identify the procedures.

_____

_____

2. Identify the imaging tests.

_____

_____

3. Define what each term listed means.

_____

_____

LO 15.4 Pathological Terms

Pathological terms are used to assign a disease to the correlating symptoms and findings of the physician. Many of the diagnoses in urology are abbreviations of longer medical terms, as you will see in the following text. One example is **UTI,** or **urinary tract infection,** which is any common infection within the urinary tract (kidneys to urethra). UTIs are common and the causes of them are many and diverse; however, most UTIs are caused from **bacteria** sneaking into the otherwise sterile urethra. See Figure 15-10 for an example of a urinalysis report.

Pathological	PRACTICE
	Provide the missing term(s) to complete the following sentences.
urinary tract infection (UTI)	Infections can occur anywhere in the urinary tract. A _____ commonly refers to a bladder or urethra infection.
nephritis [nĕ-FRĪ-tĭs] **glomerulonephritis** [glō-MĀR-yū-lō-nĕf-RĪ-tĭs] **Bright disease** **pyelitis** [pī-ĕ-LĪ-tĭs]	A number of infections and inflammations affect the urinary system. _____ is the general term for inflammation of the kidney. _____ refers to a kidney inflammation located in the glomeruli. This inflammation, known as _____, can be acute, as after a systemic infection, or may become chronic, resulting in high blood pressure, kidney failure, and other conditions. *Interstitial nephritis* is an inflammation of the connective tissue between the renal tubules. _____ is an inflammation of the renal pelvis. *Pyelonephritis* is a bacterial infection in the renal pelvis with abscesses.
nephrosis [nĕ-FRŌ-sĭs] **proteinuria** [prō-tē-NŪ-rē-ă] **edema** [ĕ-DĒ-mă] **hydronephrosis** [HĪ-drō-nĕ-FRŌ-sĭs] **polycystic kidney disease** [pŏl-ē-SĬS-tĭk KĬD-nē di-ZĒZ]	_____, or *nephrotic syndrome,* is a group of symptoms usually following or related to another illness that causes protein loss in the urine (_____). _____ (swelling) may result from this syndrome. Such swelling may adversely affect blood pressure. _____ is the collection of urine in the kidneys without release due to a blockage. _____ is a progressive, hereditary condition in which numerous kidney cysts form that can cause other conditions in adults, such as high blood pressure and excess blood and waste in the urine.
kidney (renal) failure **uremia** [yū-RĒ-mē-ă] **azotemia** [ăz-ō-TĒ-mē-ă] **end-stage renal disease (ESRD) Wilms' tumor** [vĭlmz TŪ-mŏr] **nephroblastoma** [NĔF-rō-blăs-TŌ-mă] **nephroma** [nĕ-FRŌ-mă]	*Renal hypertension* may result from other kidney or systemic diseases. _____, the loss of kidney function, may result from other conditions—some chronic, such as diabetes, and some acute, such as a kidney infection. Kidney failure can be treated with dialysis and medications. _____ and _____, excesses of urea and other nitrogenous wastes in the blood, may result from kidney failure. _____ is severe and fatal if not treated. *Renal cell carcinoma,* or kidney cancer, is usually treated by surgery. _____, or a _____, is a malignant tumor of the kidneys found primarily in children. It is usually treated with surgery, radiation, and chemotherapy. A _____ is any renal tumor.
cystitis [sĭs-TĪ-tĭs] **bladder cancer cystocele** [SĬS-tō-sēl] **cystolith** [SĬS-tō-lĭth]	_____ is an inflammation of the bladder. Aside from urinary tract infections, the bladder may be the site of _____. Various tumors can be removed or treated. In cases of extensive malignancy, the bladder may need to be surgically removed. Other bladder problems include a _____, a hernia of the bladder, and a _____, a stone in the bladder.

continued on next page

	Inflammations also can occur in the urethra (*urethritis*), the urethra and bladder together (*urethrocystitis*), or the ureters (*ureteritis*). *Urethral stenosis* is a narrowing of the urethra that causes voiding difficulties.
anuria [ăn-YŪ-rē-ă] **dysuria** [dĭs-YŪ-rē-ă] **enuresis** [ĕn-yū-RĒ-sĭs] **nocturia** [nŏk-TŪ-rē-ă] **oliguria** [ŏl-ĭ-GŪ-rē-ă] **polyuria** [pŏl-ē-YŪ-rē-ă] **incontinence** [ĭn-KŎN-tĭ-nĕns]	Difficulties in urination are often a symptom of another systemic disease, such as diabetes, or a localized infection (UTI). Such difficulties can include no urine output (_____), painful urination (_____), lack of bladder control (_____, including *nocturnal enuresis,* nighttime bed-wetting), frequent nighttime urination (_____), scanty urination (_____), excessive urination (_____), or urination during sneezing or coughing (*stress incontinence*). The general term _____ refers to the involuntary discharge of urine or feces.
albuminuria [ăl-byū-mĭ-NŪ-rē-ă] **proteinuria** [prō-tē-NŪ-rē-ă] **hematuria** [hē-mă-TŪ-rē-ă] **ketonuria** [kē-tō-NŪ-rē-ă] **pyuria** [pī-YŪ-rē-ă]	Abnormal substances or specific levels of substances in the urine indicate either urinary tract disorders or systemic disorders. Some can be minor infections or major problems. _____ or _____ indicates the presence of albumin in the urine; _____ indicates the presence of blood in the urine. _____ indicates the presence of ketone bodies in the urine. _____ indicates the presence of pus and white blood cells in the urine.
atresia [ă-TRĒ-zē-ă]	Many congenital problems can occur in the urinary system. Surgery can correct many of these. Hypospadias is a congenital problem that is a defect in which the urinary meatus opens at a place other than the distal end of the penis in males or between the clitoris and vagina in females. _____ (narrowing) of the ureters or urethra also may be present at birth.

Did you know

UTIs

UTIs, or urinary tract infections, are very common and can occur in people of all ages. However, roughly one in five women experiences a UTI in her lifetime. Girls and women are at high risk of infection because of the shorter female urethra and "wiping" incorrectly (from back to front), which can drive bacteria into the urethra.

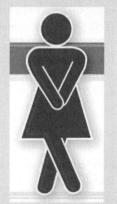

PRONOUNCE and DEFINE	Pronounce the following terms aloud and write the definition.
hematuria	[hē-mă-TŪ-rē-ă]
pyuria	[pī-YŪ-rē-ă]
cystocele	[SĬS-tō-sēl]
atresia	[ă-TRĒ-zē-ă]

SPELL	Identify if the following terms are spelled correctly. Correct the words that are spelled incorrectly. Write the definition for each word.	
	Spelling	**Definition**
pollyuria		
enuresis		
albuminouria		
oligouria		
cystitis		

UNDERSTAND Match each term on the left to its description on the right.

1. _____ atresia
2. _____ hematuria
3. _____ pyuria
4. _____ nocturia
5. _____ oliguria

a. Scanty urination
b. Blood in the urine
c. Nighttime urination
d. Narrowing
e. Pus in the urine

APPLY Read the following scenario and answer the questions.

The urinalysis report on Ms. Jana Smith (DOB: 2-2-72) comes back for the physician to review. She came in earlier today with symptoms of painful urination, scant urine, and thirst. She admitted that she has been training for a marathon and hasn't taken in very much water or food today before her run.

The partial report reads as follows:

Glucose: negative   WBC: positive-large
Ketones: trace   RBC: positive
Acetone: trace

1. When ketones are positive, what condition could be causing this?

_____

_____

2. Could there be other reasons for positive acetone and ketones?

_____

_____

3. What are the medical terms for her symptoms?

_____

_____

4. Would this be a priority for the physician?

_____

_____

Surgical Terms

Urologists, or specialists who study the urinary system, do more than just diagnose conditions. Most of them also perform surgical procedures to correct urinary structures or conditions. They may incorporate the assistance of other specialized surgeons if the procedure involves organs in another specialty. The majority of the surgical interventions are done to correct, remove, or reconstruct organs and tissues within the urinary system to improve function and quality of life.

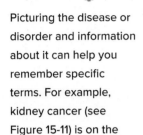

STUDY TIP

Picturing the disease or disorder and information about it can help you remember specific terms. For example, kidney cancer (see Figure 15-11) is on the rise in the United States.

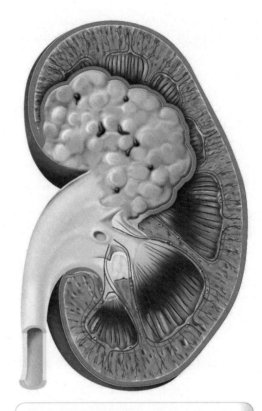

Figure 15-11 Resected kidney with cancer

In its early stages, kidney cancer rarely has any signs or symptoms, but in the later stages, the survival rate is very low. Kidney cancer signs and symptoms may include:

- Blood in your urine, which may appear pink, red, or cola colored.
- Back pain just below the ribs that doesn't go away.
- Weight loss.
- Fatigue.
- Intermittent fever.

PRACTICE

Provide the missing term(s) to complete the following sentences.

urology [yū-RŎL-ō-jē]	_____ is the practice of medicine specializing in the urinary tract. The practitioner is called a urologist. Urologists diagnose, treat, and perform surgery on the urinary system in the female and on the urinary and reproductive systems in the male.
nephrectomy [nĕ-FRĔK-tō-mē] **nephrolysis** [nĕ-FRŎL-ĭ-sĭs] **nephrostomy** [nĕ-FRŎS-tō-mē] **nephrolithotomy** [NĔF-rō-lĭ-THŎT-ō-mē] **nephropexy** [NĔF-rō-pĕk-sē] **nephrorrhaphy** [nĕf-RŌR-ă-fē]	Parts of the urinary system may be surgically removed. A person can live with only one kidney, so a diseased kidney may be removed in a _____. Diseased kidneys are removed before a kidney or renal transplant. Other surgical procedures on the kidney include _____, the removal of adhesions in the kidney; _____, the creation of an opening in the kidney leading to the outside of the body; _____, surgical removal of a kidney stone; _____, surgically affixing a floating kidney in place; and _____, suturing of a damaged kidney.
pyelotomy [pī-ĕ-LŎT-ō-mē] **pyeloplasty** [PĪ-ĕ-lō-plăs-tē] **ureteroplasty** [yū-RĒ-tĕr-ō-PLĂS-tē] **ureterorrhaphy** [yū-rē-tĕr-ŌR-ă-fē] **ureterectomy** [yū-rē-tĕr-ĔK-tō-mē]	An incision into the renal pelvis is called a _____. A _____ is the surgical repair of the renal pelvis. Surgical repair of a ureter is _____. _____ is the suture of a damaged ureter. _____ is the surgical removal of a diseased ureter.
lithotomy [lĭ-THŎT-ō-mē] **lithectomy** [lĭ-THĔK-tō-mē] **cystectomy** [sĭs-TĔK-tō-mē] **cystopexy** [SĬS-tō-pĕk-sē] **cystoplasty** [SĬS-tō-plăs-tē] **cystorrhaphy** [sĭs-TŌR-ă-fē]	The urinary bladder can be the site of stones, which are removed during a _____ or _____. A _____ is the removal of the bladder (usually when cancer is present). Surgical fixing of the bladder to the abdominal wall is _____, an operation to help correct urinary incontinence. _____ is the surgical repair of a bladder and _____ is the suturing of a damaged bladder.

continued on next page

Surgical	PRACTICE
	Provide the missing term(s) to complete the following sentences.
urethroplasty [yū-RĒ-thrō-plăs-tē] **urethropexy** [yū-RĒ-thrō-pĕk-sē] **urethrorrhaphy** [yū-rē-THRŌR-ă-fē] **urethrostomy** [yū-rē-THRŎS-tō-mē] **meatotomy** [mē-ă-TŎT-ō-mē] **urethrotomy** [yū-rē-THRŎT-ō-mē]	The urethra also may need surgical repair (_____), surgical fixation (_____), or suturing (_____). A _____ is the surgical creation of an opening between the urethra and the skin, while a _____ is the surgical enlargement of the opening of the meatus. Either of these operations may be necessary when certain birth defects are present. A narrowing in the urethra may require a _____, a surgical incision to enlarge the narrowed area.
urostomy [yū-RŎS-tō-mē] **intracorporeal** **electrohydraulic** **lithotripsy** [ĬN-tră-kōr-PŌ-rē-ăl ē-LĔK-trō-hī-DRAW-lĭk LĬTH-ō-trĭp-sē] **resectoscope** [rē-SĔK-tō-skōp]	Sometimes an opening is made to bypass diseased parts of the urinary tract. A _____ is the creation of an artificial opening in the abdomen through which urine exits the body. _____ is the use of an endoscope, an instrument for examining an interior canal or cavity, to break up stones in the urinary tract. A _____ is an endoscope used to cut and remove lesions in parts of the urinary system. An instrument called a *stone basket* may be attached to an endoscope and used for retrieving stones through a body cavity.

Did you know

Cystopexy

Cystopexy is performed to reattach the bladder to its original state after trauma, aging, or childbirth has caused it to prolapse. Sometimes the bladder can actually protrude into the vagina, causing incontinence, pain, and multiple symptoms for the female patient.

PRONOUNCE and DEFINE	Pronounce the following terms aloud and write the definition.
lithotripsy	[LĬTH-ō-trĭp-sē]
pyelotomy	[pī-ĕ-LŎT-ō-mē]
meatotomy	[mē-ă-TŎT-ō-mē]
urethrorrhaphy	[yū-rē-THRŌR-ă-fē]

SPELL	Write the correct spelling of the related term.
	Surgical creation of opening; urethra and skin
	Repair of the bladder
	Suturing of the urethra
	Opening to bypass diseased urinary parts
	Removal of a kidney

UNDERSTAND Match each term on the left to its description on the right.

1. _____ lithotripsy   a. Repair of the urethra
2. _____ urethroplasty   b. Breaking up of stones
3. _____ urostomy   c. Removal of a kidney
4. _____ nephrectomy   d. Cutting into a stone
5. _____ lithotomy   e. Creation of an artificial urinary opening

APPLY Read the following scenario and answer the questions.

You have been asked to do the surgical/procedure schedule for Shady Pines Hospital for tomorrow.

All kidney procedures are to be done first, followed with stone removal procedures, and finally all other urinary procedures.

Based on the practice list:

1. Create a list of all the kidney procedures.

_____
_____
_____
_____

2. Create a list of all the stone removal procedures.

_____
_____
_____
_____

3. Create a list of all the other urinary procedures.

_____
_____
_____
_____

4. Write their definitions behind each.

_____
_____
_____
_____

Pharmacological	PRACTICE
	Provide the missing term(s) to complete the following sentences.
antispasmodic [ĂN-tē-spăz-MŎD-ĭk] **diuretics** [dī-yū-RĔT-ĭks]	Medications for the urinary tract can relieve pain (analgesics), relieve spasms (_____), or inhibit growth of microorganisms (*antibiotics*). They also may increase (_____) or decrease (*antidiuretics*) the secretion of urine.
antihypertensives [ĂN-tē-hī-per-TEN-sivz] **ACE inhibitors**	Medications to control blood pressure related to fluid imbalance from compromised kidney function include _____ (_____).
antibiotics [ĂN-tē-bī-ŎT-ĭks]	_____ are spectrum antibacterial agents used to treat UTI bacterial infections within the urinary tract.
anticholinergics [ĂN-tē-kol-ĭ-NER-gĭcs]	Drugs that are used to treat overactive bladder are _____.

PRONOUNCE and DEFINE	Pronounce the following terms aloud and write the definition.
diuretic	[dī-yū-RĔT-ĭk]
antispasmodic	[ĂN-tē-spăz-MŎD-ĭk]
anticholinergics	[ĂN-tē-kol-ĭ-NER-gĭcs]

STUDY TIP

It is important to understand the differences in medication terms and their side effects. It will help you retain the information. For instance, ACE inhibitors are very effective in treating hypertension, but the most common side effect noted is a dry cough. Because of this irritating side effect, many patients either discontinue or change medication to treat their high blood pressure.

	Increases secretion of urine
	Antihypertensive medication related to kidney
	Relieves spasms
	Decreases secretion of urine

UNDERSTAND   Match each term on the left to its description on the right.

1. _____ antihypertensive or ACE inhibitor   a. Medication to control blood pressure
2. _____ diuretic   b. Medication to treat bacterial infections
3. _____ antibiotic   c. Medication to produce urine secretion

APPLY   Read the following scenario and answer the questions.

Ms. Kim Cardsheen presents to the physician's office complaining of trouble with bladder spasms and urinary retention (retaining urine). She is requesting medication to address these symptoms.

1. What are the medical terms for her symptoms?

_____
_____
_____
_____

2. What are the types of medication she might be prescribed?

_____
_____
_____
_____

3. What testing might the physician do to confirm which medications to give?

_____
_____
_____
_____

LO 15.7 Abbreviations

ABBREVIATION REVIEW

Abbreviation	Definition
ARF	acute renal failure
BUN	blood urea nitrogen
CRF	chronic renal failure
ESRD	end-stage renal disease
ESWL	extracorporeal shock wave lithotripsy
EUD	external urinary drainage
GFR	glomerular filtration rate
GU	genitourinary
I&O	intake and output
IVP	intravenous pyelogram
KUB	kidney/ureter/bladder
RP	retrograde pyelogram
UA, U/A	urinalysis
UTI	urinary tract infection
VCG	voiding cystogram
VCUG	voiding cystourethrogram

APPLY   **Read the following scenario and rewrite using appropriate abbreviations.**

The patient has frequent urinary tract infections, as demonstrated by urinalysis, and history of extracorporeal shock wave lithotripsy due to kidney stones. Multiple diagnostic exams including voiding cystourethrogram, retrograde pyelogram, kidney/ureter/bladder, and intravenous pyelogram. Will refer back to urologist.

_____

_____

_____

Chapter Review

	Learning Outcome	Summary
15.1	Describe the parts of the urinary system and discuss the function of each part.	The urinary system is comprised of organs and tubelike structures that function to maintain fluid balance and remove waste from the body.
15.2	Recognize the major word parts used in building words that relate to the urinary system.	Word building requires knowledge of word parts and their corresponding meanings to form medical terms within the urinary system.
15.3	Identify and understand the common diagnostic tests, laboratory tests, and clinical procedures used in testing and treating disorders of the urinary system.	Diagnostic, procedural, and laboratory findings assist the health care provider in diagnosing medical conditions. Urinalysis is often used in combination with imaging, and these tests lead to a final diagnosis and assist in treatment planning.
15.4	Define the major pathological conditions of the urinary system.	Knowledge and understanding of diseases and conditions of the urinary system, including acute and chronic diseases, structure repair and treatment to promote function, and cancer, increase critical thinking related to pathological medical terms.
15.5	Define surgical terms related to the urinary system.	Surgical procedures within the urinary system revolve closely around repair of damaged or nonfunctioning structures to restore fluid output and/or treatment of cancer with the system.
15.6	Recognize common pharmacological agents used in treating disorders of the urinary system.	Primary and common pharmacological agents used in the urinary system are symptomatic antispasmodics, antibiotics to fight bacterial infection, anticholinergics, and diuretic (antidiuretic) drugs.
15.7	Identify common abbreviations associated with the urinary system.	Abbreviations are used to describe diseases, conditions, procedures, and treatments associated with the urinary system.

1. Identify and label the major parts of the male and female urinary systems on the following figure.

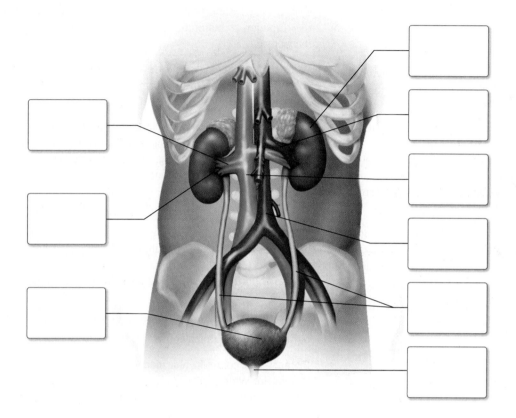

2. Describe the route of urine from production to the outside of the body.

Identify if the following terms are spelled correctly. Correct the words that are spelled incorrectly. Write the definition for each word.

	Spelling	Definition
urethrorrhea		
hematoturia		
nephroitis		
cystogram		
urinalisis		
retroperitoneal		
pyelplasty		
cystogenesis		

Pronounce the above terms aloud.

Complete the following words by using the combining forms learned in this chapter.

1. _____ scopy means viewing of the bladder.

2. _____ gram means a measure of the bladder and urethra.

3. _____ ectomy means removal of the kidney.

4. _____ itis means inflammation of the trigone.

5. _____ plegia means paralysis of the meatus.

IMPLEMENT

Complete the sentences by filling in the blanks.

1. The urinary system consists of two _____, or tubes that transport urine from the kidneys to the bladder.

2. A number of infections and inflammations affect the urinary system. _____ is the general term for inflammation of the kidney.

3. The urinary system consists of two _____, or organs that remove dissolved waste and other substances from the blood and urine.

4. _____, or *nephrotic syndrome,* is a group of symptoms usually following or related to another illness that causes protein loss in the urine.

5. _____ is the term for blood in the urine.

6. Lack of urine formation is a(n) _____.

7. _____ is the examination of urine for its physical, chemical, and microscopic properties.

8. Abnormal discharge from the urethra is _____.

9. _____ is the creation of an opening in the kidney leading to the outside of the body.

10. _____ is a substance that causes an increase in the blood pressure to maintain the filtration rate of blood.

11. Scant or small amounts of urine is _____.

12. An incision into the renal pelvis is called a(n) _____.

13. The kidneys have an outer protective portion that is called the _____.

14. _____ are the functional units of the kidney.

15. _____ relates to the urinary bladder and the abdominal wall.

16. The presence of serum protein _____ in urine may indicate a leakage of blood proteins through the renal tubules, an indicator of nephron disease.

17. Excess of urea and other nitrogenous wastes in the blood is _____.

18. _____ is the medical term for removal of a kidney.

19. Narrowing of a ureter is _____.

20. The presence of albumin in the urine is _____.

The physician records in the medical record that the patient has renal and bladder carcinoma, based on the renogram, urinalysis, cystoscope, and blood tests that have been performed recently. His options include right nephrectomy, right uretectomy, and left uretopexy, and he may need to have a cystectomy with a cystostomy placed.

Using lay terms, write what the physician has recorded in the client's medical history.

_____

_____

_____

_____

Reviewing the Terms

Pronounce each of the following terms. Write the definitions on a separate sheet of paper. This review will take you through all the words you learned in this chapter. If you have difficulty with any words, make a flash card for later study. Refer to the English-Spanish and Spanish-English glossaries in the eBook.

acetone [ĂS-ĕ-tōn]

albumin [ăl-BYŪ-mĭn]

albuminuria [ăl-byū-mĭ-NŪ-rē-ă]

antispasmodic [ĂN-tē-spăz-MŎD-ĭk]

anuria [ăn-YŪ-rē-ă]

atresia [ă-TRĒ-zē-ă]

azotemia [ăz-ō-TĒ-mē-ă]

bilirubin [bĭl-ĭ-RŪ-bĭn]

bladder [BLĂD-ĕr]

bladder cancer

Bowman's [BŌ-mănz] capsule

BUN (blood, urea, nitrogen)

cali/o, calic/o [KĀ-lē-ō, KĂL-ĭ-sō]

calices, calyces (sing., calix, calyx) [KĂL-ĭ-sēz (KĀ-lĭks)]

casts

condom catheter [KŎN-dŏm KĂTH-ĕ-tĕr]

cortex [KŌR-tĕks]

creatine [KRĒ-ă-tēn]

creatinine [krē-ĂT-ĭ-nēn]

cyst/o [SĬS-tō]

cystectomy [sĭs-TĔK-tō-mē]

cystitis [sĭs-TĪ-tĭs]

cystocele [SĬS-tō-sēl]

cystolith [SĬS-tō-lĭth]

cystopexy [SĬS-tō-pĕk-sĕ]

cystoplasty [SĬS-tō-plăs-tē]

cystorrhaphy [sĭs-TŌR-ă-fē]

cystoscope [SĬS-tō-skōp]

cystoscopy [sĭs-TŎS-kō-pē]

dialysis [dī-ĂL-ĭ-sĭs]

diuretic [dī-yū-RĔT-ĭk]

dysuria [dĭs-YŪ-rē-ă]

edema [ĕ-DĒ-mă]

end-stage renal disease (ESRD)

enuresis [ĕn-yū-RĒ-sĭs]

extracorporeal shock wave lithotripsy [ĔKS-tră-kōr-PŌR-ē-ăl shŏk wāv LĪTH-ō-trĭp-sē] (ESWL)

filtration [fĭl-TRĀ-shŭn]

Foley [FŌ-lē] catheter

glomerul/o [glō-MĂR-yū-lō]

glomerulonephritis [glō-MĂR-yū-lō-nĕf-RĪ-tĭs]

glomerulus (pl., glomeruli) [glō-MĂR-yū-lŏs (glō-MĂR-yū-lī)]

glucose [GLŪ-kōs]

hematuria [hē-mă-TŪ-rē-ă]

hemodialysis [HĒ-mō-dī-ĂL-ĭ-sĭs

hilum [HĪ-lŭm]

hydronephrosis [HĪ-drō-nĕ-FRŌ-sĭs]

incontinence [ĭn-KŎN-tĭ-nĕns]

indwelling [ĬN-dwĕ-lĭng]

intracorporeal electrohydraulic lithotripsy [ĬN-tră-kōr-PŌ-rē-ăl ē-LĔK-trō-hī-DRAW-lĭk LĪTH-ō-trĭp-sē]

ketone [KĒ-tōn]

ketonuria [kē-tō-NŪ-rē-ă]

kidney [KĬD-nē]

kidney (renal) failure

kidney, ureter, bladder (KUB)

lithectomy [lĭ-THĔK-tō-mē]

lithotomy [lĭ-THŎT-ō-mē]

meat/o [mē-Ā-tō]

meatotomy [mē-ă-TŎT-ō-mē]

meatus [mē-Ā-tŭs]

medulla [mĕ-DŪL-ă]

nephr/o [NĔF-rō]

nephrectomy [nĕ-FRĔK-tō-mē]

nephritis [nĕ-FRĪ-tĭs]

nephroblastoma [NĔF-rō-blăs-TŌ-mă]

nephrolithotomy [NĔF-rō-lĭ-THŎT-ō-mē]

nephrologist [nĕ-FRŎL-ō-jĭst]

nephrolysis [nĕ-FRŎL-ĭ-sĭs]

nephroma [nĕ-FRŌ-mă]

nephron [NĔF-rŏn]

nephropexy [NĔF-rō-pĕk-sē]

nephrorrhaphy [nĕf-RŌR-ă-fē]

nephrosis [nĕ-FRŌ-sĭs]

nephrostomy [nĕ-FRŎS-tō-mē]

nocturia [nŏk-TŪ-rē-ă]

oliguria [ŏl-ĭ-GŪ-rē-ă]

peritoneal [PĔR-ĭ-tō-NĒ-ăl] dialysis

pH

phenylketones [FĔN-ĭl-KĒ-tōnz]

polycystic [pŏl-ē-SĬS-tĭk] kidney disease

polyuria [pŏl-ē-YŪ-rē-ă]

prostate [PRŎS-tāt]

proteinuria [prō-tē-NŪ-rē-ă]

pyel/o [PĪ-ĕ-lō]

pyelitis [pī-ĕ-LĪ-tĭs]

pyeloplasty [PĪ-ĕ-lō-plăs-tē]

pyelotomy [pī-ĕ-LŎT-ō-mē]

pyuria [pī-YŪ-rē-ă]

reabsorption [rē-ăb-SŌRP-shŭn]

ren/o [RĒ-nō]

renal pelvis

renin [RĔ-nĭn]

renogram [RĒ-nō-grăm]

resectoscope [rē-SĔK-tō-skōp]

retrograde pyelogram [RĔT-rō-grād PĪ-ĕl-ō-grăm] (RP)

retroperitoneal [RĒ-trō-PĔR-ĭ-tō-NĒ-ăl]

specific gravity

trigon/o [trī-GŌ-nō]

trigone [TRĪ-gōn]

ur/o, urin/o [YŪR-ō, YŪR-ĭn-ō]

urea [yū-RĒ-ă]

uremia [yū-RĒ-mē-ă]

ureter [yū-RĒ-tĕr]

ureter/o [yū-RĒ-tĕr-ō]

ureterectomy [yū-rē-tĕr-ĔK-tō-mē]

ureteroplasty [yū-RĒ-tĕr-ō-PLĂS-tē]

ureterorrhaphy [yū-rē-tĕr-ŌR-ă-fē]

urethr/o [yū-RĒ-thrō]

urethra [yū-RĒ-thră]

urethropexy [yū-RĒ-thrō-pĕk-sē]

urethroplasty [yū-RĒ-thrō-plăs-tē]

urethrorrhaphy [yū-rē-THRŌR-ă-fē]

urethrostomy [yū-rē-THRŎS-tō-mē]

urethrotomy [yū-rē-THRŎT-ō-mē]

-uria [YŪ-rē-ă]

uric [YŪR-ĭk] acid

urinalysis [yū-rĭ-NĂL-ĭ-sĭs]

urinary [YŪR-ĭ-nār-ē] bladder

urinary system

urinary tract infection (UTI)

urine [YŪR-ĭn]

urologist [yū-RŎL-ō-jĭst]

urology [yū-RŎL-ō-jē]

urostomy [yū-RŎS-tō-mē]

vesic/o [VĔS-ĭ-kō]

voiding (urinating) cystourethrogram [sĭs-tō-yū-RĒ-thrō-grăm] (VCUG)

voiding cystogram (VCG)

Wilms' [vĭlmz] tumor

CHAPTER 16

The Male Reproductive System

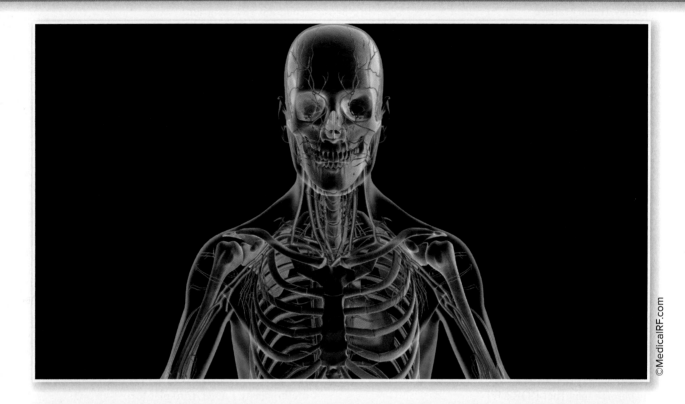

©MedicalRF.com

Learning Outcomes

After studying this chapter, you will be able to:

16.1   Recognize the parts of the male reproductive system and discuss the function of each part.

16.2   Recall the major word parts used in building words that relate to the male reproductive system.

16.3   Identify the common diagnostic tests, laboratory tests, and clinical procedures used in testing and treating disorders of the male reproductive system.

16.4   Define the major pathological conditions of the male reproductive system.

16.5   Recall the meaning of surgical terms related to the male reproductive system.

16.6   Recognize common pharmacological agents used in treating disorders of the male reproductive system.

16.7   Identify common abbreviations associated with the male reproductive system.

LO 16.1 Structure and Function of the Male Reproductive System

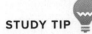
The organs of the male reproductive system (Figure 16-1) produce and maintain new sperm (male sex cells) daily; transport these cells, along with seminal fluid, to the outside; and secrete male hormones to the system. Many of the combining forms are shared with Chapter 15—The Urinary System.

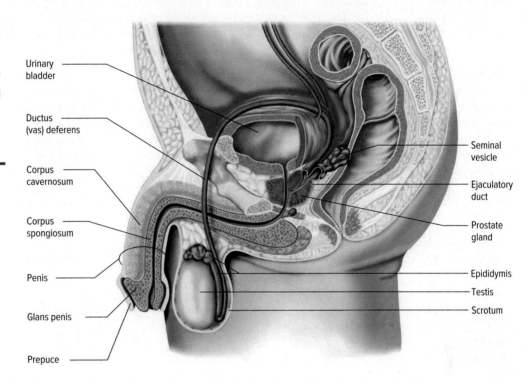

Urinary bladder
Ductus (vas) deferens
Corpus cavernosum
Corpus spongiosum
Penis
Glans penis
Prepuce

Seminal vesicle
Ejaculatory duct
Prostate gland
Epididymis
Testis
Scrotum

Figure 16-1 Sagittal view of the male reproductive organs

Structure and Function	PRACTICE
	Provide the missing term(s) to complete the following sentences.
spermatozoon [SPĔR-mă-tō-ZŌ-ŏn] **spermatozoa** [SPĔR-mă-tō-ZŌ-ă] **sperm** [spĕrm] **testes** [TĔS-tēz] **testicles** [TĔS-tĭ-klz] **scrotum** [SKRŌ-tŭm]	The sex cell, or _____ (plural, _____) or _____ , is produced in the male gonads, or _____ (singular *testis*). The testes are also called _____ and are contained within the _____ , a sac outside the body. The scrotal sac holds and protects the testes as well as regulates their temperature. If the testicles are too cold, the scrotum contracts to draw them closer to the body for warmth. If the testicles are too warm, then the scrotum relaxes to draw the testicles away from the body's heat.

continued on next page

Provide the missing term(s) to complete the following sentences.

Terms	Practice
spermatogenesis [SPĔR-mă-tō-JĔN-ĕ-sĭs] **testosterone** [tĕs-TŎS-tĕ-rōn]	The development of sperm (_____) takes place in the scrotum, where the temperature is lower than inside the body (Figures 16-2 and 16-3). The lower temperature is necessary for the safe development of sperm. Inside the testes are cells that manufacture the sperm cells. These cells are contained in *seminiferous tubules*. Between the seminiferous tubules lie endocrine cells that produce _____, the most important male hormone; it is thought to decrease during a stage of life sometimes referred to as "male menopause." See Table 16-1.
epididymis (*pl.*, **epididymes**) [ĕp-ĭ-DĬD-ĭ-mĭs (ĕp-ĭ-DĬD-ĭ-mēz)] **vas deferens** [văs DĔF-ĕr-ĕns] **prostate gland** [PRŎS-tāt glănd] **semen** [SĒ-mĕn]	At the top part of each testis is the _____, a group of ducts for storing sperm. The sperm develop to maturity and become *motile* (able to move) in the epididymis. They leave the epididymis and enter a narrow tube called the _____. The sperm then travel to the *seminal vesicles* (which secrete material to help the sperm move) and to the *ejaculatory duct* leading to the _____ and the urethra. The prostate gland also secretes *prostatic fluid,* which provides a milky color to _____ (a mixture of sperm and secretions from the seminal vesicles, Cowper's glands, and prostate), and helps the sperm move. The gland then contracts its muscular tissue during ejaculation to help the sperm exit the body.
bulbourethral glands [BŬL-bō-yū-RĒ-thrăl glăndz] **Cowper's glands** [KŎW-pĕrs glăndz] **penis** [PĒ-nĭs] **glans penis** [glănz PĒ-nĭs] **foreskin** [FŌR-skĭn] **perineum** [PĔR-ĭ-NĒ-ŭm]	Just below the prostate are the two _____ (_____) that also secrete a fluid that neutralizes the acidity of the male urethra prior to ejaculation. The urethra passes through the _____ to the outside of the body. The tip of the penis is called the _____, a sensitive area covered by the _____ (*prepuce*). Between the penis and the anus is the area called the _____.
flagellum [flă-JĔL-ŭm] **ejaculation** [ē-jăk-yū-LĀ-shŭn]	The spermatozoon is a microscopic cell, much smaller than an ovum. It has a head region that carries genetic material (*chromosomes*) and a tail (_____) that propels the sperm forward. During _____, hundreds of millions of sperm are released. Usually only one sperm can fertilize a single ovum. In rare instances, two or more ova are fertilized at a single time, resulting in twins, triplets, quadruplets, and so on. *Identical twins* result when one ovum splits after it has been fertilized by a single sperm. *Fraternal twins* are the result of two sperm fertilizing two ova.

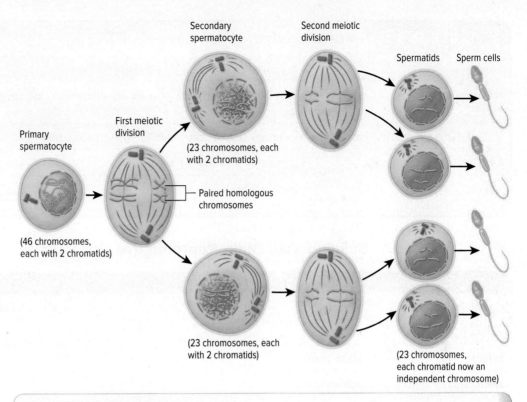

Secondary spermatocyte

Second meiotic division

Spermatids

Sperm cells

Primary spermatocyte

First meiotic division

(23 chromosomes, each with 2 chromatids)

Paired homologous chromosomes

(46 chromosomes, each with 2 chromatids)

(23 chromosomes, each with 2 chromatids)

(23 chromosomes, each chromatid now an independent chromosome)

Figure 16-2 Spermatogenesis

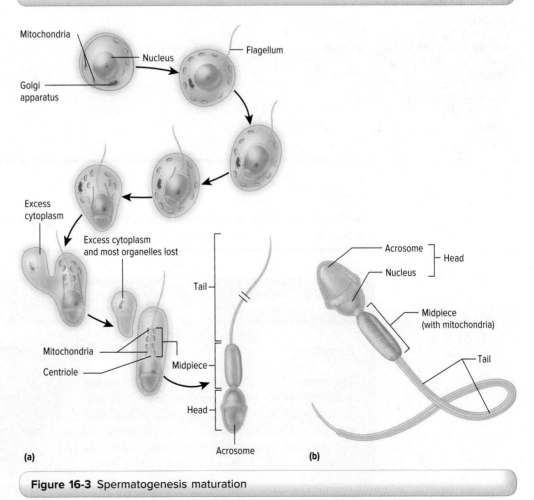

Mitochondria

Nucleus

Flagellum

Golgi apparatus

Excess cytoplasm

Excess cytoplasm and most organelles lost

Mitochondria

Centriole

Tail

Midpiece

Head

Acrosome

(a)

Acrosome

Head

Nucleus

Midpiece (with mitochondria)

Tail

(b)

Figure 16-3 Spermatogenesis maturation

TABLE 16-1	Male Reproductive Hormones	
Hormone	**Purpose**	**Source**
testosterone	stimulates development of male sex characteristics; increases sperm; inhibits LH	testes
FSH (follicle-stimulating hormone)	increases testosterone; aids in sperm production	pituitary gland
LH (luteinizing hormone)	stimulates testosterone secretion	pituitary gland
inhibin	inhibits FSH	testes

Building Your Male Reproductive Vocabulary

Combining Form	**Meaning**
andr/o	men
balan/o	glans penis
epididym/o	epididymis
orch/o, orchi/o, orchid/o	testes
prostat/o	prostate gland
scrot/o	scrotum
semin/o	semen
sperm/o, spermat/o	sperm
vas/o	vessel; ductus deferens

STUDY TIP

Spermatogenesis is the development of sperm cells and is accomplished within the walls of the seminiferous tubes in the testes.

Did you know ?

Prostate

The prostate is located just under the bladder and is responsible for making seminal fluid. A normal adult prostate is around the size of a walnut. During ejaculation, the muscles that surround the prostate and penis contract, which pushes the semen out of the penis.

Urinary bladder

Prostate gland

Urethra

PRONOUNCE and DEFINE	Pronounce the following reproductive terms aloud.
epididymis	[ĕp-ĭ-DĬD-ĭ-mĭs]
spermatozoon	[SPĔR-mă-tō-ZŌ-ŏn]
prostate gland	[PRŎS-tāt glănd]
bulbourethral	[BŬL-bō-yū-RĒ-thrăl]

SPELL and DEFINE Identify if the following terms are spelled correctly. Correct the words that are spelled incorrectly. Write the definition for each word.

	Spelling	Definition
flaggelum		
spermatogenesis		
spermatazoa		
vas deferens		

UNDERSTAND Match each term on the left to its description on the right.

1. ____________ spermatozoa
2. ____________ glans penis
3. ____________ testosterone
4. ____________ bulbourethral
5. ____________ scrotum

a. Male hormone
b. Male sex cell
c. The tip of the penis
d. Sac that contains the testes
e. Below the prostate; secretes fluid

APPLY Read the following scenario and answer the questions.

Mr. James Cocoa is the middle school health sciences teacher. He has asked you to be a guest speaker in his class, where students are studying the male reproductive system. You are to explain the male reproductive structure and function.

1. What are the main parts of the system?

____

____

2. How do they work together?

____

____

3. If this was a second grade class, how would you explain the male reproductive system?

____

____

4. What does the flagellum do?

____

____

LO 16.2 Word Building in the Male Reproductive System

Now that the male reproductive anatomy has been covered, it is time to practice word building. Following are some medical terms and combinations common to the male reproductive system.

As you work through the following practice, try to mix and match or associate various word roots with different prefixes/suffixes to extend your knowledge and vocabulary.

Word Building	PRACTICE
	Provide the correct combining form in each of the sentences.
orch-itis [ōr-KĪ-tĭs]	Inflammation of the testis is _____ itis.
andro-pathy [an-DROP-ă-thē]	Any disease peculiar to men is _____ pathy.
spermato-genesis [SPĔR-mă-tō-JĔN-ĕ-sĭs]	Sperm production is _____ genesis.
balan-itis [băl-ă-NĪ-tĭs]	Inflammation of the glans penis is _____ itis.
epididymo-plasty [ĕp-ĭ-DĬD-ĭ-mō-plăs-tē]	_____ plasty is surgical repair of the epididymis.
prostat-itis [prŏs-tă-TĪ-tĭs]	_____ itis is inflammation of the prostate.

Prostatitis is the medical term that is broken down into the word parts **prostat/o** = prostate + **itis** = inflammation. It is a generic term that can include any prostate inflammation. Benign prostatic hyperplasia (BPH), a noncancerous enlargement of the prostate gland that usually occurs in middle-age men, can cause prostatitis.

Did you know

Prostate Enlargement

For many men in their 40s, a growth of the prostate is normal. However, there is a layer of tissue that protects the prostate from outward growth. When the prostate presses on the urethra, symptoms of BPH begin to show.

PRONOUNCE and DEFINE	Pronounce the following terms aloud and write their meaning in the space provided.
balanitis	[băl-ă-NĪ-tĭs]
orchitis	[ōr-KĪ-tĭs]
epididymoplasty	[ĕp-ĭ-DĬD-ĭ-mō-plăs-tē]
andropathy	[an-DROP-ă-thē]

SPELL and DEFINE	Identify if the following terms are spelled correctly. Correct the words that are spelled incorrectly. Write the definition for each word.	
	Spelling	**Definition**
epididimitis		
balanopathy		
orchiditis		
prostatotitis		

UNDERSTAND — Match each term on the left to its description on the right.

1. _____ spermatogenesis
2. _____ epididymoplasty
3. _____ andropathy
4. _____ balanitis
5. _____ prostatitis

a. Prostate inflammation
b. Repair of the epididymis
c. Penis inflammation
d. Any disease relating to men
e. Production of sperm

APPLY — Read the following scenario and answer the questions.

Mr. Jon Meriweather is a 30-year-old Caucasian male. He has presented to the ER with symptoms of penis inflammation, testicle enlargement, and scrotal inflammation. It states in his medical record that he has a history of balanopathy and prostatitis.

1. Which reproductive parts are involved in his current problems and history?

_____

_____

2. How does each relate to the others?

_____

_____

3. What are the medical terms for each of his symptoms?

_____

_____

4. What are the lay terms for his history?

_____

_____

Diagnostic, Procedural, and Laboratory Terms

STUDY TIP

Semen analysis is a common test done to evaluate the number and quality of a male's sperm, pH of the seminal fluid, shape, and abnormalities in the fluid contents. It is mostly done when evaluating the reproductive status and ability in a couple who have been unsuccessful in conceiving a baby.

Maintenance of the male reproductive system frequently includes physical examination and testing for prostate disorders and cancer (Figure 16-4). Prostate cancer is the most common cancer in the male reproductive system. The prostate can become enlarged from either a benign or malignant condition, otherwise known as **prostatitis;** thus, a man diagnosed with an enlarged prostate will undergo a **biopsy** to evaluate prostate status, which determines treatment and outcome. Prostate cancer often goes undiagnosed and may progress to later stages, which lessens the survival rate with each stage of progression.

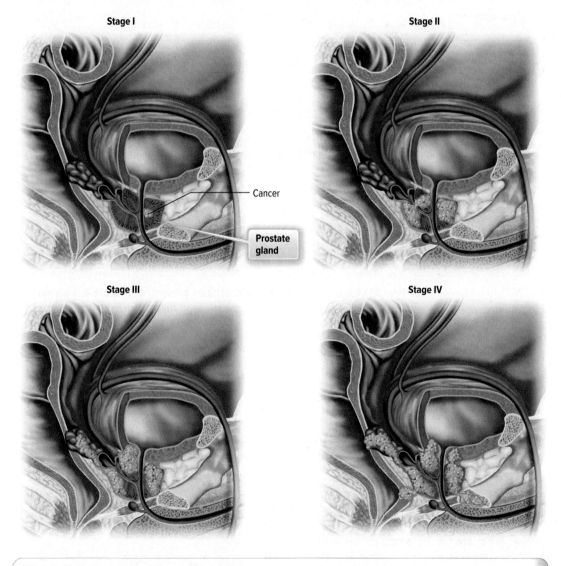

Figure 16-4 The stages of prostate cancer

Diagnostic	PRACTICE
	Provide the missing term(s) to complete the following sentences.
prostate-specific antigen (PSA) test [PRŎS-tāt spĕ-SĬF-ĭk ĂN-tĭ-jĕn]	A normal male medical checkup may include a *digital rectal exam* (*DRE*), the insertion of a finger into the rectum to check the prostate for abnormalities, tenderness, or irregularities. During the DRE, the physician can reach approximately two-thirds of the prostate. A medical checkup for males usually includes a _____, a blood test to screen for abnormal prostatic growth, which can be associated with prostate cancer.
semen analysis	If a couple is having fertility problems, a _____ is done to determine the quantity and quality of the male partner's sperm.
urethrogram [yū-RĒ-thrō-grăm]	X-ray or imaging procedures are used to further test for abnormalities or blockages. A _____ is an x-ray of the urethra and prostate.

STUDY TIP

Recent research carried out at the University of Texas Houston Health Science Center found that injections of collagen into the male urinary muscles can help men who have incontinence problems following treatment for some prostate conditions.

PRONOUNCE and DEFINE	Pronounce the following reproductive terms aloud and write their meaning.
prostate-specific antigen (PSA) test	[ĂN-tĭ-jĕn]
urethrogram	[yū-RĒ-thrō-grăm]
semen	[SĒ-mĕn]

SPELL and DEFINE	Identify if the following terms are spelled correctly. Correct the words that are spelled incorrectly. Write the definition for each word.	
	Spelling	**Definition**
prostrate		
urethogram		
prostate-specific antigen test		

UNDERSTAND	Match each term on the left to its description on the right.

1. _____ prostate-specific antigen (PSA) test   a. Tail of sperm
2. _____ semen analysis   b. X-ray of the urethra and prostate
3. _____ urethrogram   c. Test for prostate cancer
4. _____ flagellum   d. Infertility testing

Mr. Lloyd Pepper is a 48-year-old African-American male who presents to the After Hours Clinic complaining of difficulty urinating and painful urination. His record shows a history of benign prostatic hyperplasia.

1. Which reproductive organs are involved?

_____

_____

_____

2. Identify the medical terms for the symptoms he is having.

_____

_____

_____

3. What is BPH?

_____

_____

_____

4. What medical testing might the doctor order for Lloyd?

_____

_____

_____

5. List two reasons that semen analysis may be done.

_____

_____

_____

LO 16.4 Pathological Terms

STUDY TIP

New drugs to correct erectile dysfunction have become popular in recent years, giving previously impotent men an option for sexual quality. The most common uncomfortable side effect of these drugs can be priapism.

There are several male reproductive pathological conditions simply due to the male anatomy, condition of the male organs, and reproductive abnormalities at birth.

Cryptorchidism [**crypt(o)** = hidden + **-orchidism** = testicle] is a pathological condition that occurs when a testicle does not descend into the scrotal sac before birth. In the normal male infant, the testicles have descended into the scrotum by the time the child is born. Cryptorchidism occurs most often in premature babies born before 37 weeks of pregnancy or gestation.

Pathological	Provide the missing term(s) to complete the following sentences.
gynecomastia [GĪ-nĕ-kō-MĂS-tē-ă]	Swelling of the breast tissue in males is _____. It may be caused by an imbalance of hormones, medications, and liver disease.
cryptorchism [krĭp-TŌR-kĭzm] **cryptorchidism** [krĭp-TŌR-kĭ-dĭzm] **anorchism** [ăn-ŌR-kĭzm] **anorchia** [ăn-ŌR-kē-ă] **hydrocele** [HĪ-drō-sēl]	Birth or developmental defects affect the functioning of the reproductive system. An *undescended testicle* (_____ or _____) means that the normal descending of the testicle into the scrotal sac does not take place during gestation and requires surgery to place it properly. _____ or _____ is the lack of one or both testes. A _____ is a painless fluid-filled sac around one or both testicles that causes the scrotum to swell.
hypospadias [HĪ-pō-SPĂ-dē-ăs] **epispadias** [ĕp-ĭ-SPĂ-dē-ăs] **phimosis** [fī-MŌ-sĭs]	_____ is an abnormal opening of the urethra on the underside of the penis. _____ is an abnormal opening on the top side of the penis. The birth defect _____ is an abnormal narrowing of the foreskin over the glans penis (only in uncircumcised males). These conditions also are repaired by surgery (sometimes during circumcision), in which the foreskin is removed and used in the repair.
infertility [ĭn-fĕr-TĬL-ĭ-tē] **aspermia** [ā-SPĔR-mē-ă] **azoospermia** [ā-zō-ō-SPĔR-mē-ă] **oligospermia** [ŏl-ĭ-gō-SPĔR-mē-ă]	As the male matures, infections and various other medical conditions may cause _____, an inability to produce enough viable sperm to fertilize an ovum or an inability to deliver sperm to the proper location in the vagina. Several levels of sperm production may be involved in infertility. _____ is the inability to produce sperm; _____ is semen without living sperm; and _____ is the scanty production of sperm.
impotence [ĬM-pō-tĕns] **priapism** [PRĪ-ă-pĭzm] **hernia** [HĔR-nē-ă] **hydrocele** [HĪ-drō-sēl] **varicocele** [VĂR-ĭ-kō-sēl]	Medical or psychological conditions may cause _____ (*penile erectile dysfunction*), inability to maintain an erection for ejaculation. _____ is a persistent, painful erection, usually related to other medical conditions. _____, abnormal protrusions of part of a tissue or organ out of its normal space through a barrier, may occur in the male reproductive system. (Hernias are also covered in Chapter 14.) A _____ is a fluid-containing hernia in a testicle; a _____ is a group of herniated veins near the testes. This is a common cause of infertility due to the increased heat that the dilated blood vessel brings to the scrotum. It can be corrected by surgery.
prostatitis [prŏs-tă-TĪ-tĭs] **balanitis** [băl-ă-NĪ-tĭs] **epididymitis** [ĕp-ĭ-dĭd-ĭ-MĪ-tĭs]	Various inflammations occur in the male reproductive system. _____ is any inflammation of the prostate; _____ is an inflammation of the glans penis; and _____ is an inflammation of the epididymis.

continued on next page

Pathological

PRACTICE

Provide the missing term(s) to complete the following sentences.

Peyronie disease
[pā-RŌN-ē di-ZĒZ]
seminoma
[sĕm-ĭ-NŌ-mă]

_____ is a disorder with curvature of the penis caused by some hardening in the interior structure of the penis. *Prostate cancer* and *testicular cancer* are fairly common malignancies. A common tumor of the testicle is a _____.

chancroids
[SHĂNG-krŏyds]

Sexually transmitted infections (STIs) are the same for the male as for the female, with males being more susceptible to _____, venereal sores caused by a bacterial infection on the penis, urethra, or anus. More information on STIs is presented in Chapter 17.

Did you know

STIs

The six most common sexually transmitted infections in the United States today are gonorrhea, chlamydia, genital herpes, human papillomavirus (HPV), HIV/AIDS, and syphilis. Even with advances in medicine and treatments, as well as widespread education, all of them are still active and prevalent today. More information on STIs is in Chapter 17.

PRONOUNCE and DEFINE	Pronounce the following reproductive terms aloud and write their meaning.
prostatitis	[prŏs-tă-TĪ-tĭs]
phimosis	[fī-MŌ-sĭs]
hypospadias	[HĪ-pō-SPĀ-dē-ăs]
chancroids	[SHĂNG-krŏyds]

SPELL and DEFINE	Identify if the following terms are spelled correctly. Correct the words that are spelled incorrectly. Write the definition for each word.	
	Spelling	**Definition**
priaprism		
anorchism		
seminaloma		
azospermia		

1. _____ hydrocele
2. _____ varicocele
3. _____ oligospermia
4. _____ aspermia
5. _____ cryptorchidism

a. Lack of sperm production
b. Group of herniated varicose veins near the testes
c. Scanty production of sperm
d. Fluid-filled hernia within a testicle
e. Undescended testicle

APPLY   **Read the following scenario and answer the questions.**

Mr. and Mrs. Bob Schaeffer are the proud parents of a new baby boy, Robert Jr. They have requested that the baby be circumcised. The physician has done the initial evaluation and documented that Robert Jr. is healthy and okay to undergo the procedure. However, he has bilateral cryptorchidism and a varicocele.

1. Which reproductive parts are involved with this case?

_____

_____

2. What are the problems with the case?

_____

_____

3. How would you explain what the doctor has found to the parents?

_____

_____

4. Explain what Peyronie disease is and what kinds of symptoms/problems it could cause for the patient. Use medical terms for each symptom.

_____

_____

LO 16.5 Surgical Terms

STUDY TIP

Physicians agree that orchidectomy is an aggressive and primary surgical approach to treating testicular cancer. If the patient wishes to father children in the future, several semen samples are stored prior to the orchidectomy for possible future use. Castration is the term used after both testicles are removed, and usually results in impotence.

Circumcision is a common male reproductive organ surgical procedure. It is the removal of the foreskin, which is the skin that covers the tip of the penis (Figure 16-5). It is often done within the first week of the newborn boy's life. There are medical benefits and risks to circumcision. Possible benefits include a lower risk of urinary tract infections, penile cancer, and sexually transmitted diseases. The risks include pain and a low risk of bleeding or infection. These risks are higher for older babies, boys, and men. The American Academy of Pediatrics (AAP) does not recommend routine circumcision. Parents need to decide what is best for their sons, based on their religious, cultural, and personal preferences.

Penis with foreskin   Penis without foreskin

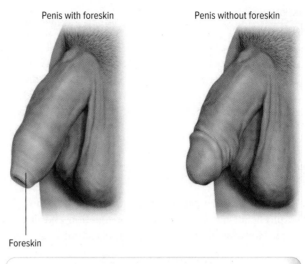

Foreskin

Figure 16-5 Uncircumcised and circumcised penis

Surgical	**PRACTICE**
	Provide the missing term(s) to complete the following sentences.
circumcision [sĭr-kŭm-SĬZH-ŭn]	The most common surgery of the male reproductive system is _____, the removal of the foreskin or prepuce. Various cultures and religions have rituals associated with this removal. Some parents prefer to have it done in the hospital immediately after birth.
epididymectomy [ĔP-ĭ-dĭd-ĭ-MĔK-tō-mē] **orchiectomy** [ōr-kē-ĔK-tō-mē] **orchidectomy** [ōr-kĭ-DĔK-tō-mē] **prostatectomy** [prŏs-tă-TĔK-tō-mē] **transurethral resection of the prostate** [trănz-yū-RĒ-thrăl rē-SĔK-shŭn] **vasectomy** [vă-SĔK-tō-mē] **vasovasostomy** [VĀ-sō-vă-SŎS-tō-mē] **castration** [kăs-TRĀ-shŭn]	Various operations to remove cancerous or infected parts of the reproductive system are an _____, removal of an epididymis; an _____ or _____, removal of a testicle; and a _____, removal of the prostate gland, which may be done through the perineum or above the pubic bone. A _____ (*TURP*) is the removal of a portion of the prostate through the urethra. _____ is the removal of part of the vas deferens as a method of birth control (Figure 16-6). A _____ is the reversing of a vasectomy so the male regains fertility. _____ is the removal of both testicles in the male.

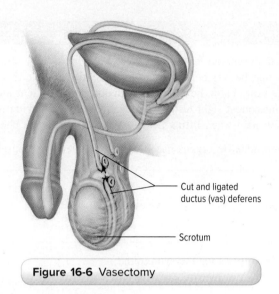

Cut and ligated
ductus (vas) deferens

Scrotum

Figure 16-6 Vasectomy

PRONOUNCE and DEFINE	Pronounce the following reproductive terms aloud and write their meaning.
epididymectomy	[ĔP-ĭ-dĭd-ĭ-MĔK-tō-mē]
prostatectomy	[prŏs-tă-TĔK-tō-mē]
orchidectomy	[ōr-kĭ-DĔK-tō-mē]
circumcision	[sĭr-kŭm-SĬZH-ŭn]

SPELL	Write the correct spelling for each related term.
	Removal of one or both testes
	Inflammation of the prostate gland
	Surgical birth control for males
	Removal of the penile foreskin

UNDERSTAND	Match each term on the left to its description on the right.

1. _____ castration
2. _____ epididymectomy
3. _____ vasectomy
4. _____ orchiectomy
5. _____ balanectomy

a. Removal of part of the vas deferens
b. Removal of the testicle
c. Removal of the epididymis
d. Removal of the penis
e. Removal of male reproductive parts

Mr. Rick Springs is a 58-year-old male who comes into the urology clinic for the first time. He relates in his surgical and medical history that he was born with an undescended testicle that required repair and had the foreskin removed at the same time. Later, he was in a skateboarding accident and ended up with penis and right testicle inflammation and consequent right testicle removal. He now is having testicle pain on the left side and inflammation of the penis and groin pain when lifting heavy objects. He wonders if he has a hernia.

1. On which male reproductive organs has Rick had problems and surgical procedures done?

_____

_____

2. What are the surgical terms for his surgical procedures?

_____

_____

3. What are the medical terms for the symptoms?

_____

_____

4. Write a medical case history of the patient's background using medical terms. (Don't forget the symptoms that he has related.)

_____

_____

5. Explain the difference between an orchidectomy and castration. List the possible reasons for each surgery.

_____

_____

LO 16.6 Pharmacological Terms

Males are sometimes treated with hormone replacement therapy (usually, testosterone). Such treatment can help with sexual problems and with some of the signs of aging. Medications for **impotence** may help some men restore sexual function. **Erectile dysfunction** also may be treated surgically or with mechanical devices. Occasionally, erectile dysfunction is a vascular problem and may be treated with medication.

Benign prostatic hyperplasia (BPH), as discussed earlier, produces uncomfortable and troublesome symptoms for the patient. There are several treatment and pharmacology options that are utilized to ease the pressure or alleviate symptoms. Many times, the condition is manageable with treatment and regular checkups (Table 16-2).

TABLE 16-2	Medical Treatments for Enlarged Prostate Gland
Surgical removal of prostate	
Radiation	
Drug (Proscar, or finasteride) to block testosterone's growth-stimulating effect on the prostate	
Alpha blocker drugs, which relax muscles near prostate, relieving pressure	
Microwave energy delivered through a probe inserted into the urethra or rectum	
Balloon inserted into the urethra and inflated with liquid	
Tumor frozen with liquid nitrogen delivered by probe through the skin	
Device (stent) inserted between lobes of prostate to relieve pressure on the urethra	

LO 16.7 Abbreviations

Abbreviation	Definition
BPH	benign prostatic hyperplasia
ED	erectile dysfunction
FSH	follicle-stimulating hormone
HPV	human papillomavirus
LH	luteinizing hormone
STI	sexually transmitted infection
TUR	transurethral resection
TURP	transurethral resection of the prostate

UNDERSTAND   **Identify the abbreviation from the definition provided.**

1. Sexually transmitted infection: _____
2. Follicle-stimulating hormone: _____
3. Human papillomavirus: _____
4. Transurethral resection: _____

Chapter Review

CHAPTER SUMMARY

	Learning Outcome	Summary
16.1	Recognize the parts of the male reproductive system and discuss the function of each part.	The male reproductive system is comprised of many anatomical structures that function to work together with the female to produce offspring, as well as share urinary functions and hormone production.
16.2	Recall the major word parts used in building words that relate to the male reproductive system.	Word building requires knowledge of word parts and their corresponding meanings to form medical terms within the male reproductive system.
16.3	Identify the common diagnostic tests, laboratory tests, and clinical procedures used in testing and treating disorders of the male reproductive system.	Diagnostic, procedural, and laboratory findings assist the health care provider in diagnosing medical conditions. Often used in combination, these tests lead to a final diagnosis and assist in treatment planning.
16.4	Define the major pathological conditions of the male reproductive system.	Knowledge and understanding of diseases and conditions of the male reproductive system, including the prostate, reproductive organs, and sexually transmitted infections, increases critical thinking related to pathological medical terms.
16.5	Recall the meaning of surgical terms related to the male reproductive system.	Surgical procedures within the male reproductive system revolve closely around repair of damaged or immature structures and treatment of cancer with the system.
16.6	Recognize common pharmacological agents used in treating disorders of the male reproductive system.	Primary and common pharmacological agents used in the male reproductive system are steroids, hormone replacement, and treatment of benign prostate symptoms.
16.7	Identify common abbreviations associated with the male reproductive system.	Abbreviations are used to describe diseases, conditions, procedures, and treatments associated with the male system.

Label the parts of the male reproductive system in the diagram provided.

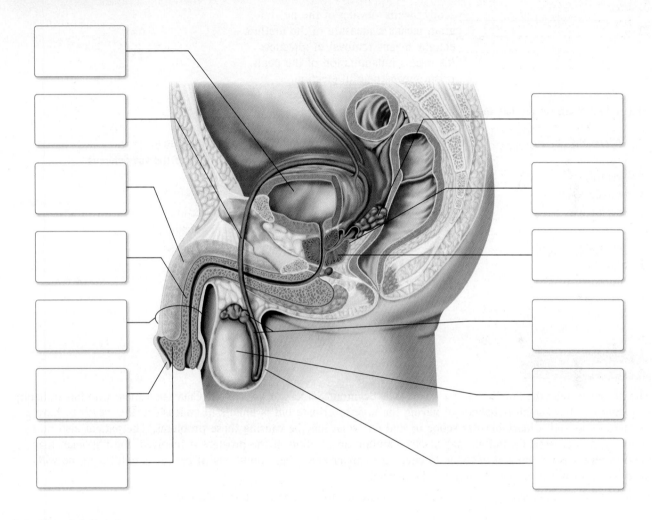

Identify if the following terms are spelled correctly. Correct the words that are spelled incorrectly. Write the definition for each word.

	Spelling	Definition
oligospermia		
azospermmia		
cryptorchism		
balanopthy		
vasovasostomy		
orchidostomy		

Pronounce each of the above terms aloud.

Complete the sentences by filling in the blanks.

1. _____ scopy means viewing of the prostate.
2. _____ gram means a measure of the urethra.
3. _____ ectomy means removal of a testicle.
4. _____ itis means inflammation of the penis.
5. _____ prism means painful erection.

Match each term on the left to its description on the right.

1. andropathy
2. prostatitis
3. priaprism
4. orchidectomy
5. cryptorchidism
6. hydrocele
7. varicocele
8. aspermia
9. oligospermia
10. vasectomy

a. Inflammation of the prostate
b. Removal of a portion of the vas deferens
c. Fluid-filled hernia
d. Tangled vein hernia
e. Scanty sperm production
f. Lack of sperm production
g. Condition of male diseases
h. Removal of a testicle
i. Undescended testicle
j. Painful erection

DECONSTRUCT

The physician tells the family that the client, Mr. Seymour Sergery, a 64-year-old Caucasian male who has difficulty urinating and has a high frequency of having the urge to urinate but is unable to "release" urine, needs to have a prostate exam and urinary bladder scope to find out what may be causing these problems. The patient also notices "pink" urine occasionally and an inability to maintain an erection. If the prostate is involved, the physician may need to take a small amount of tissue to check for cancer and other conditions. If cancer is confirmed, he will need to perform a procedure to remove the cancer.

Using medical terminology, write what the physician has told the family regarding the client.

_____

_____

_____

_____

Reviewing the Terms
Pronounce each of the following terms. Write the definitions on a separate sheet of paper. This review will take you through all the words you learned in this chapter. If you have difficulty with any words, make a flash card for later study. Refer to the English-Spanish and Spanish-English glossaries in the eBook.

andr/o [ĂN-drō]

anorchia [ăn-ŌR-kē-ă]

anorchism [ăn-ŌR-kĭzm]

aspermia [ā-SPĔR-mē-ă]

azoospermia [ā-zō-ō-SPĔR-mē-ă]

balan/o [BĂL-ă-nō]

balanitis [băl-ă-NĪ-tĭs]

bulbourethral [BŬL-bō-yū-RĒ-thrăl] gland

castration [kăs-TRĀ-shŭn]

chancroids [SHĂNG-krŏyds]

circumcision [sĭr-kŭm-SĬZH-ŭn]

Cowper's [KŎW-pĕrs] gland

cryptorchidism [krĭp-TŌR-kĭ-dĭzm]

cryptorchism [krĭp-TŌR-kĭzm]

ejaculation [ē-jăk-yū-LĀ-shŭn]

epididym/o [ĕp-ĭ-DĬD-ĭ-mō]

epididymectomy [ĔP-ĭ-dĭd-ĭ-MĔK-tō-mē]

epididymis (*pl.*, epididymes) [ĕp-ĭ-DĬD-ĭ-mĭs (ĕp-ĭ-DĬD-ĭ-mēz)]

epididymitis [ĕp-ĭ-dĭd-ĭ-MĪ-tĭs]

epispadias [ĕp-ĭ-SPĀ-dē-ăs]

flagellum [flă-JĔL-ŭm]

foreskin [FŌR-skĭn]

glans penis [glănz PĒ-nĭs]

hernia [HĔR-nē-ă]

hydrocele [HĪ-drō-sēl]

hypospadias [HĪ-pō-SPĀ-dē-ăs]

impotence [ĬM-pō-tĕns]

infertility [ĭn-fĕr-TĬL-ĭ-tē]

oligospermia [ŏl-ĭ-gō-SPĔR-mĕ-ă]

orch/o, orchi/o, orchid/o [ŌR-kō, ŌR-kē-ō, ŌR-kĭ-dō]

orchidectomy [ōr-kĭ-DĔK-tō-mē]

orchiectomy [ōr-kē-ĔK-tō-mē]

penis [PĒ-nĭs]

perineum [PĔR-ĭ-NĒ-ŭm]

Peyronie [pā-RŌN-ē] disease

phimosis [fĭ-MŌ-sĭs]

priapism [PRĪ-ă-pĭzm]

prostat/o [PRŎS-tă-tō]

prostate [PRŎS-tāt] gland

prostatectomy [prŏs-tă-TĔK-tō-mē]

prostate-specific antigen [ĂN-tĭ-jĕn] (PSA) test

prostatitis [prŏs-tă-TĪ-tĭs]

scrotum [SKRŌ-tŭm]

semen [SĒ-mĕn]

semen analysis

seminoma [sĕm-ĭ-NŌ-mă]

sperm [spĕrm]

sperm/o, spermat/o [SPĔR-mō, SPĔR-mă-tō]

spermatogenesis [SPĔR-mă-tō-JĔN-ĕ-sĭs]

spermatozoon (*pl.*, spermatozoa) [SPĔR-mă-tō-ZŌ-ŏn (SPĔR-mă-tō-ZŌ-ă)]

testicle [TĔS-tĭ-kl]

testis (*pl.*, testes) [TĔS-tĭs (TĔS-tēz)]

testosterone [tĕs-TŎS-tĕ-rōn]

transurethral resection of the prostate [trănz-yū-RĒ-thrăl rē-SĔK-shŭn]

urethrogram [yū-RĒ-thrō-grăm]

varicocele [VĂR-ĭ-kō-sēl]

vas deferens [văs DĔF-ĕr-ĕns]

vasectomy [vă-SĔK-tō-mē]

vasovasostomy [VĀ-sō-vă-SŎS-tō-mē]

The Female Reproductive System

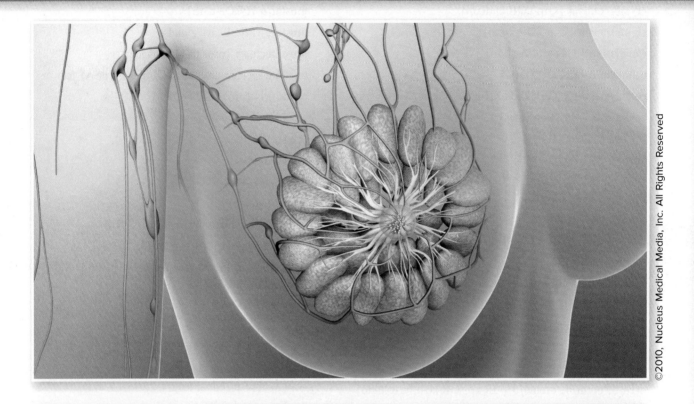

Learning Outcomes

After studying this chapter, you will be able to:

17.1   Recognize the parts of the female reproductive system and discuss the function of each part.

17.2   Recall the major word parts used in building words that relate to the female reproductive system.

17.3   Identify the common diagnostic tests, laboratory tests, and clinical procedures used in testing and treating disorders of the female reproductive system.

17.4   Define the major pathological conditions of the female reproductive system.

17.5   Recall the meaning of surgical terms related to the female reproductive system.

17.6   Recognize common pharmacological agents used in treating disorders of the female reproductive system.

17.7   Identify common abbreviations associated with the female reproductive system.

Structure and Function of the Female Reproductive System

STUDY TIP

Stress, diet, and illness can affect a woman's ability to ovulate.

Women can ovulate without menstruation, and women can menstruate without ovulation.

The average egg lives roughly 24 hours after leaving the ovary.

Reproductive Organs

The female reproductive system is responsible for providing an optimal place for fertilization and growth of another human being until birth and for providing important hormones to the body. It is comprised of the following main organs: ovaries, uterus, uterine tubes, cervix, vagina, labia, and clitoris (Figure 17-1). The mammary glands are also part of the female reproductive system. They are not involved in reproduction; their role is to nourish the fetus after birth. Mammary glands are present in both males and females but only function in the female. **Gynecology** [**gynec/o** = women + **-logy** = study of] is the study of the female systems; and **obstetrics** is the specialty that cares for the pregnant woman. There are several combining forms for structure and function that will be discussed throughout the chapter.

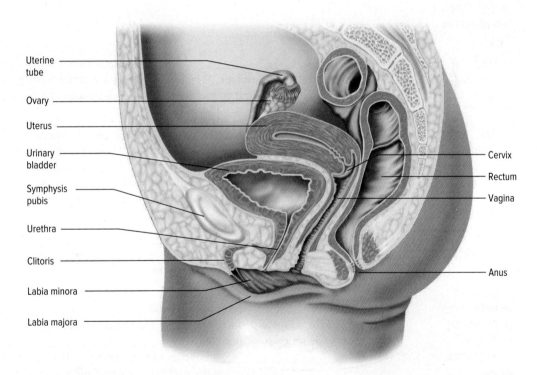

Figure 17-1 Female reproductive system; sagittal view

Structure and Function	PRACTICE
	Provide the missing term(s) to complete the following sentences.
ova [Ō-vă] **ovum** [Ō-vŭm]	The female reproductive system is a group of organs and glands that produce _____ (singular _____), or *egg cells* (female sex cells); move them to the site of fertilization; and, if they are fertilized by a sperm (male sex cell), nurture them until birth.
ovaries [Ō-vă-rēz] **gonads** [GŌ-nădz] **ova** [Ō-vă] **ovulation** [ŎV-yū-LĀ-shŭn]	The _____ (also known as the female _____) are two small, solid, oval structures in the pelvic cavity that produce _____ and secrete female hormones. The ovaries lie on either side of the uterus. In the monthly cycle of egg production, one ovary usually releases only one mature ovum. In most women, the ovaries alternate this release, called _____, each month. In rare cases, more eggs are released. In some women, the ovaries do not alternate regularly or do not alternate at all. The monthly production of ova or sex cells is fairly regular in most women. (In males, the production of sex cells is not cyclical.)
gametes [GĂM-ēts] **graafian follicle** [GRĂ-fē-ăn FŎL-ĭ-kl] **oocytes** [Ō-ō-sīts] **uterine tube** [YŪ-tĕr-ĭn tūb] **fallopian tube** [fă-LŌ-pē-ăn tūb]	Within the ovaries are sex cells, also known as _____. Before being released from an ovary, the cells develop in a part of the ovary called the _____. These sex cells have the potential to become fertilized and develop. In their immature stage, they are called _____; once mature (normally 5–7 days), they are known as ova. The ovum is then released from the graafian follicle to the _____ or _____, the tube that leads from each ovary to the uterus.
uterus [YŪ-tĕr-ŭs]	The _____ is the female reproductive organ in which a fertilized ovum implants and develops. When the ovum is not fertilized, the lining of the uterus is released during the monthly cycle, known as *menstruation*. This cycle is described later in this chapter.
vagina [vă-JĪ-nă]	The fertilized ovum attaches to the lining of the uterus, where it develops during pregnancy (discussed later in this chapter). At the end of its development, the infant is born through the _____, or birth canal (the canal leading from the uterus to the *vulva*), in a routine delivery; sometimes the infant is delivered surgically through the abdomen in a *caesarean delivery*. The organs and structures form the basic reproductive structure.
mammary gland [MĂM-ă-rē glănd]	The female breast, the _____, is also part of the female reproductive system as an *accessory organ,* providing milk to nurse the infant (*lactation*) after birth. In addition to fertilization, female reproduction is controlled by hormones, such as estrogen and progesterone.
puberty [PYŪ-bĕr-tē] **menarche** [mĕ-NĂR-kē] **menses** [MĔN-sēz] **menstruation** [mĕn-strū-Ā-shŭn] **menopause** [MĔN-ō-păwz]	At birth, most females have from 200,000 to 400,000 immature ova (oocytes) in each ovary. Many of these disintegrate before the female reaches _____, the stage at which ovulation and _____ (first menstrual flow or _____) occurs (usually between 10 and 14 years of age). _____ is the cyclical release of the uterine lining usually occurring every 28 days. Most women menstruate monthly (except during pregnancy) for about 30 to 40 years. _____ signals the end of the ovulation/menstruation cycle and, therefore, the end of the child-bearing years.

fimbriae [FĬM-brē-ē] **gestation** [jĕs-TĀ-shŭn] **fundus** [FŬN-dŭs] **placenta** [plă-SĔN-tă]	After release, the ovum next enters one of the two uterine, or fallopian, tubes, which have fingerlike ends called _____ that sweep the ovum further down into the tube, where it may be fertilized by a sperm. Fertilized or not, the ovum moves by contractions of the tube to the uterus. The uterus is pear shaped and about the size of the fist. It is wider at the top than at the bottom, where it attaches to the vagina. Once inside the uterus, a fertilized ovum attaches to the uterine wall, where it will be nourished for about 40 weeks of development (_____). The upper portion of the uterus, the _____, is where a nutrient-rich organ (the _____) grows in the uterine wall. An ovum that has not been fertilized is released along with the lining of the uterus (*endometrium*) during menstruation.
body [BŎD-ē] **isthmus** [ĬS-mŭs] **cervix** [SĔR-vĭks]	The middle portion of the uterus is called the _____. It leads to a narrow region, the _____. The neck, or lower region, of the uterus is the _____, a protective body with glands that secrete mucous substances into the vagina. The cervical canal is the opening leading to the uterine cavity. Cells from the distal part of the cervical canal are collected during a routine Pap smear. The opening of the cervical canal into the vagina is called the *cervical os*. Cervical cancers are more likely to occur in the distal third of the cervical canal and os, accessible during routine Pap smears.
hymen [HĪ-mĕn] **introitus** [ĭn-TRŌ-ĭ-tŭs]	The vagina has small transverse folds called *rugae* that can expand to accommodate an erect penis during intercourse or the passage of a baby during childbirth. A fold of mucous membranes, the _____, partially covers the external opening (_____) of the vagina. It is usually ruptured during the female's first sexual intercourse but may be broken earlier during physical activity or because of use of a tampon. It also may be congenitally absent.
perimetrium [pĕr-ĭ-MĒ-trē-ŭm] **myometrium** [MĪ-ō-MĒ-trē-ŭm] **endometrium** [ĔN-dō-MĒ-trē-ŭm]	The uterus is made up of three layers of tissue: the _____, the outer layer; the _____, the middle layer; and the _____, the inner mucous layer. The outer layer is a protective layer of membranous tissue. The middle layer is really three layers of smooth muscle that move in strong downward motions. The uterus stretches during pregnancy. The endometrium is deep and velvety, has an abundant supply of blood vessels and glands, and is built up and broken down during the ovulation/menstruation cycle.
vulva [VŬL-vă] **mons pubis** [mŏnz PYŪ-bĭs] **labia majora** [LĀ-bē-ă mă-JŌR-ă] **labia minora** [LĀ-bē-ă mĭ-NŌR-ă] **clitoris** [KLĬT-ō-rĭs] **Bartholin's glands** [BĂR-thō-lĕnz glăndz]	The external genitalia (Figure 17-2), collectively known as the _____, consist of a mound of soft tissue, the _____, which is covered by pubic hair after puberty. Two folds of skin below the mons pubis, the _____, form the borders of the vulva. Between the labia majora lie two smaller skin folds, the _____, which merge at the top to form the _____, the primary female organ of sexual stimulation. The _____ are embedded in the vaginal tissue near the vaginal os. The duct from those glands is located between the labia minora. The glands produce a lubricating fluid that bathes the vagina and surrounding vulva.
perineum [PĔR-ĭ-NĒ-ŭm]	The space between the bottom of the labia majora and the anus is called the _____. During childbirth, it is possible for the perineum to become torn. A surgical procedure (*episiotomy*) is commonly done before childbirth to avoid tearing the perineum because an even surgical incision is easier to repair.
lactiferous [lăk-TĬF-ĕr-ŭs] **sinuses** [SĪ-nŭs-ĕz] **nipple** [NĬP-l] **areola** [ă-RĒ-ō-lă] **parturition** [păr-tūr-ĬSH-ŭn]	The mammary glands, or breasts, are full of glandular tissue that is stimulated by hormones after puberty to grow and respond to the cycles of menstruation and birth. During pregnancy, hormones stimulate the _____ (milk-producing) ducts and _____ that transport milk to the _____ (or *mammary papilla*). The dark-pigmented area surrounding the nipple is called the _____. After birth (_____), the mammary glands experience a *let-down reflex*, which allows milk to flow through the nipples (lactation) when the infant suckles.

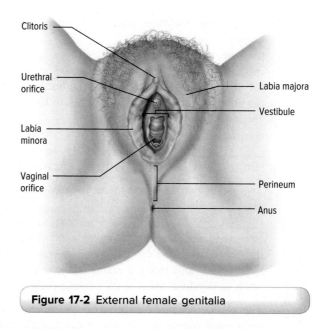

Figure 17-2 External female genitalia

Building Your Female Reproductive Vocabulary

Combining Form	Meaning
amni/o	amnion
cervic/o	cervix
colp/o	vagina
episi/o	vulva
galact/o	milk
gynec/o	female
hyster/o	uterus
lact/o, lacti	milk
mamm/o	breast
mast/o	breast
men/o	menstruation
metr/o	uterus
oo	egg
oophor/o	ovary
ov/i, ov/o	egg
ovari/o	ovary

Combining Form	Meaning
perine/o	perineum
salping/o	fallopian tube
uter/o	uterus
vagin/o	vagina
vulv/o	vulva

Did you know

Fertility

A baby girl is born with all of the egg cells (oocytes) she will ever have already in her ovaries. None develop after birth. At about 5 months of gestation, the ovaries of a female fetus contain 6 to 7 million oocytes. Most of the oocytes gradually are absorbed into the body, leaving about 1 to 2 million at birth, and by puberty, only about 300,000 are left—more than enough for a lifetime of fertility.

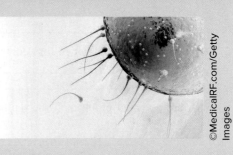

©MedicalRF.com/Getty Images

PRONOUNCE and DEFINE	Pronounce the following reproductive terms aloud and write their meaning.
endometrium	[ĔN-dō-MĒ-trē-ŭm]
menarche	[mĕ-NĂR-kē]
oocytes	[Ō-ō-sīts]
parturition	[păr-tūr-ĬSH-ŭn]

SPELL	Write the correct spelling of the related term.
	Brownish area surrounding the nipple
	Female sexual stimulation organ
	40 weeks of baby's development
	Neck of the lower region of the uterus
	Egg cells

1. _____ labia minora
2. _____ myometrium
3. _____ labia majora
4. _____ clitoris
5. _____ hymen
6. _____ endometrium

a. Smaller skin folds that merge at the top
b. Two larger folds of skin below the mons pubis
c. Female organ of sexual stimulation
d. Fold of mucous membranes
e. Inner membrane of the uterus
f. Middle layer membrane of the uterus

APPLY   Read the following scenario and answer the questions.

Ms. Jenni Takanado is a 31-year-old Asian female who comes into the clinic complaining of painful intercourse, irregular menses, and breast discomfort. She has a history of late menarche (age 16), fibrocystic breasts, and infertility.

1. Which reproductive parts may be affected?
_____
_____

2. Do any other pieces of her history contribute to her problems? How?
_____
_____

3. What are potential problems if the reproductive system is not working properly?
_____
_____

4. How would you document the above in medical terms?
_____
_____

LO 17.2 Word Building in the Female Reproductive System

Hormones and Cycles

The female reproductive system, while active, goes through a cycle termed the **menstrual cycle** (Figure 17-3). This cycle usually occurs every 28 days and consists of changes in the uterine lining that results in **menses (menorrhea),** or shedding of the lining, and a repeat of the cycle again. The purpose of the menstrual cycle is to accommodate a potential fetus. Hormones play a large part of regulation of this cycle and of the female system in general (Table 17-1).

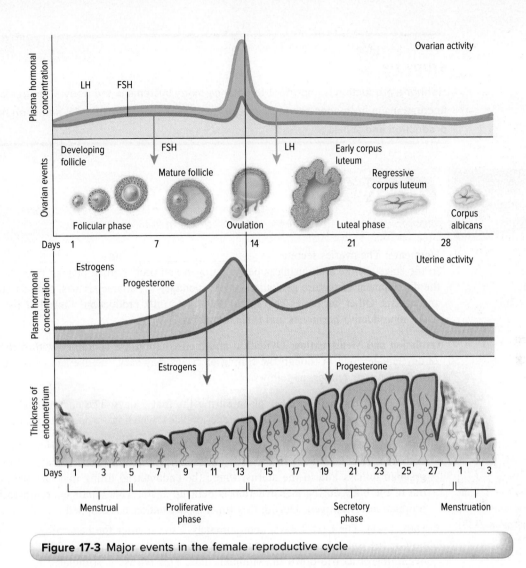

Figure 17-3 Major events in the female reproductive cycle

TABLE 17-1	Major Reproductive Hormones	
Hormone	**Purpose**	**Source**
estrogen	stimulates development of female sex characteristics and uterine wall thickening	ovarian follicle; corpus luteum
progesterone	stimulates uterine wall thickening and formation of mammary ducts	corpus luteum
prolactin	promotes lactation	pituitary gland
oxytocin	stimulates labor and lactation	pituitary gland
FSH (follicle-stimulating hormone)	stimulates oocyte maturation; increasing estrogen	pituitary gland
HCG (human chorionic gonadotropin)	stimulates estrogen and progesterone from corpus luteum	placenta, embryo

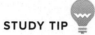
Hormone production is important to balance many systems in the body. Changes or fluctuations in hormones can increase (or decrease) acne, weight gain, and even hair production and shine.

Word Building	PRACTICE
	Provide the missing term(s) to complete the following sentences.
estrogen [ĔS-trō-jĕn] **progesterone** [prō-JĔS-tĕr-ōn]	**Hormones:** The ovaries secrete _____ and _____. In the stages before and during puberty, estrogen and progesterone play an important role in the development of mature genitalia and of secondary sex characteristics, such as pubic hair and breasts. Other hormones help in childbirth and milk production. Table 17-1 lists the major reproductive hormones and their functions.
	Ovulation and Menstruation: Ovulation and menstruation are contained within the average 28-day female cycle. Although the timing of cycles may vary, the average female cycle is divided into four phases, as follows:
	1. Days 1–5. Menstruation takes place during the first 5 days. The endometrial lining sloughs off and is released, causing generally slow bleeding through the vagina.
follicle-stimulating hormone (FSH) [FŎL-Ĭ-kl STĬM-ū-lāt-ĭng HŌR-mōn] **luteinizing hormone (LH)** [LŪ-tē-ĭ-nīz-ĭng HŌR-mōn] **corpus luteum** [KŌR-pŭs LŪ-tē-ŭm]	2. Days 6–12. The _____ is released from the anterior pituitary. The body reactions take place in the ovary, where an immature ovum is matured in the graafian follicle, and in the uterus, where the endometrial lining that has been passed out of the body during menstruation is built up again. This repair is prompted by the production of estrogen. During this time, menstruation has stopped. 3. Days 13–14. The next 2 days, approximately 2 weeks after the beginning of menstruation, is the time of ovulation, or the egg's release from the graafian follicle and the beginning of its trip down the fallopian tube. This release is stimulated by the pituitary's release of _____, which prompts the fimbriae to swell and wave to entice the newly released ovum toward the fallopian tube. Meanwhile, the graafian follicle fills with a yellow substance that secretes estrogen and progesterone. This secreting structure is known as the _____. The secreted hormones encourage the uterus to prepare for a pregnancy by growing the endometrium into a thick, nutritive layer. 4. Days 15–28. In the second 14 days of the cycle, either fertilization occurs or the built-up endometrium starts to break down as estrogen and progesterone levels drop. The symptoms (bloating, cramping, nervousness, and depression) of the hormonal changes during the phase leading to menstruation (*premenstrual syndrome [PMS]*) appear.
contraception [kŏn-tră-SĔP-shŭn] **intrauterine device (IUD)** [ĬN-tră-YŪ-tĕr-ĭn dē-VĪS] **condom** [KŎN-dŏm] **spermicide** [SPĔR-mĭ-sīd] **diaphragm** [DĪ-ă-frăm] **sponge** [spŭnj]	It is at the point of ovulation that fertilization can occur or be prevented. Prevention of fertilization is accomplished with _____. Contraceptive devices include the _____, _____ (both male and female), _____, _____, or _____ (Table 17-2 and Figure 17-4).

Did you know

Birth Control Pill

In 2010, the birth control pill celebrated its 50th birthday. The pill has gone through a lot of changes in that time. In 1965, it was illegal to take birth control pills in several states until a court decided that it was an invasion of privacy to interfere with a person's rights to family planning.

TABLE 17-2	Birth Control Methods				
	Method	**Mechanism**	**Advantages**	**Disadvantages**	**Pregnancies per Year per 100 Women***
	None				85
Barrier and Spermicidal	Condom	Worn over penis or within vagina, keeps sperm out of vagina or from entering cervix	Protection against sexually transmitted diseases (latex only)	Disrupts spontaneity, can break, reduces sensation in male	2–12
	Condom and spermicide	Worn over penis or within vagina, keeps sperm out of vagina, and kills sperm that escape	Protection against sexually transmitted infections (latex only)	Disrupts spontaneity, can break, reduces sensation in male	2–5
	Diaphragm and spermicide	Kills sperm and blocks uterus	Inexpensive	Disrupts spontaneity, messy, needs to be fitted by doctor	6–18
	Cervical cap and spermicide	Kills sperm and blocks uterus	Inexpensive, can be left in 24 hours	May slip out of place, messy, needs to be fitted by doctor	6–18
	Spermicidal film, sponge, suppository, foam, or gel	Kills sperm and blocks vagina	Inexpensive, easy to use and carry	Messy, irritates 25% of users, male and female	3–21

continued on next page

	Method	Mechanism	Advantages	Disadvantages	Pregnancies per Year per 100 Women*
Hormonal	Combination estrogen and progestin (pill, patch, ring, or injection)	Prevents follicle maturation, ovulation, and implantation	Does not interrupt spontaneity, lowers risk of some cancers, decreases menstrual flow (one pill eliminates menstruation)	Raises risk of cardiovascular disease in some women, causes weight gain and breast tenderness	3
	Minipill	Thickness; cervical mucus	Does not interrupt spontaneity	Menstrual changes	5
	Medroxyprogesterone acetate (Depo-Provera)	Prevents ovulation, alters uterine lining	Easy to use	Menstrual changes, weight gain	0.3
Behavioral	Rhythm method	No intercourse during fertile times	No cost	Difficult to do, hard to predict timing	20
	Withdrawal (coitus interruptus)	Removal of penis from vagina before ejaculation	No cost	Difficult to do	4–18
Surgical	Vasectomy	Sperm cells never reach penis	Permanent, does not interrupt spontaneity	Requires surgery	0.15
	Tubal ligation	Egg cells never reach uterus	Permanent, does not interrupt spontaneity	Requires surgery, entails some risk of infection	0.4
Other	Intrauterine device	Prevents implantation	Does not interrupt spontaneity	Severe menstrual cramps, increases risk of infection	3

TABLE 17-2   Birth Control Methods

*The lower figures apply when the contraceptive device is used correctly. The higher figures reflect human error in using birth control.

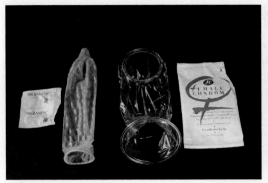

(a) Male and female condoms

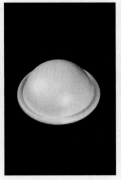

(b) Diaphragm

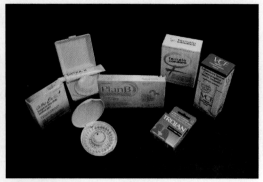

(c) Spermicide in film, sponge, suppositories, gel

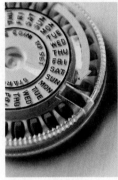

(d) Oral contraceptive

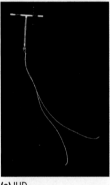

(e) IUD

(a and b): ©McGraw-Hill Education/ Jill Braaten; (c): ©McGraw-Hill Education/ Christopher Kerrigan; (d): ©Don Farrall/ Getty Images; (e): ©McGraw-Hill Education/Jill Braaten, photographer

Figure 17-4 Birth control devices

PRONOUNCE and DEFINE	Pronounce the following reproductive terms aloud and write their meaning.
intrauterine device	[ĬN-tră-YŪ-těr-ĭn dē-VĪS]
progesterone	[prō-JĚS-těr-ōn]
corpus luteum	[KŌR-pŭs LŪ-tē-ŭm]
follicle-stimulating hormone	[FŎL-Ĭ-kl STĬM-ū-lāt-ĭng HŌR-mōn]

SPELL	Write the correct spelling for each related term.
	Primary "female" hormone
	Prevention of (against) conception
	"Inside the uterus"; birth control device
	Kills sperm
	Cuplike barrier birth control device

UNDERSTAND	Match each term on the left to its description on the right.

1. _____ sponge
2. _____ corpus luteum
3. _____ luteinizing hormone (LH)
4. _____ follicle-stimulating hormone (FSH)
5. _____ intrauterine device (IUD)

a. Contraception device that is inserted right before sex
b. Contraception device that is inserted in physician's office
c. Secretes hormones estrogen and progesterone
d. Hormone that triggers ovulation
e. Released by the anterior pituitary

Mrs. Beth Meyers is a 24-year-old Caucasian female who has come into her family physician for a yearly recheck and wants to discuss birth control options. She has been taking birth control pills for 4 years and is experiencing break-through bleeding. She states that she "forgets" sometimes to take her daily pill. She also relates that she has only one sex partner and is currently taking a 21-day birth control prescription.

1. Which structures of the female reproductive system are involved in her cycle?

   _____
   _____
   _____

2. What other options would she have for contraception, based on her history?

   _____
   _____
   _____

3. Based on her history of "forgetting" or noncompliance, which birth control method might be the best option?

   _____
   _____

4. Which of the following are barrier contraceptives? List only the barrier contraceptives.

   - IUD _____
   - Condom _____
   - Diaphragm _____
   - Birth control pills _____
   - Sponge _____
   - Spermicide _____
   - Rhythm _____

   _____
   _____
   _____

Did you know ?

Pregnancies

Every pregnancy is different for a mother. Her first pregnancy may have been uneventful without many symptoms or problems and the second or third may be the complete opposite. Also, many women have cravings during pregnancy for certain foods (or even nonfood items), but not all pregnant women experience cravings.

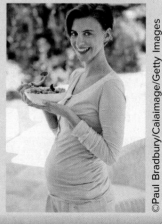
©Paul Bradbury/Caiaimage/Getty Images

Pregnancy and Menopause

Pregnancy is comprised of three trimesters (40 weeks) that mark the fetus's (and eventual baby's) development before birth. Conception occurs when a female egg (**oocyte**) and male sperm (**spermatocyte**) unite after intercourse. Child-bearing time frames vary, depending on menses, but the age span for pregnancy to occur is usually between 13 and 45.

Perimenopause [peri = around + **menopause** = stop child-bearing] is the transition period between the later child-bearing years and the full onset of menopause. It usually occurs between the ages of 35 and 50, but medications and surgery can begin the process earlier. Perimenopause symptoms are similar to menopause, but to a lesser and nonconsistent extent.

Menopause occurs after child-bearing years, when the reproductive hormones begin to decline, usually between the ages of 45 and 55. These changes cause irregular menses, before periods stop altogether. Common symptoms of menopause are:

- Irregular periods
- Decreased fertility
- Hot flashes
- Sleep disturbances
- Night sweats
- Mood swings
- Increased abdominal fat
- Thinning hair
- Vaginal dryness
- Loss of breast fullness

The onset of perimenopause and menopause is different for each woman, just as the onset of menses is different for each girl. It is largely related and dependent on hereditary factors.

Word Building

coitus
[KŌ-ĭ-tŭs]
copulation
[kŏp-yū-LĀ-shŭn]
gravida
[GRĂV-ĭ-dă]

PRACTICE

Provide the missing term(s) to complete the following sentences.

Pregnancy: As a result of contact between the sperm and an ovum, usually through sexual intercourse (_____ or _____), fertilization may occur. Fertilization should take place soon after ovulation and high in the fallopian tube to ensure the cells are at the proper stage of development when entering the uterus. If fertilized, implantation in the uterus takes place, the placenta forms, and pregnancy begins. Fertilization also may take place through artificial insemination. This can take place either by mechanical insertion of sperm from a sperm donor or by in vitro fertilization, which occurs in a laboratory that harvests ova and fertilizes them in the laboratory before implanting them into the uterus. A pregnant woman is known as a _____, with gravida I being the first pregnancy, gravida II being the second, and so on.

continued on next page

	Provide the missing term(s) to complete the following sentences.
umbilical cord [ŭm-BĬL-ĭ-kăl kōrd] **chorion** [KŌ-rē-ŏn] **amnion** [ĂM-nē-ŏn] **amniotic fluid** [ăm-nē-ŎT-ĭk FLŪ-ĭd]	An _____ connects the placenta to the navel of the fetus so that the mother's blood and the fetal blood do not mix, but nutrients and waste products are exchanged. The fetus develops in a sac containing the _____, the outermost membrane covering the fetus, and the _____, the innermost membrane next to the fluid surrounding the fetus (_____). The birth process usually begins when the sac breaks naturally or is broken by medical intervention.
afterbirth [ĂF-tĕr-bĕrth] **para** [PĂ-ră]	The placenta separates from the uterus after delivery and is expelled from the body as the _____. The umbilical cord is then severed and tied so that the infant is physically separated from its mother. At the end of this process, the woman is known as a _____ (one who has maintained a pregnancy to the point of viability). Para I refers to the first such pregnancy, para II the second, and so on.
climacteric [klī-MĂK-tĕr-ĭk, klī-măk-TĔR-ĭk] **perimenopause** [pĕr-ĭ-MĔN-ō-păws]	**Menopause:** Menopause, the cessation of menstruation, takes place after levels of estrogen decline. Most women experience menopause between the ages of 45 and 55. The period of hormonal changes leading up to menopause is called the _____. The 3 to 5 years of decreasing estrogen levels prior to menopause is called _____. The hormonal changes cause symptoms in some women that can be uncomfortable, such as night sweats, fatigue, irritability, or vaginal dryness. Hormone replacement therapy is sometimes used. Some women find relief from increasing their intake of natural plant estrogens found in such products as soy.

Did you know ?

Uterus Expansion

A full-term pregnancy is 36 to 40 weeks from conception, and during that time the uterus expands up to 500 times its normal size. Breast feeding helps speed up the process of the uterus contracting back to normal, usually within 4 to 6 weeks after delivery.

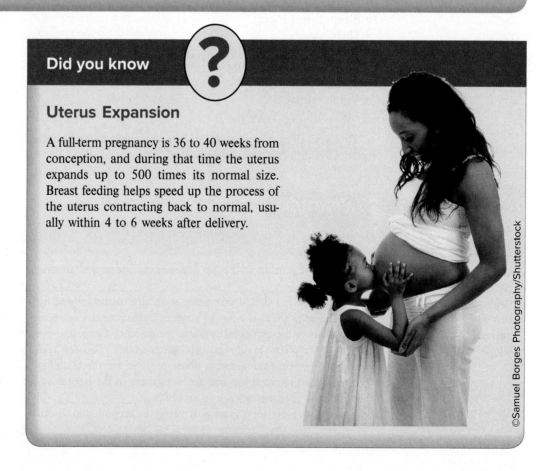

©Samuel Borges Photography/Shutterstock

PRONOUNCE and DEFINE	Pronounce the following reproductive terms aloud and write their meaning.
chorion	[KŌ-rē-ŏn]
coitus	[KŌ-ĭ-tŭs]
climacteric	[klī-MĂK-tĕr-ĭk, klī-măk-TĔR-ĭk]
gravida	[GRĂV-ĭ-dă]

SPELL and DEFINE	Identify if the following terms are spelled correctly. Correct the words that are spelled incorrectly. Write the definition for each word.	
	Spelling	Definition
amnion		
paremenopause		
coppulation		
amneotic fluid		

UNDERSTAND — Match each term on the left to its description on the right.

1. _____ climacteric
2. _____ chorion
3. _____ amnion
4. _____ copulation
5. _____ gravida

a. Another name for a pregnant woman
b. Period of changes before menopause
c. Outermost membrane
d. Innermost membrane
e. Intercourse leading to pregnancy

APPLY — Read the following scenario and answer the questions.

Ms. Heidi Red Feather is a 47-year-old Native American female who presents to the ER with night sweating, bleeding in between periods, feeling hot then cold, depression, and weight gain.

1. What could be occurring? Why?

_____

_____

2. What is the period leading up to this called?

_____

_____

3. What would the terms be for the symptoms she is having?

_____

_____

4. What would you anticipate that the doctor may want to do to help this patient?

_____

_____

Constructing Words for the Female Reproductive System

Now that the female anatomy, hormone cycles, pregnancy, and menopause have been covered, it is time to practice word building. Following are some medical terms and combinations common to the female reproductive system.

As you work through the practice, try to mix and match or associate various word roots with different prefixes/suffixes to extend your knowledge and vocabulary.

Word Building	PRACTICE
	Provide the correct combining form to complete each of the sentences.
metro-pathy [mē-TRŎP-ă-thē]	Disease of the uterus is _____ pathy.
episio-tomy [ĕ-pĭz-ē-ŎT-ō-mē]	Surgical incision into the perineum to prevent tearing during childbirth is an _____ tomy.
mast-itis [măs-TĪ-tĭs]	Inflammation of the breast is _____ itis.
colpo-rrhagia [kol-pō-RĀ-jē-ă]	Vaginal hemorrhage is _____ rrhagia.
vulv-itis [vŭl-VĪ-tĭs]	Inflammation of the vulva is _____ itis.
salpingo-plasty [săl-PĬNG-gō-plăs-tē]	_____ plasty is surgical repair of a fallopian tube.
amnio-centesis [ĂM-nē-ō-sĕn-TĒ-sĭs]	Test of amniotic fluid by insertion of a needle into the amnion is _____ centesis.
utero-plasty [YŪ-tĕr-ō-plăs-tē]	_____ plasty is surgical repair of the uterus.
oophor-itis [ō-ŏf-ōr-Ī-tĭs]	_____ itis is inflammation of an ovary.
galacto-poiesis [gă-LĂK-tō-poy-Ē-sĭs]	_____ poiesis relates to milk production.
hyster-ectomy [hĭs-tĕr-ĔK-tō-mē]	_____ ectomy is surgical removal of the uterus.
ovario-cele [ō-VĂR-ē-ō-sēl]	Hernia of an ovary is _____ cele.
oo-genesis [ō-ō-JĔN-ĕ-sĭs]	_____ genesis is production of eggs.
gyneco-logy [gī-nĕ-KŎL-ō-jē]	Medical specialty that diagnoses and treats disorders of the female reproductive system is _____ logy.
cervic-itis [sĕr-vĭ-SĪ-tĭs]	_____ itis is inflammation of the cervix.
meno-rrhea [mĕn-ōr-Ē-ă]	Menstrual discharge is _____ rrhea.

Chapter 17

mammo-graphy [mă-MŎG-ră-fē]	Imaging of the breast is _____ graphy.
ov-oid [Ō-voyd]	_____ oid is egg shaped.
lacto-genesis [lăk-tō-JĔN-ĕ-sĭs]	Milk production is _____ genesis.
vagin-itis [văj-ĭ-NĪ-tĭs]	Inflammation of the vagina is _____ itis.
meno-pause [MĔN-ō-păwz]	Cessation of menstruation is _____ pause.

Did you know

Breast Milk Bank

Established in 1985, the Human Milk Banking Association of North America (HMBANA) is a professional association for milk banks across the United States, Canada, and Mexico. Mothers who cannot supply enough milk for their babies can acquire donated human milk via milk banks. The HMBANA establishes guidelines and standards for human milk banks across North America.

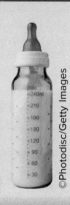

©Photodisc/Getty Images

PRONOUNCE and DEFINE	Pronounce the following reproductive terms aloud and write their meaning.
mastitis	[măs-TĪ-tĭs]
oophoritis	[ō-ŏf-ōr-Ī-tĭs]
metropathy	[mē-TRŎP-ă-thē]
lactogenesis	[lăk-tō-JĔN-ĕ-sĭs]

SPELL	Write the correct spelling for each related term.
	Inflammation of the cervix
	Repair of the fallopian tube
	Removal of an ovary
	Puncture into the amnion to draw fluid
	Imaging of the breast

Match each term on the left to its description on the right.

1. _____ galactopoiesis
2. _____ gynecology
3. _____ hysterectomy
4. _____ colporrhagia
5. _____ perineocele

a. Vaginal hemorrhage
b. Relates to milk production
c. The study of the female reproductive system
d. Hernia of the perineum
e. Surgical removal of the uterus

APPLY   **Read the following scenario and answer the questions.**

Ms. Pamela Kline is a 40-year-old African-American female who is a new patient in the Fairview Gynecology Clinic. She is relaying her past medical, surgical, and social history for the doctor's review. She states that she has had five pregnancies with removal of fluid from the last one; inflammation of the vagina and cervix; hernia of the uterine (fallopian) tubes with repair; and surgical removal of her uterus, ovaries, and fallopian tubes.

1. List all of the medical terms for her history.

_____
_____

2. How many surgeries has she relayed?

_____
_____

3. She is still in child-bearing years; could another pregnancy be an option for her?

_____
_____

4. Write exactly how you would relay this history to the physician using medical terminology.

_____
_____
_____

LO 17.3 Diagnostic, Procedural, and Laboratory Terms

STUDY TIP

Approximately 40 million women undergo a mammogram to screen for breast cancer each year in the United States. The National Cancer Institute recommends that every woman have an initial mammogram at the age of 40 (Figure 17-5).

The female reproductive system is its own specialty, and therefore has multiple diagnostic, procedural, and laboratory testing terms and options that span from nonpregnant to pregnant, disease states, and menopausal conditions. Because of the vast span and its effect on every female, it makes **gynecology** one of the most utilized diagnostic testing specialties.

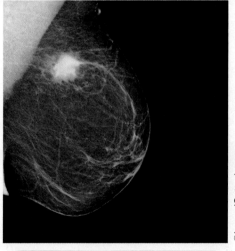

©ksass/Getty Images

Figure 17-5 Mammogram of breast with tumor

Many women use their **gynecologist** as their primary care physician. This is usually because most women of child-bearing age need only a physician trained around the female system and/or **obstetrics;** therefore, they are comfortable with one physician taking care of all their needs.

In most practices, a gynecologist is also an obstetrician. The difference is that a gynecologist treats nonpregnant female disorders and an obstetrician treats only pregnant women.

Diagnostic	**PRACTICE** Provide the missing term(s) to complete the following sentences.
gynecologist [gī-nĕ-KŎL-ō-jĭst] **obstetrician** [ŏb-stĕ-TRĬSH-ŭn]	The major function of the female reproductive system is to bear children. There are several basic tests for pregnancy. Diagnosis of fertility problems involves more sophisticated technology. Aside from pregnancy, the health of the female reproductive system is monitored on a regular basis by a _____, a physician who diagnoses and treats disorders of the female reproductive system. An _____ diagnoses and treats both normal and abnormal pregnancies and childbirths.
Papanicolaou (Pap) smear [pă-pă-NĒ-kō-lū (păp)] **colposcopy** [kŏl-PŎS-kō-pē]	A routine gynecological exam usually includes a _____, a gathering of cells from the cervix to detect cervical or vaginal cancer or other anomalies. The vagina is held open by a vaginal *speculum,* a device that holds open any cavity or canal for examination. The cervix and vagina also may be examined by _____, use of a lighted instrument (a *colposcope*) for viewing into the vagina. The colposcope is used for almost all vaginal examinations and is a very common instrument in a gynecological or obstetrical office.
hysteroscopy [hĭs-tĕr-ŎS-kō-pē] **culdoscopy** [kŭl-DŎS-kō-pē]	_____ is the use of a *hysteroscope,* a lighted instrument for examination of the interior of the uterus. _____ is the use of an endoscope to examine the contents of the pelvic cavity. These tests can determine whether masses, tumors, or other abnormalities are present. Some abnormalities are caused by sexually transmitted infections. A Venereal Disease Research Laboratory (VDRL) slide test can show the presence of a sexually transmitted infection.
mammography [mă-MŎG-ră-fē]	Depending on a woman's age, a routine gynecological exam usually includes a prescription for a *mammogram,* a cancer screening test for the breasts that can detect tumors before they can be felt. _____ is a procedure that produces radiograms of the breasts. The age recommended for routine mammography differs according to family history, physical condition, and the recommending body. (Recommendations from the American Medical Association, American Cancer Society, and the National Institutes of Health vary.)
	A pregnancy test is a blood or urine test to detect *human chorionic gonadotropin (HCG),* a hormone that stimulates growth during the first trimester of pregnancy.
hysterosalpingography [HĬS-tĕr-ō-săl-pĭng-GŎG-ră-fē]	Several tests for fertility problems include _____, a procedure to x-ray the uterus and uterine tubes after a contrast medium is injected; *pelvic ultrasonography,* imaging of the pelvic region using sound waves (used both for detection of tumors and for examination of the fetus); and *transvaginal ultrasound,* also a sound wave image of the pelvic area but done with a probe inserted into the vagina.
pelvimetry [pĕl-VĬM-ĕ-trē]	During pregnancy, the dimensions of the pelvis are measured during _____, the taking of a measurement to see if the pelvis is large enough to allow delivery. Fetal monitoring records an infant's heart rate and other functions during labor. There is also a simple blood test recently developed to detect pregnant women at risk for preeclampsia (see the Pathological Terms section), a potentially fatal condition.

Did you know

Pap Smear

The Pap smear test was developed and named after Dr. George Papanicolaou in the 1930s. A Pap smear is a scraping of the cells of the cervix to see if they are normal. It is the number one way of catching and diagnosing cervical cancer early. With early detection, the chance of survival increases significantly.

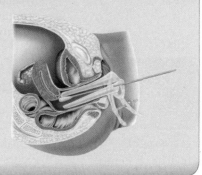

PRONOUNCE and DEFINE	Pronounce the following reproductive terms aloud and write their meaning.
Papanicolaou smear	[pă-pă-NĒ-kō-lū smēr]
culdoscopy	[kŭl-DŎS-kō-pē]
pelvimetry	[pĕl-VĬM-ĕ-trē]
colposcopy	[kŏl-PŎS-kō-pē]

SPELL and DEFINE	Identify if the following terms are spelled correctly. Correct the words that are spelled incorrectly. Write the definition for each word.	
	Spelling	**Definition**
mammogography		
pelvimetry		
hystroscopy		
gynecologist		

UNDERSTAND	Match each term on the left to its description on the right.

1. _____ hysterosalpingography
2. _____ pelvimetry
3. _____ colposcopy
4. _____ hysteroscopy
5. _____ culdoscopy

a. Scope procedure of the uterus
b. Scope procedure of the pelvic contents
c. X-ray of the uterus and uterine (fallopian) tubes
d. Scope procedure of the vagina
e. Measurement of the pelvis

Miss Charity Peterson is a 29-year-old African-American female who recently had a hysteroscopy with a biopsy. The biopsy came back suspicious for cancer. The physician ordered further testing as follows: culdoscopy, colposcopy, and hysterosalpingography.

1. On which reproductive parts is the physician ordering tests?

_____

_____

2. What is a biopsy?

_____

_____

3. What are the test instruments that are going to be used?

_____

_____

4. How would you explain what the physician has ordered to the patient?

_____

_____

5. What is the difference between a hysteroscopy and a colposcopy?

_____

_____

LO 17.4 Pathological Terms

Pathology in the female reproductive system is very important due to the many potential concerns possible and the number of patients that each of these affects. The range is so large and depends on the child-bearing state, age, and preexisting conditions that the woman may have. Whether it is sexually transmitted, structural, or a pregnancy, most women have some type of female pathological diagnosis in their lifetime.

STUDY TIP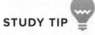

HPV (<u>h</u>uman <u>p</u>apilloma <u>v</u>irus) is the most common female sexually transmitted infection in the United States today. It is otherwise called genital warts, but the majority of cases affect the cervix and, therefore, many women do not even know that they have it. There are currently more than 40 different strains and it is the leading cause of cervical cancer. Regular Pap smears can detect the condition. There is also a vaccine that may prevent HPV.

Pathological	PRACTICE
	Provide the missing term(s) to complete the following sentences.
abortion [ă-BŎR-shŭn] **miscarriage** [mĭs-KĂR-ăj]	Pregnancy is a normal process, with gestation taking about 40 weeks and ending in the birth of an infant. Some pregnancies are not in themselves normal and spontaneously end in _____. Abortion is a controversial term in public discourse, but in medicine, it simply means the premature end of a pregnancy, whether spontaneously during a _____ or surgically.

continued on next page

Pathological	Provide the missing term(s) to complete the following sentences.
abruptio placentae [ăb-RŬP-shē-ō plă-SĔN-tē] **placenta previa** [plă-SĔN-tă PRĒ-vē-ă] **preeclampsia** [prē-ē-KLĂMP-sē-ă]	The placenta may break away from the uterine wall (_____) and require immediate delivery of the infant. _____ is a condition in which the placenta blocks the birth canal, and usually requires a caesarean delivery. Even though a pregnancy appears normal, a *stillbirth,* birth of a dead fetus, may occur. The typical pregnancy lasts from 37 to 40 weeks. An infant may be born *prematurely,* before 37 weeks of gestation. A toxic condition during pregnancy is called _____.
	**Abnormalities in the Female Cycle**
amenorrhea [ă-mĕn-ō-RĒ-ă] **dysmenorrhea** [dĭs-mĕn-ōr-Ē-ă] **menorrhagia** [mĕn-ō-RĀ-jē-ă] **oligomenorrhea** [ŎL-ĭ-gō-mĕn-ō-RĒ-ă] **menometrorrhagia** [MĔN-ō-mē-trō-RĀ-jē-ă] **metrorrhagia** [mē-trō-RĀ-jē-ă]	Menstrual abnormalities sometimes occur. _____, the absence of menstruation, may result from a normal condition (pregnancy or menopause) or an abnormal condition (excessive dieting or extremely strenuous exercise). It also may occur for no apparent reason. _____ is painful cramping associated with menstruation. _____ is excessive menstrual bleeding. _____ is a scanty menstrual period. _____ is irregular and often excessive bleeding during or between menstrual periods. _____ is uterine bleeding between menstrual periods.
anovulation [ăn-ŏv-yū-LĀ-shŭn] **oligoovulation** [ŎL-ĭ-gō-ŎV-ū-LĀ-shŭn] **leukorrhea** [lū-kō-RĒ-ă]	Other abnormal conditions in the female cycle also occur: _____ is the absence of ovulation. _____ is irregular ovulation. _____ is an abnormal vaginal discharge.
	**Abnormalities and Infections in the Reproductive System**
dyspareunia [dĭs-pă-RŪ-nē-ă]	_____ is painful sexual intercourse, usually due to some condition, such as dryness, inflammation, or other disorder in the female reproductive system.
anteflexion [ăn-tē-FLĔK-shŭn] **retroflexion** [rĕ-trō-FLĔK-shŭn] **retroversion** [rĕ-trō-VĔR-zhŭn]	The uterus normally sits forward over the bladder. Abnormal positioning of the uterus includes _____, a bending forward. _____ is a bending backward of the uterus so that it is angled and _____ is a backward turn of the uterus (sometimes called a *tipped uterus*) so that it faces toward the back.
cervicitis [sĕr-vĭ-SĪ-tĭs] **mastitis** [măs-TĪ-tĭs] **salpingitis** [săl-pĭn-JĪ-tĭs] **vaginitis** [văj-ĭ-NĪ-tĭs]	Various inflammations and infections occur in the female reproductive system. _____ is an inflammation of the cervix. _____ is a general term for inflammation of the breast, particularly during lactation. _____ is an inflammation of the fallopian tubes. _____ is an inflammation of the vagina. *Toxic shock syndrome* is a rare, severe infection that occurs in menstruating women and is usually associated with tampon use. *Pelvic inflammatory disease (PID)* is a bacterial infection anywhere in the female reproductive system.
Kegel exercises [KĒ-gĕl ĔK-sĕr-sīz-ĕs]	Organs of the reproductive system may suffer from muscle weakness. A *prolapsed uterus* is a condition where the uterine muscles cause the cervix to protrude into the vaginal opening. Perineal muscles can be strengthened using _____, alternately contracting and releasing the perineal muscles.

condyloma [kŏn-dĭ-LŌ-mă] **fibroids** [FĪ-broydz] **endometriosis** [ĔN-dō-mē-trē-Ō-sĭs]	A _____ is a growth on the outside of the genitalia that may be a result of an infection by the human papilloma virus (HPV). An *ovarian cyst* develops on or in the ovaries. _____ are common benign tumors found in the uterus. They may cause pain and bleeding. Some growths occur when normal tissue is found in abnormal areas; for example, _____ is an abnormal condition in which uterine lining tissue (endometrium) is found in the pelvis or on the abdominal wall. This results in the endometrial cells growing and shedding with each menstrual cycle, making the problem worse with each passing month. Any symptom that is new or unusual should be watched and checked with a health care provider.
carcinoma in situ [kăr-sĭ-NŌ-mă ĭn SĪ-tū]	Malignant growths found in the reproductive system can be fatal unless detected early. Cervical cancer is often detected early with Pap smears before having spread (_____). *Endometrial cancer* occurs in the endometrium. *Ovarian cancer* is a potentially fatal cancer of the ovary; it is difficult to diagnose in its earliest stages and often spreads to other organs before it is detected.
	**Sexually Transmitted Infections**
syphilis [SĬF-ĭ-lĭs] **gonorrhea** [gŏn-ō-RĒ-ă] **chlamydia** [klă-MĬD-ē-ă]	*Sexually transmitted infections (STIs)* are infections that are transmitted primarily through sexual contact. Some common sexually transmitted infections include _____, an infectious disease treatable with antibiotics; _____, a contagious infection of the genital mucous membrane; *herpes II,* a contagious and recurring infection with lesions on the genitalia; *human papilloma virus (HPV),* a contagious infection that causes genital warts; _____, a microorganism that causes several sexually transmitted diseases; and *HIV* (which leads to *AIDS*). HPV is sometimes associated with cervical cancer. *Trichomoniasis,* an infection often in the vaginal tract, also may be transmitted through sexual contact (Table 17-3).

TABLE 17-3 — Sexually Transmitted Infections

Disease	Cause	Symptoms	Estimated New Cases (U.S)*	Effects on Fetus	Treatment	Complications
acquired immune deficiency syndrome	human immunodeficiency virus	fever, weakness, infections, cancer	40,000	exposure to HIV and other infections	drugs to treat or delay symptoms; no cure	body overrun by infection and cancer
chlamydia infection	*Chlamydia trachomatis* bacteria	painful urination and intercourse, mucous discharge from penis or vagina	1.2 million (most cases go undiagnosed)	premature birth, blindness, pneumonia	antibiotics	pelvic inflammatory disease, infertility, arthritis, ectopic pregnancy
genital herpes	herpes simplex 2 virus	genital sores, fever	>700,000	brain damage, stillbirth	antiviral drug (acyclovir)	increased risk of cervical cancer

continued on next page

TABLE 17-3	Sexually Transmitted Infections					
Disease	Cause	Symptoms	Estimated New Cases (U.S)*	Effects on Fetus	Treatment	Complications
genital warts	human papilloma virus	warts on genitals	>350,000 human papilloma virus: 14 million	none known	chemical or surgical removal	increased risk of cervical cancer
gonorrhea	*Neisseria gonorrhoeae* bacteria	in women, usually none; in men, painful urination	>800,000	blindness, stillbirth	antibiotics	arthritis, rash, infertility, pelvic inflammatory disease
syphilis	*Treponema pallidum* bacteria	initial chancre sore usually on genitals or mouth; rash 6 months later; several years with no symptoms as infection spreads; finally damage to heart, liver, nerves, brain	>80,000	miscarriage, premature birth, birth defects, stillbirth	antibiotics	dementia

*2016 CDC statistics, Centers for Disease Control and Prevention

Did you know

Syphilis

Syphilis is a serious STI that is passed from contact with an affected person. The disease itself is very similar, in a basic way, to rabies. It can be treated if caught early (same as rabies) and it eventually affects the brain and causes insanity before death (same as rabies). Al Capone, the famous mobster, died of syphilis complications.

PRONOUNCE and DEFINE	Pronounce the following reproductive terms aloud and write their meaning.
amenorrhea	[ă-mĕn-ō-RĒ-ă]
carcinoma in situ	[kăr-sĭ-NŌ-mă ĭn SĪ-tū]
dyspareunia	[dĭs-pă-RŪ-nē-ă]
abruptio placentae	[ăb-RŬP-shē-ō plă-SĔN-tē]

	Spelling	Definition
preclampsia		
gonorrhea		
endometriosis		
leukarrhea		

| UNDERSTAND | Read the following scenario and answer the questions. |

1. _____ menorrhagia
2. _____ retroversion
3. _____ retroflexion
4. _____ anovulation
5. _____ dysmenorrhea

a. Difficult menstrual flow
b. Absence of ovulation
c. "Tipped" uterus
d. Bending backward of the uterus (angled)
e. Excessive menstrual bleeding

| APPLY | Read the following scenario and answer the questions. |

Mrs. Rosie McConnell is a pregnant 33-year-old Caucasian female. She has been referred to New Hope Obstetrics Clinic for the first time and brought her previous records with her for review. They read as follows:

6-10-2018:   Patient seen; diagnosis: menorrhagia and dysmenorrhea.

6-15-2018:   Patient scheduled for hysteroscopy for dysmenorrhea on 7-09-2018.

7-1-2018:   Results given to patient per Dr. Candy's orders. Relayed to patient that she has a retroverted uterus and fibroids.

7-3-2018:   Patient calls and states that she has done a home pregnancy test that has shown positive. Appt. with New Hope Obstetrics Clinic scheduled due to her history of preeclampsia with previous pregnancies per Dr. Candy's verbal order.

1. What was Rosie seen for at the previous clinic?

_____

_____

2. What kind of test was performed? On which female part?

_____

_____

3. What are the lay terms for all of her diagnoses?

_____

_____

4. How could the position of her uterus present problems?

_____

_____

5. Based on her history, would she need special care and monitoring during her pregnancy? Why?

_____

_____

Postpartum Depression

Most women experience some form of postpartum depression after giving birth. Many factors play a part in this condition, including extreme fluctuations in hormone levels, body changes, and lack of sleep from caring for a newborn. Postpartum depression can be managed with the care of a physician, medication, and/or counseling.

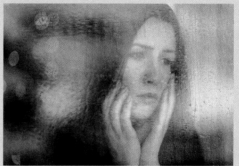

©Bojan Kontrec/Getty Images

LO 17.5 Surgical Terms

STUDY TIP

One in eight women, or approximately 12% of all women, will get breast cancer in her lifetime, and it is estimated that 40,000 women in the United States will die this year from it. About 50,000 women have mastectomies each year as a result of breast cancer directly or as a prophylactic measure for those with high risk of breast cancer.

Abnormalities in menses, pathological conditions, and preventive measures have made a **hysterectomy** one of the most common surgical procedures today. Advances in techniques have helped to alleviate many of the **postoperative** pain and open wound healing issues. **Laparoscopic hysterectomy** and **vaginal hysterectomy** have decreased many of the risks and fears patients have with an open abdominal surgery (Figure 17-6).

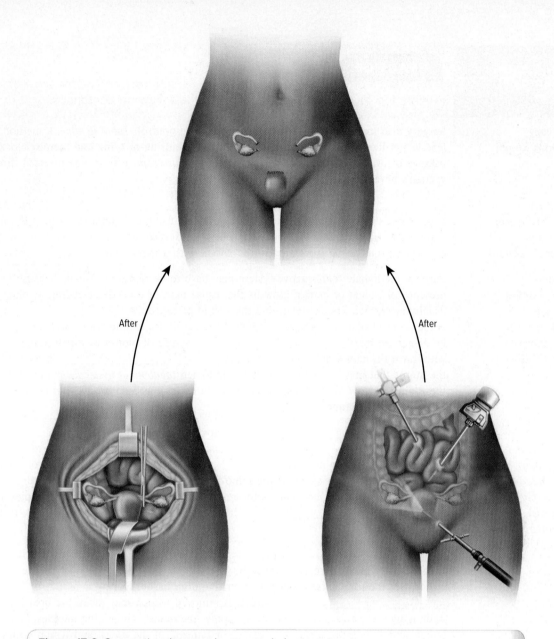

After

After

Figure 17-6 Conventional versus laparoscopic hysterectomy

Surgical	PRACTICE
	Provide the missing term(s) to complete the following sentences.
amniocentesis [ĂM-nē-ō-sĕn-TĒ-sĭs] **culdocentesis** [KŬL-dō-sĕn-TĒ-sĭs]	Surgery of the female reproductive system is performed for a variety of reasons. During pregnancy, it may be necessary to terminate a pregnancy prematurely (*abortion*), to remove a fetus through an abdominal incision (*caesarean birth*), to open and scrape the lining of the uterus (*dilation and curettage* [*D&C*]), or to puncture the amniotic sac to obtain a sample of the fluid for examination (_____). In _____, a sample of fluid from the base of the pelvic cavity may show if an ectopic pregnancy has ruptured. An ectopic pregnancy can be removed through a *salpingotomy,* an incision into one of the fallopian tubes.

continued on next page

laparoscopy [lăp-ă-RŎS-kō-pē]	Surgery also may be performed as a form of birth control. *Tubal ligation,* a method of female sterilization, blocks the fallopian tubes by cutting or tying and thereby blocking the passage of ova. It is usually performed using a *laparoscope,* a thin tube inserted through a woman's navel during _____.
cryosurgery [KRĪ-ō-SĔR-jĕr-ē] **cauterization** [kăw-tĕr-ĭ-ZĀ-shŭn]	_____ (freezing) and _____ (burning) are two methods of destroying tissue (such as polyps), using cold temperatures in the former and burning in the latter. A loop electrosurgical excision procedure (LEEP) is the removal of precancerous tissue from around the cervix with a wirelike instrument.
conization [kō-nĭ-ZĀ-shŭn] **aspiration** [ăs-pĭ-RĀ-shŭn] **hysterectomy** [hĭs-tĕr-ĔK-tō-mē]	Parts of the female reproductive system may have to be removed, usually because of the presence of cancer or benign growths that cause pain or excessive bleeding. A biopsy is usually performed first to determine the spread of cancer. A _____ is the removal of a cone-shaped section of the cervix for examination. Breast cancer may be diagnosed by _____, a type of biopsy in which fluid is withdrawn through a needle by suction. A _____ is removal of the uterus that may be done through the abdomen (*abdominal hysterectomy*) or through the vagina (*vaginal hysterectomy*). New procedures such as *laparoscopic hysterectomies* are reducing recovery time.
myomectomy [mī-ō-MĔK-tō-mē] **oophorectomy** [ō-ŏf-ōr-ĔK-tō-mē] **salpingectomy** [săl-pĭn-JĔK-tō-mē] **salpingotomy** [săl-pĭng-GŎT-ō-mē]	A _____ is the removal of fibroid tumors. An _____ is the removal of an ovary. An *ovarian cystectomy* is the removal of an ovarian cyst. A _____ is the removal of a fallopian tube. A *salpingo-oophorectomy* is the removal of one ovary and one fallopian tube. A *bilateral salpingo-oophorectomy* is the removal of both ovaries and both fallopian tubes. A _____ is an incision into the fallopian tubes (usually to remove blockages).
lumpectomy [lŭm-PĔK-tō-mē] **mastectomy** [măs-TĔK-tō-mē]	Breast cancer may be treated surgically. A _____ is the removal of the tumor itself along with surrounding tissue. During a _____, a breast is removed, which may mean the breast and underlying muscle as in a simple mastectomy; the breast, underlying muscles, and the lymph nodes, as in a *radical mastectomy;* or removal of the breast and lymph nodes, as in a *modified radical mastectomy.*
mammoplasty [MĂM-ō-plăs-tē] **mastopexy** [MĂS-tō-pĕk-sē]	Breast surgery may include plastic surgery after mastectomy (_____) or reduction of the size of the breast (*reduction mammoplasty*). Some women have pendulous breast tissue raised (_____) or have small breasts augmented by surgical insertion of implants (*augmentation mammoplasty*).

Did you know

Endometriosis

Endometriosis affects more women than cancer or AIDS. Nearly 5 million women are affected by endometriosis.

In the United States, endometrial cancer is the most common cancer of the female reproductive organs.

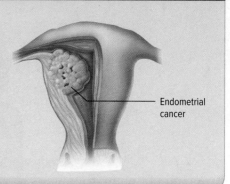

Endometrial cancer

PRONOUNCE and DEFINE	Pronounce the following reproductive terms aloud and write their meaning.
cryosurgery	[KRĪ-ō-SĔR-jĕr-ē]
cauterization	[kăw-tĕr-ĭ-ZĀ-shŭn]
aspiration	[ăs-pĭ-RĀ-shŭn]
culdocentesis	[KŬL-dō-sĕn-TĒ-sĭs]

SPELL	Write the correct spelling for each related term.
	Repair of a fallopian tube
	Scope procedure of the abdomen
	Freezing treatment for destroying tissue
	Removal of fibroid tumors
	Cone-shaped biopsy

UNDERSTAND

Match each term on the left to its description on the right.

1. _____ lumpectomy
2. _____ mastectomy
3. _____ myomectomy
4. _____ culdocentesis
5. _____ amniocentesis

a. Procedure to obtain fluid from pelvic contents
b. Procedure to obtain fluid from sac surrounding fetus
c. Removal of only tumor and surrounding tissue
d. Removal of an entire breast
e. Removal of fibroid tumors

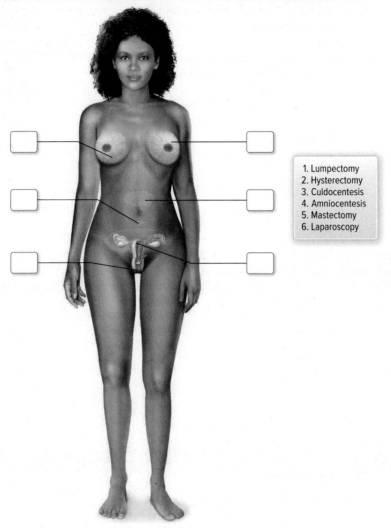

1. Lumpectomy
2. Hysterectomy
3. Culdocentesis
4. Amniocentesis
5. Mastectomy
6. Laparoscopy

The local continuing medical educational society president, Dr. John Schaefer, has asked you to give an informative presentation on certain procedures. Specifically, he has asked that you cover mammography, lumpectomy, bilateral mastectomy, mastopexy, and mammoplasty.

1. Which part of the body is the focus of your presentation?

_____

_____

2. Which of the medical terms are procedures?

_____

_____

3. Which are surgeries?

_____

_____

4. List the lay terms for each of the topics Dr. Schaefer has asked you to discuss.

_____

_____

5. List the order in which these procedures would normally occur on a patient.

_____

_____

LO 17.6 Pharmacological Terms

Medications and prescriptions written from a gynecology practice usually revolve around the female cycle, sexual activity, conception/prevention, and drugs to induce and ease the pain of labor. Practitioners treat a variety of other illnesses and symptoms, and several over-the-counter herbal and vitamin therapies are popular to relieve symptoms such as bloating and PMS that accompany menses.

Pharmacological	PRACTICE
	Provide the missing term(s) to complete the following sentences.
birth control pills **implants** **abortifacients** [ă-bŏr-tĭ-FĀ-shĕnts] **morning-after pills**	Various forms of birth control are pharmacological agents. Spermicides destroy sperm in the vagina; _____, patches, and _____ control the flow of hormones to block ovulation; and _____ or _____ prevent implantation of an ovum.
hormone replacement **therapy (HRT)** **oxytocin** [ŏk-sē-TŌ-sĭn] **tocolytic** [tō-kō-LĬT-ĭk]	_____ is used during and after natural or surgical menopause to alleviate symptoms, such as hot flashes. _____, another hormone, is used to induce labor. A _____ agent stops labor contractions.

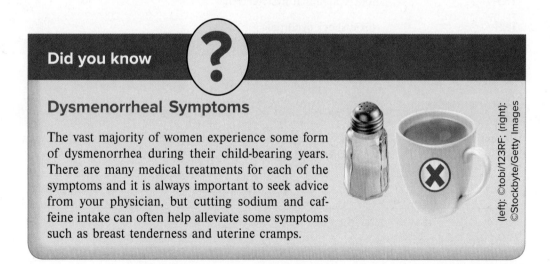

Did you know ?

Dysmenorrheal Symptoms

The vast majority of women experience some form of dysmenorrhea during their child-bearing years. There are many medical treatments for each of the symptoms and it is always important to seek advice from your physician, but cutting sodium and caffeine intake can often help alleviate some symptoms such as breast tenderness and uterine cramps.

(left): ©tobi/123RF; (right): ©Stockbyte/Getty Images

Abbreviations

ABBREVIATION REVIEW

Abbreviation	Definition
Cx	cervix
D&C	dilation and curettage
FSH	follicle-stimulating hormone
GYN	gynecology, gynecologist
HCG	human chorionic gonadotropin
HRT	hormone replacement therapy
IUD	intrauterine device
LH	luteininzing hormone
LMP	last menstrual period
Pap	Papanicolaou test/smear
PID	pelvic inflammatory disease
PMS	premenstrual syndrome
STI	sexually transmitted infection
TAH	total abdominal hysterectomy
TSS	toxic shock syndrome

APPLY   Read the following scenario and rewrite using the medical term for each abbreviation.

Patient has a history of TSS and STIs—believed IUD would prevent. Here for Pap, Cx inflamed, symptoms of PID. Will refer to GYN for possible D&C and may need TAH.

_____

_____

_____

CHAPTER SUMMARY

	Learning Outcome	Summary
17.1	Recognize the parts of the female reproductive system and discuss the function of each part.	The female reproductive system is comprised of structures that work to regulate hormones associated with the menstrual cycle, produce offspring in pregnancy, and cease reproduction in menopause.
17.2	Recall the major word parts used in building words that relate to the female reproductive system.	Word building requires knowledge of word parts and their corresponding meanings to form medical terms within the female reproductive system.
17.3	Identify the common diagnostic tests, laboratory tests, and clinical procedures used in testing and treating disorders of the female reproductive system.	Diagnostic, procedural, and laboratory findings assist the health care provider in diagnosing medical conditions. Often used in combination, these tests lead to a final diagnosis and assist in treatment planning.
17.4	Define the major pathological conditions of the female reproductive system.	Knowledge and understanding of diseases and conditions of the female reproductive system, including the nonpregnant and pregnant states, reproductive organs, and sexually transmitted infections, increase critical thinking related to pathological medical terms.
17.5	Recall the meaning of surgical terms related to the female reproductive system.	Surgical procedures of the female reproductive system focus on repair of structures and cancer, including biopsy and staging of cancer.
17.6	Recognize common pharmacological agents used in treating disorders of the female reproductive system.	The primary and common pharmacological agents of the female reproductive system include birth control, hormone replacement and regulation agents, and treatment for sexually transmitted infections.
17.7	Identify common abbreviations associated with the female reproductive system.	Abbreviations are used to describe diseases, conditions, procedures, and treatments associated with the female reproductive system.

1. Identify and label the parts of the female reproductive system.

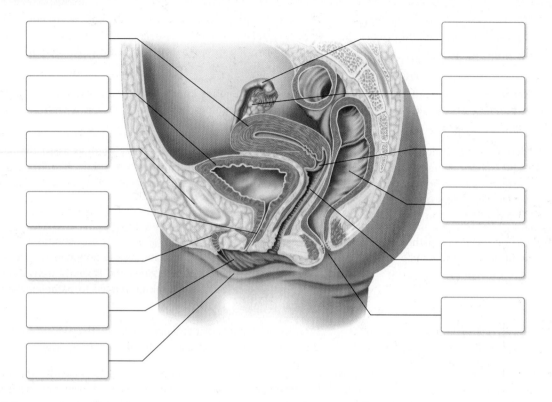

2. Identify and list the main female reproductive hormones and where they are produced.

_____

_____

_____

Identify if the following terms are spelled correctly. Correct the words that are spelled incorrectly. Write the definition for each word.

	Spelling	Definition
preclampsia		
progesterone		
corpus		
luteum		
conezation		
ariola		
vulva		
prolacten		
spermicide		

Pronounce each of the above terms aloud.

IMPLEMENT

Complete the sentences by filling in the blanks.

1. _____ scopy means viewing of the uterine (fallopian) tubes.
2. _____ gram means a measure of the breast tissue.
3. _____ ectomy means removal of the ovaries.
4. _____ itis means inflammation of the vagina.
5. _____ plegia means paralysis of the uterus.

Match each term on the left to its description on the right.

1. lumpectomy
2. menorrhagia
3. myomectomy
4. culdocentesis
5. amniocentesis
6. oocytes
7. labia minora
8. colporrhagia
9. labia majora
10. ova

a. Procedure to obtain fluid from sac surrounding fetus
b. Two larger folds of skin below the mons pubis
c. Removal of only tumor and surrounding tissue
d. Vaginal bleeding
e. Removal of fibroid tumors
f. Smaller skin folds that merge at the top
g. Excessive menstrual bleeding
h. Immature egg cells
i. Procedure to obtain fluid from pelvic contents
j. Mature eggs

DECONSTRUCT

The physician tells the family that the client, Ms. Vanessa Redburn, a 64-year-old, white female who is menopausal, has had some unexplained excessive vaginal bleeding, and he will need to perform a scope procedure going from the vagina through the uterus to the fallopian tubes to find out what may be causing the bleeding. If it is coming from the uterus itself, he may need to take a small amount of tissue to check for cancer and other conditions. If cancer is confirmed, he will need to perform a complete removal of all female reproductive organs.

Using medical terminology, write what the physician has told the family regarding the client.

_____

_____

_____

_____

Reviewing the Terms

Pronounce each of the following terms. Write the definitions on a separate sheet of paper. This review will take you through all the words you learned in this chapter. If you have difficulty with any words, make a flash card for later study. Refer to the English-Spanish and Spanish-English glossaries in the eBook.

abortifacient [ă-bŏr-tĭ-FĀ-shĕnt]

abortion [ă-BŎR-shŭn]

abruptio placentae [ăb-RŬP-shē-ō plă-SĔN-tē]

afterbirth [ĂF-tĕr-bĕrth]

amenorrhea [ă-mĕn-ō-RĒ-ă]

amni/o [ĂM-nē-ō]

amniocentesis [ĂM-nē-ō-sĕn-TĒ-sĭs]

amnion [ĂM-nē-ŏn]

amniotic [ăm-nē-ŎT-ĭk] **fluid**

anovulation [ăn-ŏv-yū-LĀ-shŭn]

anteflexion [ăn-tē-FLĔK-shŭn]

areola [ă-RĒ-ō-lă]

aspiration [ăs-pĭ-RĀ-shŭn]

Bartholin's [BĂR-thō-lĕnz] **gland**

birth control pills or implants
body
carcinoma in situ [kăr-sĭ-NŌ-mă ĭn SĪ-tū]
cauterization [kăw-tĕr-ĭ-ZĀ-shŭn]
cervic/o [SĔR-vĭ-kō]
cervicitis [sĕr-vĭ-SĪ-tĭs]
cervix [SĔR-vĭks]
chlamydia [klă-MĬD-ē-ă]
chorion [KŌ-rē-ŏn]
climacteric [klī-MĂK-tĕr-ĭk, klī-măk-TĔR-ĭk]
clitoris [KLĬT-ō-rĭs]
coitus [KŌ-ĭ-tŭs]
colp/o [KŎL-pō]
colposcopy [kŏl-PŎS-kō-pē]
condom [KŎN-dŏm]
condyloma [kŏn-dĭ-LŌ-mă]
conization [kō-nĭ-ZĀ-shŭn]
contraception [kŏn-tră-SĔP-shŭn]
copulation [kŏp-yū-LĀ-shŭn]
corpus luteum [KŌR-pŭs LŪ-tē-ŭm]
cryosurgery [KRĪ-ō-SĔR-jĕr-ē]
culdocentesis [KŬL-dō-sĕn-TĒ-sĭs]
culdoscopy [kŭl-DŎS-kō-pē]
diaphragm [DĪ-ă-frăm]
dysmenorrhea [dĭs-mĕn-ōr-Ē-ă]
dyspareunia [dĭs-pă-RŪ-nē-ă]
endometriosis [ĔN-dō-mē-trē-Ō-sĭs]
endometrium [ĔN-dō-MĒ-trē-ŭm]
episi/o [ĕ-PĬZ-ē-ō]
estrogen [ĔS-trō-jĕn]
fallopian [fă-LŌ-pē-ăn] tube
fibroid [FĪ-broyd]
fimbriae [FĬM-brē-ē]
follicle [FŎL-Ĭ-kl]-stimulating hormone (FSH)
fundus [FŬN-dŭs]
galact/o [gă-LĂK-tō]
gamete [GĂM-ēt]
gestation [jĕs-TĀ-shŭn]
gonad [GŌ-năd]
gonorrhea [gŏn-ō-RĒ-ă]
graafian follicle [GRĂ-fē-ăn FŎL-ĭ-kl]

gravida [GRĂV-ĭ-dă]
gynec/o [GĪ-nĕ-kō]
gynecologist [gī-nĕ-KŎL-ō-jĭst]
hormone [HŌR-mōn]
hormone replacement therapy (HRT)
hymen [HĪ-mĕn]
hyster/o [HĬS-tĕr-ō]
hysterectomy [hĭs-tĕr-ĔK-tō-mē]
hysterosalpingography [HĬS-tĕr-ō-săl-pĭng-GŎG-ră-fē]
hysteroscopy [hĭs-tĕr-ŎS-kō-pē]
intrauterine [ĬN-tră-YŪ-tĕr-ĭn] device (IUD)
introitus [ĭn-TRŌ-ĭ-tŭs]
isthmus [ĬS-mŭs]
Kegel [KĒ-gĕl] exercises
labia majora [LĀ-bē-ă mă-JŌR-ă]
labia minora [mī-NŌR-ă]
lact/o, lacti [LĂK-tō, LĂK-tĭ]
lactation [lak-TĀ-shun]
lactiferous [lăk-TĬF-ĕr-ŭs]
laparoscopy [lăp-ă-RŎS-kō-pē]
leukorrhea [lū-kō-RĒ-ă]
lumpectomy [lŭm-PĔK-tō-mē]
luteinizing [LŪ-tē-ĭ-nīz-ĭng] hormone (LH)
mamm/o [MĂM-ō]
mammary [MĂM-ă-rē] glands
mammography [mă-MŎG-ră-fē]
mammoplasty [MĂM-ō-plăs-tē]
mast/o [MĂS-tō]
mastectomy [măs-TĔK-tō-mē]
mastitis [măs-TĪ-tĭs]
mastopexy [MĂS-tō-pĕk-sē]
men/o [MĔN-ō]
menarche [mĕ-NĂR-kē]
menometrorrhagia [MĔN-ō-mē-trō-RĀ-jē-ă]
menopause [MĔN-ō-păwz]
menorrhagia [mĕn-ō-RĀ-jē-ă]
menses [MĔN-sēz]
menstruation [mĕn-strū-Ā-shŭn]
metr/o [MĒ-trō]
metrorrhagia [mē-trō-RĀ-jē-ă]
miscarriage [mĭs-KĂR-ăj]

mons pubis [mŏnz PYŪ-bĭs]

morning-after pill

myomectomy [mī-ō-MĔK-tō-mē]

myometrium [MĪ-ō-MĒ-trē-ŭm]

nipple [NĬP-l]

obstetrician [ŏb-stĕ-TRĬSH-ŭn]

oligomenorrhea [ŎL-ĭ-gō-mĕn-ō-RĒ-ă]

oligoovulation [ŎL-ĭ-gō-ŎV-ū-LĀ-shŭn]

oo [Ō-ō]

oocytes [Ō-ō-sīts]

oophor/o [ō-ŎF-ōr-ō]

oophorectomy [ō-ŏf-ōr-ĔK-tō-mē]

ov/i, ov/o [Ō-vĭ, Ō-vō]

ova (sing., ovum) [Ō-vă (Ō-vŭm)]

ovari/o [ō-VĂR-ē-ō]

ovary [Ō-vă-rē]

ovulation [ŎV-yū-LĀ-shŭn]

oxytocin [ŏk-sē-TŌ-sĭn]

Papanicolaou [pă-pă-NĒ-kō-lū] (Pap [păp]) smear

para [PĂ-ră]

parturition [păr-tūr-ĬSH-ŭn]

pelvimetry [pĕl-VĬM-ĕ-trē]

perimenopause [pĕr-ĭ-MĔN-ō-păws]

perimetrium [pĕr-ĭ-MĒ-trē-ŭm]

perine/o [PĔR-ĭ-NĒ-ō]

perineum [PĔR-ĭ-NĒ-ŭm]

placenta [plă-SĔN-tă]

placenta previa [plă-SĔN-tă PRĒ-vē-ă]

preeclampsia [prē-ĕ-KLĂMP-sē-ă]

progesterone [prō-JĔS-tĕr-ōn]

puberty [PYŪ-bĕr-tē]

retroflexion [rĕ-trō-FLĔK-shŭn]

retroversion [rĕ-trō-VĔR-zhŭn]

salping/o [săl-PĬNG-gō]

salpingectomy [săl-pĭn-JĔK-tō-mē]

salpingitis [săl-pĭn-JĪ-tĭs]

salpingotomy [săl-pĭng-GŎT-ō-mē]

sinus [SĪ-nŭs]

spermicide [SPĔR-mĭ-sīd]

sponge [spŭnj]

syphilis [SĬF-ĭ-lĭs]

tocolytic [tō-kō-LĬT-ĭk]

umbilical [ŭm-BĬL-ĭ-kăl] cord

uter/o [YŪ-tĕr-ō]

uterine [YŪ-tĕr-ĭn] tube

uterus [YŪ-tĕr-ŭs]

vagin/o [VĂJ-ĭ-nō]

vagina [vă-JĪ-nă]

vaginitis [văj-ĭ-NĪ-tĭs]

vulv/o [VŬL-vō]

vulva [VŬL-vă]

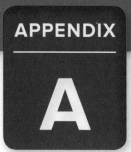

APPENDIX A

Combining Forms, Prefixes, and Suffixes

Listed here are the combining forms, prefixes, and suffixes used in building medical terms.

A

a-, an- *prefix.* not, without, lacking

ab-, abs- *prefix.* from; away; off

abdomin, abdomino *combining form.* abdomen

acanth *combining form.* thorny or having spines

acetabul, acetabulo *combining form.* acetabulum

-acousis, -acusis *suffix.* hearing

acromi, acromio *combining form.* end point of the scapula

actin, actino *combining form.* ray, beam; having raylike structures

ad- *prefix.* to, toward; near the midline

-ad *suffix.* toward; in the direction of

aden, adeno *combining form.* gland or glandular

adenoid, adenoido *combining form.* adenoid

adipo *combining form.* fat, fatty

adren, adreno, adrenal, adrenalo *combining form.* adrenal gland

aero *combining form.* air

agglutin, agglutino *combining form.* agglutinin; adhere or combine

-algesia *suffix.* pain

algesio, algi, alg *combining form.* pain

-algia *suffix.* pain or a specific painful condition

alveol, alveolo *combining form.* alveolus

ambi- *prefix.* **1.** around, on all sides; **2.** both, double

amnio *combining form.* amnion

amylo *combining form.* starch

an- *prefix.* **1.** not; **2.** up; upward; back; backward

andr, andro *combining form.* masculine

angi, angio *combining form.* blood or lymph vessel

ankyl, anklyo *combining form.* bent; crooked

ant-, anti- *prefix.* against, opposite

ante- *prefix.* **1.** before: *for example,* antepartum; **2.** in front of

anterio *combining form.* front

antero- *prefix.* anterior

aort, aorto *combining form.* aorta

apo- *prefix.* separated from; derived from

arteri, arterio *combining form.* artery

arthr, arthro *combining form.* joint

-asthenia *suffix.* weakness

ather, athero *combining form.* soft fatty deposit

atri, atrio *combining form.* atrium

audio, audito *combining form.* sound; hearing

aur, auro, auricul, auriculo *combining form.* hearing

auto- *prefix.* self, same

B

bacilli *combining form.* bacilli; bacteria

bacteri, bacterio *combining form.* bacteria

balan, balano *combining form.* glans penis

bar, baro *combining form.* weight, pressure

bas, basio *combining form.* base; foundation

bi- *prefix.* twice; double

bio *combining form.* life, living

blast, blasto *combining form.* immature cell

-blast *suffix.* immature, forming

blephar, blepharo *combining form.* eyelid

brachi, brachio *combining form.* arm

brachy- *prefix.* short

brady- *prefix.* slow

bronch, bronchi, broncho *combining form.* bronchus, bronchi

bronchiol *combining form.* bronchiole

burs, burso *combining form.* bursa, bursae

C

calcaneo *combining form.* heel

calco, calcio *combining form.* calcium

calic, calico, calio *combining form.* calyx

capno *combining form.* carbon dioxide

carcin, carcino *combining form.* cancer

card, cardi, cardio *combining form.* heart

-cardia *suffix.* the condition of having a specific kind of heart or heartbeat

carp, carpo *combining form.* wrist

cata- *prefix.* down

-cele *suffix.* hernia

cephal, cephalo *combining form.* head

cerebell, cerebello *combining form.* cerebellum

cerebr, cerebro *combining form.* cerebrum

cerumin, cerumino *combining form.* wax

cervic, cervico *combining form.* neck; cervix

cheil, cheilo *combining form.* lips

chemo *combining form.* chemical

chlor, chloro *combining form.* **1.** green; **2.** chlorine

chol, chole, cholo *combining form.* bile

cholecyst, cholecysto *combining form.* gallbladder

chondr, chondro *combining form.* cartilage

chrom, chromat, chromo *combining form.* color

chron, chrono *combining form.* time

chyl, chylo *combining form.* chyle

chym *combining form.* chyme, semifluid production of chyme in the stomach

-cidal *suffix.* killing; destroying

-cide *suffix.* killing; destroying

circum- *prefix.* around

-clasis *suffix.* breaking

-clast *suffix.* breaking instrument

co-, col-, com-, con-, cor- *prefix.* together

cochle, cochleo *combining form.* cochlea

colon, colono *combining form.* colon

colp, colpo *combining form.* vagina

com- *prefix.* with, together

con- *prefix.* with, together

condyl *combining form.* rounded, knoblike, condyle

conio *combining form.* dust

conjunctiv, conjunctivo *combining form.* conjunctiva

contra- *prefix.* opposed, against

cor-, core-, coreo- *combining form.* pupil

corne, corneo *combining form.* cornea

cost, costo *combining form.* rib

crani, cranio *combining form.* skull; cranium

-crine *suffix.* secreting

crino *combining form.* secrete

-crit *suffix.* separate

cryo *combining form.* cold

crypt, crypto *combining form.* hidden or obscure

cutaneo *combining form.* skin

cyan *combining form.* blue

cycl, cyclo *combining form.* circle; cycle; ciliary body

cyst, cysto *combining form.* **1.** the bladder; **2.** cyst

cyt, cyto *combining form.* a cell

-cyte *suffix.* a cell

-cytosis *suffix.* condition of cells

D

dactyl, dactylo *combining form.* fingers; toes

de- *prefix.* away from

dent, dento *combining form.* teeth

derm, derma, dermo *combining form.* skin

-derma *suffix.* skin

dermat, dermato *combining form.* skin

-desis *suffix.* binding

dextro *combining form.* right; on the right side

di-, dif-, dir-, dis- *prefix.* not; separated

dia- *prefix.* through; throughout; completely

dipl, diplo *combining form.* double, twofold

dips, dipso *combining form.* thirst

dors, dorsi, dorso *combining form.* back

duoden, duodeno *combining form.* duodenum

dyna, dynamo *combining form.* strength or force; energy

-dynia *suffix.* pain

dys- *prefix.* abnormal, difficult; painful

E

echo *combining form.* reflected sound

-ectasia, -ectasis *suffix.* dilation, expansion

ecto- *prefix.* outer, on the outside

-ectomy *suffix.* excision, removal

-edema *suffix.* swelling

electro *combining form.* electrical; electricity

-emesis *suffix.* vomit

-emia *suffix.* blood

-emic *suffix.* relating to blood

encephal, encephalo *combining form.* brain

end, endo *combining form.* within, inner, absorbing, containing

enter, entero *combining form.* intestines

eosin, eosino *combining form.* red; eosinophil

epi- *prefix.* over

epididym, epididymo *combining form.* epididymis

epiglott, epiglotto *combining form.* epiglottis

episi, episio *combining form.* vulva

erythro *combining form.* red, redness

esophag, esophago *combining form.* esophagus

-esthesia *suffix.* sensation, perception

ethm *combining form.* ethmoid bone

eti, etio *combining form.* cause

eu- *prefix.* well, good, normal

ex-, exo- *prefix.* external; out of; away from

extra- *prefix.* without, on the outside

F

fasci, fascio *combining form.* a band of fibrous tissue

femor, femoro *combining form.* relating to the femur or thigh

fibr, fibro *combining form.* fiber

fluor, fluoro *combining form.* **1.** fluorine; **2.** light; **3.** luminous

-form *suffix.* in the shape of

fung, fungi, fungo *combining form.* fungus

G

galact, galacto *combining form.* milk

gangli, ganglio *combining form.* ganglion

gastr, gastro *combining form.* stomach

-gen *suffix.* producer

-genesis *suffix.* origin

-genic *suffix.* produced by

geno *combining form.* producing; being born

gero, geronto *combining form.* old age

gingiv, gingivo *combining form.* gum

gli, glia, glio *combining form.* neuroglia

-globin *suffix.* protein

-globulin *suffix.* protein

glomerul, glomerulo *combining form.* glomerulus

gloss, glosso *combining form.* tongue

gluc, gluco *combining form.* glucose

glyc, glyco *combining form.* sugar, glycogen

gonad, gonado *combining form.* sex glands

gonio *combining form.* angle

-gram *suffix.* a recording

granul, granulo *combining form.* granule or granular

-graph *suffix.* recording instrument

-graphy *suffix.* process of recording

gyn, gyne, gyneco *combining form.* women

H

hem, hemo *combining form.* blood

hemangi, hemangio *combining form.* blood vessel

hemat, hemato *combining form.* blood

hemi- *prefix.* half

hepat, hepato *combining form.* liver

hidr, hidro *combining form.* sweat; sweat glands

homeo, homo *combining form.* like; similar; consistent

humer, humero *combining form.* humerus

hydr, hydro *combining form.* hydrogen, water, liquid

hymen, hymeno *combining form.* membrane

hyper- *prefix.* excessive or above normal

hypn, hypno *combining form.* sleep

hypo- *prefix.* low, below normal

hyster, hystero *combining form.* uterus

I

-iasis *suffix.* pathological condition or state; presence of

-ic *suffix.* of, pertaining to

ichthy, ichthyo *combining form.* dry; scaly; fishy

-ics *suffix.* treatment; practice; body of knowledge

idio *combining form.* unknown; distinct

ile, ileo *combining form.* ileum

ilio *combining form.* ilium

immuno *combining form.* safe; immune; immunity

in- *prefix.* **1.** into; **2.** not

infra- *prefix.* positioned beneath

inter- *prefix.* between; within

intra- *prefix.* within

ir, iro, irid, irido *combining form.* iris

ischi, ischio *combining form.* ischium

-ism *suffix.* condition of; disease

iso- *prefix.* equal; same

-itis *suffix.* inflammation or disease of

J

jejun, jejuno *combining form.* jejunum

K

kerat, kerato *combining form.* **1.** the cornea; **2.** horny tissue or cells

ket, keto *combining form.* ketone; acetone or ketone group

kin, kine *combining form.* movement

kinesi, kines *combining form.* movement

-kinesia *suffix.* movement

-kinesis, *suffix.* movement or activation

kyph, kypho *combining form.* abnormal curvature of the spine; humpback

L

labi, labio *combining form.* lips

lacrim, lacrimo *combining form.* tears

lact, lacti, lacto *combining form.* milk

lamino *combining form.* lamina

laparo *combining form.* abdomen, abdominal wall

laryng, laryngo *combining form.* the larynx

later, latero *combining form.* to one side; lateral

leiomy, leiomyo *combining form.* smooth muscle

-lepsy *suffix.* seizure

-leptic *suffix.* pertaining to seizures

leuk, leuko *combining form.* white

lingu, linguo *combining form.* tongue

lip, lipo *combining form.* fat (outside of a blood vessel)

lith, litho *combining form.* stone, calculus, calcification

-lith *suffix.* stone, calculus, calcification

-lithiasis *suffix.* presence of stones

lob, lobo *combining form.* lobe of the lung

-logist *suffix.* one who studies

logo *combining form.* speech; words; thought

-logy *suffix.* study; practice

lumb, lumbo *combining form.* lumbar

lymph, lympho *combining form.* lymph

lymphaden, lymphadeno *combining form.* lymph node.

lymphangi, lymphangio *combining form.* lymphatic vessels

lys, lyso *combining form.* dissolution; destruction

-lysis *suffix.* destruction of

-lytic *suffix.* pertaining to destruction

M

macro- *prefix.* large; long

mal- *prefix.* bad; inadequate; abnormal

-malacia *suffix.* softening

mamm, mamma, mammo *combining form.* breast

-mania *suffix.* obsession; madness

mast, masto *combining form.* breast

mastoid, mastoido *combining form.* mastoid process

maxill, maxillo *combining form.* maxilla; upper jaw

meat, meato *combining form.* meatus

medi, medio *combining form.* middle; central

mediastin, mediastino *combining form.* mediastinum

mega, megalo *combining form.* large; million

mega-, megalo- *prefix.* **1.** very large; huge; **2.** abnormally large; enlarged

melan, melano *combining form.* melanin; black; dark

mening, meningi, meningo *combining form.* meninges; membrane

meno *combining form.* menses; menstruation

mes, meso *combining form.* **1.** middle; central; **2.** intermediate; in between; **3.** mesentery

mes-, meso- *prefix.* middle; median

meta- *prefix.* after, behind, altered

metacarpo *combining form.* metacarpal

-meter *suffix.* instrument for or method of measuring

metr-, metri-, metro- *prefix.* uterus

-metry *suffix.* process or method of measuring something

micro- *prefix.* small; tiny

mid- *prefix.* middle

mio *combining form.* smaller; less

mon, mono *combining form.* single; alone

mon-, mono- *prefix.* single

morpho *combining form.* form, shape, or structure

muc, muci, muco *combining form.* mucus; mucous.

multi- *prefix.* many

my-, myo- *prefix.* muscle.

myc, myco *combining form.* fungus

myel, myelo *combining form.* **1.** bone marrow; **2.** the spinal cord and medulla oblongata; **3.** the myelin sheath enclosing nerve fibers

myo *combining form.* muscle

myocardi, mycardio *combining form.* myocardium

myring, myringo *combining form.* eardrum; middle ear

N

narc, narco *combining form.* sleep; numbness or drowsiness

nas, naso *combining form.* nose

necr, necro *combining form.* death; dying

neo- *prefix.* new, recent

nephr, nephro *combining form.* kidney

neur, neuri, neuro *combining form.* nerve, nervous system

noct, nocti, nocto *combining form.* night

norm, normo *combining form.* normal

nucle *combining form.* nucleus

nyct, nycto *combining form.* night

O

ocul, oculo *combining form.* eye

odont, odonto *combining form.* tooth, teeth

-odynia *suffix.* pain

-oid *suffix.* like, resembling

-oma (*pl.,* **-omas** or **-omata**) *suffix.* tumor, neoplasm

onch, oncho, onc, onco *combining form.* tumor, mass, swelling

onych, onycho *combining form.* nail

oo *combining form.* egg

oophor, oophoro *combining form.* ovary

ophthalm, ophthalmo *combining form.* eye

-opia *suffix.* vision

-opsia *suffix.* vision

-opsy *suffix.* view of

opt, opto, optic, optico *combining form.* vision

or, oro *combining form.* mouth

orch, orchi, orchid, orchido, orchio *combining form.* testicle

orth, ortho *combining form.* straight, correct

-ose *suffix.* **1.** full of; **2.** carbohydrate

-osis *suffix.* condition; state; process

ossicul, ossiculo *combining form.* ossicle

ost, oste, osteo *combining form.* bone

-ostomy *suffix.* opening

ot, oto *combining form.* ear

ov, ovi, ovo *combining form.* egg

ovari, ovario *combining form.* ovary

ox, oxo, oxi, oxy *combining form.* **1.** oxygen; **2.** pointed

-oxia *suffix.* oxygen

P

pachy *combining form.* thick

pan-, panto- *prefix.* all; entire; the whole

pancreat, pancreato *combining form.* pancreas

par-, para- *prefix.* **1.** near; beside. **2.** beyond; outside. **3.** assistant; associate. **4.** abnormal

-para *suffix.* bearing

parathyroid, parathyroido *combining form.* parathyroid

-paresis *suffix.* slight paralysis; feeling of numbness and tingling

-parous *suffix.* producing; bearing.

patell, patello *combining form.* knee

-pathic *suffix.* of or pertaining to disease

patho *combining form.* disease

-pathy *suffix.* disease or diseased condition

ped, pedi, pedo *combining form.* **1.** child; **2.** foot or feet

pelv, pelvi *combining form.* pelvis

-penia *suffix.* small; deficiency; fewer

-pepsia *suffix.* digestion.

per- *prefix.* **1.** through; **2.** intensely

peri- *prefix.* about, around, near

pericardi, pericardio *combining form.* near the heart; pericardium

perine, perineo *combining form.* perineum

-pexy *suffix.* fixation; usually done surgically

phac, phaco *combining form.* shaped like a lens; birthmark

phag, phago *combining form.* swallowing; eating; devouring

-phage, -phagia, -phagy *suffix.* consuming, eating; swallowing

phalang, phalango *combining form.* finger, toe

pharmaco *combining form.* drugs; medicine

pharyng, pharyngo *combining form.* pharynx

-phasia *suffix.* speaking

-pheresis *suffix.* removal

-phil, -phile, -philic, -philia *suffix.* love; desire for

phleb, phlebo *combining form.* vein

-phobia *suffix.* fear

phon, phono *combining form.* sound, voice

-phonia *suffix.* sound

-phoresis *suffix.* carrying

-phoria *suffix.* feeling; carrying

phot, photo *combining form.* light

phren, phreno *combining form.* diaphragm

-phrenia *suffix.* of the mind

-phthisis *suffix.* wasting away, shriveling

-phylaxis *suffix.* protection, prevention

phys *combining form.* air, gas, growing

physio *combining form.* physical; natural

physis- *suffix.* growing

phyto *combining form.* plant

pilo *combining form.* hair

-plakia *suffix.* plaque (small patch on skin)

-plasia *suffix.* formation; development; growth

-plasm *suffix.* thing formed

plasma, plasmo *combining form.* formative; plasma

-plastic *suffix.* forming

-plasty *suffix.* surgical repair

-plegia *suffix.* paralysis

-plegic *suffix.* pertaining to paralysis; one who is paralyzed

pleur, pleuro *combining form.* **1.** pleura; **2.** rib, side

pluri- *prefix.* several; more

-pnea *suffix.* breath

pneum, pneuma, pneumat, pneumato, pneumo *combining form.* **1.** breath; **2.** air

pneumon, pneumono *combining form.* breath; lung.

pod *combining form.* foot

-poiesis *suffix.* formation, production

-poietic *suffix.* pertaining to production

-poietin *suffix.* substance that produces

poly- *prefix.* many; multiple

-porosis *suffix.* lessening in density

post- *prefix.* after, following

pre- *prefix.* before

primi- *prefix.* first

pro- *prefix.* before, forward

proct, procto *combining form.* anus, rectum

prostate, prostat, prostato *combining form.* prostate gland

pseud, pseudo *combining form.* false

-ptosis *suffix.* falling down; drooping

pub, pubo *combining form.* pubic, pubis

pulmon, pulmono *combining form.* the lungs

pupill, pupillo *combining form.* pupil

py, pyo *combining form.* plant; pus

pyel, pyelo *combining form.* renal pelvis

pylor, pyloro *combining form.* the pylorus (outlet of the stomach)

pyr, pyro *combining form.* fever

Q

quadra-, quadri- *prefix.* four

R

rach, rachi, rachio *combining form.* spine

radi, radio *combining form.* **1.** forearm, radius; **2.** radiation; **3.** xray

radicul, radiculo *combining form.* relating to the root, as of a nerve or tooth

re- *prefix.* **1.** again; **2.** backward

rect, recto *combining form.* rectum

ren, reni, reno *combining form.* kidney

retin, retino *combining form.* retina

retro- *prefix.* **1.** backward; **2.** located behind

rhabd, rhabdo *combining form.* rod shaped

rhabdomy, rhabdomyo *combining form.* striated muscle

rheumat, rheumato *combining form.* joint

rhin, rhino *combining form.* the nose, nasal

-rrhage *suffix.* discharging heavily

-rrhagia *suffix.* excessive bleeding (amount and/or frequency)

-rrhaphy *suffix.* surgical suturing

-rrhea *suffix.* flow or discharge

-rrhexis *suffix.* rupture

S

sacr, sacro *combining form.* sacrum

saliv, salivo *combining form.* salivary glands

salping, salpingi, salpingo *combining form.* tube; salpinx

sarc, sarco *combining form.* flesh

scapulo *combining form.* scapula

-schisis *suffix.* splitting

schisto *combining form.* split; cleft

scler, sclero *combining form.* **1.** hard; **2.** sclera; **3.** white of the eye

-sclerosis *suffix.* hardening

scoli, scolio *combining form.* twisted; bent; crooked

-scope *suffix.* an instrument used for viewing or examining

-scopy *suffix.* viewing; seeing; observing

scot, scoto *combining form.* darkness

seb, sebo *combining form.* sebum; sebaceous glands

semi- *prefix.* half; partial; similar to

semin, semino *combining form.* semen

sidero *combining form.* iron

sigmoid, sigmoido *combining form.* sigmoid colon

sinistr, sinistro *combining form.* left

sinus, sinuso *combining form.* sinus

socio *combining form.* social

somat, somato *combining form.* body

-some *suffix.* body

-somnia *suffix.* sleep

somno, somni *combining form.* sleep

sono *combining form.* sound

-spasm *suffix.* contraction

spasmo *combining form.* spasm; contraction

sperm, spermat, spermato, spermo *combining form.* sperm

spher, sphero *combining form.* round; spherical

sphygm, sphygmo *combining form.* pulse

spin, spino *combining form.* spine, spinous

spir, spiro *combining form.* breath; breathe; breathing, respiration

splen, spleno *combining form.* spleen

spondyl, spondylo *combining form.* vertebra, vertebrae

squam *combining form.* scale; squamous (meaning scaly)

-stalsis *suffix.* contraction

staphyl, staphylo *combining form.* **1.** relating to *staphylococci*; **2.** relating to the uvula (of the soft palate of the mouth); **3.** grapelike clusters

-stasis *suffix.* stopping; constant

-stat *suffix.* agent to maintain a state of equilibrium

-static *suffix.* maintaining a state

steat, steato *combining form.* fat

steno *combining form.* narrowness

-stenosis *suffix.* narrowing

stereo *combining form.* threedimensional

stern, sterno *combining form.* sternum

steth, stetho *combining form.* chest

stomat, stomato *combining form.* mouth; stoma

-stomy *suffix.* surgical opening in an organ or body part

strepto *combining form.* streptococcus; twisted chains

sub- *prefix.* **1.** less than; **2.** under; **3.** inferior

supra- *prefix.* above; over

syl-, sym-, syn-, sys *prefix.* **1.** together; united; **2.** same; similar

synov, synovo *combining form.* synovial membrane

syring *combining form.* tube

T

tachy- *prefix.* speedy; fast; rapid

tars, tarso *combining form.* tarsus

tel, tele, telo *combining form.* **1.** distant; **2.** end

ten, teno, tendino *combining form.* tendon

terat, terato *combining form.* grossly deformed fetus or part

tetr, tetra *combining form.* four

thalam, thalamo *combining form.* thalamus

therm, thermo *combining form.* heat

thorac, thoraco *combining form.* chest or thorax

thromb, thrombo *combining form.* blood clot

thym, thymo *combining form.* thymus

thyr, thyro *combining form.* thyroid

thyroid *combining form.* thyroid gland

tibi, tibio *combining form.* tibia

-tome *suffix.* **1.** cutting instrument; **2.** part, segment.

-tomy *suffix.* incision

tono *combining form.* tone; pressure; tension

tonsill, tonsillo *combining form.* tonsil

topo *combining form.* place; topical

tox, toxi, toxic, toxico, toxo *combining form.* poison; toxin

trache, tracheo *combining form.* trachea

trachel, trachelo *combining form.* neck, usually of the uterus; uterine cervix

trans- *prefix.* across; through

tri- *prefix.* three

trich, tricho *combining form.* hair; thread

trigon, trigono *combining form.* trigone

-tripsy *suffix.* crushing; pulverizing

troph-, tropho- *combining form.* food; nutrition

-trophic *suffix.* relating to nutrition

-trophy *suffix.* nutrition; growth

-tropia *suffix.* turning

-tropic *suffix.* turning toward

-tropy *suffix.* attracted to target structures

tympan, tympano *combining form.* middle ear, eardrum

U

ulno *combining form.* ulna

ultra- *prefix.* **1.** beyond; **2.** excessive

un- *prefix.* not

uni- *prefix.* one; single

ur, uro *combining form.* urine; urinary tract; urination

-uresis *suffix.* **1.** urination; **2.** excretion in the urine (of the substance indicated)

ureter, uretero *combining form.* ureter

urethr, urethro *combining form.* urethra

-uria *suffix.* urine

urin, urino *combining form.* urine

utero *combining form.* uterus

uve, uveo *combining form.* uvea

V

vag, vago *combining form.* vagus nerve

vagin, vagino *combining form.* vagina

valvul, valvulo *combining form.* valve

vas, vaso *combining form.* **1.** blood vessel; **2.** vessel; **3.** vas deferens

ven, veni, veno *combining form.* vein

ventricul, ventriculo *combining form.* ventricle

-version *suffix.* turning (of the type specified)

vertebr, vertebro *combining form.* vertebra or vertebrae

vesic, vesico *combining form.* bladder

vulv, vulvo *combining form.* vulva

X

xanth, xantho *combining form.* yellow

xeno *combining form.* strange; foreign matter

xer, xero *combining form.* dryness

xiph, xipho *combining form.* sword shaped

Common Medical Abbreviations

A

a 1. before; **2.** area; **3.** asymmetric; **4.** artery

A 1. adenine; **2.** alanine; **3.** as a subscript, used to refer to alveolar gas

AA, aa 1. amino acid; **2. AA** Alcoholics Anonymous (www.alcoholics-anonymous.org)

AAA abdominal aortic aneurysm

AAMA American Association of Medical Assistants (www.aama-ntl.org)

AAMT American Association for Medical Transcription (www.aamt.org)

A&P 1. auscultation and percussion; **2.** anterior and posterior

AB antibiotic

ABC airway, breathing, and circulation; used in cardiac life support

ABCD airway, breathing, circulation, and defibrillation; used in cardiac life support

ABCDE airway, breathing, circulation and cervical spine, disability, and exposure; used in advanced trauma life support

ABG arterial blood gas

ABR auditory brainstem response

ABR test auditory brainstem response test

a.c. Latin *ante cibum,* before meals

AC air conduction

ACE angiotensin-converting enzyme

ACE2 angiotensin-converting enzyme 2

AcG, ac-g accelerator globulin

Ach acetylcholine

ACL anterior cruciate ligament

ACR American College of Radiology

ACTH adrenocorticotropic hormone

AD Alzheimer disease

A.D. Latin *auris dextra,* right ear

ad lib. Latin *ad libitum,* freely

ADA 1. American Dental Association (www.ada.org); **2.** Americans with Disabilities Act

ADAA American Dental Assistants Association (www.dentalassistants.org)

ADD attention deficit disorder

ADH antidiuretic hormone

ADHD attention deficit hyperactivity disorder

ADLs activities of daily living

Adm admission

ADR adverse drug reaction

AF atrial fibrillation

AFB acid-fast bacillus

AFO ankle-foot orthotic

Ag silver

A/G albumin: globulin ratio

AGN 1. acute glomerulonephritis; **2.** acute necrotizing gingivitis

AHD atherosclerotic heart disease

AHIMA American Health Information Management Association (www.ahima.org)

AI aortic insufficiency

AID artificial insemination by donor

AIDS acquired immunodeficiency syndrome or acquired immunodeficiency disease

AIH artificial insemination, homologous (using the donor's semen)

AK actinic keratosis

A-K above the knee

AKA above-the-knee amputation

ALL 1. acute lymphoblastic leukemia; **2.** acute lymphocytic leukemia

ALS amyotrophic lateral sclerosis

ALT alanine aminotransferase

a.m., AM Latin *ante meridiem,* before noon

AMA 1. against medical advice; **2.** American Medical Association (www.ama-assn.org)

AMC arthrogryposis multiplex congenita

AMI acute myocardial infarction

AML 1. acute myelogenous lymphocytic leukemia; **2.** acute myeloblastic leukemia; **3.** acute myelocytic leukemia; **4.** acute myeloid leukemia

ANA antinuclear antibody titer, elevated in connective tissue disease

ANUG acute necrotizing ulcerative gingivitis

AP 1. angina pectoris; **2.** arterial pressure; **3.** anterior pituitary; **4.** anteroposterior

AP & LAT anteroposterior and lateral

AP view anteroposterior view

APC **1.** acetylsalicylic acid, phenacetin, and caffeine, combined to make an analgesic; **2.** antigen-presenting cells

APTT activated partial thromboplastin time

aq. water

ARB angiotensin II receptor blocker

ARC AIDS-related complex

ARDS **1.** adult respiratory distress syndrome; **2.** acute respiratory distress syndrome

ARF **1.** acute renal failure; **2.** acute respiratory failure

Arg arginine

AROM active range of motion

ART **1.** antiretroviral therapy; **2.** assisted reproductive technology

A.S. Latin *auris sinister,* left ear

ASA (drug caution code) abbreviation of acetylsalicylic acid (aspirin), placed on the label of a medication as a warning that it contains acetylsalicylic acid, which can cause complications for someone with specific medical conditions

ASD atrial septal defect

ASL American Sign Language

ASP aspartic acid

AST aspartate aminotransferase

ATL **1.** adult T-cell leukemia; **2.** adult T-cell leukemia/lymphoma; **3.** adult T-cell lymphoma

ATP adenosine triphosphatase

A.U. Latin *auris unitas,* both ears

AUL acute undifferentiated leukemia

AV atrioventricular

AVM arteriovenous malformation

AZT azidothymidine, also known as zidovudine, a drug used in the treatment of HIV

B

Ba barium

BaE, Ba enema, BE barium enema

BAEP brainstem auditory evoked potentials

BAER brainstem auditory evoked response

baso basophil

BBB blood–brain barrier

BC bone conduction

BCG bacillus of Calmette and Guerin (vaccination for tuberculosis)

BIA biological impedance analysis

b.i.d., bid, BID Latin *bis in die,* two times a day (on prescriptions)

B-K below the knee

BKA below-knee amputation

BM bowel movement

BMD **1.** bone mass density; **2.** bone mineral density

BMI body mass index

BMR basal metabolic rate

BMT bone marrow transplant

BP, bp blood pressure

BPH **1.** benign prostatic hyperplasia; **2.** benign prostatic hypertrophy

BSA body surface area

BSE bovine spongiform encephalopathy

BUN blood urea nitrogen

bx, BX, Bx, Bx. biopsy

BZD benzodiazepine

C

c **1.** small calorie (gram calorie); **2.** centi-; **3.** curie

C **1.** calorie (kilocalorie); **2.** carbon; **3.** Celsius/centigrade; **4.** cervical vertebra/vertebrae; **5.** cytosine

Ca calcium

CA **1.** (also ca) cancer/carcinoma; **2.** chronological age; **3.** coronary artery

CA-125 cancer antigen 125

CABG coronary artery bypass graft

CAD coronary artery disease

CAM complementary and alternative medicine

cap capsule

CAPD continuous ambulatory peritoneal dialysis

CAT computerized axial tomography

Cath, cath catheter

CBC, cbc complete blood count

CBT cognitive behavioral therapy

cc cubic centimeter

CC chief complaint

CCS certified coding specialist (hospital)

CCS-P certified coding specialist–physician

CCU coronary care unit

CDA certified dental assistant

CDC Centers for Disease Control and Prevention

CEA carcinoembryonic antigen

CHF congestive heart failure

CIC completely in the canal (said of hearing aids)

CIS carcinoma in situ

CJD Creutzfeldt-Jakob disease

CK creatinine kinase

Cl chlorine

CLL chronic lymphocytic leukemia

cm centimeter

CMA certified medical assistant

CMI cell-mediated immunity

CML chronic myelogenous leukemia

CMS Centers for Medicare and Medicaid Services (www.cms.gov)

CMT certified medical transcriptionist

CMV cytomegalovirus

CNS central nervous system

C/o complaining of

CO cardiac output

CO₂ carbon dioxide

CoA coarctation of the aorta

COBRA U.S. Federal Consolidated Omnibus Budget Reconciliation Act

COLD chronic obstructive lung disease

COPD chronic obstructive pulmonary disease

CP cerebral palsy

CPAP continuous positive airway pressure

CPC certified professional coder

CPC-H certified professional coder–hospital

CPD cephalopelvic disproportion

CPK creatine phosphokinase

CPR cardiopulmonary resuscitation

CPT Current Procedural Terminology

CRF 1. corticotropin-releasing factor; 2. chronic renal failure

CRH corticotropin-releasing hormone

CRNA Certified Registered Nurse Anesthetist

CRP 1. cAMP receptor protein; 2. C-reactive protein

CSF 1. cerebrospinal fluid; 2. colony-stimulating factor

CT computed tomography

CTS carpal tunnel syndrome

CVA 1. cerebrovascular attack; 2. cerebrovascular accident

CVC central venous catheter

CVD cardiovascular disease

CVP central venous pressure

Cx cervix

CXR chest x-ray

D

D (drug caution code) found on the label of some medications, indicating that it may cause drowsiness

D&C, D and C dilation and curettage

D&E dilation and evacuation

dB decibel

D/c discontinue

DC 1. (also d.c.) direct current; 2. Doctor of Chiropractic

DDS 1. Doctor of Dental Surgery; 2. Denver Developmental Screening Test

def, DEF decayed, extracted, and filled; said of teeth

derm dermatology

DES diethylstilbestrol

DEXA scan the image or data produced by a special x-ray machine, used to measure bone density [dual-energy x-ray absorptiometry]

DHEA dehydroepiandrosterone

DHF dengue hemorrhagic fever

DI diabetes insipidus

diff differential

diff dx differential diagnosis

DLE discoid lupus erythematosus

DM diabetes mellitus

DNA deoxyribonucleic acid

DNR do not resuscitate

D.O. Doctor of Osteopathy

DOA dead on arrival

DOB date of birth

Dr, Dr. doctor

DRE digital rectal exam

DRG diagnosis-related group, payment categories used by hospitals to charge fees to insurers

DRI dietary reference intake

DSA digital subtraction angiography

DSM *Diagnostic and Statistical Manual*

DT 1. duration tetany, the spasm of degenerated muscle upon application of electrical current; 2. diphtheria tetanus, a vaccine used for immunization of diphtheria and tetanus

DTs delirium tremens

DV daily value, as the recommended intake of a nutrient

DVT deep vein thrombosis

dx, DX diagnosis

DXA dual x-ray absorptiometry

E

EBCT electron beam computerized tomography

EBV Epstein-Barr virus

ECG, EKG electrocardiogram

ECHO echocardiogram

ECMO extracorporeal-membrane oxygenation, a complex therapeutic tool used in extreme ICU conditions where lung function has failed but is expected to recover within a few days

ECT electroconvulsive therapy, formerly called electroshock therapy

ED 1. effective dose; 2. emergency department; 3. erectile dysfunction

EDC estimated date of confinement

EEE eastern equine encephalitis

EEG electroencephalogram

EENT eye, ear, nose, and throat; *see also* ENT

EF ejection fraction

EGD esophagogastroduodenoscopy

EIA enzyme immunoassay

EKG, ECG electrocardiogram

ELISA enzyme-linked immunosorbent assay

elix. elixir

EMG electromyogram

EMR electronic medical record

EMT emergency medical technician

ENT ear, nose, throat; *see also* EENT

eos eosinophil

EPO erythropoietin

ER 1. emergency room; 2. estrogen receptor

ERCP endoscopic retrograde cholangiopancreatography

ERT estrogen replacement therapy

ESP extrasensory perception

ESR erythrocyte sedimentation rate

ESRD end-stage renal disease

ESWL extracorporeal shock wave lithotripsy

EUD external urinary drainage

F

F Fahrenheit

FAE fetal alcohol effects

FAP 1. familial adenomatous polyposis; 2. functional ambulation profile (analysis of a patient's ability to walk)

FAS fetal alcohol syndrome

FBG fasting blood glucose

FBS fasting blood sugar

FDA Food and Drug Administration (www.fda.gov)

FEF forced expiratory flow

FET forced expiratory time

FEV1 forced expiratory volume measured during first second of expiration, useful in quantifying pulmonary disability

FHR fetal heart rate

FHT fetal heart tone

fMRI functional magnetic resonance imaging, a type of magnetic resonance imaging that demonstrates the correlation between physical changes and mental functioning

FNA fine needle aspiration biopsy

FP 1. freezing point; 2. family physician; 3. family practice

FSH follicle-stimulating hormone

ft. foot; feet

FTT failure to thrive

FUO fever of unknown origin

FVC forced vital capacity

Fx fracture

G

g gram; grams

G 1. (drug caution code) abbreviation of glaucoma, placed on the label of a medication as a warning that it can cause complications for someone with the disease 2. gravida

GB gallbladder

GC gas chromatography

g-cal gram calorie

G-CSF granulocyte colony-stimulating factor

GDM gestational diabetes mellitus

GERD gastroesophageal reflux disease

GFR glomerular filtration rate

GH growth hormone

GHB gamma hydroxybutyrate

GHz gigahertz

GI gastrointestinal

GI series gastrointestinal series

GI tract gastrointestinal tract

GIFT gamete intrafallopian transfer

GLC gas-liquid chromatography

gm gram; grams

GM-CSF granulocyte-macrophage colony-stimulating factor

GOT glutamic-oxaloacetic transaminase

GSR galvanic skin response

gtt Latin *guttae,* drops

GTT glucose tolerance test

GU genitourinary

GYN gynecology; gynecologist

H

h 1. height 2. hour

H 1. hyperopia; hyperopic; 2. hydrogen; 3. (drug caution code) found on the label of medication indicating that it can be habit forming

H&P history and physical

HAV hepatitis A virus, the RNA virus that causes hepatitis A

Hb, Hgb hemoglobin

HB hepatitis B vaccine

HBIG hepatitis B immune globulin

HBV hepatitis B virus, the DNA virus that causes hepatitis B

HCFA Health Care Finance Administration, now the Centers for Medicare and Medicaid Services

HCG human chorionic gonadotropin

hct, HCT hematocrit

HCV hepatitis C virus, the RNA virus that causes hepatitis C

HD Hodgkin disease

HDL high-density lipoprotein

HDN hemolytic disease of the newborn

HDV hepatitis D virus, the RNA virus that causes hepatitis D

HEENT head, ears, eyes, nose, throat

HEV hepatitis E virus, the RNA virus that causes hepatitis E

Hg mercury

HGB, Hgb, HB hemoglobin

HGH human growth hormone

HHS U.S. Department of Health and Human Services (www.hhs.gov)

HIPAA Health Insurance Portability and Accountability Act

His histidine

HIV human immunodeficiency virus

HMD hyaline membrane disease

HMO health maintenance organization

h/o history of

HPV human papilloma virus

HRR high-risk register

HRT hormone replacement therapy

hs at bedtime

HSG hysterosalpingography

HSV herpes simplex virus

HTLV human T-cell leukemia virus

HTN hypertension

hx history

Hz hertz

I

I (drug caution code) a symbol placed on the label of a medication, indicating possible adverse interaction if taken with other drugs

I&D incision and drainage

I&O intake and output

IBD inflammatory bowel disease

IBS irritable bowel syndrome

ICD-10-CM title of *International Classification of Diseases, 10th Revision, Clinical Modification;* system for diagnosis classification now in use for medical coding; ICD-11 is under review and was expected to be adopted by 2018 but is delayed as it is still in testing.

ICF **1.** intermediate care facility; **2.** intracellular acid

ICP intracranial pressure

ICU intensive care unit

IDDM insulin-dependant diabetes mellitus

Ig immunoglobulin

IgA immunoglobulin A

IgD immunoglobulin D

IgE immunoglobulin E

IGF insulin-like growth factor(s)

IgG immunoglobulin G

IgM immunoglobulin M

IL interleukin

IM intramuscular

IOL intraocular lens

IOP intraocular pressure

IPPB intermittent positive pressure breathing

IPPV intermittent positive pressure ventilation

IPV inactivated polio vaccine

IQ intelligence quotient

IU international unit

IUD intrauterine contraceptive device

IUI intrauterine insemination

IV **1.** *adj.* intravenous; **2.** *n.* intravenous injection; **3.** *n.* intravenous drip

IVF in vitro fertilization

IVP intravenous pyelogram

K

K potassium

kg kilogram; kilograms

KUB kidneys, ureter, and bladder

L

l, L **1.** liter; liters; **2.** left

LAC laceration

LASIK laser-assisted in situ keratomileusis

lat lateral

lb pound; pounds

LD lethal dose, often LD50 or LD95, used to describe the dose at which 50% or 95% of the subjects (usually lab animals) die

LDH lactate dehydrogenase

LDL low-density lipoprotein

LE **1.** left eye (usually abbreviated OS or o.s.); **2.** lupus erythematosus (usually abbreviated SLE)

LEEP loop electrosurgical excision procedure

LES lower esophageal sphincter

LFT liver function test

LH luteinizing hormone

LI large intestine

LLQ left lower quadrant

LMP last menstrual period

LOC level of consciousness

LP **1.** latency period; **2.** lipoprotein/low protein; **3.** lumbar puncture

LPN licensed practical nurse

LR **1.** labor room; **2.** lactated Ringer (injection or solution); **3.** lateral rectus; **4.** light reaction or light reflex

LRM left radical mastectomy

LRT lower respiratory tract

LS **1.** left side; **2.** liver and spleen; **3.** lumbosacral; **4.** lymphosarcoma

LSH lutein-stimulating hormone

LTC long-term care

LUL **1.** left upper limb; **2.** left upper lobe (of lung)

LUQ left upper quadrant

LV **1.** left ventricle; **2.** leukemia virus; **3.** live virus

LVAD left ventricular assist device

LVN licensed vocational/visiting nurse

LVRS lung volume reduction surgery

Lys lysine

M

Mb myoglobin

MBC maximum breathing capacity

mcg microgram; micrograms

MCH 1. mean corpuscular hemoglobin; **2.** maternal and child health (services)

MCHC mean corpuscular hemoglobin concentration

MCP metacarpophalangeal

MCS multiple chemical sensitivity

MCV mean corpuscular volume

MD 1. (*also* **M.D.**) Doctor of Medicine; **2.** muscular dystrophy

MDI metered-dose inhaler

ME medical examiner

MEP maximum expiratory pressure

MET 1. metabolic equivalent; **2.** muscle energy technique

mets metastasis

mg milligram

MG myasthenia gravis

Mg magnesium

mGy milligray

mh, MHz megahertz

MI 1. myocardial infarction; **2.** mitral incompetence or inadequacy

MIS medical information system

ml, mL milliliter; milliliters

mm millimeter; millimeters

MMPI Minnesota Multiphasic Personality Inventory

Mn Manganese

mono monocyte

MP mentoposterior position

MPD 1. multiple personality disorder; **2.** medical program director

MR mitral regurgitation

MRA magnetic resonance angiography

MRI magnetic resonance imaging

MS 1. multiple sclerosis; **2.** mitral stenosis

MUGA multiple-gated acquisition scan

MVP mitral valve prolapse

N

N nitrogen

Na sodium

NARP neuropathy, ataxia, and retinitis pigmentosa, a genetic disease inherited from the mother, featuring weakness of the muscles near the trunk, ataxia (wobbliness), seizures, disease of the retina, and sometimes retardation or developmental delay

ND Doctor of Naturopathic Medicine

NEC not elsewhere classified (used in medical coding)

neg, neg. negative

neut neutrophil

NG nasogastric

NHL non-Hodgkin lymphoma

NICU neonatal intensive care unit

NIDDM non-insulin-dependent diabetes mellitus

NK cell natural killer cell

NKDA no known drug allergies

NMR nuclear magnetic resonance

noc. Latin *nocte,* at night

noc, n.o.c. not otherwise classified

NOS not otherwise specified (used in medical coding)

NPC Niemann-Pick disease

NPO, n.p.o. Latin *nil per os,* nothing by mouth

NREM sleep or **nonREM sleep** non-rapid eye movement sleep

NSAID nonsteroidal anti-inflammatory drug

NTD neural tube defect

O

O_2 oxygen

OB obstetrics; obstetrician

OB/GYN obstetrics and gynecology

OBS organic brain syndrome

OCD obsessive-compulsive disorder

OD 1. *n.* an overdose; **2.** *v.* to overdose

o.d. Latin *oculus dexter,* the right eye (in optometry)

oint, oint. ointment

OR operating room

orth orthopedic surgeon

OS, o.s. Latin *oculus sinister,* the left eye (in optometry)

OSA obstructive sleep apnea

OSHA Occupation Safety and Health Administration (www.osha.gov)

OT occupational therapy; occupational therapist

OTC over the counter (for sale without a prescription)

OU, o.u. Latin *oculus uterque,* each eye (in prescriptions)

oz, oz. ounce; ounces

P

PA 1. physician assistant; **2.** posteroanterior (as in a typical chest x-ray); **3.** pulmonary artery

PAC premature atrial contraction

PACU postanesthesia care unit

Pap 1. Papanicolaou('s); **2.** (*also* **pap**) Pap test; **3.** (*also* **pap**) Pap smear

PAP 1. positive airway pressure; **2.** pulmonary artery pressure

Pb lead

p.c. Latin *post cibum,* after meals

PCA 1. patient-controlled analgesia; **2.** posterior cerebral artery

PCL posterior cruciate ligament

PCN penicillin

PCP 1. *Pneumocystis carinii* pneumonia; **2.** primary care physician; primary care provider

PCR polymerase chain reaction, commonly used in medical testing to amplify particular sequences of DNA

PCT patient care technician

PCV packed cell volume

PD peritoneal dialysis

PDR 1. *Physicians' Desk Reference;* **2.** primary drug resistance

PDT photodynamic therapy

PE 1. physical examination; **2.** pleural effusion; **3.** pulmonary edema; **4.** pulmonary embolism

PED pediatric emergency department

peds pediatrics

PEEP positive end-expiratory pressure

PEFR peak expiratory flow rate

PEG percutaneous endoscopic gastrostomy

PERRL or **PERRLA** pupils equally round and reactive to light or pupils equally round and reactive to light and accommodation

PET positron emission tomography

PFT pulmonary function test

PICU pediatric intensive care unit

PID pelvic inflammatory disease

PIP proximal interphalangeal joints

PKD polycystic kidney disease

PKU phenylketonuria

Pl platinum

PLT platelet count

PM, p.m. Latin *post meridian,* at night

PMN polymorphonucleated cells

PMS premenstrual syndrome

PN parenteral nutrition

PNS peripheral nervous system

p.o., PO Latin *per os,* by mouth

polio poliomyelitis

POS point of service

PPD 1. postpartum depression; **2.** purified protein derivative, used in a skin test for tuberculosis

PPMA postpolio muscular atrophy

PPO preferred provider organization

PPS postpolio syndrome

PR per rectum

PRBC packed red blood cells

preop preoperative

primip primipara

PRK photorefractive keratectomy

PRN, p.r.n. Latin *pro re nata,* as needed (in prescriptions)

PROM passive range of motion

PSA prostate-specific antigen, a protein produced by the prostate gland that is used in the diagnosis of prostate cancer

PSG polysomnography

pt patient

PT 1. physical therapy; **2.** physical therapist; **3.** prothrombin time

PTA percutaneous transluminal angioplasty

PTCA percutaneous transluminal coronary angioplasty

PTSD posttraumatic stress disorder

PTT partial thromboplastin time

PUBS percutaneous umbilical blood sampling, a technique used for diagnosing and treating a fetus in which a blood sample is taken from the umbilical vein by inserting a needle through the mother's abdominal and uterine walls

PUD peptic ulcer disease

pulv. powder (used in prescriptions)

PUVA psoralen and UVA, a treatment for psoriasis that combines the medication psoralen with carefully timed UVA (ultraviolet light of A wavelength) exposure

PV 1. polycythemia vera; **2.** peripheral vascular

PVC premature ventricular contraction

PVD peripheral vascular disease

PVS persistent vegetative state

Q

q, q. every

qam, q.a.m. every morning

q.d., qd Latin *quaque die,* every day

q.h., qh Latin *quaque hora,* every hour

q.2h. every 2 hours

q.3h. every 3 hours

q.i.d., qid Latin *quatuor in die,* four times a day

q.n.s., QNS quantity not sufficient; used by a laboratory when an insufficient amount of specimen is received to perform a requested test

qod, q.o.d. every other day

qoh, q.o.h. every other hour

qpm, q.p.m. every evening

q.s., QS quantity sufficient; quantity required

qt 1. (*also* qt.) quart; quarts; **2.** interval in QRS complex

R

R, r roentgen

Ra radium

RA rheumatoid arthritis

rad radiation absorbed dose

RAST radioallergosorbent test

RBC **1.** red blood cells; **2.** red blood count

RD registered dietitian

RDA **1.** Recommended Daily Allowance; **2.** Recommended Dietary Allowance

RDS respiratory distress syndrome

rehab rehabilitation

REM rapid eye movements

RES reticuloendothelial system

RF rheumatoid factor

Rh rhesus

RIA radioimmunoassay

RLL right lower lobe

RLQ right lower quadrant

RMSF Rocky Mountain spotted fever

Rn radon

RN registered nurse

RNA ribonucleic acid

ROM range of motion

RP **1.** retinitis pigmentosa; **2.** retrograde pyelogram

RT, rt **1.** radiologic technologist; **2.** reaction time; **3.** recreational therapy; **4.** respiratory therapist

RUQ right upper quadrant

RV **1.** residual volume; **2.** right ventricle

Rx, RX **1.** medical prescription; **2.** treatment

S

s without

S sulfur

SA sinoatrial

SA node sinoatrial node, the natural pacemaker of the heart

SAD seasonal affective disorder

SARS severe acute respiratory syndrome

SBC systolic blood pressure

SBS shaken baby syndrome

sc, SC subcutaneous

Sc scandium

SCI spinal cord injury

Se selenium

SERM selective estrogen receptor modulator

SGOT serum glutamic oxaloacetic transaminase

SGPT serum glutamic pyruvic transaminase

SIADH syndrome of inappropriate ADH (antidiuretic hormone)

SIDS sudden infant death syndrome

SL sublingual

SLE systemic lupus erythematosus

SLS Sjogren-Larsson syndrome

SNOMED Systematized Nomenclature of Medical Terms, an international standardized system of medical terminology gradually being instituted worldwide

SOB shortness of breath

sol, sol. solution

SPECT single photon emission computed tomography

SPF sun protection factor

sq subcutaneous

Sr strontium

SR **1.** sedimentation rate; **2.** sinus rhythm

SSPE subacute sclerosing panencephalitis

SSRI selective serotonin reuptake inhibitor

staph *staphyloccocus*

STD sexually transmitted disease

STH somatrophic hormone

STI sexually transmitted infection

STM short-term memory

strep streptococcus

supp. supplement

susp. suspension

SV stroke volume

syr. syrup

sz seizure

T

T **1.** thymine; **2.** temperature; **3.** time; **4.** tablespoon; tablespoons

t. teaspoon; teaspoons

T3, T$_3$ triiodothyronine

T4, T$_4$ thyroxine

TAH total abdominal hysterectomy

tab. tablet

TB tuberculosis

TBI **1.** traumatic brain injury; **2.** total body irradiation

Tbsp, tbsp. tablespoon; tablespoons

TBV total blood volume

TCA tricyclic antidepressant

TCM traditional Chinese medicine

TDD telecommunications device for the deaf

TDM therapeutic drug monitoring

temp, temp. temperature

TENS transcutaneous electrical nerve stimulation

THC tetrahydrocannabinol

Thr threonine

THR **1.** target heart rate; **2.** threshold heart rate; **3.** total hip replacement; **4.** thyroid hormone receptor

Ti titanium

TIA transient ischemic attack

tid, t.i.d. three times a day, used in writing prescriptions

TJC The Joint Commission (TJC), an organization that inspects hospitals and reviews and gives accreditation to health care organizations (www.jointcommission.org)

TL thallium

TLC total lung capacity

TMJ temporomandibular joint

TNF tumor necrosis factor

TNM tumor-node-metastasis

tPA, TPA tissue plasminogen activator

TPN total parenteral nutrition

TPR temperature, pulse, respiration

Trp tryptophan

TSE 1. transmissible spongiform encephalopathy, any of a group of brain diseases, such as kuru or Creutzfeldt-Jakob disease, in which the brain matter deteriorates; **2.** testicular self-examination

TSH thyroid-stimulating hormone

tsp. teaspoon; teaspoons

TSS toxic shock syndrome

TTP thrombotic thrombocytopenic purpura

TUR transurethral resection

TURP transurethral resection of the prostate

U

u atomic mass unit

U 1. uranium; **2.** unit; units; **3.** uracil; **4.** urine

UA, U/A urinalysis

UBT urea breath test

UGI upper gastrointestinal

ung, ung. ointment

UNOS United Network for Organ Sharing

URI upper respiratory infection

URTI upper respiratory tract infection

USDA United States Department of Agriculture (www.usda.gov)

USFDA United States Food and Drug Administration (www.fda.gov)

USP *United States Pharmacopeia*

USP-NF *United States Pharmacopeia–National Formulary*

UTI urinary tract infection

UV ultraviolet

UVR ultraviolet radiation

V

VA 1. vertebral artery; **2.** Veterans Administration; **3.** visual acuity; **4.** volt-ampere

VAD 1. vascular access device; **2.** vascular assist device; **3.** ventricular assist device

Val valine

VATS video-assisted thoracoscopy

VC 1. vital capacity; **2.** vocal cord; vocal cords

VCU voiding cystourethrography

VCUG voiding cystourethrogram/cystourethrography

VD venereal disease

VF 1. visual field; **2.** ventricular fibrillation

Vfib ventricular fibrillation

VHDL very-high-density lipoprotein

VLDL very-low-density lipoprotein

V/Q ventilation-perfusion

VS vital sign; vital signs

VSD ventricular septal defect

VT, V-tach ventricular tachycardia

W

WAIS Wechsler Adult Intelligence Scale

WBC 1. white blood cell; **2.** white blood (cell) count

WBC count white blood cell count

WBC differential white blood cell differential

WC wheelchair

WHO World Health Organization (www.who.int)

WISC Wechsler Intelligence Scale for Children

WNL within normal limits

w/o without

wt, wt. weight

X

XRT radiation therapy

Z

ZIFT zygote intrafallopian transfer

Laboratory Testing

Health care professionals order laboratory tests to diagnose diseases and conditions, and to assess the general health and functioning of various parts of the body. The basic types of tests are blood tests, urinalyses, stool tests, and spinal taps, which analyze spinal fluid to look for diseases, such as meningitis.

Blood Tests

The two most common blood tests are the complete blood count (CBC) and the blood culture. The CBC measures levels of substances in the blood as described in the following paragraphs. The blood culture is a test for bacteria or yeast. Blood is cultured in the laboratory and if bacteria or yeast is present, it is analyzed for what type it is and which infection it indicates.

The CBC

The CBC tests for electrolytes by measuring levels of sodium, potassium, chloride, and bicarbonate in the body. It also measures other substances, such as blood urea, nitrogen, glucose, and sugars. In addition, it measures the red blood cells, white blood cells, and platelets to look for signs of anemia or infection.

- **Sodium** plays a major role in regulating the amount of water in the body. Also, sodium is necessary for many body functions, like transmitting electrical signals in the brain. The test determines whether there's the right balance of sodium and liquid in the blood to carry out important bodily functions. High levels of sodium can lead to certain conditions, such as high blood pressure.
- **Potassium** is essential to regulate how the heart beats. When potassium levels are too high or too low, it can increase the risk of an abnormal heartbeat. Low potassium levels are also associated with muscle weakness.
- **Chloride** also helps maintain a balance of fluids in the body.
- **Bicarbonate** prevents the body's tissues from getting too much or too little acid. The kidney and lungs balance the levels of bicarbonate in the body. So if bicarbonate levels are abnormal, it might indicate that there is a problem with those organs.
- **Blood urea nitrogen (BUN)** is a measure of how well the kidneys are working.
- **Creatinine** levels in the blood that are too high can indicate that the kidneys are not working properly. The kidneys filter and excrete creatinine. Both dehydration and muscle damage also can raise creatinine levels.
- **Glucose** is the main type of sugar in the blood. Glucose levels that are too high or too low can cause problems and are often indicative of diabetes.

Three tests that are part of a CBC measure red blood cell (RBC) count, hemoglobin, and mean (red) cell volume (MCV). These studies test for anemia, a common condition that occurs when there aren't enough red blood cells.

- The red blood cell count is a measure of the number of RBCs in the body.
- Hemoglobin is the oxygen-carrying protein in red blood cells. RBCs carry oxygen to all parts of the body.
- MCV measures the average size of the red blood cells.

Other tests include the **hematocrit (HCT),** which determines the percentage of red blood cells in the blood sample. This is also a test for anemia.

Also part of the CBC is the blood differential test that measures the relative number of different types of white blood cells (WBCs) in the blood. WBCs (also called leukocytes) help the body fight infection. An abnormal white blood cell count may indicate that there is an infection, inflammation, or other stress in the body. There are five types of white blood cells: neutrophils, lymphocytes, eosinophils, basophils, and monocytes.

Platelets are the smallest blood cells and are important to blood clotting and the prevention of excessive bleeding. If the platelet count is too low, a person can be in danger of bleeding in any part of the body.

Blood Cultures

Blood is cultured when an infection or the condition of sepsis is suspected. Bacteria or yeast will show up in the blood culture if such conditions exist. Blood cultures are usually done twice if there is a positive result because false positives can lead to unnecessary treatment.

Urinalysis

The kidneys make urine as they filter wastes from the bloodstream while leaving substances in the blood that the body needs, like protein and glucose. Urinalysis checks for the presence of protein and glucose in the urine as well as other substances that can indicate infection, poor function of a body part, or the presence of illegal drugs. The urine is checked for blood as well as many other substances and is an important diagnostic tool.

Stool Test

The most common reason to collect stool is to determine whether a type of bacteria or parasite may be infecting the intestine. Stool is also checked for occult blood, possibly indicative of internal bleeding. Stool samples also are sometimes analyzed for the substances they contain. Some substances may indicate digestive disorders.

Spinal Tap

A spinal tap or lumbar puncture (LP) is a procedure in which a small amount of the fluid that surrounds the brain and spinal cord, called the cerebrospinal fluid (CSF), is removed and examined. The fluid is examined for meningitis and other diseases of the central nervous system.

Normal Values

Note that "normal" values can vary depending on a variety of factors, including the patient's age or gender, time of day test was taken, and so on. In addition, as new medical advances are made, the understanding of what is the ideal range for some readings has changed.

Index

eructation, 443
erythro/o, 18, 19, 274, 284
erythroblastosis fetalis, 288
erythrocyte sedimentation rate
        (ESR), 286
erythrocytes, 277, 279, 281, 282
erythrocytopenia, 288
erythropenia, 288
erythropoietin, 277, 279
esophagitis, 441
esophago/o, 412, 416
esophagoplasty, 455
esophagoscope, 435
esophagoscopy, 435
esophagus, 413
    diameter of, 441
    disorders of, 440–442
esotropia, 79, 229
ESR (erythrocyte sedimentation
        rate), 286
ESRD (end-stage renal disease), 486
essential hypertension, 323
-esthesia, 62
esthesio/o, 15, 16
estrogen, 250, 252, 529, 530
ESWL (extracorporeal shock wave
        lithotripsy), 482, 483
ethmo/o, 13, 14
ethmoid bone, 141, 142
ethmoidal sinuses, 141
etio/o, 28, 29
eu-, 53, 54
EUD (external urinary drainage)
        catheters, 479
eupnea, 366
eustachian tubes, 219, 220
eversion, 151
ex-, 48, 49
excitability, 177
excoriation, 112, 114
exhalation, 353, 356
exo-, 48, 49
exocrine glands, 107, 244
exophthalmos, 230, 258
exophthalmus, 230
exotropia, 229
expectorants, 376
expiration, 353, 357
extension, 151
external auditory meatus, 220
external ear, 219
external fixation devices, 163
external nares, 351
external respiration, 348
external urinary drainage (EUD)
        catheters, 479
extra-, 48, 49
extracorporeal circulation, 332
extracorporeal shock wave lithotripsy
        (ESWL), 482, 483

extremities, bones of, 147–148
exudates, 110
eye, 215–218
eye color, 218
eye disorders, 228–231
eyebrows, 217
eyelashes, 217
eyelid, 216
eyestrain, 229

F

facial nerves, 185
factor, word roots and combining forms
        that relate to, 17–18
Factor VIII, 288
fainting, 202
fallopian tube, 524
false ribs, 145
farsightedness, 229
fascia, 151
fascio/o, 136
fasting blood sugar, 255
fatty acids, 413
feces, 425, 426
feelings, 15, 62–64
female reproductive organs,
        523–528
femoral, 6
femoral artery, 306
femoral hernia, 454
femoro/o, 136
femur, 147, 148
fertility, 527
fetal circulation, 312–313
FEV (forced expiratory volume), 361
fever blister, 118
fibrillation, 321
fibrin clot, 275
fibrinogen, 274, 275
fibro/o, 28, 30, 136, 152
fibula, 147, 148
filtration, 471
fimbriae, 525
first-degree burns, 120
fissures, 112, 114, 180
fistulas, 450, 452
flaccid, 160
flagellum, 502
flat bones, 140
flatulence, 443
flatus, 453
flexion, 151
fluorescein angiography, 227
fluoro/o, 28, 30
flutter, 321
Foley catheter, 479, 480
follicle-stimulating hormone (FSH), 504,
        529, 530
fontanelles, 142

foramen magnum, 142
foramen ovale, 312, 313
forced expiratory volume (FEV), 361
forced vital capacity (FVC), 361
foreskin, 502
-form, 78
forms, 560–567
fossae, 32
fractures, 158
    avulsion, 158
    intracapsular, 158
fraternal twins, 502
free edge, 104, 105
frenulum, 418
frontal, 92
frontal bone, 141, 142
frontal lobe, 180
frontal sinus, 141
FSH (follicle-stimulating hormone), 504,
        529, 530
fulguration, 124
fundus, 422, 525
fungi, 28, 29
furuncle, 116
FVC (forced vital capacity), 361
Fx, 35

G

gait, 194
galacto/o, 28, 30, 526, 538
gallbladder, 428, 429
    disorders of, 445–449
gallop, 316, 321
gallstones, 445, 446
gametes, 524
gamma globulins, 275
gangliitis, 198
ganglio/o, 176, 187
ganglion, 32, 200
gangrene, 116
gastralgia/gastrodynia, 443
gastrectomy, 456
gastric bypass, 455, 456
gastric resection, 456
gastritis, 443
gastro/o, 9, 412, 421
gastroenteritis, 443
gastroenterology, 411
gastropathy, 421
gastroscope, 435
gastroscopy, 435
-gen, 75
gender identity, 501
gene, 3
-genesis, 75
-genic, 75
genital herpes, 118, 512, 545
genital warts, 546
geno/o, 25

lymph, 387, 388, 389
lymph nodes, 385, 386, 387, 388, 389, 390
  dissection of, 403
  surgery on, 403
lymphadenectomy, 403
lymphadeno/o, 389
lymphadenopathy, 399
lymphadenotomy, 403
lymphangio/o, 389
lymphangiogram, 395
lymphatic, 86
lymphatic and immune systems, 86,
    384–409
  allergic response and autoimmune
    disorders, 400–402
  diagnostic, procedural, and laboratory
    terms, 395–396
  pathological terms, 396–402
  pharmacological terms, 403–404
  structure and function of, 385–393
  surgical terms, 402–403
lymphatic pathways, 388, 389
lympho/o, 389
lymphocytes, 277, 278, 279, 388, 391, 578
lymphocytic lymphoma, 399
lymphoid system, 390
lymphoma, 399
-lysis, 9, 72
lyso/o, 28, 30
-lytic, 72

M

macro/o, 18, 20
macrophages, 279, 391
macroscopic phase, 479
macular degeneration, 229
macule, 112, 113
magnetic resonance angiography
    (MRA), 189
magnetic resonance imaging (MRI)
    scans, 53, 189, 317
MAI (mycobacterium avium-
    intracellulare), 398
mal-, 53, 54
-malacia, 68
male menopause, 502
male reproductive hormones, 504
malignant melanoma, 122
mammary gland, 524
mammary papilla, 525
mammo/o, 526, 539
mammogram, 540, 541
mammography, 541
mammoplasty, 550
mandible, 141, 142
mandibular bone, 142
-mania, 64
Mantoux test, 109–110
marrow, 140

mast, 538
mastectomy, 550
mastication, 416, 418
masticatory muscles, 149
mastitis, 544
masto/o, 526
mastoid process, 220
mastoido/o, 215, 224
mastopexy, 550
matrix, 104, 105
maxilla, 141
maxillary bones, 142
maxillary sinus, 141
maxillo/o, 136, 152
mcg, 35
mean (red) cell volume (MCV), 577
meato/o, 469, 475
meatotomy, 490
meatus, 467
medial, 90
mediastino/o, 347
mediastinoscopy, 362
mediastinum, 353
medical coder/biller, 254
medical lab technician, 113
medical record, 36
medical terminology, 2–41
  abbreviations, 35–36
  derivation of, 2–3
  forming, 8–10
  pluralizing terms, 31–33
  pronunciation of, 6–8
  SNOMED(r) (Systematized
    Nomenclature of Medicine), 36–37
  spelling of, 6–8
  surgical, pathological, pharmacological
    terms, 34
medio/o, 23, 24
medroxyprogesterone acetate (Depo-
    Provera), 532
medulla, 471
medulla oblongata, 179
meg(a), 18, 45, 46
megakaryocytes, 280
megalo/o, 18, 20
-megaly, 9, 64
melanin, 103
melano/o, 18, 19, 101, 108
melanocytes, 103, 104, 105, 108, 218
melanoma, 108, 122
melatonin, 245
melena, 453
membranous labyrinth, 220
menarche, 524
Ménière disease, 231
meninges, 181–184
meningioma, 200
meningitis, 198
meningo/o, 176, 187
meningocele, 192

meningomyelocele, 192
meno/o, 526, 538, 539
menometrorrhagia, 544
menopause, 502, 524, 535, 536
menorrhagia, 544
menorrhea, 528
menses, 524, 528
menstrual cycle, 528
menstruation, 524, 530
mesentery, 425
meso/o, 23, 48
mesothelioma, 371
meta-, 55, 56
metabolism, 249
metacarpals, 147, 148
metacarpo/o, 136, 152
metastasis, 399
metatarsals, 147
metatarsophalangeal, 147
-meter, 75
metro/o, 526, 538
metrorrhagia, 544
-metry, 76
MG (myasthenia gravis), 195
MI (myocardial infarction), 326, 327
micro/o, 18, 45, 46
microphages, 391
microscopic capillaries, 386, 388
microscopic phase, 479
midbrain, 179
middle ear, 219
middle lobe, 355
midsagittal, 92
minipill, 532
mio/o, 18, 20
miotic, 234
miscarriage, 543
miscellaneous combining forms, 27–28
mitral insufficiency, 329
mitral reflux, 329
mitral stenosis, 329
mitral valve, 302
mitral valve prolapse, 329
modern imaging, 53
modified radical mastectomy, 550
Mohs' surgery, 124
mono/o, 45, 46
monocytes, 277, 278, 279, 578
mononuclear phagocytic system, 390
mons pubis, 525
morbid obesity, 438
morning-after pills, 553
morpho/o, 18, 19
motion sickness, 222
mouth, 413, 417
  disorders of, 440–442
MRA (magnetic resonance
    angiography), 189
MRI (magnetic resonance imaging) scans,
    53, 189, 317

pericardial cavity, 299
pericardial fluid, 299
pericardio/o, 298, 314
pericarditis, 327
pericardium, 299
perimenopause, 535, 536
perimetrium, 525
perineo/o, 527
perineum, 502, 525
peripheral nervous system, 175, 184–187
peripheral vascular disease, 324
peristalsis, 413
peritoneal dialysis, 482, 483
peritoneoscope, 435
peritoneoscopy, 435
peritonitis, 450
pernicious anemia, 287
pertussis, 370
PET (positron emission tomography), 190, 317
petechiae, 112, 115, 116, 288, 324
petit mal seizures, 196
-pexy, 72
Peyronie disease, 512
pH, 479
phaco/o, 215, 223
-phage, 68
-phagia, 68
phago/o, 25, 26, 274, 284
phagocytic system, 390
phagocytosis, 391
phako/o, 215
phalanges, 147, 148
phalango/o, 136
phalanx, 105
pharmaco, 28, 30
pharmacological terms, 125–127, 376–377
pharmacology, 37
pharyngeal tonsils, 352
pharyngitis, 364
pharyngo/o, 348, 412, 416
pharynx, 352, 364, 413, 417, 418
    disorders of, 440–442
-phasia, 68
phenylketones, 479
-pheresis, 76
-phil, 76
-philia, 64
phimosis, 511
phlebitis, 324
phlebo/o, 298
phlebograms, 317
phlebography, 317
phlebotomy, 3, 287, 333
-phobia, 9, 62
-phonia, 62
phono/o, 15, 16, 348
-phoresis, 68
-phoria, 62
phosphorus, 137

photo/o, 15, 16
photophobia, 229
-phrenia, 64
phreno/o, 348
-phthisis, 64
-phylaxis, 78
physical phase, 479
physio/o, 18, 19
-physis, 64
phyto/o, 28, 29
pia mater, 181, 183
PID (pelvic inflammatory disease), 544
pilo/o, 101, 108
pilonidal cyst, 113, 115
pimple, 113
pineal gland, 243, 245
pinkeye, 230
pinna, 220
pituitary disorders, 256–260
pituitary glands, 245, 246, 256
placenta, 525
placenta previa, 544
-plakia, 70
planes of body, 91–93
plantar flexion, 151
plantar wart, 118
plaque, 112, 113, 324
-plasia, 68, 71
-plasm, 71
plasma, 13, 274, 281, 282, 387
plasma cells, 392
plasmapheresis, 275
plasmo/o, 13, 14
-plastic, 68
plastic surgery, 74, 123
-plasty, 72
platelet count (PLT), 286
platelets, 275
-plegia, 64
-plegic, 65, 78
pleura, 355
pleurae, 355
pleural cavity, 355
pleural effusion, 371
pleurisy, 364
pleuritis, 364
pleuro/o, 348
pleurocentesis, 374
PLT (platelet count), 286
pluralizing terms, 31–33
pluri-, 45, 46
PMN (polymorphonucleated cells), 391
PMS (premenstrual syndrome), 530
-pnea, 68
pneumatic otoscope, 227
pneumo/o, 348
pneumoconiosis, 371
Pneumocystis carinii, 397
Pneumocystis jirovecii (P. carinii), 397, 398
pneumonectomy, 374

pneumonia, 370
pneumonitis, 364
pneumono/o, 348
pneumothorax, 371
po, 36
podagra, 161
podiatrists, 154
podo/o, 136
-poiesis, 68
-poietic, 68
-poietin, 68
polarization, 310
poly-, 44, 45, 46
polycystic kidney disease, 486
polycystic ovarian disease, 44
polycythemia, 288
polydipsia, 258
polymorphonucleated cells (PMN), 391
polyp, 113
polypectomy, 456
polyposis, 450
polyps, colon, 436
polysomnography (PSG), 189
polyuria, 258, 487
pons, 179
popliteal artery, 306
popping, of ears, 219
pores, 107
-porosis, 68
position, prefixes related, 47–51
position or location, combining forms that refer to, 23
positron emission tomography (PET), 190, 317
post-, 51, 52
posterior, 90, 92
posthemorrhagic anemia, 288
postoperative, 548
postpartum depression, 548
postprandial blood sugar, 255
potassium, 577
PPD test, 110
pre-, 51, 52
preeclampsia, 544
prefixes, 9, 11, 42–58, 560–567
    miscellaneous medical, 55–56
    related to location, 47–51
    related to position, 47–51
    related to presence, 53–55
    related to quality, 53–55
    related to quantity, 45–47
    related to size, 45–47
    related to time, 51–52
pregnancy, 534
premature atrial contractions (PACs), 321
premature ventricular contractions (PVCs), 321
premenstrual syndrome (PMS), 530
prepuce, 502
presbyo/o, 215

retro-, 9, 48, 49
retroflexion, 544
retrograde pyelogram (RP), 482
retroperitoneal, 470
retroversion, 544
retrovirus, 397
Rh blood types, 282
Rh factor, 283
Rh negative, 283
Rh positive, 283
rhabdo/o, 137
rhabdomyo/o, 137
rheumatic heart disease, 329
rheumatoid arthritis, 160, 161
rheumatoid factor test, serum, 155
rheumatologists, 154
rhinitis, 364
rhino/o, 9, 348
rhinoplasty, 73, 374
rhinorrhea, 370
rhonchi, 367
rhythm method, 532
RIA (radioactive immunoassay), 255
ribs, 145, 146
rickets, 156
right atrium, 299
right lower quadrant, 94, 95
right upper quadrant, 94, 95
right ventricle, 299
rigidity, 160
rigor, 160
ringworm, 116
Rinne test, 227
risk factors, 321
RNs (registered nurses), 203
rods, 217
rosacea, 116
roseola, 116
rotation, 151
RP (retrograde pyelogram), 482
-rrhage, 68
-rrhagia, 65
-rrhaphy, 72
-rrhea, 65, 68
-rrhexis, 65
rub, 321
rubella, 15, 116
rubeola, 116
rugae, 418, 422
rule of nines, 119

S

SA (sinoatrial) node, 308, 309
sacral, 185
sacroiliac, 147
sacrum, 143, 144
safety, sun, 122
sagittal, 93
saliva, 418

salivary glands, 418
salivo/o, 412
salpingectomy, 549, 550
salpingitis, 544
salpingo/o, 13, 215, 527, 538
salpingo-oophorectomy, 550
salpingotomy, 550
saphenous veins, 306
sarcoidosis, 399
SARS (severe acute respiratory
    syndrome), 372
saturated fats, 318
scabies, 121
scale, 28, 112, 114
scanning electron micrograph, 395
scapula, 145, 146, 147
scapulo/o, 137
-schisis, 68
schisto/o, 21, 22
schizo/o, 21, 22
sciatica, 156, 198
sclera, 216
scleritis, 230
sclero/o, 18, 20, 215, 223
scleroderma, 120
scolio/o, 18, 19, 137
scoliosis, 162
-scope, 76
-scopy, 76
scoto/o, 215, 224
scratch test, 110
scroto/o, 504
scrotum, 501
sebaceous cyst, 113
sebaceous glands, 101, 102, 104, 106, 107
sebo/o, 101, 108
seborrhea, 120
seborrheic dermatitis, 120
sebum, 107
secondary hypertension, 323
secondary lesions, 112, 113, 114
second-degree burns, 121
sedatives, 204
sedimentation rate (SR), 286
semen, 502
semen analysis, 508, 509
semi-, 53, 54
semicircular canals, 220
semilunar valve, 302
seminal vesicles, 502
seminiferous tubules, 502
semino/o, 504
seminoma, 512
sensations, 15, 62-64
sensorineural hearing loss, 231
sensory, 86
sensory (afferent) neurons, 177
sensory organs, 214
sensory receptors, 214
sensory system, 213-240

diagnostic, procedural, and laboratory
    terms, 226-228
function and structure of, 214-223
hearing and equilibrium-the ear,
    218-222
pathological terms, 228-232
pharmacological terms, 234-235
smell and taste, 222-223
surgical terms, 232-234
touch, pain, and temperature-the skin,
    222, 223
septa, 299
septal defect, 329
septoplasty, 374
septostomy, 374
septum, 299, 353
serous otitis media, 231
serum calcium, 155
serum enzyme test, 318
serum phosphorus, 155
sesamoid bones, 140
sessile polyp, 113
severe acute respiratory syndrome
    (SARS), 372
sexually transmitted diseases (STDs), 512,
    545-546
shaken baby syndrome, 192
shave biopsy, 124
shin, 148
shingles, 118, 198
short bones, 140
SIADH (syndrome of inappropriate
    ADH), 258
sialoadenitis, 441
sickle cell anemia, 288
sidero/o, 13, 14
sight, 215-218
sigmoid colon, 426
sigmoido/o, 412, 424
sigmoidoscope, 435
sigmoidoscopy, 435
simple (closed) fracture, 158
sinoatrial (SA) node, 308, 309
sinus, 3, 141, 525
sinus rhythm, 310
sinusitis, 364
sinusotomy, 374
size, prefixes related to, 45-47
skeletal muscle, 150
skeleton, 135, 137
skin, 101-104, 222
    cancer of, 108, 122-123
    cross-section of, 102
    pathological conditions of, 112-123
    touch, pain, and temperature, 222, 223
    treatment of disorders of, 125-127
    viral disease of, 118
skin graft, 123
skin surgery, 123-125
sleep apnea, 189

Tx, 36
tympanic cavity, 220
tympanic membrane, 220
tympano/o, 215, 224
tympanoplasty, 232
Type I diabetes, 261
Type II diabetes, 261

U

ulcer, 112, 114
ulcerative colitis, 449, 450
ulna, 147, 148
ulno/o, 137
ultra-, 53, 54
ultradian rhythms, 247
ultrasonography, 317, 435
ultrasound, 53, 482
ultraviolet light, 126
umbilical, 94
umbilical cord, 536
umbilical hernia, 454
un-, 53, 54
uni-, 45, 46
universal donors, 283
universal recipients, 283
upper respiratory infection, 369
upper respiratory tract, 349
ur-, 475
urea, 468, 471
uremia, 486
ureterectomy, 490
ureteritis, 486
uretero/o, 469, 473, 476
ureteroplasty, 490
ureterorrhaphy, 490
ureters, 467, 473–474
urethra, 467, 473–474
urethral stenosis, 486
urethritis, 486
urethro/o, 469, 475
urethrocystitis, 486
urethrogram, 509
urethropexy, 490
urethroplasty, 490
urethrorrhaphy, 490
urethrostomy, 490
urethrotomy, 490
-uria, 71, 469, 475
uric acid, 471
uric acid test, 155
urinalysis, 477, 478, 479, 578
urinary, 86
urinary bladder, 467, 473, 474
urinary catheterization, 479
urinary system, 466–499
    diagnostic, procedural, and laboratory
        terms, 477–484
    function and structure of,
        467–474

imaging tests and urinary tract
    procedures, 482–484
pathological terms, 485–488
pharmacological terms,
    492–493
surgical terms, 489–492
urinary tract infection (UTI), 476, 485,
    486, 487
urine, 470, 471
urine sugar, 255
urino/o, 469
uro/o, 469
urologists, 489
urology, 467, 482, 490
urostomy, 491
urticaria, 116
uterine tube, 524
utero/o, 527, 538
uterus, 524
uterus expansion, 536
UTI (urinary tract infection), 476, 485,
    486, 487
uvea, 216
uveo/o, 215, 224
uvula, 418

V

vaccinations, 50, 392
vaccine, 392
vagina, 524
vaginal hysterectomy, 548, 550
vaginitis, 544
vagino/o, 527, 539
vago/o, 176, 187
vagotomy, 203
vagus nerves, 185
valve conditions, 329–330
valve replacement, 333
valves, 302
valvotomy, 333
valvulitis, 329
valvuloplasty, 333
varicella, 116
varicocele, 511
varicose veins, 324
vas deferens, 502
vascular disorders, 201–203
vascular lesions, 112, 113
vasectomy, 32, 514, 532
vaso/o, 298, 314, 504
vasoconstrictors, 335
vasodilators, 335
vasovasostomy, 514
VCG (voiding cystogram), 482
VCUG (voiding (urinating)
    cystourethrogram), 482
VDRL (Venereal Disease Research
    Laboratory), 541
vegetation, 329

veins, 3, 102, 302, 304
vena cava, 306
venae cavae, 306
Venereal Disease Research Laboratory
    (VDRL), 541
venipuncture, 285, 287, 333
veno/o, 298, 314
venograms, 317
venography, 317
ventilation/perfusion (V/Q)
    scan, 362
ventilators, 376
ventral, 88, 92
ventral thalamus, 180
ventricles, 180, 299
ventriculo/o, 176, 187
ventriculogram, 317
venules, 306
vermiform appendix, 425
verruca, 118
-version, 79
vertebrae, 143, 144
vertebral column, 144
vertebro/o, 137, 152
vertigo, 231
very low-density lipoproteins
    (VLDLs), 318
vesicle, 112, 113
vesico/o, 469, 476
vestibule, 220
vestibulocochlar nerves, 185
villi, 425
villus, 425
viral diseases, 118
viral enteritis, 443
viral meningitis, 198
viral skin disease, 118
virilism, 259
virus Type 1, 118
virus Type 2, 118
visceral, 151
visceral pericardium, 299
visceral pleura, 355
visual field examination, 227
vitamin D, 137
VLDLs (very low-density lipoproteins),
    318
vocal chords, 350
vocal cords, 352
voice box, 352
voiding cystogram (VCG), 482
voiding (urinating) cystourethrogram
    (VCUG), 482
voluntary muscle, 151
volvulus, 450
von Willebrand disease, 288
V/Q (ventilation/perfusion)
    scan, 362
vulva, 525
vulvo/o, 527, 538